Workbook and Competency Evaluation Review for Mosby's Textbook for Long-Term Care Nursing Assistant

Ninth edition

Christine M. Sorensen RN, BSN
Adjunct Instructor Nurse Aide,
Des Moines Area Community College,
Ames, Iowa
Clinic Nurse,
Boone County Family Medicine,
Boone, Iowa

MOSBY

ELSEVIER

Elsevier
3251 Riverport Lane
St. Louis, Missouri 63043

WORKBOOK AND COMPETENCY EVALUATION REVIEW FOR MOSBY'S TEXTBOOK
FOR LONG-TERM CARE NURSING ASSISTANTS, NINTH EDITION   ISBN: 978-0-323-87512-7

Notice

Practitioners and researchers must always rely on their own experience and knowledge in evaluating and using any information, methods, compounds or experiments described herein. Because of rapid advances in the medical sciences, in particular, independent verification of diagnoses and drug dosages should be made. To the fullest extent of the law, no responsibility is assumed by Elsevier, authors, editors or contributors for any injury and/or damage to persons or property as a matter of products liability, negligence or otherwise, or from any use or operation of any methods, products, instructions, or ideas contained in the material herein.

Previous editions copyrighted 2020, 2015, 2011, 2007, and 2003.

Executive Content Strategist: Sonya Seigafuse
Content Development Manager: Danielle Frazier
Senior Content Development Specialist: Maria Broeker
Publishing Services Manager: Deepthi Unni
Project Manager: Sheik Mohideen K

Printed in the United States of America

Last digit is the print number: 9   8   7   6   5   4   3   2   1

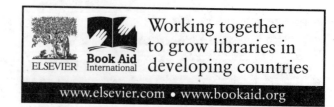

To my husband Curtis; for his constant love and encouragement.

To my children Isaac, Olivia, Cecilia, and Elijah; for their patience and support.

To my mom, for her guidance and having faith in me.

To my dad, for his knowledge and advice

Preface

This workbook is written to be used with *Mosby's Textbook for Long-Term Care Nursing Assistants*, Ninth Edition. You will not need other resources to complete the exercises in this workbook.

It is designed to help you apply what you have learned in each chapter of the textbook. You are encouraged to use this book as a study guide. Each chapter is thoroughly covered in the multiple-choice questions, which will help prepare you to take the NATCEP test. In addition, other exercises such as fill-in-the-blank, matching, and crossword puzzles are used in many chapters. Independent Learning Activities at the end of each chapter may be used to apply the information you will learn in a practical setting. The section titled Optional Learning Activities may be used as an alternative exercise to give you more practice in studying the materials.

In addition, Procedure Checklists that correspond with the procedures in the textbook are provided. These checklists are designed to help you become skilled at performing procedures that affect quality of care. In addition to NATCEP skills being identified for you, icons in the checklists indicate skills that are in Mosby's Nursing Assistant Video Skills 4.0, and on the Evolve student learning resources website (video clips).

The Competency Evaluation Review includes a general review section and two practice exams to help you prepare for the written certification exam. A skills review guide to help you practice procedures required for certification as well as answers to the two practice exams can be found on the Evolve student learning resources website.

Assistive personnel are important members of the health team. Completing the exercises in this workbook will increase your knowledge and skills. The goal is to prepare you to provide the best possible care and to encourage pride in a job well done.

Contents

1 The Nursing Assistant Working in Long-Term Care

FILL IN THE BLANKS: KEY TERMS

Accountable
Acute illness
Alzheimer disease (AD)
Assisted living residence (ALR)
Board and care home
Case management
Chronic illness
Delegate
Group home

Hospice
Independence
Interdisciplinary team
Job description
Licensed practical nurse (LPN)
Licensed vocational nurse (LVN)
Medicaid
Medicare
Nursing assistant

Nursing center
Nursing facility (NF)
Nursing home
Nursing task
Nursing team
Registered nurse (RN)
Responsibility
Skilled nursing facility (SNF)

1. A person who has completed a 1-year nursing program and passed a licensing test is a _____ _____.

2. A _____ provides health care to persons who need regular or continuous care.

3. Another name for a nursing center or a nursing facility is a _____.

4. _____ means a person is not relying on or requiring care from others.

5. A sudden illness from which the person should recover is an _____.

6. A facility that provides nursing care for residents who have many or severe health problems or who need rehabilitation is called a _____ _____.

7. A _____ is an ongoing illness, slow or gradual in onset, that has no cure; the illness can be controlled and complications can be prevented with proper treatment.

8. An _____ provides housing, personal care, supportive services, health care, and social activities in a home-like setting.

9. Being responsible for one's actions and the actions of others who performed tasks is being _____ _____.

10. RNs, LPNs/LVNs, and nursing assistants provide nursing care as part of the _____.

11. _____ is a disease that affects the brain tissue; there is increasing memory loss and confusion.

12. To _____ is to authorize another person to perform a nursing task in a certain situation.

13. _____ is a federal health insurance plan for persons 65 years of age or older and younger people with certain disabilities.

14. A _____ provides rooms, meals, laundry, and supervision to a few independent residents, often in a home setting.

15. A nursing center or nursing home may be called a _____.

16. A _____ is a document that describes what the center expects you to do.

17. A person who has completed a 2-, 3-, or 4-year nursing program and who has passed a licensing test is a _____.

18. Nursing care that can be delegated to nursing assistants when it does not require an RN's professional knowledge or judgment is a _____ _____.

19. A nursing care pattern where an RN coordinates a person's care is _____.

20. A _____ gives basic nursing care under the supervision of a licensed nurse.

21. Another name for a licensed practical nurse is _____ _____.

22. The many health care workers whose skills and knowledge focus on the person's total care are the _____.

23. _____ is a health care payment program sponsored by state and federal governments.

24. A health care agency or program for persons who are dying is a _____.

25. Another name for a board and care home is a _____.

26. The duty or obligation to perform some act or function is _____.

27. Residents who live in a board and care home
    A. Receive care that meets the person's basic needs
    B. Stay there for a short time while recovering from an illness or surgery
    C. Are in a program for persons who are dying
    D. Are in a closed unit that provides a safer environment

28. Some assisted living facilities are part of
    A. A hospital
    B. A retirement community or nursing center
    C. A hospice
    D. A skilled care facility

29. Skilled nursing facilities provide
    A. Supportive care
    B. More complex care than nursing centers do
    C. A closed unit for residents who have Alzheimer disease or other dementia
    D. Care for persons who are dying

30. Nursing centers provide health care and nursing care to
    A. Cure an acute illness
    B. Persons who need regular or continuous care
    C. Help the person recover after surgery
    D. Cure a chronic illness

31. Colds and influenza can cause major health problems for older and disabled persons. These are called
    A. Chronic illnesses
    B. Communicable diseases
    C. Emotional illnesses
    D. Disabilities

32. Rehabilitation or restorative care helps
    A. The person to have a complete return of all functions
    B. To provide supportive care that meets basic physical needs
    C. To keep the person safe
    D. Persons return to their highest possible level of physical and mental function

33. Children and pets usually can visit when a dying person is in
    A. A memory care unit
    B. A hospital
    C. A hospice
    D. A subacute care center

34. A memory care unit is a closed unit that provides
    A. A safer environment for residents to wander freely
    B. A program for persons who are dying
    C. A place for residents who suffer from deconditioning after an acute illness
    D. A program for residents with a communicable disease

35. Which of these workers or areas in a health care center is under the director of nursing in the organizational chart?
    A. Nursing assistant
    B. Medical director
    C. Case manager
    D. Social worker

36. The director of nursing is responsible for
    A. Coordinating resident care for a certain shift
    B. Planning and presenting educational programs
    C. The entire nursing staff
    D. All resident care and the actions of the nursing staff on a unit

37. Who coordinates care for a certain shift in the nursing center?
    A. Doctor
    B. Staff nurse
    C. Shift manager
    D. Director of nursing

38. Which of the following describes an RN?
    A. Completes a 1-year nursing program and passes a licensing test
    B. Completes studies that qualify the person to become the medical director of the nursing center
    C. Has formal training to give care and passes a competency examination
    D. Completes a 2-, 3-, or 4-year nursing program and has passed a licensing test

39. The nursing assistant gives basic nursing care under the supervision of
    A. The center administrator
    B. The director of nursing
    C. A licensed nurse
    D. Another nursing assistant

40. Medicare is a federal health insurance plan that has benefits for
    A. Persons 65 years of age and older
    B. Families with low income
    C. Individuals and families who buy the insurance
    D. Groups of individuals who buy the insurance

41. Part B of Medicare
    A. Pays for hospital costs and some SNF costs
    B. Benefits only persons 65 years of age and older
    C. Is administered by the Social Security Administration
    D. Helps pay for doctor's visits, outpatient hospital care, physical and occupational therapists, and some home care

42. A MS-DRG (Medicare severity-adjusted diagnosis-related group) plan
    A. Covers only persons 65 years of age and older
    B. Is used for hospital costs
    C. Pays for care in an SNF
    D. Limits the choice of where to go for care

43. If a person has managed care, the insured person will have costs covered based on
   A. Health care available in the community
   B. The age of the person
   C. His or her physical needs
   D. The pre-approval process used by the person's insurer

44. Nursing centers require certification to
   A. Signal quality and excellence
   B. Receive Medicare and Medicaid funds
   C. Operate and provide care
   D. Meet state and federal standards

45. A nursing assistant could prevent common nursing center deficiencies by
   A. Protecting residents from abuse, mistreatment, and neglect when giving care
   B. Hiring only people with no legal history of abusing, neglecting, or mistreating residents
   C. Applying physical restraints to keep residents safe
   D. Ignoring other caregivers who may be abusing or neglecting residents

46. Until the 1980s, nursing assistants
   A. Attended nursing assistant classes approved by the state
   B. Were not used in giving basic nursing care
   C. Received on-the-job training from nurses
   D. Worked only in hospitals

47. State laws that regulate nursing assistant roles and functions are determined by
   A. OBRA
   B. The Nurse Practice Act
   C. The state medical society
   D. Insurance companies

48. If you do something beyond the legal limits of your role, you could be
   A. Protected by the Nurse Practice Act
   B. Practicing nursing without a license
   C. Protected by the nurse who supervises your work
   D. Accused of a criminal act

49. OBRA requires that the nursing assistant training and competency evaluation program have at least _____ hours of instruction.
   A. 16
   B. 75
   C. 120
   D. 200

50. Which of these areas of study is included in a training program for nursing assistants?
   A. Giving feedings through the naso-gastric tube
   B. Changing sterile dressings independently
   C. Phlebotomy (drawing blood)
   D. Elimination procedures

51. The competency evaluation for nursing assistants has two parts. They are
   A. A written test and a skills test
   B. A multiple-choice test and a true-false test
   C. A skills test and a complete bed bath demonstration
   D. A written test and an oral question-and-answer test

52. If you fail the competency evaluation the first time it is taken, you
   A. Can retest one more time
   B. Must repeat your training program
   C. Can retest two more times (for a total of three times)
   D. Can retest as often as necessary free of charge

53. Which of the following information is contained in the nursing assistant registry?
   A. Every place you have worked
   B. Date of birth
   C. Number of dependents
   D. A credit report

54. OBRA requires that retraining and a new competency evaluation test must be taken if you have not worked as a certified nursing assistant for
   A. 24 months
   B. 5 years
   C. 1 consecutive year
   D. 6 months

55. If you wish to work as a CNA in another state, you should
   A. Present your certificate to the nursing center where you wish to work
   B. Apply to that state's nursing board for endorsement, reciprocity, or equivalency
   C. Never tell that state that you lost your certification in another state
   D. Take a nursing assistant course and pass the NATCEP in that state

56. Your work as a nursing assistant is supervised by
   A. A licensed nurse
   B. The doctor
   C. The director of nursing
   D. A nursing assistant with more experience

57. When in-service programs or training is scheduled, the nursing assistant
   A. Must attend those that are required
   B. Needs to attend only if the program is scheduled on a day he or she is scheduled to work
   C. Cannot attend if the program is scheduled during the workday
   D. Does not need to attend if it means he or she must come to work early or stay late

58. You are alone in the nurses' station and you answer the phone. Dr. Cruz begins to give you verbal orders. You should
    A. Hang up the phone
    B. Politely give him your name and title and ask him to wait while you get the nurse
    C. Quickly write down the orders and give them to the nurse
    D. Politely give him your name and title and ask him to call back later when the nurse is there

59. As a nursing assistant you may give medications if
    A. The nurse is busy and asks you to give them
    B. The resident is in the shower and the nurse leaves the medications at the bedside
    C. You have completed a state-required medication and training program on giving medications
    D. You are feeding the resident and the nurse asks you to mix the medications with the food

60. The nurse asks you to carry out a task you do not know how to do. You should
    A. Ignore the order since it is something you cannot do
    B. Perform the task as well as you can
    C. Ask another nursing assistant to show you how to carry out the task
    D. Promptly explain to the nurse why you cannot carry out the task

61. The nurse asks you to assist him as he changes sterile dressings. You should
    A. Assist him as needed
    B. Tell him you cannot assist with performing any sterile procedures
    C. Tell him this is something you cannot do
    D. Report his request to the supervisor

62. Who can tell the person or the family a diagnosis or prescribe treatments?
    A. The director of nursing
    B. The RN
    C. The doctor
    D. An experienced nursing assistant

63. When you read a job description, you should not take a job if it requires you to
    A. Carry out duties you do not like to do
    B. Maintain required certification
    C. Attend in-service training
    D. Function beyond your training limits

64. Which of the following would be wrong?
    A. An RN delegates a task to an LPN/LVN.
    B. An LPN/LVN delegates a task to a nursing assistant.
    C. An RN delegates a task to a nursing assistant.
    D. A nursing assistant delegates a task to another nursing assistant.

65. When a nurse considers delegating tasks, the decision
    A. Should always result in the best care for the person at the time
    B. Depends on whether the nurse likes the nursing assistant
    C. Depends on how busy the nurse is that day
    D. Depends on how well the nurse likes the person.

66. You have been caring for Mr. Watson for several weeks. The nurse tells you she will give his care today. Her delegation decision is based primarily on
    A. How well you performed his care yesterday
    B. Changes in Mr. Watson's condition
    C. Whether the nurse knows you or not
    D. How much supervision you need

67. Which of the following is one of the five rights of delegation?
    A. The right task
    B. The right delegation
    C. The right time
    D. The right team members

68. You may refuse to carry out a task if
    A. The team members you like cannot help you
    B. You do not know how to use the supplies or equipment
    C. You are too busy
    D. You do not like the resident

FILL IN THE BLANKS

Write out the meaning of each abbreviation.

69. CNA_____

70. LNA_____

71. LPN/LVN_____

72. AD_____

73. UAP_____

74. SNF_____

75. DON_____

76. ALR_____

77. RNA_____

78. STNA_____

79. HMO_____

80. PPO_____

81. OBRA_____

82. NATCEP_____

83. NCSBN_____

84. RN_____

MATCHING

Match the types of health care service with the correct example.

85. _____ Provides health care and nursing care for residents who have many or severe health problems or who need rehabilitation.

86. _____ Provides rooms, meals, laundry, and supervision to independent residents.

87. _____ Provides a unit closed off from the rest of the center. This provides a safe setting for residents to wander freely.

88. _____ Health care agency or program for people who are dying.

89. _____ Provides housing, personal care, supportive services, health care, and social activities in a home-like setting.

A. Skilled care facility
B. Hospice unit
C. Board and care home
D. Memory care unit
E. Assisted living residence

OPTIONAL LEARNING EXERCISES

Comparing Long-Term Care Centers

90. A board and care home provides care in a home-like setting. What is the resident usually able to do with little help? _____
_____

91. What happens if the person has an emergency in the middle of the night? _____

92. An assisted living residence provides care in a home-like setting. Help given includes _____
_____. There is access to _____
_____.

93. A nursing center provides health care to persons _____. The facility is required to employ _____ nurses on the staff.

94. A skilled nursing facility provides health and nursing care for residents who have _____.

95. Long-term care centers help and encourage residents to
A. Focus on _____.
B. Do as much _____.
C. Change habits _____.
D. Understand and accept the limits of _____
_____.

96. A hospice is an agency or program for _____
_____. What needs are met by a hospice? _____
_____

97. A memory care unit is designed for persons with _____. A memory care unit is closed off from the rest of the center because these residents may _____.

98. Persons on a rehabilitation or subacute care unit often stay there for _____.

Health Team Members (Table 1-1)

Name the health team member who provides the service described.

99. Mr. Chen needs assistance to regain skills to dress, shave, and feed himself (ADL). He is assisted by the _____.

100. The nurse has a concern about a drug action, so calls the _____.

101. Mrs. Young needs the corns on her feet treated. The nurse notifies the _____.

102. Ms. Sharma has the responsibility of doing physical examinations, health assessments, and health education in the center where she works. She is a _____.

103. Mr. Gomez keeps turning up the volume on his TV. His hearing is tested by the _____.

104. The _____ meets with a new resident and his family to discuss his nutritional needs.

105. Mr. Mohamed had a stroke and has weakness on his left side. The _____ assists him by developing a plan that focuses on restoring function and preventing disability from his illness.

106. The doctor orders x-rays after Mr. Jackson falls. The x-rays are done by the _____.

107. Mr. Schwartz has chronic lung disease and needs respiratory treatments. These are given by the _____.

108. Ms. Walker plans the recreational needs of a nursing center. She is an _____.

109. After a stroke, Mr. Saito has difficulty swallowing. He is evaluated by the _____.

110. When the doctor orders blood tests, the samples are collected by the _____.

OBRA Requirements Related to the Nursing Assistant

111. The nursing assistant must meet federal and state training and competency requirements in order to work in _____.

112. OBRA requires _____ hours of instruction. _____ hours of supervised practical training are required. Where can the practical training take place? _____ or _____.

113. OBRA requires 15 areas of study. Write the area of study where you learn the skill for each example.
A. You make a bed. _____
B. You close Mr. Smith's door to give him privacy. _____
C. You tell Mrs. Nguyen the time of day and the day of week frequently during the day. _____
D. You apply lotion to a resident's dry skin. _____
E. You assist a resident to put on his shirt. _____
F. When assigned to a new unit, you find the location of the fire alarm. _____
G. You wash your hands before and after giving care. _____
H. You get help to move a resident from his bed to the chair. _____
I. When speaking to Mr. Eriksson, you maintain good eye contact. _____
J. The nurse tells you to exercise a resident's extremities (limbs). _____
K. You shave Mr. Garcia. _____
L. You position a urinal for a resident in bed. _____
M. You assist Mrs. Markovic to walk in the hall. _____
N. You notice Mrs. Liu has an elevated temperature and her skin is warm. _____
O. You cut up the meat on Mr. Johnson's plate before helping him to eat. _____

INDEPENDENT LEARNING ACTIVITIES

Gather the following information about long-term care centers in your area.

- How many board and care homes are located in your area? Choose one home and answer the following questions.
  - Is this home attached to a nursing center or is it a separate center?
  - What services are provided?
  - How many residents are in the home?
  - How many staff members work there? How many staff members are RNs? LPNs? Nursing assistants? What care is provided by nursing assistants?
- How many nursing centers are located in your area? Choose one center and answer the following questions.
  - What types of residents are accepted in the center? (For example, does the center consider level of care needed, the resident's disease, or method of payment?)
  - How many residents live in the center?
  - How many staff members work there? How many staff members are RNs? LPNs? Nursing assistants? What care is provided by nursing assistants?
- How many nursing centers in your area provide skilled nursing care? Choose one center and answer the following questions.
  - How many residents live in the center?
  - How many staff members work there? How many staff members are RNs? LPNs? Nursing assistants? What care is provided by nursing assistants?
- How many assisted living facilities are located in your area? Choose one facility and answer the following questions.
  - Is this facility independent or part of a long-term care center?
  - How many residents live in the facility?
  - What kind of living quarters do the residents have? (For example, does each resident have an apartment or studio? Do residents share kitchen facilities or does each person have a kitchen?)
  - How many staff members work there? How many staff members are RNs? LPNs? Nursing assistants? What care is provided by nursing assistants?
- Find a nursing center that has a memory care unit and answer the following questions.
  - How is the unit identified? Is it a separate wing? Separate floor? Is the unit closed off?
  - How is the unit different from other units in the center?
  - Do the staff members who work on this unit receive special training? If so, what extra training are they given? What duties are assigned to nursing assistants on this unit?
- Does your area have a hospice program? If so, answer the following questions about the program.
  - Is this program located within a center or does it provide care in the person's facility or home?
  - What type of care is provided?
  - What special training is given to the staff? What duties can be performed by a nursing assistant?
- Obtain a copy of the Nurse Practice Act for your state. How are nursing assistant roles, functions, education, and certification requirements addressed? Are there separate laws for nursing assistants? What rules and regulations apply to nursing assistants?
- Obtain a job description for a nursing assistant. You may be able to ask for this at the facility where you had your clinical experience. What information is contained in the job description about:
  - Who will direct or supervise the nursing assistant?
  - What set of competencies is the nursing assistant expected to have?
  - What professional requirements are listed?
  - What other skills or requirements are listed?

2 Resident Rights, Ethics, and Laws

FILL IN THE BLANKS: KEY TERMS

Abuse
Assault
Battery
Boundary crossing
Boundary sign
Boundary violation
Civil law
Crime
Criminal law
Defamation
Ethics

False imprisonment
Fraud
Invasion of privacy
Involuntary seclusion
Law
Libel
Malpractice
Neglect
Negligence
Ombudsman
Professional boundary

Professional sexual misconduct
Protected health information
Representative
Self-neglect
Slander
Standard of care
Tort
Treatment
Vulnerable adult
Will

1. Separating a person from others against his or her will, keeping the person in a certain area, or keeping the person from his or her room without consent is _____.

2. A _____ is a person 18 years of age or older who has a disability or condition that makes him or her at risk for being wounded, attacked, or damaged.

3. When an act, behavior, or thought warns of a boundary crossing or violation it is a _____.

4. _____ is negligence by a professional person.

5. Saying or doing something to trick, fool, or deceive another person is _____.

6. _____ is concerned with offenses against the public and society in general.

7. A _____ is a legal statement about how a person wishes to have property distributed after death.

8. _____ is identifying information and information about the person's health care that is maintained or sent in any form.

9. A brief act or behavior outside of the helpful zone is _____.

10. An _____ is someone who supports or promotes the needs and interests of another person.

11. A rule of conduct made by a government body is a _____.

12. _____ is the touching of a person's body without the person's consent.

13. The willful infliction of injury, unreasonable confinement, intimidation, or punishment that results in physical harm, pain, or mental anguish is _____.

14. _____ is making false statements orally.

15. Injuring a person's name and reputation by making false statements to a third person is _____.

16. _____ is knowledge of what is right and wrong conduct.

17. Intentionally attempting or threatening to touch a person's body without the person's consent is _____.

18. A _____ is a wrong committed against a person or the person's property.

19. _____ are laws concerned with relationships between people.

20. A _____ is any person who has the legal right to act on the resident's behalf when he or she cannot do so for himself or herself.

21. _____ is an act, behavior, or comment that is sexual in nature.

22. An act or behavior that meets your needs, not the person's, is a _____.

23. Violating a person's right not to have his or her name, photograph, or private affairs exposed or made public without giving consent is _____.

7

24. _____ is the skills, care, and judgment required by the health team member under similar circumstances.

25. _____ separates helpful behaviors from behaviors that are not helpful.

26. An act that violates a criminal law is a _____ _____.

27. _____ is the unlawful restraint or restriction of a person's movement.

28. Defamation through written statements is _____.

29. A _____ is an unintentional wrong in which a person does not act in a reasonable and careful manner and causes harm to a person or to the person's property.

30. The care provided to maintain or restore health, improve function, or relieve symptoms is _____ _____.

31. _____ is the failure to provide the person with goods or services needed to avoid physical harm, mental anguish, or mental illness.

32. A person's behaviors that threaten his or her health or safety is _____.

CIRCLE THE BEST ANSWER

33. A resident in long-term care has the right to
    A. Have a private room in which to live
    B. Have personal choice in what to wear and how to spend his or her time
    C. Have all meals delivered from outside the facility
    D. Have friends live with him or her at the facility

34. Under OBRA, if a resident is incompetent (not able) to exercise his or her rights, who can exercise these rights for the person?
    A. The doctor
    B. A responsible party such as a partner, adult child, or court-appointed guardian
    C. The charge nurse
    D. A neighbor

35. If a resident refuses treatment, what should you do?
    A. Avoid giving any care to the person and move on to other duties
    B. Report the refusal to the nurse
    C. Tell the resident the treatment must be done and continue to carry out the treatment
    D. Tell the resident's family so they can make him accept the treatment

36. A student wants to observe a treatment but the resident does not want her to be present. What is the correct action?
    A. The student cannot watch, as this violates the resident's right to privacy.
    B. The student may observe from the doorway, where the resident cannot see her.
    C. The staff nurse tells the resident he must allow the student to watch.
    D. The nurse calls the resident's wife to get her permission.

37. The resident should be given personal choice whenever it
    A. Is safely possible
    B. Does not interfere with scheduled activities
    C. Is approved by the director of nursing
    D. Is ordered by the doctor

38. If a resident voices concerns about care and the center promptly tries to correct the situation, this action meets the resident's right to
    A. Participate in a resident group
    B. Voice a grievance
    C. Personal choice
    D. Freedom from abuse, mistreatment, and neglect

39. When a resident volunteers to take care of houseplants at the center, this is an acceptable part of
    A. The care plan
    B. A requirement to receive care or care items
    C. Paying the cost of his care
    D. The doctor's orders

40. When a resident and the family plan activities together, this meets the resident's right to
    A. Privacy
    B. Freedom from restraint
    C. Freedom from mistreatment
    D. Take part in resident and family groups

41. The resident you are caring for has many old holiday decorations covering her night-stand. If you throw away these items without her permission you are denying her right to
    A. Privacy
    B. Work
    C. Keep and use personal items
    D. Freedom from abuse

42. A staff member tells a resident he cannot leave his room because he talks too much. This action denies the resident
    A. The right to be free from involuntary seclusion
    B. Freedom from restraint
    C. Care and security of personal possessions
    D. Personal choice

43. When a resident is given certain drugs that affect his mood, behavior, or mental function, it may deny his right to
    A. Freedom from abuse, mistreatment, and neglect
    B. Personal choice
    C. Privacy
    D. Freedom from restraint

44. Which of these actions will promote courteous and dignified care?
    A. Calling the resident by a nickname he does not choose
    B. Assisting with dressing the resident in clothing appropriate for the time of day
    C. Changing the resident's hairstyle without her permission
    D. Leaving the bathroom door open so you can see the person

45. You ask a resident if you may touch him. This is an example of
    A. Courteous and dignified interactions
    B. Courteous and dignified care
    C. Providing privacy and self-determination
    D. Maintaining personal choice and independence

46. Assisting a resident to ambulate without interfering with his independence is an example of
    A. Courteous and dignified interaction
    B. Courteous and dignified care
    C. Providing privacy and self-determination
    D. Maintaining personal choice and independence

47. You provide privacy and self-determination for a resident when you
    A. Knock on the door before entering and wait to be asked in
    B. Allow the resident to smoke in designated areas
    C. Listen with interest to what the person is saying
    D. Groom his beard as he wishes

48. You allow the resident to maintain personal choice and independence when you
    A. Obtain her attention before interacting with her
    B. Provide extra clothing for warmth, such as a sweater or lap robe
    C. Assist him to take part in activities according to his interests
    D. Use curtains or screens during personal care and procedures

49. Which of these activities would be carried out by an ombudsman?
    A. Organize activities for a group of residents
    B. Accompany residents to a religious service at a house of worship
    C. Investigate and resolve complaints made by a resident
    D. Assist the resident to choose friends

50. Which of the following is part of the code of conduct for a nursing assistant?
    A. Carry out any task assigned to you
    B. Take a coworker's medication for a headache
    C. Know the limits of your role and your knowledge
    D. Plan your work so you can go to lunch with your friend

51. Which of the following is an example of boundary crossing?
    A. You avoid caring for a friend or family member.
    B. You hug a person every time you see him or her.
    C. You share information about your personal relationships or problems.
    D. You protect the person's privacy.

52. A boundary violation would be
    A. Keeping secrets with the person
    B. Giving a person a brief hug when he or she is upset
    C. Trading assignments with other staff so you can care for a person
    D. Changing how you dress when you work with a person

53. If a person or family member offers you a gift, you maintain professional boundaries by
    A. Accepting the gift and thanking the person
    B. Refusing the gift by saying: "I don't need this"
    C. Thanking the person but explaining that you cannot accept gifts from those you care for
    D. Giving the gift to someone else

54. A nurse failed to do what a reasonable and careful nurse would have done. Legally, this is called
    A. Fraud
    B. A tort
    C. Negligence
    D. Malpractice

55. You may be accused of negligence if you
    A. Fail to test the temperature of a hot soak and the person is burned
    B. Imply or suggest that a person is stealing from the staff
    C. Threaten to restrain a person
    D. Tell the person or the family that you are a nurse

56. If you fail to identify a person properly and perform a treatment on him intended for another, you are
    A. Committing a crime
    B. Legally responsible (liable) for your actions
    C. Not responsible legally but are unethical
    D. Guilty of an intentional tort

57. A nursing assistant writes a note to a friend that injures the name and reputation of a person by making false statements. This is called
    A. Libel
    B. Slander
    C. Malpractice
    D. Negligence

58. The nursing assistant would violate the Health Insurance Portability and Accountability Act of 1996 (HIPAA) if he or she
    A. Says or does something that tricks or deceives a person
    B. Gives out information about the person's health care
    C. Signs a legal document for a resident
    D. Makes false statements about a resident to a third person

59. A nursing assistant tells a resident she is a nurse. She has committed
    A. Fraud
    B. Libel
    C. Slander
    D. Negligence

60. When a caregiver threatens to "tie down" a person, the caregiver is guilty of
    A. Physical abuse
    B. Assault
    C. Invasion of privacy
    D. Battery

61. If a resident says he does not want you to dress him and you go ahead and touch him, you can be accused of
    A. Fraud
    B. Battery
    C. Assault
    D. False imprisonment

62. If you are asked to obtain a resident's signature on an informed consent, you should
    A. Make sure the resident is mentally competent
    B. Refuse. You are never responsible for obtaining a written consent
    C. Make sure the resident understands what he is signing
    D. Ask a family member to witness the signed consent

63. If a person is confused or unconscious, informed consent
    A. Is not necessary
    B. Cannot be obtained and so no treatments can be given
    C. Can be given by a husband, wife, son, daughter, or legal representative
    D. Can be given by the director of nursing

64. You can refuse to sign a will if
    A. You are named in the will
    B. You do not believe the person is of sound mind
    C. Your nursing center has policies that do not allow employees to witness wills
    D. All of the above

65. Which of the following is a form of abuse?
    A. Assisting the person to take a shower
    B. Telling the person he or she will never see family members again
    C. Expecting a person to feed and dress himself within his abilities
    D. Feeding the person in a dining room

66. When a person refuses medical treatment for a serious illness or is not taking needed drugs, this may be a warning sign of
    A. Elder abuse
    B. Physical abuse
    C. Self-neglect
    D. Involuntary seclusion

67. What kind of abuse occurs when an elderly person is left to sit in urine or feces?
    A. Neglect
    B. Involuntary seclusion
    C. Mental abuse
    D. Sexual abuse

68. An example of verbal abuse can be
    A. Failing to answer a call light
    B. Locking a person in a room
    C. Oral or written statements that speak badly of a person
    D. Making threats of harm to a person

69. Depriving a person of a basic need is
    A. Physical abuse
    B. Involuntary seclusion
    C. Emotional or mental abuse
    D. Sexual abuse

70. Which of the following may be a sign of elder abuse?
    A. The person answers questions openly.
    B. The family makes sure the hearing aids have new batteries.
    C. A caregiver is present during all conversations.
    D. All medications are taken as scheduled.

71. If you suspect an elderly person is being abused, you should
    A. Call the police
    B. Discuss the matter and your observations with the nurse
    C. Discuss the situation with the family
    D. Notify community agencies that investigate elder abuse

72. You have an assignment sheet with residents' names in your pocket. You have recorded information about personal care that was given during your shift. Before you leave the unit you should
    A. Discard in a wastebasket
    B. Place it in the secure document disposal bin
    C. Leave it on the counter to be used as scratch paper
    D. Leave it in a resident's room

FILL IN THE BLANKS: ABBREVIATIONS

73. DON _____

74. HIPAA _____

75. OBRA _____

MATCHING

Match the examples with the correct tort.

76. _____ While cleaning a resident's dentures, the nursing assistant drops and breaks them.

77. _____ A nursing assistant opens a resident's mail and reads it without permission.

78. _____ Instead of allowing the resident a choice, the nursing assistant tells him he will have a shower whether he wants one or not.

79. _____ An individual touches a person's body without the person's consent.

80. _____ An individual tricks or fools another person.

81. _____ An individual restrains or restricts a resident's freedom of movement without a physician's order.

82. _____ A nurse gives a treatment to the wrong person.

83. _____ A nursing assistant injures the name and reputation of a resident by making false statements to a third person.

84. _____ A nursing assistant writes notes falsely accusing another nursing assistant of stealing her purse.

A. Negligence
B. Malpractice
C. Libel
D. Slander
E. False imprisonment
F. Assault
G. Battery
H. Fraud
I. Invasion of privacy

OPTIONAL LEARNING EXERCISES

OBRA-Required Actions That Promote Dignity and Privacy (Box 2-2)

Match the action to promote dignity and privacy with the examples.

85. _____ File fingernails and apply polish as resident requests

86. _____ Cover the resident with a blanket during a bath

87. _____ Gain the person's attention before giving care

88. _____ Show interest when a person tells stories about the past

89. _____ Open containers and arrange food at meal times

90. _____ Close the door when the person asks for privacy

91. _____ Allow a resident to smoke in a designated area

92. _____ Take the resident to his weekly card game

A. Courteous and dignified interaction
B. Courteous and dignified care
C. Privacy and self-determination
D. Maintain personal choice and independence

Code of Conduct for Nursing Assistants (Box 2-3)

Fill in the blank with the correct code of conduct.

93. You cover the person and close the door when giving care. _____

94. You delay going on break when you find a person has soiled, wet linens that need to be changed. _____

95. A classmate offers to share her antibiotic prescription with you, but you refuse. _____

96. You report to the nurse that you gave a treatment to the wrong person. _____

97. You refuse to share information with your mother about a person in your care. _____

98. You return the person's shampoo to his room after a shower. _____

INDEPENDENT LEARNING ACTIVITIES

- Visit a nursing center and ask for a copy of the Resident Rights. Compare it to the information in this chapter. What is the same? What is different?
- When you visit a nursing center, ask if they have an ombudsman. If so, ask for an appointment to meet with this person. Ask the ombudsman the following questions.
  - What are the primary responsibilities he or she has in the center?
  - How often does he or she meet with residents?
  - What kind of problems has he or she helped to resolve?
- Make a list of tasks that would conflict with your moral or religious beliefs.
  - How would you feel about performing these tasks in your job?
  - What would you say about these tasks to your employer or coworkers?

- Role-play a situation in which you are asked to perform one of the tasks you identified in the previous activity. Have one student play the person asking you to perform the task. Have a second student observe and answer these questions.
  - What was your reaction when asked?
  - In what way did you communicate your discomfort?
  - What suggestions did you offer to make sure the task was done?

3 Work Ethics

FILL IN THE BLANKS: KEY TERMS

Confidentiality   Harassment   Stress
Courtesy   Priority   Stressor
Gossip   Professionalism   Work ethics

1. A _____ is the event or factor that causes stress.

2. Trusting others with personal and private information is _____.

3. _____ are behaviors in the workplace.

4. _____ is to spread rumors or talk about the private matters of others.

5. The response or change in the body caused by any emotional, physical, social, or economic factor is _____.

6. _____ is a polite, considerate, or helpful comment or act.

7. _____ means to trouble, torment, offend, or worry a person by one's behavior or comments.

8. A _____ is the most important thing at the time.

9. _____ is following laws, being ethical, having good work ethics, and having the skills to do your work.

CIRCLE THE BEST ANSWER

10. Work ethics involves
    A. How well you do your skills
    B. What religion you practice
    C. How you treat and work with others
    D. Cultural beliefs and attitudes

11. Your diet will maintain your weight if
    A. You avoid salty and sweet foods
    B. You take in fewer calories than your energy needs require
    C. It includes foods with fats and oils
    D. The number of calories taken in equals your energy needs

12. Most adults need about _____ hours of sleep daily.
    A. 7
    B. 10
    C. 4
    D. 12

13. Exercise is needed for
    A. Rest and sleep
    B. Muscle tone, circulation, and weight loss
    C. Good body mechanics
    D. Good nutrition

14. Smoking odors
    A. Disappear quickly when the person finishes smoking
    B. Can be covered up by chewing gum
    C. Are noticed only by the smoker
    D. Stay on the person's breath, hands, clothing, and hair

15. The most important reason why a person must not work under the influence of alcohol or drugs is that it
    A. Affects the person's safety
    B. Causes the person to be disorganized
    C. Makes coworkers angry
    D. Is not allowed by your nursing center

16. Which of these is part of good personal hygiene for work?
    A. Bathe every other day to prevent dry skin
    B. Brush your teeth once a day
    C. Cut toenails straight across
    D. Keep fingernails long and polished

17. Tattoos should be covered when working because they
    A. May offend others
    B. Can become infected
    C. May spread infection
    D. Increase the risk of skin injuries

18. When working, the nursing assistant usually may wear
    A. Jewelry in a pierced eyebrow, nose, lip, or tongue
    B. Wedding and engagement rings
    C. Multiple earrings in each ear
    D. Nail polish

19. When working, the nursing assistant may wear
    A. Sandals or open-toed shoes
    B. Hair that is off the collar and away from the face
    C. Perfume, cologne, or after-shave
    D. Colored or patterned underwear

20. What is a common reason for losing a job?
    A. Not knowing how to perform a task
    B. Frequent absences or tardiness
    C. Being disorganized
    D. Lacking self-confidence

21. If you are scheduled to begin work at 3 PM, you should arrive
    A. At 3 PM
    B. At 2:30 PM
    C. Early enough to be ready to work at 3 PM
    D. As close to 3 PM as you can

22. You can avoid being part of gossip by
    A. Remaining quiet when you are in a group where gossip is occurring
    B. Talking about residents and family members only to coworkers
    C. Repeating comments only in writing
    D. Removing yourself from a group or situation where gossip is occurring

23. Privacy and confidentiality for residents are rights protected by
    A. Your job description
    B. Resident rights under OBRA
    C. An agreement between the resident and the nurse
    D. Doctor's orders

24. When you are working, you should not wear
    A. Clothing that is wrinkled or needs to be mended
    B. A loose-fitting shirt
    C. A shirt with the top button open
    D. White socks

25. Slang or swearing should not be used at work because
    A. Words used with family and friends may offend residents and family members
    B. The resident may not understand you
    C. The resident may have difficulty hearing
    D. Coworkers may overhear it

26. You should say "please" and "thank you" to others because
    A. Courtesies mean so much to people; they can brighten someone's day
    B. It shows respect to the person
    C. It is required by your job
    D. It shows you like the person

27. When you are working, it is acceptable to
    A. Take a pen to use at home
    B. Sell cookies for your child's school project
    C. Use your cell phone on your break to make a call
    D. Make a copy of a letter on the copier in the nurses' station

28. When you leave and return to the unit for breaks or lunch, you should
    A. Tell each resident
    B. Tell any family members present
    C. Tell the nurse
    D. All of the above

29. Safety practices are important to follow because
    A. They help you to be more organized
    B. Negligent behavior affects the safety of others
    C. They save the center money
    D. You will get promoted more quickly

30. When setting priorities, which of these is not important?
    A. Planning care so you can have breaks and lunch with your friends
    B. Giving care to the person who has the greatest or most life-threatening needs
    C. Finding out what tasks need to be done at a set time
    D. Finding out what tasks need to be done at the end of your shift

31. Which of the following is not a healthy method to cope with stress
    A. Exercise regularly
    B. Getting enough rest
    C. Have a sense of humor
    D. Attempting to perform many tasks at one time

32. What physical effects of stress can be life-threatening?
    A. High blood pressure, heart attack, strokes, ulcers
    B. Increased heart rate, faster and deeper breathing
    C. Anxiety, fear, anger, depression
    D. Headaches, insomnia, muscle tension

33. Which of these actions is harassment?
    A. Offending others with gestures or remarks
    B. Offending others with jokes or pictures
    C. Making a sexual advance or requesting sexual favors
    D. All of the above

34. Good work ethics helps residents to
    A. Feel safe, secure, loved, and cared for
    B. Receive adequate care
    C. Recover from their illnesses
    D. Have more freedom to go to activities

OPTIONAL LEARNING EXERCISES

Qualities and Traits for Good Work Ethics (Box 3-2)

Match the qualities and traits for good work ethics with the examples.

35. _____ While working with Mr. Smith, you try to understand and feel what it must be like to be paralyzed on one side.

36. _____ You realize you are very good at giving basic care. You know you need to improve your communication skills.

37. _____ When caring for elderly residents, you try to do small things to make them happy or to find ways to ease their pain.

38. _____ You thank coworkers when they help you and remember to wish residents happy birthday as appropriate.

39. _____ When Mrs. Gibson is upset and angry, you remember to respect her feelings and to be kind.

40. _____ You report blood pressure and temperature readings accurately to the nurse.

41. _____ You realize that giving care to residents is important and you are excited about your work.

42. _____ Your supervisor tells you she knows she can count on you because you are always on time and perform delegated tasks as assigned.

43. _____ Even though Mr. Acevado has different cultural and religious views than yours, you value his feelings and beliefs.

44. _____ Before you left home today, you had an argument with your child. When you get to work, you make every effort to put that aside and be pleasant and happy.

45. _____ The nurse discusses a resident problem with you and says she knows you will keep the information confidential.

46. _____ When you are assigned to give care to a resident, you make sure his care is done thoroughly and exactly as instructed.

47. _____ Your coworker says she needs help to turn her resident and you cheerfully offer to help.

A. Caring
B. Dependable
C. Considerate
D. Cheerful
E. Empathetic
F. Trustworthy
G. Respectful
H. Courteous
I. Conscientious
J. Honest
K. Cooperative
L. Enthusiastic
M. Self-aware

INDEPENDENT LEARNING ACTIVITIES

- How well do you take care of your own health? What can you do to improve your health practices?
  - Do you maintain a healthy weight by eating calories adequate for your energy needs? What can you do to improve your diet?
  - How much sleep do you get each night?
  - How do you practice good body mechanics at all times, not just at work?
  - How many hours do you exercise each week? What type of exercise do you do?
  - When did you last have your eyes checked? Do you wear glasses if they were prescribed?
  - Do you smoke? How much? Have you considered any smoking cessation programs?
  - Are you taking any drugs that affect your thinking, feeling, behavior, and function? Did a doctor prescribe them or are you self-medicating? Have you talked with your doctor about the effects of any drugs you are taking?
  - Do you drink alcohol? How much? Have you been told it affects your behavior? Have you considered finding a program to help you quit drinking alcohol?
  - What activities or hobbies do you engage in to relieve stress?

CROSSWORD

Use the terms in Box 3-2 in the textbook to complete the crossword.

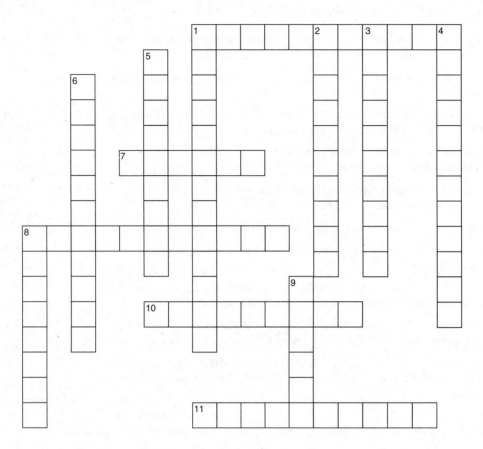

Across

1. Respect the person's physical and emotional feelings
7. Have concern for the person
8. Willing to help and work with others
10. Be polite and courteous to residents, families, and visitors
11. See things from the person's point of view

Down

1. Be careful, alert, and exact in following directions
2. Report to work on time and when scheduled
3. Do not judge or condemn residents and treat them with dignity and respect
4. Be eager, interested, and excited about your work
5. Know your feelings, strengths, and weaknesses
6. Residents and staff have confidence in you. They trust you to keep information confidential.
8. Greet and talk to people in a pleasant manner
9. Accurately report the care given, your observations, and any errors

Chapter 3 **Work Ethics**

4 Communicating with the Health Team

FILL IN THE BLANKS: KEY TERMS

Abbreviation
Chart
Communication
Conflict
Diagnosis

Kardex
Medical record
Prefix
Progress note
Recording

Reporting
Root
Suffix
Word element

1. A _____ is a word element placed before the root; it changes the meaning of the word.

2. An _____ is a shortened form of a word or phrase.

3. _____ is the exchange of information—a message sent is received and interpreted by the intended person.

4. A _____ is a clash between opposing interests and ideas.

5. A type of card file that summarizes information found in the medical record is a _____.

6. A _____ is the term used when symptoms, signs, or reasons for a problem are identified

7. The _____ is another name for the medical record.

8. _____ is a verbal account of care and observations.

9. A written description of the care given and the person's response and progress is the _____ _____.

10. A word element placed after a root that changes the meaning of the word is a _____.

11. A word element containing the basic meaning of the word is the _____.

12. A _____ is a written or electronic document of a person's condition and response to the treatment and care.

13. The written account of care and observations is _____.

14. A part of the word is the _____.

CIRCLE THE BEST ANSWER

15. For communication to be effective
    A. Use words that have the same meaning for the sender and the receiver
    B. Use terms that are unfamiliar to residents and families
    C. Add unrelated information to the message
    D. Answers should not be specific

16. The medical record will include
    A. Physical examination results
    B. The Kardex
    C. Change-of-shift reports
    D. Hospital records

17. To prevent errors and improper placement of records, the medical record is
    A. Kept in the resident's room
    B. Placed in a locked cabinet
    C. Stamped with the person's name, room number, and other identifying information on each page
    D. Printed on colored paper

18. Before a nursing assistant reads a person's chart, he should
    A. Know the center's policy
    B. Ask the nurse for permission
    C. Ask the doctor's permission
    D. Sign a sheet to get permission

19. If a resident asks to see the chart, you should
    A. Give it to him or her because the person always has a right to see the chart
    B. Read the chart and tell the person what it says
    C. Report the request to the nurse
    D. Tell the person that residents are not allowed to see their charts

20. The admission sheet is used to
    A. Find out the person's physical condition
    B. Help the person become familiar with the center
    C. Learn identifying information about a person
    D. Carry out a physical examination

21. Progress notes are usually written
    A. Every shift
    B. When there is a change in the person's condition
    C. Each day
    D. Once a year

22. OBRA requires that summaries of care be written
    A. Once a day
    B. Once every month
    C. At least every 3 months
    D. Once a year

23. Which of these is included on the activities of daily living flow sheet?
    A. Doctor's orders
    B. Vital signs
    C. Care plan
    D. Old records

24. Information in an electronic flow sheet
    A. Cannot be entered by the nursing assistant
    B. Is not confidential
    C. Is often faster and easier than paper charting
    D. Is entered only at the end of the shift

25. If you make an error when recording in a paper chart, you should follow center policy. Many centers require you to
    A. Erase it
    B. Use correction fluid to cover it
    C. Throw away the page and start over
    D. Draw a line through the incorrect part and date and initial the line

26. The resident and family can
    A. Attend any resident care conference held on the unit
    B. Accompany the staff on walking rounds
    C. Refuse actions suggested by the health team at a conference
    D. Add written notes to the chart

Choose the word that is spelled correctly for each of the definitions in questions 27 to 36.

27. Slow heart rate
    A. Bradecardia
    B. Bradycardia
    C. Bradacordia
    D. Bradicardia

28. Difficulty urinating
    A. Dysuria
    B. Dysurya
    C. Dysuira
    D. Disuria

29. Paralysis on one side of the body
    A. Hemyplegia
    B. Hemaplegia
    C. Hemoplega
    D. Hemiplegia

30. Opening into the ileum
    A. Ileostomie
    B. Ileostomy
    C. Ileastoma
    D. Illiostomy

31. Blue color or condition
    A. Cyonosis
    B. Cyinosis
    C. Cyanosis
    D. Cianosys

32. Opening into the trachea
    A. Tracheastomy
    B. Trachiostomy
    C. Tracheostome
    D. Tracheostomy

33. Pain in a nerve
    A. Neuralgia
    B. Neurolgia
    C. Nourealgia
    D. Neurilegia

34. Examination of a joint with a scope
    A. Arthoscopie
    B. Arthroscopy
    C. Arethroscopy
    D. Artheroscope

35. Rapid breathing
    A. Tachepnea
    B. Tachypinea
    C. Tachypnea
    D. Tachypnia

36. Removal of the gallbladder
    A. Cholecystectomy
    B. Cholcystectomy
    C. Cholicystetomy
    D. Cholecistectomy

37. When you are given a computer password, you
    A. Must never change it
    B. Can share it with a coworker
    C. Should never tell anyone your password
    D. Can use another person's password when entering the computer

38. Computers should not be used to
    A. Send messages and reports to the nursing unit
    B. Store resident records and care plans
    C. Send emails that require immediate reporting
    D. Monitor blood pressure, temperatures, and heart rates

39. When you answer the telephone, do not put callers on hold if
    A. The person has an emergency
    B. It is a doctor
    C. The call needs to be transferred to another unit
    D. You are too busy to find the nurse

40. If you have a conflict with a coworker, you should
    A. Ask the nurse in charge to schedule you at different times
    B. Ignore the person
    C. Identify the problem and try to resolve it
    D. Talk to other coworkers to explain your side of the story

41. When a conflict occurs, what is the first step you should take?
    A. Talk with other coworkers to see if they also have a conflict with the person.
    B. Confront the person and demand that he or she meets with you.
    C. Identify or define the real problem.
    D. Assume that the conflict will resolve itself if you ignore it.
42. Why is it important to resolve a conflict at work?
    A. Unkind words or actions may occur.
    B. The work environment becomes unpleasant.
    C. Care is affected.
    D. All of the above.

FILL IN THE BLANKS: ABBREVIATIONS

43. ADL_____

44. EHR_____

45. EMR_____

46. EPHI_____

47. HIPAA_____

48. MDS_____

49. OBRA_____

50. PHI_____

51. POC_____

MATCHING
Match each common health care term with the correct definition.

52. _____ Urinating

53. _____ Part of a call system that allows persons to signal the nurses' station for help

54. _____ A semi-sitting position; the head of the bed is raised between 45 and 60 degrees

55. _____ Difficult, labored, or painful breathing

56. _____ Lack of joint mobility caused by abnormal shortening of a muscle

57. _____ Not being able to control urination or defecation

58. _____ Involves memory, thinking, reasoning, ability to understand, judgment, and behavior

59. _____ Decrease in size or wasting away of tissue

60. _____ Temperature, pulse, respirations, and blood pressure

61. _____ Activities usually done during a normal day in a person's life

62. _____ Head of bed is raised 30 degrees, or head of bed is raised 30 degrees and knee portion is raised 15 degrees

63. _____ Written guide about the person's care; provides staff with approaches to reach the resident's goals

64. _____ Semi-solid mass of waste products in the colon that is expelled through the anus

65. _____ Loss of cognitive and social function caused by changes in the brain

66. _____ Localized injury to skin and/or underlying tissue, usually over a bony prominence

67. _____ Difficulty swallowing

68. _____ Back-lying or dorsal recumbent position

69. _____ Any item used by the person or staff to promote the person's function or safety

70. _____ Lying on the abdomen with the head turned to one side

71. _____ Elevated body temperature

A. Activities of daily living
B. Assist device
C. Atrophy
D. Call light
E. Care plan
F. Cognitive function
G. Contracture
H. Dementia
I. Dysphagia
J. Dyspnea
K. Feces
L. Fever
M. Fowler position
N. Incontinence
O. Pressure injury
P. Prone
Q. Semi-Fowler position
R. Supine
S. Vital signs
T. Voiding

FILL IN THE BLANKS

72. Next to each time, write the time using the 24-hour clock.

   A. 11:00 AM _____

   B. 8:00 AM _____

   C. 4:00 PM _____

   D. 7:30 AM _____

   E. 6:45 PM _____

   F. 12 NOON _____

   G. 3:00 AM _____

   H. 4:50 AM _____

   I. 5:30 PM _____

   J. 10:45 PM _____

   K. 11:55 PM _____

   L. 9:15 PM _____

Write the definition of each prefix.

73. auto- _____

74. brady- _____

75. dys- _____

76. ecto- _____

77. leuk- _____

78. macro- _____

79. neo- _____

80. supra- _____

81. uni- _____

Write the definition of each root word.

82. adeno _____

83. angio _____

84. broncho _____

85. cranio _____

86. duodeno _____

87. entero _____

88. gyneco _____

89. masto _____

90. pyo _____

Write the definition of each suffix.

91. -asis _____

92. -genic _____

93. -megaly _____

94. -oma _____

95. -phasia _____

96. -plegia _____

97. -ptosis _____

98. -scopy _____

99. -stasis _____

Using the abbreviations listed on the inside back cover of the textbook, write the correct abbreviations for each phrase below.

100. _____ Before meals

101. _____ After meals

102. _____ With

103. _____ Cancer

104. _____ Nothing by mouth

105. _____ Lower left quadrant

106. Every 2 hours, every 3 hours, every 4 hours

   _____

107. _____ Range of motion

LABELING

Convert the times from standard to military time and from military time to standard time. Use textbook Figure 4-9 as a guide.

108. _____ 2:00 AM

109. _____ 10:30 AM

110. _____ 5:00 AM

111. _____ 9:30 AM

112. _____5:45 PM

113. _____10:45 PM

114. _____0600 AM/PM

115. _____1145 AM/PM

116. _____1800 AM/PM

117. _____2200 AM/PM

118. Identify the four abdominal regions. Use RUQ, LUQ, RLQ, and LLQ as labels.

A. _____

B. _____

C. _____

D. _____

OPTIONAL LEARNING EXERCISES

- Class Experiment: It is often difficult to describe fluids in a clear and precise manner. Set up the following examples that imitate situations where you need to describe intake, output, or drainage.
  - Bloody drainage: Mix a teaspoon of ketchup and a teaspoon of water. Pour on the center of a paper napkin.
  - Urine: Pour a tablespoon of tea on the center of a paper towel.
  - Bleeding: Smear a teaspoon of red jelly on the center of a paper towel.
  - Broth: Pour 4 ounces of tea into a bowl.
    - Describe as accurately as possible what you see in terms of amounts, colors, and textures.
    - Compare your notes with classmates to see if you are using words that all have the same meaning.
    - What words were used that were clear to understand? What words were used that had more than one meaning?

Class Experiment	
Substance	**Observations**
Bloody drainage	
Urine	
Bleeding	
Broth	

- Case Study: *Mr. Larsen was admitted to a subacute care center after his abdominal surgery 1 week ago. This morning the nursing assistant gave Mr. Larsen a shower and assisted him to sit in a comfortable chair. The nursing assistant noticed that he sat very still and held his arms across his abdomen. He asked for a pillow and held it tightly against his abdomen.*
- Imagine you are the patient and answer the following questions.
  - What would you like the nursing assistant to ask you?
  - How would you communicate your feelings to the nursing assistant?
  - How could you let the nursing assistant know that you have pain without telling him or her?
- Imagine you are the nursing assistant and answer the following questions.
  - As the nursing assistant, what observations would be important to make about Mr. Larsen?
  - What questions could you ask Mr. Larsen?
  - What nonverbal communication would give you information about Mr. Larsen?
- Case Study: *Mrs. Miller was admitted to the health care center since you last worked 3 days ago. You have just started your shift and have been assigned to Mrs. Miller.*
  - What information would you need to know before giving care? Why?
  - What information would be important to provide to the on-coming shift?
  - What methods would you use to communicate this information?

INDEPENDENT LEARNING ACTIVITIES

Answer These Questions About Situations in Which You May Need to Communicate With Others

- When have you had a problem with communicating?
  - Why was it difficult? How did you handle this?
- Think about a situation in which you feel you communicated your point well.
  - What made the communication successful? How could you use a similar technique in caring for residents?
- How would you communicate with a person who speaks a language that you do not speak or understand?
  - What methods could you use to explain what you are going to do?
  - How would you communicate with a person from a different culture?

- Make flash cards of the prefixes, suffixes, and root words listed in Chapter 4.
  - Put the meaning of each one on the back of the appropriate card.
  - Work alone or with a partner. By looking at the cards, practice identifying the correct meaning of each term.
- The next time you visit a healthcare professional and receive a summary of care, look at the medical terms and abbreviations used. Have you ever accessed your own electronic medical record?
- Do you see any abbreviations or medical terms that you learned in this chapter? What do they mean? How did this chapter help you understand what was written?

5 Assisting with the Nursing Process

Assessment
Comprehensive care plan
Evaluation
Goal
Implementation
Interdisciplinary team (IDT)

Medical diagnosis
Nursing diagnosis
Nursing intervention
Nursing process
Objective data
Observation

Planning
Signs
Skilled care
Subjective data
Symptoms
Triggers

1. Daily services provided by the RN and/or therapist for rehabilitation or other complex services is _____.

2. _____ are things a person tells you about that you cannot observe through your senses.

3. _____ is to perform or carry out measures in the care plan; a step in the nursing process.

4. The method that RNs use to plan and deliver nursing care is the _____.

5. Another name for subjective data is _____.

6. A written guide about the care a person should receive is the _____.

7. _____ is collecting information about the person; a step in the nursing process.

8. Another name for objective data is _____.

9. The _____ describes a health problem that can be treated by a nursing measure; a step in the nursing process.

10. Information that is seen, heard, felt, or smelled is _____ or signs.

11. A step in the nursing process that is used to measure whether goals in the planning step were met is called _____.

12. _____ is setting priorities and goals; a step in the nursing process.

13. A _____ is an action or measure taken by the nursing team to help the person reach a goal.

14. A _____ is that which is desired in or by the person as a result of nursing care.

15. Using the senses of sight, hearing, touch, and smell to collect information is _____.

16. The identification of a disease or condition by a doctor is a _____.

17. _____ is information that is collected from the MDS for the Care Area Assessments (CAAs).

18. The _____ are the members of departments found in a nursing home.

CIRCLE THE BEST ANSWER

19. Which of these is one of the steps in the nursing process?
    A. Subjective data
    B. Objective data
    C. Observation
    D. Evaluation

20. The nursing process focuses on
    A. The doctor's orders
    B. The person's nursing needs
    C. Tasks and procedures that are needed
    D. Reducing the cost of health care

21. The nursing process
    A. Helps all nursing team members to do the same things for the person
    B. Stays the same from admission to discharge
    C. Cannot be used in home care
    D. Can be used only for adults

22. When you observe by using your senses, you assist the nurse to
    A. Assess the person
    B. Plan for care
    C. Implement care for the person
    D. Evaluate the person

23. Which of these is an example of objective data?
    A. Mrs. Hewitt complains of pain and nausea.
    B. Mr. Rodriguez tells you he has a dull ache in his stomach.
    C. You are taking Mrs. Wong's blood pressure and notice her skin is hot and moist.
    D. Mrs. Murano tells you she is tired because she could not sleep last night.

24. A Minimum Data Set (MDS) is used
    A. For nursing center residents
    B. In all health care settings
    C. In acute care settings
    D. In home care

25. The MDS is completed and updated
    A. Shortly after admission
    B. Each quarter
    C. Annually
    D. All of the above

26. Information is recorded in a point of care (POC) module to
    A. Record care given and observations made
    B. Assess the resident
    C. Document the doctor's orders
    D. List medications ordered and given to the person

27. A nursing diagnosis
    A. Identifies a disease or condition
    B. Helps to identify drugs or therapies used by the doctor
    C. Describes a health problem that can be treated by nursing measures
    D. Identifies only physical problems

28. When a nurse uses the nursing process, the person is given
    A. Only one nursing diagnosis
    B. No more than five nursing diagnoses
    C. As many nursing diagnoses as are needed
    D. Nursing diagnoses that involve only physical needs

29. Planning involves
    A. Setting priorities and goals
    B. Choosing nursing interventions to help the person reach a goal
    C. Revising the care plan as a person's needs change
    D. All of the above

30. OBRA requires an interdisciplinary care planning conference
    A. For each person
    B. To meet agency guidelines
    C. To assess the person
    D. To implement the care plan

31. What part of the nursing process is being carried out when you give personal care to a person?
    A. Assessment
    B. Planning
    C. Implementation
    D. Evaluation

32. An assignment sheet usually includes information about
    A. Each person's care
    B. Evaluation of the goals for care
    C. An assessment of the person
    D. The nursing diagnoses for the person

33. Nurses measure which goals have been met in the _____ part of the nursing process.
    A. Assessing
    B. Planning
    C. Implementation
    D. Evaluation

FILL IN THE BLANKS: ABBREVIATIONS

34. ADL_____

35. CAA_____

36. IDT_____

37. MDS_____

38. NANDA-I_____

39. OBRA_____

40. POC_____

41. RN_____

FILL IN THE BLANKS

42. When you make observations while you give care, what senses are used?

    A. _____

    B. _____

    C. _____

    D. _____

43. Each of the following is either subjective or objective data. In the blank next to each statement, place an "S" for subjective or an "O" for objective.

    A. _____ Sleepy

    B. _____ Chest pain

    C. _____ Skin cool

    D. _____ Cyanosis of nails

    E. _____ Labored breathing

    F. _____ Gas pain

    G. _____ Pain when urinating

    H. _____ Productive cough

    I. _____ Breath has fruity odor

    J. _____ Pulse rapid

44. Name the area involved in each of these examples that you would note when making basic observations (Box 5-1).

    A. Is the abdomen firm or soft?

    _____

    B. Is the person sensitive to bright lights?

    _____

C. Are sores or reddened areas present?

_____

D. What is the frequency of the person's cough?

_____

E. Can the person bathe without help?

_____

F. Can the person swallow food and fluids?

_____

G. What is the position of comfort?

_____

H. Does the person answer questions correctly?

_____

I. Does the person complain of stiff or painful joints?

_____

45. When planning care, needs that are required for life and survival (oxygen, water, food) must be met before _____.

46. A comprehensive care plan is

A. Developed for _____.

B. Suggestions are welcomed from all _____
_____.

C. It tells the health team members what care _____
_____.

47. The assignment sheet tells you about

A. _____

B. _____

C. _____

List at least three nursing interventions for each of these nursing diagnoses and goals.

48. Nursing Diagnosis: Feeding Self-Care Deficit related to weakness in right arm
Goal: Patient will eat 75% of each meal by 2/1.
Nursing Interventions:

A. _____

B. _____

C. _____

49. Nursing Diagnosis: Hygiene Self-Care Deficit related to forgetfulness
Goal: Patient will be assisted to maintain good hygiene throughout hospital stay.
Nursing Interventions:

A. _____

B. _____

C. _____

INDEPENDENT LEARNING ACTIVITIES

- Ask permission to look at the nursing care plans used at the agency where you had your clinical experience. Answer the following questions about the nursing care plans.
  ○ How do the nurses develop the plans? What resources do they use?
  ○ How often are the plans reviewed and revised?
  ○ How are the plans used by the nursing assistants?
  ○ How do nursing assistants help to develop and revise nursing interventions?
  ○ How do the nurses communicate the information on the nursing care plan?

Understanding the Resident

FILL IN THE BLANKS: KEY TERMS

Body language
Comatose
Culture
Disability
Esteem

Holism
Need
Nonverbal communication
Optimal level of function
Paraphrasing

Religion
Self-actualization
Self-esteem
Verbal communication

1. Experiencing one's potential is called _____ _____.

2. _____ is thinking well of oneself, seeing oneself as useful, and being well thought of by others.

3. A person's highest potential for mental and physical performance is the _____.

4. A _____ is that which is necessary or desirable for maintaining life and mental well-being.

5. Communication that uses the written or spoken word is called _____.

6. _____ is lost, absent, or impaired physical or mental function.

7. _____ is communication that does not involve words.

8. The characteristics of a group of people—language, values, beliefs, habits, likes, dislikes, customs—passed from one generation to the next is called _____.

9. The worth, value, or opinion one has of a person is _____.

10. _____ is spiritual beliefs, needs, and practices.

11. A person who is _____ has an inability to respond to stimuli.

12. Restating the person's message in your own words is called _____.

13. _____ sends messages through facial expressions, gestures, posture, and body movements.

14. _____ is a concept that considers the whole person.

CIRCLE THE BEST ANSWER

15. Who is the most important person in the nursing center?
    A. The director of nursing
    B. The resident
    C. The doctor
    D. The nurse

16. Which of these losses may have happened to an older resident?
    A. Loss of home and family members
    B. Loss of the person's role in the family or community
    C. Loss of body functions
    D. All of the above

17. When speaking about the resident, which of these statements is best?
    A. "Mrs. Jones in 135 needs a pain pill."
    B. "Granny Jones needs something for pain."
    C. "135 needs a pain pill."
    D. "Janie is complaining of pain."

18. What is the main reason you call a resident by a title such as Mr., Mrs., or Miss?
    A. It best identifies the person.
    B. It gives the person dignity and respect.
    C. It is polite.
    D. It shows the person you are in charge.

19. When is it acceptable to call a person by his or her first name or another name?
    A. You have cared for the person for several months.
    B. The person is confused.
    C. The person asks you to use the name.
    D. The person has difficulty hearing.

20. Which of these needs is affected when the person has a disability or illness?
    A. Physical
    B. Social
    C. Psychological
    D. All of the above

21. What needs are most important for survival?
    A. Physical
    B. Safety and security
    C. Love and belonging
    D. Self-esteem

22. It is important for the person to know what to expect when care is given because the person will
    A. Be combative
    B. Feel safer and more secure
    C. Have a more meaningful relationship
    D. Experience his or her potential

23. What need is rarely, if ever, totally met?
    A. Physiological
    B. Safety and security
    C. Self-esteem
    D. Self-actualization

24. Mrs. Young is a new resident. She will feel more secure when you
    A. Give her explanations of routines and procedures only one time
    B. Spend as little time as possible in her room
    C. Use new equipment without telling her what it is
    D. Listen to her concerns and explain all routines and procedures as often as needed

25. Mrs. Russo never has visitors and is becoming weaker and unable to care for herself. What need is not being met?
    A. Physiological
    B. Safety and security
    C. Love and belonging
    D. Self-esteem

26. A person who is ill and disabled is often very angry because
    A. The care he or she is receiving is poor
    B. He or she is angry at the situation
    C. He or she does not like you
    D. He or she has a bad temper

27. How can you help Mr. Diakos maintain his optimal level of functioning?
    A. Give him complete care.
    B. Encourage him to be as independent as possible.
    C. Avoid staying with him to visit.
    D. Do not respond promptly when he asks for help.

28. Mrs. Nelson is alert and oriented. Why would she require care in a nursing center?
    A. She has trouble remembering where she is.
    B. She cannot tell you what she needs or wants.
    C. She has physical problems, so she requires help.
    D. She does not know who she is.

29. Which of these is a reason why confusion and disorientation may be temporary?
    A. The person has a disabling disease.
    B. The person has recently been admitted to the nursing center.
    C. The person needs complete help with all activities of daily living (ADL).
    D. The person is terminally ill.

30. Mrs. Hayashi is admitted to the nursing center. The nurse tells you she will only be here short term. You know the reason for most short-term admissions is to
    A. Provide quality care to dying residents
    B. Give complete care to the resident
    C. Help the resident recover from fractures, acute illness, or surgery
    D. Prevent injury of the resident

31. Respite care provides
    A. Time to recover from surgery or acute illness
    B. Recovery from temporary confusion
    C. Care for a dying person
    D. The caregiver a chance to take a vacation, tend to business, or rest

32. A person who needs life-long care has a disability that occurs
    A. Due to birth defects or childhood illnesses or injuries
    B. Because of mental illness
    C. Because of the aging process
    D. Because the person is dying

33. If a resident is comatose, how would you know the person is in pain?
    A. The person cries and lies very still.
    B. The person asks for pain medications.
    C. Pain is shown by grimacing and groaning.
    D. You cannot tell if the person is in pain.

34. Which of these ways to deal with a person with behavior issues would be helpful?
    A. Argue with the person to show him he is wrong.
    B. Avoid going into the room unless you must give care.
    C. Carry out care and tasks without talking to the person.
    D. Stay calm and professional if the anger and hostility is directed at you.

35. Which of these would help effective communication?
    A. Use words that have the same meaning to both you and the person.
    B. Give long, detailed explanations to questions.
    C. Change the subject when the person seems confused.
    D. Use medical terminology when talking to the person.

36. Mrs. Stevens cannot speak. Which of these would be an example of her verbal communication?
    A. She may use touch.
    B. Her body language sends messages.
    C. She uses gestures to communicate.
    D. She writes messages on a notepad.

37. When you go to Mrs. Hart's room, you can tell she is not happy or not feeling well because
    A. Her hair is well-groomed
    B. She has a slumped posture
    C. She smiles when you enter the room
    D. She is watching TV and does not carry on a conversation

27

38. You show that you listen effectively when you
    A. Look across the room to avoid eye contact
    B. Lean away from the person with your arms folded
    C. Change the subject if the person seems upset
    D. Respond to the person by nodding your head
39. Which of these is an example of paraphrasing?
    A. "You don't know how long you will be here."
    B. "Do you want to take a tub bath or a shower?"
    C. "Tell me about living on a farm."
    D. "Can you explain what you mean?"
40. When you say "Mr. Patel, have you taken a shower this morning?," you are
    A. Paraphrasing his thoughts
    B. Asking a direct question
    C. Focusing his thoughts
    D. Asking an open-ended question
41. Responses to open-ended questions generally are
    A. Longer and give more information than responses to direct questions
    B. "Yes" or "no" answers
    C. Able to make sure you understand the message
    D. Focused on dealing with a certain topic
42. Mr. Parker often rambles and tells long stories in which his thoughts wander. You need to know if he had a bowel movement today, so you will
    A. Make a clarifying statement
    B. Ask an open-ended question
    C. Make a focusing statement
    D. Paraphrase his thoughts
43. What is best if the person takes long pauses between statements?
    A. You do not need to talk. Just being there helps.
    B. Try to cheer the person up by talking.
    C. Leave the room.
    D. Find another resident to talk with the person.
44. A statement that is a communication barrier is:
    A. "You do not know why your wife was crying after she talked to the doctor."
    B. "Did you have a bowel movement today?"
    C. "What do you like about being retired?"
    D. "Don't worry. Everything will be fine."
45. Mrs. MacBride has visitors and you need to give care. What would you do?
    A. Give the care while visitors are present.
    B. Politely ask the visitors to leave the room.
    C. Tell the visitors to give the care.
    D. Tell the visitors they must leave the nursing center.

FILL IN THE BLANKS: BASIC NEEDS

46. List the basic needs for life as described by Maslow, from the lowest level to the highest level.

    A._____

    B._____

    C._____

    D._____

    E._____

Basic Needs
Physical needs

47. What are the six physical needs required for survival?
    _____, _____,
    _____, _____,
    _____, _____

48. The lower-level needs must be met before the _____ needs.

Safety and security

49. Safety and security needs relate to feeling safe from, and _____, _____, and _____.

50. Why do many people feel a loss of safety and security when admitted to a nursing center?

    A._____

    B._____

    C._____

    D._____

Love and belonging

51. The need for love and belonging relates to _____, _____, and _____.

52. These needs also involve _____ _____.

53. How can you help a resident feel loved and accepted? _____

Self-esteem

54. What does self-esteem relate to?_____, _____, and _____

55. Why is it important to encourage residents to do as much as possible for themselves? _____ _____

Self-actualization

56. What does self-actualization involve? _____ _____, _____, and _____

57. What happens if self-actualization is postponed? _____

Case Study

You have completed your duties for the morning and have some free time. Mr. Donal is a resident in the nursing center. He rarely has visitors and you try to spend time with him when you can. Fill in the blanks in the following statements about communication techniques you use when you visit with Mr. Donal.

58. You sit in a chair next to Mr. Donal so you can see each other. This position will help you to be at his _____.

59. You should lean _____ Mr. Donal to show interest.

60. Mr. Donal says, "I know this is the best place for me but I miss my flower garden at home." You respond, "You miss your home." This is an example of _____.

61. You ask Mr. Donal, "You told me you did not sleep well last night. Can you tell me why?" He replies: "There was a lot of noise in the hall." This is an example of a _____.

62. You say to Mr. Donal, "Tell me about your flower garden at home." This is an _____ question.

63. When you ask, "Can you explain what that means?" you are asking a person to _____.

64. Mr. Donal says that he "hurts all over" and then begins to talk about the weather. You say, "Tell me more about where you hurt. You said you hurt all over." This statement helps in _____ the topic.

65. Mr. Donal begins to cry when he talks about his flower garden. How can you show caring and respect for his situation and feelings? _____ _____.

66. When Mr. Donal begins to cry, you quickly begin to talk about the activities planned this morning. Changing the subject is a _____ _____.

INDEPENDENT LEARNING ACTIVITIES

- Refer to the discussion about basic needs in Chapter 6. Think about how well you are meeting your own needs.
  - Do you smoke? What need may be affected by smoking?
  - What kinds of foods and fluids do you eat? Is your diet meeting your basic needs for food and water?
  - How much rest and sleep do you get each day? How much sleep do you need to feel well rested?
  - How safe do you feel at home? At school? In your community? How do your feelings affect your ability to hold a job or attend school?
  - Who are the people who make you feel loved? Who helps you when you have problems?
  - What are you doing that helps you meet the need for self-actualization?
- Answer the following questions about your personal health care practices.
  - What health care practices are followed in your family? How do these practices help or interfere with good health?
  - How often do you go to the doctor? For regular check-ups? Only when ill?
  - When do you go to the dentist? Once or twice a year for cleaning and check-ups? Only when you have a toothache?
  - When a family member is in a health care center, how does your family respond? Does someone stay with the person and do all of the care? Or do family members visit for brief periods and let health care workers provide all of the care? Is the family response related to any cultural or religious practices?
- Look at your answers to both sets of questions above.
  - How well are you meeting your basic needs? How could you improve in meeting your needs? What changes would be the most beneficial?

Culture, Religion, and Spirituality

FILL IN THE BLANKS: KEY TERMS

Agnostic
Atheist
Bias
Cleric
Culture
Ethnicity

Extended family
Fast
Nuclear family
Personal space
Prejudice

Race
Religion
Sensitivity
Spirituality
Stereotyping

1. A person who believes it is impossible to know if a god exists is _____.

2. _____ is a person's need to find meaning and purpose in life.

3. A _____ is a family consisting of parents and their children.

4. A leader or representative from an organized religion is a _____.

5. A family comprised of parents, their children, grandparents, aunts, uncles, and cousins is an _____ _____.

6. A person who denies the existence of a god or deity is an _____.

7. _____ is a classification of persons based on physical and biological characteristics.

8. To prefer something or someone, often without sound judgment, is _____.

9. Spiritual beliefs, needs, and practices comprise _____.

10. The ability to appreciate the personal characteristics of others is _____.

11. Forming an opinion without having facts or information is _____.

12. _____ is the name for the beliefs, practices, customs, and language of a group of people that is passed on between generations.

13. The distance that people require to comfortably communicate is _____.

14. _____ is the classification of people based on national origin or culture.

15. To refrain from consuming food (and sometimes food and drink) is to _____.

16. _____ is believing that everyone in a group is the same.

CIRCLE THE BEST ANSWER

17. When you are caring for persons from a culture that is different from yours, you should
    A. Expect them to accept new cultural practices
    B. Ignore them if they speak a different language
    C. Asked to be assigned to people of the same culture as yours
    D. Set aside any values, biases, and attitudes that are judgmental.

18. When caring for a person from Vietnam who has died, you may see the family
    A. Pour water into the person's mouth
    B. Prepare to have the body cremated
    C. Have a priest tie strings around the deceased persons neck or wrist
    D. Place coins or rice in the person's mouth

19. A person from certain cultures may not make eye contact because he or she is
    A. Not interested in the conversation
    B. From a culture that feels eye contact shows disrespect
    C. Uncomfortable with the care he is receiving
    D. Shy and afraid of others

20. A Muslim patient may ask the time several times during the day in order to
    A. Take communion
    B. Conduct prayers
    C. Read the Bible
    D. Apply healing oils

21. When you wish a person a "Happy Birthday," she tells you her religion does not celebrate birthdays. One possibility is that she is
    A. Hindu
    B. Buddhist
    C. Jehovah's Witness
    D. Catholic

22. When the family asks to give care to a dying person, you should
    A. Ask the nurse if you are unsure this is permitted
    B. Tell them that this is against facility policy
    C. Tell them it is your assignment and you will be fired if you do not give the care
    D. Record that the care is done and go on to other duties

23. When a person asks to see a spiritual leader or adviser, you should
    A. Tell the person that no one is available to see him or her until the Sabbath
    B. Ignore the request because a visit is not on the schedule
    C. Tell the person to have family members get in touch with the spiritual leader
    D. Report the request to the nurse at once

24. Persons often have special religious objects that have special meaning to them. It would be correct to
    A. Move these objects out of the way to keep the area neat
    B. Allow the person to light a candle whenever it is needed for their beliefs

C. Never place an object on top of a Bible, Koran, Torah, or other holy books
D. Tell the family to take these objects home to avoid clutter in the room

25. The person's cultural, spiritual, and religious practices are found in the
    A. Doctor's orders
    B. Care plan
    C. Assignment sheet
    D. Nurse's notes

FILL IN THE BLANKS: ABBREVIATIONS

26. RN_____

27. CNA_____

28. OBRA_____

29. CMS_____

MATCHING

30. _____ Believe that Jesus is the son of God

31. _____ Often abstain from meat on Fridays during Lent

32. _____ Conduct prayers five times a day

33. _____ Do not celebrate birthdays or many Christian holidays

34. _____ Observe Sabbath from sundown on Friday until sundown on Saturday

35. _____ Follow a diet that is strictly vegetarian, and fasting is common

36. _____ May fast on the first Sunday of the month and do not consume alcohol or caffeine

37. _____ After death, may keep the body as still as possible for a certain period of time

A. Christian
B. Catholic
C. Jehovah's Witness
D. Mormon (Latter Day Saints)
E. Hindus
F. Jewish
G. Muslim (Islam)
H. Buddhism

OPTIONAL LEARNING EXERCISES

38. How can you help a resident to observe religious practice if services are held in the nursing center?
    _____

39. If a person wants to have a visit from a spiritual leader, you should tell _____.

40. If the person wants a spiritual leader or adviser to visit in the room, you should _____, _____, and _____ _____.

41. If a person has religious objects in the room, you should treat the items with _____ and should not _____ without permission.

42. If a person refuses a particular food due to a religious custom, you should offer _____.

43. A person tells you he has no belief in a god. This person is an _____.

44. An _____ does not deny that a god exists but does not believe it can be _____.

INDEPENDENT LEARNING ACTIVITIES

After studying this chapter, answer these questions related to your own cultural and religious backgrounds to identify how they influence your life and how to relate to others.

- What health care practices are followed in your family? How are these practices related to your cultural, spiritual or religious beliefs? Identify whether any of these beliefs are different than some of the health information you are learning in class.
- How do your cultural, spiritual, or religious practices influence your caring for others? What beliefs could interfere with you giving to care to others (for example, caring for a person of the opposite sex, a person of a different religion, a person of a different race)? How will you deal with these situations as you work as a health care giver?
- Have a discussion with friends or classmates about different beliefs or cultural practices among the group. Discuss how these practices may influence your caring for others.
- Have a discussion about various foods that certain cultures enjoy. Are some associated with particular religious or spiritual holidays?

8 Body Structure and Function

FILL IN THE BLANKS: KEY TERMS

Artery
Capillary
Cell
Digestion
Hemoglobin

Hormone
Immunity
Menstruation
Metabolism
Organ

Peristalsis
Respiration
System
Tissue
Vein

1. The substance in red blood cells that carries oxygen and gives blood its color is _____.

2. _____ is protection against a disease or condition.

3. The process of supplying the cells with oxygen and removing carbon dioxide from them is called _____.

4. The process of physically and chemically breaking down food so it can be absorbed for use by the cells is _____.

5. _____ is the burning of food for heat and energy by the cells.

6. A blood vessel that carries blood away from the heart is the _____.

7. _____ is the involuntary muscle contractions in the digestive system that move food through the alimentary canal.

8. Organs that work together to perform special functions form a _____.

9. The basic unit of body structure is a _____.

10. Groups of tissues with the same function form an _____.

11. A _____ is a tiny blood vessel.

12. A group of cells with similar function is _____.

13. _____ is the process in which the lining of the uterus breaks up and is discharged from the body through the vagina.

14. A chemical substance secreted by the glands into the bloodstream is a _____.

15. A _____ is a blood vessel that carries blood back to the heart.

CIRCLE THE BEST ANSWER

16. A cell is
    A. Found only in muscles
    B. The basic unit of body structure
    C. Able to live without oxygen
    D. A group of tissues

17. The control center of a cell is the
    A. Membrane
    B. Protoplasm
    C. Cytoplasm
    D. Nucleus

18. Genes control
    A. Cell division
    B. Tissues
    C. Traits inherited by children
    D. Organs

19. Connective tissue
    A. Covers internal and external body surfaces
    B. Receives and carries impulses to the brain and back to body parts
    C. Anchors, connects, and supports other body tissues
    D. Allows the body to move by stretching and contracting

20. Living cells of the epidermis contain
    A. Blood vessels and many nerves
    B. Sweat and oil glands
    C. Pigment that gives skin its color
    D. Hair roots

21. Sweat glands help
    A. The body to regulate temperature
    B. To keep the hair and skin soft and shiny
    C. To protect the nose from dust, insects, and other foreign objects
    D. The skin to sense pleasant and unpleasant sensations

22. Long bones
    A. Allow skill and ease in movement
    B. Bear the weight of the body
    C. Protect organs
    D. Allow various degrees of movement and flexion

23. Blood cells are manufactured in
    A. The heart
    B. The liver
    C. Blood vessels
    D. Bone marrow
24. Joints move smoothly because of the
    A. Cartilage
    B. Synovial fluid
    C. Muscle
    D. Ligaments
25. A joint that moves in all directions is a
    A. Ball and socket
    B. Hinge
    C. Pivot
    D. All of the above
26. Voluntary muscles are
    A. Found in the stomach and intestines
    B. Attached to bones
    C. Cardiac muscle
    D. Tendons
27. Muscles produce heat by
    A. Contracting
    B. Relaxing
    C. Maintaining posture
    D. Working automatically
28. The central nervous system (CNS) consists of
    A. A myelin sheath
    B. Nerves throughout the body
    C. The brain and spinal cord
    D. Cranial nerves
29. The medulla controls
    A. Muscle contraction and relaxation
    B. Heart rate, breathing, blood vessel size, and swallowing
    C. Reasoning, memory, and consciousness
    D. Hearing and vision
30. Cerebrospinal fluid
    A. Cushions shocks that could injure the structure of the brain and spinal cord
    B. Controls voluntary muscles
    C. Lubricates movement
    D. Controls involuntary muscles
31. The cranial nerves conduct impulses between the
    A. Brain and the head, neck, chest, and abdomen
    B. Brain and the skin and extremities
    C. Brain and internal body structures
    D. Spinal cord and lower extremities
32. When you are frightened, the _____ nervous system is stimulated.
    A. Sympathetic
    B. Parasympathetic
    C. Central
    D. Cranial
33. Receptors for vision and nerve fibers of the optic nerve are found in the
    A. Sclera
    B. Choroids
    C. Retina
    D. Cornea

34. What structure of the ear is involved in balance?
    A. Malleus
    B. Auditory canal
    C. Tympanic membranes
    D. Semicircular canals
35. Hemoglobin in red blood cells gives blood its red color and carries
    A. Oxygen
    B. Food to cells
    C. Waste products
    D. Water
36. Red blood cells live for
    A. About 9 days
    B. 3 or 4 months
    C. 4 days
    D. A year
37. White blood cells or leukocytes
    A. Protect the body against infection
    B. Are necessary for blood clotting
    C. Carry food, hormones, chemicals, and waste products
    D. Pick up carbon dioxide
38. The left atrium of the heart
    A. Receives blood from the lungs
    B. Receives blood from the body tissues
    C. Pumps blood to the lungs
    D. Pumps blood to all parts of the body
39. Arteries
    A. Return blood to the heart
    B. Pass food, oxygen, and other substances into the cells
    C. Pick up waste products, including carbon dioxide, from the cells
    D. Carry blood away from the heart
40. In the lungs, oxygen and carbon dioxide are exchanged
    A. In the epiglottis
    B. Between the right bronchus and the left bronchus
    C. By the bronchioles
    D. Between the alveoli and capillaries
41. The lungs are protected by
    A. The diaphragm
    B. The pleura
    C. A bony framework of the ribs, sternum, and vertebrae
    D. The lobes
42. Food is moved through the alimentary canal (gastrointestinal tract) by
    A. Chyme
    B. Peristalsis
    C. Swallowing
    D. Bile
43. Water is absorbed from chyme in the
    A. Small intestine
    B. Stomach
    C. Esophagus
    D. Large intestine

44. Digested food is absorbed through tiny projections called
    A. Jejunum
    B. Ileum
    C. Villi
    D. Colon
45. A function of the urinary system is to
    A. Remove waste products from the blood
    B. Rid the body of solid waste
    C. Rid the body of carbon dioxide
    D. Burn food for energy
46. A person usually feels the need to urinate when the bladder contains about
    A. 1000 mL of urine
    B. 500 mL of urine
    C. 250 mL of urine
    D. 125 mL of urine
47. Testosterone is needed for
    A. Male secondary sex characteristics
    B. Female secondary sex characteristics
    C. Sperm to be produced
    D. Ova to be produced
48. The prostate gland lies
    A. In the scrotum
    B. In the testes
    C. Just below the bladder
    D. In the penis
49. The ovaries secrete progesterone and
    A. Estrogen
    B. Testosterone
    C. Ova
    D. Semen
50. When an ovum is released from an ovary, it travels first through the
    A. Uterus
    B. Fallopian tube
    C. Endometrium
    D. Vagina
51. Menstruation occurs when
    A. The hymen is ruptured
    B. An ovum is released by the ovary
    C. The endometrium breaks up
    D. Fertilization occurs

52. A fertilized cell implants in the
    A. Ovary
    B. Fallopian tubes
    C. Endometrium
    D. Vagina
53. The master gland is the
    A. Thyroid gland
    B. Parathyroid gland
    C. Adrenal gland
    D. Pituitary gland
54. Thyroid hormone regulates
    A. Growth
    B. Metabolism
    C. Proper functioning of nerves and muscles
    D. Energy produced during activity
55. If too little insulin is produced by the pancreas, the person has
    A. Tetany
    B. Slow growth
    C. Diabetes
    D. Slowed metabolism
56. When antigens (an unwanted substance) enter the body, white blood cells called lymphocytes increase the production of
    A. Antibodies
    B. Phagocytes
    C. B cells
    D. T cells

FILL IN THE BLANKS: ABBREVIATIONS

57. CNS_____

58. GI_____

59. mL_____

60. RBC_____

61. WBC_____

MATCHING

Match the musculoskeletal term with the correct description.

62. _____ Connective tissue at the end of long bones

63. _____ Skeletal muscle

64. _____ Membrane that covers bone

65. _____ Connects muscle to bone

66. _____ The point at which two or more bones meet

67. _____ Muscle found only in heart

68. _____ Involuntary muscle

69. _____ Acts as a lubricant so the joint can move smoothly

A. Periosteum
B. Joint
C. Cartilage
D. Synovial fluid
E. Striated muscle
F. Smooth muscle
G. Cardiac muscle
H. Tendons

Match the nervous system term with the correct description.

70. _____ Contains eustachian tubes and ossicles
71. _____ Has 12 pairs of cranial nerves and 31 pairs of spinal nerves
72. _____ White of the eye
73. _____ Outside of the cerebrum; controls highest function of brain
74. _____ Inner layer of eye; receptors for vision are contained here
75. _____ Controls involuntary muscles, heartbeat, blood pressure, and other functions
76. _____ Light enters the eye through this structure
77. _____ Contains the midbrain, pons, and medulla
78. _____ Waxy substance secreted in the auditory canal
79. _____ Contains the semicircular canal and cochlea

A. Sclera
B. Cornea
C. Retina
D. Cerumen
E. Middle ear
F. Inner ear
G. Brainstem
H. Cerebral cortex
I. Autonomic nervous system
J. Peripheral nervous system

Match the circulatory system term with the correct description.

80. _____ The part of blood that is mostly water
81. _____ The thin sac covering the heart
82. _____ Very tiny blood vessels
83. _____ The substance in blood that picks up oxygen
84. _____ Carry blood away from the heart
85. _____ White blood cells
86. _____ Carry blood toward the heart
87. _____ Red blood cells
88. _____ The thick muscular portion of the heart
89. _____ Platelets; necessary for clotting
90. _____ The membrane lining the inner surface of the heart

A. Plasma
B. Erythrocytes
C. Hemoglobin
D. Leukocytes
E. Thrombocytes
F. Pericardium
G. Myocardium
H. Endocardium
I. Arteries
J. Veins
K. Capillaries

Match the respiratory system term with the correct description.

91. _____ Air passes from the larynx into this structure
92. _____ A two-layered sac that covers the lungs
93. _____ Piece of cartilage that acts like a lid over the larynx
94. _____ Separates the lungs from the abdominal cavity
95. _____ The voice box
96. _____ Several small branches that divide from the bronchus
97. _____ Tiny one-celled air sacs

A. Epiglottis
B. Larynx
C. Bronchiole
D. Trachea
E. Alveoli
F. Diaphragm
G. Pleura

Match the digestive system term with the correct description.

98. _____ Structure in which more digestive juices are added to chyme
99. _____ Semi-liquid food mixture formed in the stomach
100. _____ Portion of the GI tract that absorbs food
101. _____ Stores bile
102. _____ Portion of the GI tract that absorbs water
103. _____ Produces bile
104. _____ Moistens food particles in the mouth
105. _____ Produces digestive juices

A. Liver
B. Chyme
C. Colon
D. Duodenum
E. Jejunum
F. Saliva
G. Pancreas
H. Gallbladder

Match the urinary system term with the correct description.

106. _____ Basic working unit of the kidney

107. _____ Bean-shaped structure that produces urine

108. _____ A cluster of capillaries in the tubule

109. _____ Structure that allows urine to pass from the bladder

110. _____ A tube attached to the renal pelvis of the kidney

111. _____ Hollow muscular sac that stores urine

112. _____ Opening at the end of the urethra

113. _____ Fluid and waste products form urine in this structure

A. Bladder
B. Glomerulus
C. Kidney
D. Meatus
E. Nephrons
F. Tubules
G. Ureter
H. Urethra

Match the reproductive system term with the correct description.

114. _____ Male sex glands

115. _____ Two folds of tissue on each side of the vagina

116. _____ Sac between the thighs that contains the testes

117. _____ External genitalia of female

118. _____ Testicles; sperm are produced here

119. _____ Attached to uterus; ova travel through this structure

120. _____ Stores sperm and produces semen

121. _____ Tissue lining the uterus

A. Scrotum
B. Testes
C. Seminal vesicle
D. Gonads
E. Fallopian tube
F. Endometrium
G. Labia
H. Vulva

Match the endocrine system term with the correct description.

122. _____ Released by the pancreas; regulates sugar in blood

123. _____ Sex hormone secreted by the testes

124. _____ Sex hormone secreted by the ovaries

125. _____ Regulates metabolism

126. _____ Regulates calcium levels in the body

127. _____ Stimulates the body to produce energy during emergencies

A. Epinephrine
B. Estrogen
C. Insulin
D. Parathormone
E. Testosterone
F. Thyroxine

Match the immune system term with the correct description.

128. _____ Normal body substances that recognize abnormal or unwanted substances

129. _____ Type of cell that destroys invading cells

130. _____ Type of white blood cell that digests and destroys microorganisms

131. _____ Type of cell that causes production of antibodies

132. _____ An abnormal or unwanted substance

133. _____ Type of white blood cell that produces antibodies

A. Antibodies
B. Antigens
C. Phagocytes
D. Lymphocytes
E. B cells
F. T cells

134. Name the parts of the cell.

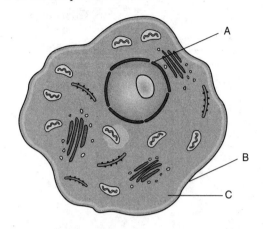

A. _____

B. _____

C. _____

135. Name each type of joint.

A. _____

B. _____

C. _____

136. Name the parts of the brain.

A. _____

B. _____

C. _____

137. Name the four chambers of the heart.

A. _____

B. _____

C. _____

D. _____

138. Name the structures of the respiratory system.

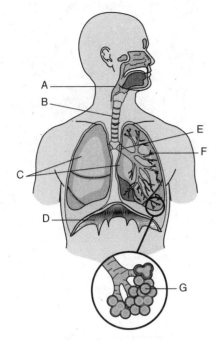

A. _____

B. _____

C. _____

D. _____

E. _____

F. _____

G. _____

139. Name the structures of the digestive system.

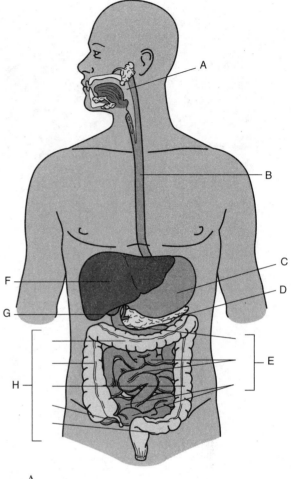

A. _____

B. _____

C. _____

D. _____

E. _____

F. _____

G. _____

H. _____

140. Name the structures of the urinary system.

A. _____

B. _____

C. _____

D. _____

141. Name the structures of the male reproductive system.

A. _____

B. _____

C. _____

D. _____

E. _____

F. _____

G. _____

H. _____

142. Name the external female genitalia.

A. _____

B. _____

C. _____

D. _____

E. _____

F. _____

143. Explain the function of each part of the cell.

    A. Cell membrane _____

    _____

    B. Nucleus _____

    _____

    C. Cytoplasm_____

    _____

    D. Protoplasm _____

    _____

    E. Chromosomes _____

    _____

    F. Genes _____

    _____

144. List the structures contained in the two skin layers.

    A. Epidermis_____

    _____

    B. Dermis _____

    _____

145. Explain the function of the types of bone.

    A. Long bones _____

    _____

    B. Short bones _____

    _____

    C. Flat bones _____

    _____

    D. Irregular bones _____

    _____

146. Describe how each type of joint moves and give an example of each type.

    A. Ball and socket _____

    _____

    Example: _____

    _____

    B. Hinge _____

    _____

    Example: _____

    _____

    C. Pivot _____

    _____

    Example: _____

    _____

147. Explain what happens when muscles contract.

    _____

    _____

    _____

    _____

148. Explain the function of the three main parts of the brain. Include the function of the cerebral cortex and the midbrain, pons, and medulla.

    A. Cerebrum _____

    _____

    Cerebral cortex _____

    _____

    B. Cerebellum _____

    _____

    C. Brainstem _____

    _____

    Midbrain and pons _____

    _____

    Medulla _____

    _____

149. Explain how the sympathetic and parasympathetic nervous systems balance each other.

    _____

    _____

    _____

    _____

150. Explain what happens to each of these structures when light enters the eye.

    A. Choroid _____

    _____

    B. Cornea _____

    _____

    C. Lens _____

    _____

    D. Retina _____

    _____

151. Explain how each of these structures helps to carry sound in the ear.

A. Ossicles _____

_____

B. Cochlea _____

_____

C. Auditory nerve _____

_____

152. Where are red blood cells destroyed as they wear out? _____

153. When an infection occurs, what do white blood cells do? _____

154. Explain the function of the four atria (chambers) of the heart.

A. Right atrium _____

_____

B. Left atrium _____

_____

C. Right ventricle _____

_____

D. Left ventricle _____

_____

155. Explain where each of these veins carries blood.

A. Inferior vena cava _____

_____

B. Superior vena cava _____

_____

156. _____ Explain what happens in the alveoli.

_____

_____

157. After food is swallowed, explain what happens in each of these parts of the digestive tract.

A. Stomach _____

_____

B. Duodenum _____

_____

C. Jejunum and ileum _____

_____

D. Colon _____

_____

E. Rectum _____

_____

F. Anus _____

_____

158. Explain what happens in these structures of the kidney.

A. Glomerulus _____

_____

B. Collecting tubules _____

_____

C. Ureters _____

_____

D. Urethra _____

_____

E. Meatus _____

_____

159. Sperm is produced in the testicles. What happens to the sperm in each of these structures?

A. Testes _____

_____

B. Vas deferens _____

_____

C. Seminal vesicle _____

_____

D. Ejaculatory duct _____

_____

E. Prostate gland _____

_____

F. Urethra _____

_____

160. What is the function of the endometrium? _____

_____

161. Menstruation occurs about every _____ days. Ovulation usually occurs on or about the _____ day of the cycle.

162. What is the function of each of these pituitary hormones?

    A. Growth hormone _____

    _____

    B. Thyroid-stimulating hormone _____

    _____

    C. Adrenocorticotropic hormone _____

    _____

    D. Antidiuretic hormone _____

    _____

    E. Oxytocin_____

    _____

163. _____ What is the function of insulin?

    _____

    What happens if too little insulin is produced?

    _____

164. What happens when the body senses an antigen?

    _____

INDEPENDENT LEARNING ACTIVITIES

- Listen to a friend's chest with a stethoscope.
  - What sounds do you hear?
  - What body systems are making the sounds?
  - Are you able to count any of the sounds you hear? What are you counting?
- Listen to your lower abdomen with a stethoscope.
  - What sounds can you hear?
  - What causes sound in the abdomen? What body system is involved in this activity?
- Look at a friend's eyes in a dimly lit area and observe the size of the pupils.
  - What size are the pupils? Are they both the same size?
  - Shine a flashlight in one eye. What happens to the pupil?
  - What happens when you move the light away? If you see a change, how quickly does it occur?

43

9 The Older Person

FILL IN THE BLANKS: KEY TERMS

Development
Developmental task
Dysphagia
Dyspnea

Geriatrics
Gerontology
Growth
Menopause

Podiatrist
Presbyopia

1. When menstruation stops it is called _____ _____.

2. _____ is a skill that must be completed during a stage of development.

3. Difficult, labored, or painful breathing is _____ _____.

4. _____ is difficulty swallowing.

5. The care of aging people is _____ _____.

6. The study of the aging process is _____ _____.

7. _____ is age-related farsightedness.

8. Changes in mental, emotional, and social function are _____.

9. Physical changes that are measured and that occur in a steady, orderly manner are called _____ _____.

10. A medical professional who treats disorders of the foot and ankle is _____.

CIRCLE THE BEST ANSWER

11. Most older people live
    A. In a nursing center
    B. Alone
    C. In a family setting
    D. With nonrelatives
12. A stage of growth and development in late adulthood is
    A. Adjusting to aging parents
    B. Developing new friends and relationships
    C. Developing a satisfactory sex life
    D. Developing leisure time activities
13. In 2019, how many people were 65 years of age or older?
    A. 3,200,000
    B. 17,500,000
    C. 33,000,000
    D. 54,100,000

14. As aging occurs
    A. Illness and disability always result
    B. Physical changes are slow
    C. The person is lonely and isolated
    D. Most persons live in nursing centers
15. Social changes include
    A. A decline in mental function
    B. Physical disabilities
    C. A need to find activities to replace the work role
    D. Decreased physical strength
16. It may be difficult to meet all self-esteem needs when retired because
    A. The person can do whatever he or she wants
    B. Work helps meet love, belonging, and self-esteem needs
    C. A retired person develops new relationships
    D. Physical strength decreases
17. Retired people may feel fulfilled and useful when they
    A. Travel
    B. Work part-time or do volunteer work
    C. Live alone
    D. Live with adult children
18. Money problems can result with retirement because
    A. Income is reduced
    B. The person lives alone
    C. The person is unable to work
    D. The person plans for retirement with savings and investments
19. Loneliness in an older person may be reduced when the person
    A. Is allowed to eat meals alone in his or her room
    B. Has family members who live far away and call infrequently
    C. Is able to join community group activities
    D. Spends quiet time watching TV or reading
20. An older person can adjust to social relationship changes by
    A. Avoiding visits with family members
    B. Developing hobbies and church and community activities
    C. Asking for a private room and having meals in his or her room
    D. Staying at home alone to save money

21. When children care for older parents
    A. The older person may feel unwanted and useless
    B. The older person may feel more secure
    C. Tension may develop among the children and the family
    D. All of the above
22. What causes wrinkles to appear on an older person?
    A. Decreases in oil and sweat gland secretions
    B. Fewer nerve endings
    C. Loss of elasticity, strength, and fatty tissue layer
    D. Poor circulation
23. Skin breakdown may heal slowly in older people because
    A. Older people eat a poor diet
    B. Blood vessels are fragile
    C. The skin has more nerve endings
    D. Secretions from oil and sweat glands decrease
24. Bones may break easily because
    A. Joints become stiff and painful
    B. Joints become slightly flexed
    C. Bones lose strength and become brittle
    D. Vertebrae shorten
25. Older persons can prevent bone loss and loss of muscle strength by
    A. Staying active, exercising, and eating a healthy diet
    B. Taking hormones
    C. Resting with their feet elevated
    D. Taking vitamins
26. Dizziness may increase in older people because
    A. They have difficulty sleeping
    B. Blood flow to the brain is decreased
    C. Nerve cells are lost
    D. Brain cells are lost
27. Painful injuries and diseases may go unnoticed because
    A. The person is confused
    B. Touch and sensitivity to pain are reduced
    C. Memory is shorter
    D. Blood flow is reduced
28. Eyes are irritated easily because
    A. The lens yellows
    B. The eye takes longer to adjust to changes in light
    C. Tear secretion is less
    D. The person becomes farsighted
29. If severe circulatory changes occur, the person
    A. May be encouraged to walk long distances
    B. May need to rest during the day
    C. May not do any kind of exercise
    D. Should exercise only once a week
30. A person with dyspnea can breathe more easily when
    A. Lying flat in bed
    B. Covered with heavy bed linens
    C. Allowed to stay in one position on bedrest
    D. Resting in the semi-Fowler position
31. Dulled taste and smell decreases
    A. Peristalsis
    B. Appetite
    C. Saliva
    D. Swallowing
32. Older persons need
    A. Fewer calories
    B. Less fluids
    C. More calories
    D. A low-protein diet
33. Many older persons have to urinate several times during the night because
    A. Bladder infections are common
    B. Urine is more concentrated
    C. Bladder muscles weaken and bladder size decreases
    D. Urinary incontinence may occur
34. Sexual activity in older persons changes because
    A. Orgasms for men and women are less intense or forceful
    B. The vaginal secretions increase
    C. An erection lasts longer
    D. Sex hormones increase
35. An advantage of an older person living with family is that
    A. The person and family are together all of the time
    B. The family can provide care during illness or disability
    C. The person is with others who are of same age
    D. The person will have a private bedroom
36. Most adult day care centers
    A. Require that the person performs some self-care
    B. Accept only persons capable of self-care
    C. Provide complete care
    D. Provide respite care
37. A common dining room and meals usually are not provided when the person lives in
    A. An apartment building
    B. Congregate housing
    C. A board and care home
    D. A residential hotel
38. Assisted living residences provide
    A. Nursing care
    B. A place for family members to live with the person
    C. Shared household chores and expenses
    D. Social contact with other residents
39. Continuing care retirement communities (CCRCs) may have
    A. Independent living units
    B. Food service and help nearby
    C. Additional services as the person's needs change
    D. All of the above
40. Nursing centers are housing options for older persons who
    A. Need only companionship
    B. Cannot care for themselves
    C. Need care during the daytime while the family works
    D. Are developmentally disabled
41. Moving to a nursing center
    A. Is an exciting change for the older person
    B. Can cause a loss of identity
    C. Is always a permanent move
    D. Allows the person to have more personal freedom

45

42. A quality nursing center is
    A. Approved by the medical society
    B. Medicare-certified and Medicaid-certified
    C. Licensed by the state board of nursing
    D. Operated by the local health department
43. A quality nursing center is required to have
    A. An area with hot tubs and saunas
    B. All common areas, residents' rooms, and door-ways designed for wheelchair use
    C. Toilet facilities that are shared by all residents
    D. A private room for each resident
44. OBRA's environment requirements include
    A. Handrails, assist devices, and surfaces in good repair
    B. A private bathroom for each resident
    C. Requiring residents to provide furniture for their rooms
    D. Using tablecloths and cloth napkins in the dining room

FILL IN THE BLANKS: ABBREVIATIONS

45. CCRC _____

46. CMS _____

47. OBRA _____

MATCHING

Match the physical change during the aging process with the body system affected.

48. _____ Reduced blood flow to kidneys

49. _____ Arteries narrow and become stiffer

50. _____ Forgetfulness

51. _____ Gradual loss of height

52. _____ Decreased strength for coughing

53. _____ Decreased secretion of oil and sweat glands

54. _____ Difficulty digesting fried and fatty foods

55. _____ Heart pumps with less force

56. _____ Bladder muscles weaken

57. _____ Problems seeing green and blue colors

58. _____ Difficulty swallowing

59. _____ Lung tissue less elastic

60. _____ Bone mass decreases

61. _____ Testosterone level decreases

62. _____ Facial hair in some women

A. Integumentary
B. Musculoskeletal
C. Nervous
D. Circulatory
E. Respiratory
F. Digestive
G. Urinary
H. Reproductive

OPTIONAL LEARNING EXERCISES

Nursing Concerns Related to Physical Changes

63. When bathing an older person, what kind of soap should be used? _____

    Often no soap is used on the _____.

64. If a nick or cut occurs on the feet, it can lead to a _____. This can happen because the feet usually have _____.

65. Skin disorders rarely cause death if they are _____.

66. When bone mass decreases, why is it important to turn an older person carefully? _____ _____

67. Why does an older person often have a gradual loss of height? _____

68. What types of exercise help prevent bone loss and loss of muscle strength? _____ _____

69. Older persons have changes in the nervous system. When the changes listed below happen, what physical problems occur?

    a. Nerve conduction and reflexes are slower _____ _____

    b. Blood flow to the brain is reduced _____ _____

    c. Changes in brain cells _____ _____

70. When you are eating with an older person, you notice she puts salt on vegetables that taste fine to you. What may be a reason she does this?_____ _____

71. A female nurse has a high-pitched voice and several residents seem to have difficulty hearing her. They do not complain about hearing the male charge nurse. What may be a reason for the difference? _____ _____ _____

72. How can you help the circulation of persons confined to bed? _____ What other body system will be helped by this activity? _____ _____

73. What can the nursing assistant do to prevent respiratory complications from bedrest? _____ _____

74. The stomach and colon empty slower and flatulence and constipation are common in the older person. What causes these problems? _____ _____

75. How does good oral hygiene and denture care improve food intake? _____

76. Why should you plan to give most fluids to the older person before 1700 (5:00 PM)? _____ _____

INDEPENDENT LEARNING ACTIVITIES

- Interview an older person who lives independently. Use the following questions to find out what concerns the person has about remaining independent.
  - What physical problems does the person have, if any?
  - What activities are more difficult now than when the person was younger?
  - What does the person use to provide safety? (Walkers, canes, alarms, daily phone calls, etc.)
  - What comfort measures are needed to decrease pain or help the person sleep?
  - What are transportation needs? Does the person drive? How does the person grocery shop? Visit with family and friends? Attend social functions?
  - How are social needs met? How often does the person go out to socialize? How often does the person have visitors?
- Interview an older person and talk about life when the person was young.
  - Observe facial expression and tone of voice when the person talks about events remembered. What changes do you see?
  - Compare how well the person remembers events of long ago with those that happened recently.
  - How do you feel differently about the person after hearing about his or her youth?

10 Sexuality

FILL IN THE BLANKS: KEY TERMS

Bisexual
Erectile dysfunction (ED)
Heterosexual
Homosexual

Impotence
LGBTQ+
Mastectomy
Natal sex

Sex
Sexuality
Transgender

1. _____ is a broad term used to describe people who self-identify as a gender that does not match their natal sex.

2. Another name for impotence is _____ _____.

3. _____ is the physical, psychological, social, cultural, and spiritual factors that affect a person's feelings and attitudes about his or her sex.

4. _____ is a person's genital anatomy that is present at birth.

5. A person attracted to both sexes is _____ _____.

6. _____ is a community of people who do not identify as heterosexual, but instead may identify as lesbian, gay, bisexual, transgender, queer, or questioning.

7. A _____ is a person who is attracted to members of the same sex.

8. The physical activities involving the reproductive organs that are done for pleasure or to have children are called _____.

9. A person who is attracted to members of the other sex is _____.

10. The inability of the male to have an erection is erectile dysfunction or _____.

11. The surgical removal of a breast is a _____ _____.

CIRCLE THE BEST ANSWER

12. Sexuality
    A. Involves the personality and the body
    B. Is the name for physical activities involving reproductive organs
    C. Is unimportant in old age
    D. Is done for pleasure or to have children

13. A woman who is attracted to men is
    A. Homosexual
    B. Heterosexual
    C. Lesbian
    D. Bisexual

14. Transgender
    A. Is a term used to describe an individual's sexual orientation.
    B. Describes a person who is only attracted to women.
    C. Is a person who may receive hormone therapy or surgery for sexual reassignment.
    D. Is a person who self-identifies as the gender that matches their natal sex.

15. Diabetes, spinal cord injuries, and multiple sclerosis may cause
    A. Impotence
    B. Menopause
    C. Sexual aggression
    D. Heterosexuality

16. Which of these is true about sexuality and older persons?
    A. An orgasm is more forceful in older persons than in younger persons.
    B. Older persons are unable to have intercourse.
    C. Older persons do not lose sexual needs and desires.
    D. Love and affection become less important as the person ages.

17. When older adult couples live in a nursing center, OBRA requires that they
    A. Are allowed to share the same room
    B. Are placed in separate rooms
    C. Are not encouraged to be intimate
    D. Cannot share a bed

18. If a person in a nursing center becomes sexually aroused, you should
    A. Report this to the nurse immediately
    B. Tell the person that the behavior is not allowed
    C. Stay with the person
    D. Allow for privacy

19. If a person touches you in a way that feels uncomfortable or inappropriate, you should
    A. Ignore it and realize that the person is not responsible
    B. Tell the person you do not like him or her
    C. Tell the person that those behaviors make you uncomfortable
    D. Refuse to give care to the person

48

20. If you do not share a person's sexual attitudes, values, practices, or standards, you should
    A. Not judge or gossip about the person
    B. Avoid the person
    C. Tell him or her your feelings
    D. Discuss the person's relationships with other staff members

FILL IN THE BLANKS

21. Sexuality develops when the baby's _____ _____.

22. Children know their own sex at age _____ _____.

23. Bisexuals often _____ and have _____ _____.

24. Sexual function may be affected by chronic illnesses such as
    A. _____
    B. _____
    C. _____
    D. _____

25. What reproductive surgeries may affect sexuality?
    A. Men _____
    _____
    B. Women _____
    _____

26. Some older people do not have intercourse. They may express their sexual needs or desires by _____
    _____
    _____.

27. When you are assisting persons, what grooming practices will promote sexuality for residents?
    A. Men _____
    _____
    B. Women _____
    _____

28. What can you do to allow privacy for a person and a partner?
    A. Close _____.
    B. Remind the person about _____
    _____.
    C. Tell other _____
    _____.
    D. Knock _____
    _____.

29. Masturbation is a normal _____.

30. What health-related problems may cause a person to touch his or her genitals?
    A. _____ or _____ system disorders
    B. Poor _____
    C. Being _____ or _____ from urine and feces

OPTIONAL LEARNING EXERCISES

Mr. and Mrs. Davis are 78-year-old residents in a nursing center, where they share a room. They need assistance with ADL but are mentally alert. They are an affectionate couple and care deeply for each other. Answer these questions about meeting their sexual needs.

31. Mr. Davis has diabetes and high blood pressure. What effect can these disorders have on sexuality?
    _____

32. What is an important thing you could do when Mr. and Mrs. Davis ask for privacy? _____
    _____

INDEPENDENT LEARNING ACTIVITIES

- Consider this situation about a sexually aggressive person. Answer the questions about how you would respond.

SITUATION: *John James is 72 years old and has paraplegia because of an accident several years ago. His caregivers report that recently he has begun to make sexually suggestive remarks. While you are giving his morning care, he touches you several times in private areas and makes frequent sexually suggestive remarks. The other nursing assistants tell you they just ignore him or joke with him about the actions.*

  ○ What would you say to Mr. James when he touches you in private areas?
  ○ How would you respond to his suggestive remarks?
  ○ What would you say to your colleagues who suggest you ignore or joke with Mr. James?
  ○ Has this type of situation ever happened to you? How did you handle it then? What would you do differently after studying this chapter?

SITUATION: *Bobbie Freeman is 45 years old and has had gallbladder surgery. While assisting her to ambulate, she begins to talk about her friend Judy. She tells you that they have been lovers for 15 years.*

  ○ What would you say to a person who tells you she is gay? Do you understand the importance of being nonjudgmental with the care you offer?
  ○ What effect would this information have on the care you provide for the person?
  ○ Has this type of situation ever happened when you were caring for a person? How did you respond? How would you respond differently after studying this chapter?

49

11 Safety

FILL IN THE BLANKS: KEY TERMS

Anti-coagulant
Coma
Dementia
Disaster
Electrical shock
Ground

Hazard
Hazardous substance
Hemiplegia
Hemorrhage
Incident
Paralysis

Paraplegia
Quadriplegia
Suffocation
Tetraplegia
Workplace violence

1. The loss of cognitive and social function caused by changes in the brain is _____.

2. Anything in the person's setting that may cause injury or illness is a _____.

3. Paralysis in the arms, legs, and trunk or tetraplegia is called _____.

4. A _____ is any chemical in the workplace that can cause harm.

5. A _____ is a sudden catastrophic event in which many people are injured and killed and property is destroyed.

6. _____ occurs when breathing stops from the lack of oxygen.

7. Paralysis on one side of the body is _____.

8. A _____ is a state of being unaware of one's surroundings and being unable to react or respond to people, places, or things.

9. That which carries leaking electricity to the earth and away from an electrical appliance is a _____.

10. _____ is paralysis in the legs and lower trunk.

11. _____ occurs when electrical current passes through the body.

12. Violent acts directed toward persons at work or while on duty is _____.

13. An _____ is any event that has harmed or could harm a resident, staff member, or visitor.

14. _____ means loss of muscle function, loss of sensation, or loss of both muscle function and sensation.

15. Another name for quadriplegia is _____ _____.

16. An _____ is a blood-thinning medication.

17. _____ is the excessive loss of blood in a short time.

CIRCLE THE BEST ANSWER

18. To protect the person from harm you need to
    A. Use restraints
    B. Follow the person's care plan
    C. Limit mobility
    D. Lock all doors

19. A person's risk of accidents increases because of
    A. Obesity
    B. Poor diet
    C. Age
    D. Carelessness

20. People with dementia are at risk of injury because they
    A. No longer know what is safe and what is dangerous
    B. Are in a coma
    C. Have problems sensing heat and cold
    D. Have poor vision

21. Medications can be a risk factor for accidents because side effects can
    A. Affect hearing
    B. Reduce the ability to sense heat and cold
    C. Cause loss of balance or lack of coordination
    D. Cause hemiplegia

22. Identifying the person is most important because
    A. You must give the right care to the right person
    B. Visitors may ask for your help to find someone
    C. You need to call the person by the right name
    D. You will have to give care to two people if you give it to the wrong person first

50

23. Which of these is a reliable way to identify the person?
    A. Look at the name above the bed.
    B. Use the person's ID bracelet given by the center.
    C. Ask the person's roommate to identify him or her.
    D. Just call the person by name.
24. Burns from smoking can be prevented if
    A. Smoking is allowed when the person is in bed
    B. Residents are allowed to smoke only in smoking areas
    C. No smoking is allowed
    D. Smoking materials are kept at each person's bedside
25. It is most important to store personal care items according to center policy because
    A. This keeps the person's unit tidy
    B. Everyone will be able to find the items
    C. These items can cause harm when swallowed
    D. It maintains privacy for the resident
26. Suffocation can be caused by
    A. Cutting food into small, bite-sized pieces
    B. Making sure dentures fit properly and are in place
    C. Giving oral food and fluids to a person with a feeding tube
    D. Checking the care plan for swallowing problems
27. If a person clutches the throat and is unable to speak, he or she has a
    A. Sore throat
    B. Dangerous level of carbon monoxide
    C. Severe airway obstruction
    D. Mild airway obstruction
28. During a tornado warning, you should
    A. Transport residents to the lowest level by using the elevator.
    B. Move residents to an interior hallway.
    C. Open windows and doors.
    D. Continue giving residents their baths.
29. An electrical appliance owned by the resident cannot be used if it
    A. Has a three-pronged plug
    B. Is connected directly to a wall outlet
    C. Has not been checked by the maintenance staff
    D. The cord is in good repair
30. An electrical shock is especially dangerous because it can
    A. Start a fire
    B. Damage equipment
    C. Affect the heart and cause death
    D. Violate OBRA regulations
31. If you are shocked by electric equipment, you should
    A. Report it at once
    B. Try to see what is wrong with the equipment
    C. Make sure it has a ground prong
    D. Test the equipment in a different outlet

32. Wheelchair brakes are locked when
    A. Transporting the person
    B. Taking a wheelchair up or down stairs
    C. A person is transferring to or from the wheelchair
    D. Storing the wheelchair
33. When moving a person on a stretcher, it is correct to
    A. Use safety straps or side rails only when the person is confused
    B. Unlock the stretcher before transferring the person
    C. Leave the person alone if he or she is alert
    D. Stand at the head of the stretcher. Your coworker stands at the foot
34. An example of a health hazard caused by chemicals would be
    A. A burn from an explosion
    B. Damage to the kidneys, nervous system, lungs, skin, eyes, or mucous membranes
    C. Using oxygen in a room
    D. An ungrounded electrical plug
35. What should be done if a label is missing from a hazardous substance?
    A. Take the container to the nurse
    B. Return the container to the cupboard or shelf
    C. Use the substance as usual
    D. Leave the container where you found it and go for help
36. Where will you find information about a hazardous substance?
    A. The nurse
    B. The care plan
    C. SDS (Safety Data Sheet)
    D. The doctor's orders
37. When you are cleaning up a hazardous substance, you should
    A. Work from dirty areas to clean areas using circular motions
    B. Wear personal protective equipment when instructed to do so by the nurse
    C. Dispose of hazardous waste in sealed bags or containers
    D. Use paper towels and discard them in the regular trash
38. _____ requires a hazard communication program so that employees know how to handle hazardous substances.
    A. Omnibus Budget Reconciliation Act of 1987 (OBRA)
    B. Occupational Safety and Health Administration (OSHA)
    C. Joint Commission on Accreditation of Healthcare Organizations (JCAHO)
    D. Safety Data Sheet (SDS)
39. Where would you find the Safety Data Sheets (SDSs) for hazardous materials?
    A. Attached to the substance
    B. In the administrator's office
    C. In a binder at a certain place in each nursing unit
    D. In the patient's chart

40. If a resident is receiving oxygen, he or she is at special risk for
    A. Burns
    B. Suffocation
    C. Poisoning
    D. Electrical shock
41. A person receiving oxygen should wear
    A. Fireproof clothing
    B. Disposable clothing
    C. Cotton gown or pajamas
    D. Clothing made with wool or synthetic fabrics
42. If a fire occurs, what should you do first?
    A. Rescue people in immediate danger.
    B. Sound the nearest fire alarm and call the switchboard operator.
    C. Close doors and windows to confine the fire.
    D. Use a fire extinguisher on a small fire that has not spread to a larger area.
43. When using a fire extinguisher, the "P" in the word *PASS* means
    A. Pull the fire alarm
    B. Pull the safety pin
    C. Rescue person in immediate danger
    D. Push the handle or lever down
44. If evacuating is necessary, residents who are
    A. Closest to the outside door are rescued first
    B. Able to walk are rescued last
    C. Closest to the fire are taken out first
    D. Helpless are rescued last
45. If there is a disaster, you
    A. Are expected to go to your nursing center immediately
    B. Should follow procedures for the nursing center
    C. Should stay away or leave to get out of the way
    D. May go home to check on your family
46. Why is workplace violence a big concern in health care?
    A. Nurses and nursing assistants have the most contact with residents and families.
    B. Acutely disturbed and violent persons may seek health care.
    C. Agency pharmacies are a source of drugs and therefore a target for robberies.
    D. All of the above.
47. Which of these would be effective in dealing with an agitated or aggressive person?
    A. Stand away from the person at a safe distance so he cannot hit or kick you.
    B. Close the door to keep the person away from others.
    C. Sit quietly with the person in her room. Hold her hand to calm her.
    D. Tell the person that his behavior is unacceptable.

48. Which of these could *not* be used as a weapon by an aggressive person?
    A. Your jewelry or scarf
    B. Long hair that is worn up and off the collar
    C. Keys, scissors, or other items
    D. Tools or items left by maintenance staff
49. Risk management involves
    A. Training the staff to understand SDSs
    B. Identifying and controlling risks and safety hazards
    C. Firing employees who have accidents
    D. Hiring security staff to prevent injuries
50. When you are filling out a valuables list or envelope, which of these would be the best description?
    A. "A diamond in a gold setting"
    B. "A one-carat diamond in a 14K gold setting"
    C. "A white stone in a yellow setting"
    D. "A white diamond-like stone in a gold-like setting"
51. Which of these would *not* be reported as an accident or error?
    A. Forgetting to give care
    B. Giving the wrong care
    C. Assisting a coworker to give care
    D. Losing a resident's dentures

FILL IN THE BLANKS: ABBREVIATIONS

52. AED _____

53. C _____

54. CPR _____

55. EMS _____

56. F _____

57. FBAO _____

58. ID _____

59. NOAA _____

60. OSHA _____

61. PASS _____

62. RACE _____

63. SDS _____

MATCHING

Match each safety measure with the risk of injury it prevents.

64. _____ Do not let the person use an electric blanket

65. _____ Keep soap and shampoo in a safe place

66. _____ Be sure that residents smoke only in smoking areas

67. _____ Keep electrical items away from water

68. _____ Make sure that casters face forward

69. _____ Do not leave the person alone

70. _____ Do not give the resident a shower or tub bath when there is an electrical storm

71. _____ Keep matches away from confused and disoriented persons

72. _____ Report loose teeth or dentures to the nurse

73. _____ Do not let the person stand on the footplates of a wheelchair

74. _____ Do not touch a person who is experiencing an electrical shock

75. _____ Move all residents from the area if you smell gas or smoke

76. _____ Do not allow smoking near oxygen tanks or concentrators

77. _____ Fasten safety straps when the person is positioned properly

A. Burns
B. Suffocation
C. Poisoning
D. Fire
E. Electrical
F. Wheelchair Safety
G. Stretcher Safety

FILL IN THE BLANKS

78. Before giving care, use the _____ to identify the person.

79. _____ is a gas produced by the burning of fuel.

80. It is important to be familiar where the _____ are located in case any hazardous substance is splashed in the eye.

81. If a person is on an _____ medication, bleeding may be harder to control.

82. If a ground (three-pronged) plug is not used, it can cause _____ and possible _____.

83. Before using a hazardous substance, you check the _____ for safety information.

84. If a person is receiving oxygen therapy, _____ _____ signs are placed on the door and near the bed.

85. Color-coded wristbands are used to promote the person's safety and prevent harm. Explain what these colors mean:
    A. Red _____
    B. Yellow _____
    C. Purple _____
    D. Pink _____

86. If an incident that has harmed a person occurs, you should _____ at once.

OPTIONAL LEARNING EXERCISES

87. What factors related to age make older persons more at risk for accidents?
    A. _____ strength
    B. Poor balance makes it hard to avoid _____ _____
    C. Less sensitive to _____ and _____

88. How does impaired smell and touch increase accident risks?
    A. Person may not detect _____ or _____ odors.
    B. Person has problems sensing _____ and _____.
    C. Decreased sense of _____

89. When identifying a person, why is just calling the name not enough? _____ _____

90. Warning labels on hazardous substances identify
    A. _____
    B. _____
    C. _____
    D. _____
    E. _____

91. If a person is receiving oxygen therapy, why are wool blankets and synthetic fabrics removed from the room? _____ _____

92. What does RACE mean when a fire occurs?

A. R _____

B. A _____

C. C _____

D. E _____

93. When using a fire extinguisher, what does the word **PASS** stand for?

A. P _____

B. A _____

C. S _____

D. S _____

92. What kinds of threats are considered workplace violence?

A. _____

B. _____

C. _____

92. What information is required on an incident report?

A. _____

B. _____

C. _____

D. _____

E. _____

F. _____

Indicate the related safety measure from textbook Box 11-4, Safety Measures to Prevent Equipment Accidents, and Box 11-5, Wheelchair and Stretcher Safety.

96. The nursing assistant tells the resident that his shower will be delayed until the storm passes.

_____

97. The nursing assistant tells the nurse that she has never used the portable foot bath before.

_____

98. The nursing assistant dries her hands carefully before plugging in a razor.

_____

99. An electric fan will not work and the staff member follows the correct procedure to have it repaired.

_____

100. The nursing assistant moves an electrical cord that is lying across a heat vent.

_____

101. The nursing assistant makes sure that the person has both feet on the wheelchair footplates.

_____

102. The nursing assistant notices that one wheel is flat on a wheelchair and reports it to the nurse.

_____

103. The nursing assistant locks the wheelchair when the person is sitting in it next to her bed.

_____

Indicate the safety measures you should follow when handling hazardous materials (Box 11-6).

104. When cleaning up a hazardous material, how do you know what equipment to wear?

_____

105. When a spill occurs, what is the correct way to wipe it up?

_____

106. The nurse tells the nursing assistant that the resident is having an x-ray done in her room.

_____

107. The staff opens the windows when cleaning up a hazardous material.

_____

What fire prevention measure is being practiced in each of these examples? (Box 11-7)

108. The resident is taken to the smoking area in his wheelchair.

_____

109. When cleaning the smoking area, the staff uses a metal can partially filled with sand.

_____

110. When heating food for a resident, the nursing assistant remains in the kitchen.

_____

Answer how each of these is related to preventing or controlling workplace violence (Box 11-8).

111. How can jewelry serve as a weapon?

_____

112. Why is long hair worn up?

_____

113. Why are few pictures, vases, and other items kept in some areas?

_____

_____

114. What type of glass protects nurses' stations, reception areas, and admitting areas?

_____

115. What clothing items should be worn by staff to assist the ability to run?

_____

Answer how each of these practices will help affect personal safety (Box 11-9).

116. Where should you park your car in a parking garage?

_____

117. What items should you keep in the car for safety?

_____

118. Why is a "dry run" important?

_____

119. If you think someone is following you, what should you do?

_____

_____

120. If someone wants your wallet or purse, what should you do?

_____

121. How can you use your car keys as a weapon?

_____

122. How can you use your thumbs as a weapon?

_____

123. What part of the body can you attack on either a man or a woman?

_____

INDEPENDENT LEARNING ACTIVITIES

- Safety is important to everyone and needs to be practiced at all times. Check the following items or areas in your own home to determine whether they are safe.
  - What areas are adequately lighted for safety? What areas need improved lighting?
  - Check electrical cords and plugs on appliances and lamps. How many have frayed cords? Ungrounded plugs? Other problems that make them unsafe to use?
  - How many smoke detectors do you have in your home? When were the batteries last replaced? How can you check the smoke detector to make sure it is working correctly?
  - Is there a fire extinguisher available on each level of your home? Would all family members know how to operate it?
  - How many scatter rugs are used on slippery surfaces? How many have some type of backing to prevent slipping?
  - Where are hazardous materials (medications, cleaning solutions, painting supplies, etc.) stored? Which of these could be reached by children? What could be done to store them more safely?
- Make a list of good safety practices in your home. Make a list of safety practices that could be improved.
- Develop a plan for your home and family that helps everyone know how to escape if a fire occurs.
- Make sure every person knows at least two escape routes from the sleeping area.
- Practice how to check a door for heat before opening it.
- Arrange a place to meet once you are outside the building.

12 Preventing Falls

FILL IN THE BLANKS: KEY TERMS

Bed rail   Orthostatic hypotension
Gait belt   Transfer belt

1. A device used to support a person who is unsteady or disabled is a _____.

2. A _____ is a device that serves as a guard or barrier along the side of the bed.

3. Another name for a transfer belt is a _____ _____.

4. A form of low blood pressure that happens when standing up from sitting or lying position is called _____.

CIRCLE THE BEST ANSWER

5. Most falls occur in
   A. Hallways
   B. Resident rooms and bathrooms
   C. Outside areas
   D. Dining areas

6. Falls are more likely to occur
   A. After midnight
   B. During shift changes
   C. At meal time
   D. In the morning after breakfast

7. Which of these would help to prevent falls?
   A. Answer call light promptly.
   B. Take the person to the bathroom once per shift.
   C. Always keep side rails up.
   D. Have the person wear socks to walk in his or her room.

8. What can be done to prevent falls when assisting a person in the shower?
   A. Support the person with your hand while he or she is standing in the shower.
   B. Make sure that grab bars are secure and the person can reach them.
   C. Always use a gait belt when giving a shower.
   D. Only give tub baths to prevent falls in the shower.

9. Bed rails
   A. Are used for all older persons
   B. Are considered restraints by OBRA
   C. Prevent falls
   D. Are never used when giving care

10. When giving care, the bed wheels are
    A. Unlocked
    B. Locked
    C. Unlocked on the side of the bed where you are working
    D. Locked when moving the bed

11. A transfer belt is
    A. Always applied over clothing
    B. Applied with the buckle over the spine
    C. Applied very loosely
    D. Always applied next to the skin

12. If a person begins to fall, you should
    A. Try to prevent the fall
    B. Call for help and hold the person up
    C. Ease the person to the floor
    D. Stand back and let the person fall

FILL IN THE BLANKS

13. Most falls occur between _____ and _____.

14. Meeting basic needs may help to _____ _____.

15. Grab bars are in _____ and by _____ and _____.

16. Tubs and showers may be made safer if they have _____ surfaces.

17. Alarms are used on the bed, chair, door, floor mat, and belt to sense _____.

18. The need for bed rails is noted in the person's _____ _____ and _____.

19. You raise the bed to give care. What safety measures are taken during care to prevent the person from falling?
    A. For the person who uses side rails, _____ _____.
    B. If you need to leave the bedside for any reason, raise _____.
    C. For the person who does not use bed rails, a coworker stands _____.
    D. Never leave the person _____.
    E. Always lower the bed _____.

20. Handrails in hallways and stairways give support to persons who are _____.

21. When a transfer belt is applied, you should be able to slide your _____ under the belt.

22. The transfer belt buckle is never applied over the _____.

23. When a person starts to fall, you should protect the person's _____ as you ease the person to the floor.

OPTIONAL LEARNING EXERCISES

24. Why are falls more likely to happen during shift changes? The staff members are _____
_____.
Confusion can occur about _____
_____.

25. Why should floor coverings be one color in areas where older persons are living? _____
_____
_____.

26. Why are falls prevented when the person's phone, lamp, and personal belongings are at the bedside?
_____
_____.

27. Before using a transfer/gait belt, check with the nurse and the care plan to determine if the person has any of these conditions:

    A. _____
    B. _____
    C. _____
    D. _____
    E. _____
    F. _____
    G. _____
    H. _____

28. What kind of footwear and clothing will help to prevent falls?

    A. Footwear _____
    _____

    B. Clothing _____
    _____

29. Why is it important to answer call lights promptly?
_____

30. If a person needs bed rails, keep them up at all times except _____.

31. For a person who uses bed rails, always raise the far bed rail if you _____.

32. If a person does not use bed rails and you are giving care, how do you protect the person from falling?
_____
_____.

33. Wheels are locked at all times except when _____.

34. If a person starts to fall, you _____
_____. This lets you control _____
_____.

INDEPENDENT LEARNING ACTIVITIES

- Look at the nursing center where you are assigned to answer these questions about safety.
  - How quickly are call lights answered? How does the staff know who should answer each light?
  - If you are there during a shift change, how does the staff make sure that residents do not fall?
  - What safety measures do you see being used? (Use Box 12-2 as a guide to check for these measures.)
  - How many residents use bed rails? What are the reasons these residents need bed rails?
- Practice easing a falling person to the floor with a classmate.
  - How did you support the person?
  - How did using the transfer/gait belt help to control the fall?
  - What was easy and what was difficult about this practice?
  - How did this practice help you to feel more confident about helping a falling person?

13 Restraint Alternatives and Safe Restraint Use

Chemical restraint   Medical symptom   Remove easily
Freedom of movement   Physical restraint

1. Any change in place or position of the body or any part of the body that the person is physically able to control is _____ _____.

2. A _____ is any manual method or mechanical device, material, or equipment attached to or near the person's body that he or she cannot remove easily and that restricts freedom of movement or normal access to one's body.

3. Any drug that is used for discipline or convenience and not required to treat medical symptoms is a _____ _____.

4. A _____ is an indication or characteristic of a physical or psychological condition.

5. _____ is when the manual method, device, material, or equipment used to restrain the person can be removed intentionally by the person in the same manner it was applied by the staff.

CIRCLE THE BEST ANSWER

6. Restraints may be used
   A. Whenever the nurse feels they are necessary
   B. For the immediate physical safety of the person or others
   C. To make sure the person does not fall
   D. To decrease work for the staff
7. The decision to find ways to meet the person's safety needs is made by
   A. The doctor
   B. The nurse and family
   C. The health team at a resident care conference
   D. The nursing assistants giving care
8. Research shows that restraints
   A. Prevent falls
   B. Cause falls
   C. Are used whenever the nurse decides
   D. Are necessary protective devices
9. A person's harmful behaviors may be caused by
   A. Being afraid of a new setting
   B. Being too hot or too cold
   C. Being hungry or thirsty
   D. All of the above

10. Guidelines about using restraints are part of
    A. FDA regulations
    B. State agencies
    C. OBRA and CMS regulations
    D. All of the above
11. The Centers for Medicare & Medicaid Services (CMS) rules for restraint use say they
    A. May be used to discipline or punish a person
    B. Must be discontinued at the earliest possible time
    C. May be as restrictive as needed as decided by the staff
    D. May be used to keep a person confined to the bed or room
12. Which of these can be a physical restraint?
    A. A soft chair with a footstool to elevate the feet
    B. A bed without rails
    C. A chair with a laptop tray attached
    D. A drug that helps a person function at his or her highest level
13. The most serious risk from restraints is
    A. Cuts, bruises, and fractures
    B. Death from strangulation
    C. Falls
    D. Depression, anger, and agitation
14. After receiving instructions about the correct use of a restraint, you should
    A. Ask for help to apply it to a person
    B. Demonstrate proper application before using it on a person
    C. Watch someone else apply it to a person
    D. Apply it to the person independently
15. Which of these is a chemical restraint?
    A. A vest restraint
    B. A chair with an attached tray
    C. A drug that affects the person's mental function
    D. Sheets tucked in so tightly they restrict movement
16. In order to use a restraint, the nurse must
    A. Get permission from the family
    B. Have a doctor's order
    C. Get permission from the health care team
    D. Receive OBRA permission
17. Unnecessary restraint is
    A. False imprisonment
    B. Needed to give good care
    C. Acceptable if the person does not resist
    D. Acceptable if used for short periods of time

18. An informed consent must be obtained after necessary information is provided by the
    A. Person's legal representative
    B. Doctor or nurse
    C. Person
    D. Nursing assistant
19. When restraining a combative and agitated person, it should be done
    A. Slowly by only one person
    B. By the nurse
    C. With enough help to protect the person and staff from injury
    D. In a public area so the person is distracted
20. The person who is restrained must be observed at least every
    A. 5 minutes
    B. 15 minutes or more often
    C. Hour
    D. 2 hours
21. Wrist restraints are used when a person
    A. Tries to get out of bed
    B. Moves his wheelchair without permission
    C. Pulls at tubes used in medical treatments
    D. Slides out of a chair easily
22. Belt restraints
    A. Are more restrictive than other restraints
    B. May allow the person to turn from side to side
    C. Must be released by the staff
    D. Can be used only in bed
23. A vest restraint
    A. Always crosses in the front
    B. Is applied next to the skin under clothing
    C. Must be secured very tightly to be safe
    D. Crosses in the back
24. When applying wrist restraints
    A. Tie the straps to the bed rail
    B. Tie firm knots in the straps
    C. Place the restraints over clothing
    D. Place the soft part toward the skin

25. When you apply mitt restraints
    A. Make sure the person's hand is clean and dry
    B. Pad the mitt with soft material
    C. Make sure the mitt is securely tied so the hand cannot move
    D. Make sure you can slide three or four fingers between the wrist and the restraint
26. When using a vest restraint in bed the
    A. Straps are buckled or tied to the movable part of the bed frame
    B. Straps are secured to the bed rail
    C. Vest crosses in the back
    D. Person can turn over
27. How can you improve the quality of life for a person with restraints?
    A. Provide water or other fluids frequently.
    B. Check often to make sure breathing and circulation are normal.
    C. Treat the person with kindness, caring, respect, and dignity.
    D. All of the above.

FILL IN THE BLANKS: ABBREVIATIONS

Write out the meaning of each abbreviation.

28. CMS _____

29. FDA _____

30. OBRA _____

31. TJC _____

MATCHING

Match each legal aspect of restraint use with the correct statement.

32. _____ The person must understand the reason for the restraints.

33. _____ Restraints are not used to punish or penalize uncooperative persons.

34. _____ The care plan must include measures to protect the person and to prevent the person from harming others.

35. _____ The doctor gives the reason for the restraint, what to use, and how long to use the restraint.

36. _____ The restraint allows the greatest amount of movement or body access possible.

37. _____ If told to apply a restraint, you must clearly understand the need.

A. Restraints must protect the person.
B. A doctor's order is required.
C. The least restrictive method is used.
D. Restraints are used only after other measures fail to protect the person.
E. Unnecessary restraint is false imprisonment.
F. Informed consent is required for restraint use

59

Match each safety guideline with the correct example.

38. _____ The nurse gives you the printed instructions about applying and securing the restraint safely.

39. _____ When the restraint is removed, range of motion exercises are done or the person is ambulated.

40. _____ Some people become more confused because they do not know what is happening to them.

41. _____ Persons in immediate danger of harming themselves or others are restrained quickly.

42. _____ Restraints are used for as short a time as possible.

43. _____ Injuries and deaths have occurred from improper restraint and poor observation.

A. Observe for increased confusion and agitation.
B. Protect the person's quality of life.
C. Follow the manufacturer's instructions.
D. Apply restraints with enough help to protect the person and staff from injury.
E. Observe the person at least every 15 minutes or more often as noted in the care plan.
F. Remove or release the restraint, re-position the person, and meet basic needs at least every 2 hours.

FILL IN THE BLANKS

44. When using restraints, what information is reported and recorded?

A. _____

B. _____

C. _____

D. _____

E. _____

F. _____

G. _____

H. _____

I. _____

J. _____

K. _____

45. Persons restrained in a supine position must be monitored constantly because they are a great risk for _____.

46. You should carry scissors with you because in an emergency _____.

LABELING

47. Explain what is being done in the figure.

_____

_____

Restraint

OPTIONAL LEARNING EXERCISES

48. Drugs or drug dosages are chemical restraints if they

A. _____

B. _____

49. How does a restraint increase incontinence?

_____

50. What life-long habits and routines could be included in the nursing care plan as alternatives to restraints?

_____

_____

51. Why would a person in restraints be at risk for dehydration? _____

52. Why would videotapes of family and friends or visiting with family be good alternatives to restraints?

_____

_____

INDEPENDENT LEARNING ACTIVITIES

- **_Role play:_** One person is a nursing assistant and one is a person who is restrained. An active physical restraint is applied as the person sits in a chair or wheelchair. Once the restraint is in place, the nursing assistant leaves and does not return for 15 minutes. Discuss the following questions after the experiment.
  - How did the person feel when the restraints were applied? What did the nursing assistant tell the person about the restraints?
  - Did the nursing assistant ask the person if toileting was needed? If the person was thirsty?
  - Was the chair comfortable? Was there any padding? Did the nursing assistant check for wrinkles? Could the person move around to re-position himself or herself for comfort?
  - How was the person able to get help during the 15 minutes of being alone?
  - What diversions were offered while the person was restrained? TV or radio? Reading materials? A window with a pleasant view? If any of these were provided, who chose the channel, station, book, or view?
  - Was the person told someone would return in 15 minutes? Was a clock or watch available to see the time? How long did it seem?
  - What was learned from this experience by both people?

14 Preventing Infection

FILL IN THE BLANKS: KEY TERMS

Asepsis
Biohazardous waste
Carrier
Clean technique
Communicable disease
Contagious disease
Contamination
Disinfection
Epidemic
Germicide

Healthcare-associated infection
   (HAI)
Immunity
Infection
Infection control
Medical asepsis
Microbe
Microorganism
Non-pathogen
Normal flora
Norovirus

Pandemic
Pathogen
Reservoir
Spore
Sterile
Sterile field
Sterile technique
Sterilization
Surgical asepsis
Vaccination
Vaccine

1. A human or animal that is a reservoir for microbes but does not have signs and symptoms of infection is a _____.

2. A _____ is a small living plant or animal seen only with a microscope.

3. Protection against a certain disease is _____ _____.

4. A preparation that contains dead or weakened microbes and is given to produce immunity against an infectious disease is a _____.

5. A work area free of all pathogens and nonpathogens is a _____.

6. _____ is items contaminated with blood, body fluids, secretions, and excretions that may be harmful to others.

7. _____ is the administration of a vaccine to produce immunity against an infectious disease.

8. _____ is the practices used to remove or destroy pathogens and to prevent their spread from one person or place to another person or place.

9. A communicable disease is also called a _____ _____.

10. An _____ is a disease state resulting from the invasion and growth of microorganisms in the body.

11. _____ is the practice that keeps equipment and supplies free of all microbes.

12. A _____ is a disease caused by pathogens that spread easily.

13. The process of destroying pathogens is _____ _____.

14. A _____ is an infection acquired in a health care agency.

15. _____ is being free of disease-producing microbes.

16. Another name for a microorganism is a _____ _____.

17. The environment in which microbes live and grow is a _____ or host.

18. Medical asepsis is also called _____ _____.

19. The process of becoming unclean is _____ _____.

20. The absence of all microbes is _____ _____.

21. Surgical asepsis is also called _____ _____.

22. A bacterium protected by a hard shell that forms around microbes is a _____.

23. _____ are microbes that usually live and grow in a certain location.

24. A disinfectant applied to the skin, tissue, or non-living objects is a _____.

25. A microbe that does not usually cause an infection is a _____.

26. _____ is a process of destroying all microbes.

27. A microbe that is harmful and causes an infection is a _____.

28. Practices and procedures that prevent the spread of infection are called _____.

29. A sudden outbreak of disease in a certain geographical area is called a(n) _____.

30. An outbreak of disease that spreads easily and extends across several countries or continents is called a(n) _____.

31. _____ is a very contagious virus that causes vomiting and diarrhea.

CIRCLE THE BEST ANSWER

32. Germs are a type of microbe called
    A. Protozoa
    B. Fungi
    C. Viruses
    D. Bacteria

33. *Rickettsiae* are transmitted to humans by
    A. Plants
    B. Other humans
    C. Insect bites
    D. One-celled animals

34. In order to live and grow, all microbes need
    A. Oxygen
    B. A reservoir
    C. A hot environment
    D. Plenty of light

35. Normal flora
    A. Are always pathogens
    B. Are always non-pathogens
    C. Become pathogens when transmitted from their natural site to another site
    D. Cause signs and symptoms of an infection

36. Multidrug-resistant organisms
    A. Are killed easily by antibiotics
    B. Are normal flora
    C. Can resist the effects of antibiotics
    D. Are not a serious problem

37. If a person has an MRSA infection, this means the person
    A. Is infected with normal flora and is not infectious
    B. Has a methicillin-resistant staphylococcus infection
    C. Has a vancomycin-resistant enterococcus infection
    D. Can be cured easily with antibiotics

38. When caring for a person with a *C. difficile* infection, it is important to
    A. Wear a face mask and gown
    B. Use only alcohol-based hand sanitizers
    C. Wash hands with soap and warm water
    D. Make sure the person eats all of the meals served

39. Which of these is a sign or symptom of infection?
    A. Normal vital signs (temperature, pulse, and respirations)
    B. Increased activity and energy
    C. Sores on mucous membranes
    D. Increased appetite

40. The source of infection is
    A. A break in the skin
    B. A human or animal
    C. Poor nutritional status
    D. A pathogen

41. In the chain of infection, one portal of exit is
    A. Blood
    B. Humans and animals
    C. A pathogen
    D. A carrier

42. Healthcare-associated infections often occur when
    A. Insects are present
    B. Hand washing is poor
    C. Medical asepsis is used correctly
    D. A person is in isolation

43. The practice that keeps equipment and supplies free of all microbes is
    A. Medical asepsis
    B. Clean technique
    C. Contamination
    D. Surgical asepsis

44. What is the easiest and most important way to prevent the spread of infection?
    A. Sterilize all equipment
    B. Use only disposable equipment
    C. Keep all residents in isolation
    D. Practice good hand washing (hand hygiene)

45. When washing hands you should
    A. Use hot water
    B. Keep hands lower than the elbows
    C. Turn off faucets after lathering
    D. Keep hands higher than elbows

46. Clean under fingernails by rubbing your fingers against your palms
    A. Each time you wash your hands
    B. If you have long nails
    C. Only for the first hand washing of the day
    D. For at least 10 seconds

47. To avoid contaminating your hands, turn off the faucets
    A. After soap is applied
    B. Before drying hands
    C. With clean, dry paper towels
    D. With your elbows

48. When cleaning dirty equipment
    A. Wear personal protective equipment (PPE)
    B. Rinse in hot water first
    C. Use the clean utility room
    D. Remove any organic materials with a paper towel

49. What should be done with non-disposable equipment when a resident leaves a facility?
    A. Send it home with the family
    B. Discard it
    C. Clean, disinfect, and then sterilize it
    D. Give it to another resident

50. How are reusable items such as wheelchairs or commodes disinfected?
    A. Sterilized using surgical asepsis
    B. Cleaned with germicides
    C. Boiling water or steam is used
    D. Dusted with a dry cloth
51. Residents with dementia are protected from infection when the staff
    A. Keep the person confined to his or her room
    B. Wear gloves when in contact with the person
    C. Practice isolation precautions when caring for the person
    D. Assist them with hand washing
52. Isolation precautions are used
    A. For all residents
    B. During a sterile procedure
    C. To prevent the spread of communicable or contagious diseases
    D. When cleaning a room after a resident is discharged
53. You can make a person in isolation more comfortable if you
    A. Organize your work so you can stay to visit with the person
    B. Avoid going to the room to allow the person to rest
    C. Keep the room dark and quiet
    D. Make sure no visitors enter the room
54. When you don personal protective equipment (PPE), you
    A. May go in and out of the room to get supplies
    B. Must remove it before leaving the room
    C. May take it off and keep it in the room to don later
    D. Hang it up to dry it if becomes wet while giving care
55. Standard Precautions are used
    A. For a person with a respiratory infection
    B. For a person with a wound infection
    C. For a person with tuberculosis
    D. In the care of all residents
56. A person placed in airborne precautions may have
    A. Meningitis, pneumonia, or influenza
    B. A wound infection
    C. Mumps, rubella, or pertussis
    D. Measles, chicken pox, or tuberculosis
57. Health team members are restricted from the room when the person has an airborne infection if
    A. The person has skin lesions
    B. The team member is susceptible to the infection
    C. The person is sneezing or coughing
    D. The skin lesions are not covered
58. When a person has contact precautions, a gown should be worn
    A. At all times
    B. When making a safety check of the person
    C. When you are delivering a food tray
    D. When clothing may have direct contact with the person

59. Gloves worn in Standard Precautions
    A. Do not need to be changed when performing several tasks for the same person
    B. Do not need to be changed as you care for different persons
    C. Should be changed before giving care to a different person
    D. Are worn only when the person has an infection
60. If you are allergic to latex gloves, you should
    A. Wash hands each time you remove the gloves
    B. Make sure the gloves have powder inside
    C. Report the allergy to the nurse
    D. Never wear any gloves
61. When wearing gloves you know that
    A. The inside of the glove is contaminated
    B. Slightly used gloves can be saved and re-used
    C. You may need more than one pair of gloves for a task
    D. Gloves are easier to put on when hands are damp
62. When removing gloves
    A. Pull the glove down over your hand so it is inside out
    B. Pull off the gloves by the fingers
    C. Reach inside one glove with the other gloved hand to pull it off
    D. Hold the discarded gloves tightly in your hands
63. Hands are washed or decontaminated
    A. After removing gloves
    B. For 5 minutes between residents
    C. Only when moving between residents
    D. Only if gloves were not worn
64. When donning a gown, what is tied first?
    A. Strings at the back of the neck
    B. The waist strings at the back
    C. Mask ties
    D. It does not matter
65. When removing protective apparel, which of these is done first?
    A. Remove the goggles or face shield
    B. Remove the gloves
    C. Remove the gown
    D. Untie the gown
66. When removing a mask, touch only the ties or elastic bands because
    A. The front of the mask is contaminated
    B. The front of the mask is sterile
    C. Your gloves are contaminated
    D. Your hands are contaminated
67. Reusable eyewear is contaminated after use and
    A. Should be discarded
    B. Should be autoclaved
    C. Is washed with soap and water and then a disinfectant
    D. Is rinsed in cool running water
68. How are contaminated items identified when sent to the laundry or trash collection?
    A. Bags are transparent so materials are visible
    B. They are labeled as "contaminated"
    C. They are always double-bagged
    D. They are labeled with a BIOHAZARD symbol

69. How are specimen containers handled in an isolation room?
    A. All are double-bagged
    B. They are put in the biohazard bag
    C. Testing must be done in the room
    D. Special specimen containers are needed
70. If a resident in isolation precautions must be transported to another area
    A. The person wears a mask as required by Transmission-Based Precautions
    B. The person wears PPE as required
    C. The elevator is disinfected before anyone else can use it
    D. The wheelchair or stretcher stays with the person and is used only for him or her
71. Which of these will help a person in isolation meet the need for love, belonging, and self-esteem?
    A. Avoid the room so you do not disturb the person
    B. Let the person see your face before putting on the mask
    C. Discourage the person from using the telephone to contact friends
    D. Remind the person often that he or she has a contagious disease
72. Persons with dementia in isolation may have increased confusion and agitation because
    A. The infection increases confusion
    B. Personal protective equipment may increase these behaviors
    C. They feel dirty and undesirable
    D. They do not receive any visitors
73. What viruses are bloodborne pathogens?
    A. Influenza and pneumococcus
    B. Measles and chicken pox
    C. HIV and HBV
    D. Staphylococcus and streptococcus
74. Which of these items can transmit bloodborne pathogens?
    A. Laundry soiled with blood or other potentially infectious materials
    B. Items caked with dried blood
    C. Contaminated sharps
    D. All of the above
75. How do staff members know what to do if exposed to a bloodborne pathogen?
    A. Training and information must be provided upon employment and yearly by employers
    B. Information is provided on the Internet
    C. They may attend classes offered at colleges or hospitals
    D. The nurse tells them what they need to know
76. The hepatitis B (HBV) vaccine
    A. Requires only one vaccination
    B. Must be given every year
    C. Involves three injections
    D. Is required by law

77. Which of these is a work practice control to reduce exposure risks?
    A. Discard contaminated needles and sharp instruments in regular trash containers
    B. Shear (break) contaminated needles before discarding them
    C. Do not store food or drinks where blood or potentially infectious materials are kept
    D. Wash hands only if you have not worn gloves
78. Personal protective equipment
    A. Is free to employees
    B. Is purchased by staff members
    C. Must be worn by all employees instead of regular uniforms
    D. Must be laundered by the employee
79. If glass is broken
    A. It can be picked up carefully with gloved hands
    B. It is cleaned up with a brush and dustpan
    C. A person specially trained to remove biohazardous materials is required to clean it up
    D. It is wiped up with wet paper towels
80. When discarding regulated waste, the containers are
    A. Colored red and labeled with the BIOHAZARD symbol
    B. Labeled as "contaminated" in red letters
    C. Meltaway bags
    D. Cloth reusable bags
81. If an exposure incident occurs
    A. Report it only if you had a skin break or needlestick
    B. You can have free medical evaluation and follow-up
    C. Wait at least 90 days before having a blood test
    D. See your own doctor to maintain confidentiality in the workplace
82. If a sterile item touches a clean item
    A. It can still be used
    B. It is no longer sterile
    C. It should be handled with sterile gloves
    D. It can be placed on the sterile field
83. When working with a sterile field, you should
    A. Always wear a mask
    B. Keep items within your vision and above your waist
    C. Keep the door open
    D. Wear clean gloves
84. When arranging the inner package of sterile gloves
    A. Have the right glove on the left and the left glove on the right
    B. Have the fingers pointing toward you
    C. Have the right glove on the right and the left glove on the left
    D. Straighten the gloves to remove the cuff
85. When picking up the first sterile glove
    A. Touch only the cuff and inside of the glove
    B. Reach under the cuff with your fingers
    C. Grasp the edge of the glove with your hand
    D. Slide your hand into the glove without touching it with the other hand

65

FILL IN THE BLANKS: ABBREVIATIONS

Write out the meaning of each abbreviation.

86. ABHR _____

87. AIIR _____

88. CDC _____

89. *C. diff* _____

90. cm _____

91. COVID-19 _____

92. HAI _____

93. HBV _____

94. HIV _____

95. MDRO _____

96. MRSA _____

97. NIOSH _____

98. OPIM _____

99. OSHA _____

100. PPE _____

101. SARS _____

102. TB _____

103. VRE _____

104. WHO _____

MATCHING

Match the kind of asepsis being used to each example.

105. _____ An item is placed in an autoclave.

106. _____ Each person has his or her own toothbrush, towel, washcloth, and other personal care items.

107. _____ Hands are washed before preparing food.

108. _____ Non-disposable items are cleaned, disinfected, and then sterilized.

109. _____ All pathogens, including spores, are destroyed.

110. _____ Hands are washed every time you use the bathroom.

A. Medical asepsis (clean technique)
B. Surgical asepsis (sterile technique)

Match each statement to the link in the chain of infection it would control.

111. _____ Provide the person with tissues to use when coughing or sneezing.

112. _____ Make sure linens are dry and wrinkle-free to protect the skin.

113. _____ Use leak-proof plastic bags for soiled tissues, linens, and other materials.

114. _____ Wear protective equipment.

115. _____ Hold equipment and linens away from your uniform.

116. _____ Assist with cleaning or clean the genital area after elimination.

117. _____ Clean from cleanest area to the dirtiest.

118. _____ Label bottles.

119. _____ Follow the care plan to meet the person's nutritional and fluid needs.

120. _____ Make sure drainage tubes are properly connected.

121. _____ Do not use items that are on the floor.

122. _____ Assist the person with coughing and deep-breathing exercises as directed.

123. _____ Do not sit on a person's bed. You will pick up microorganisms and transfer them.

A. Reservoir (host)
B. Portal of exit
C. Method of transmission
D. Portal of entry
E. Susceptible host

Match each practice to the correct principle for surgical asepsis.

124. _____ Consider any item as contaminated if unsure of its sterility.

125. _____ Wear a mask if you need to talk during the procedure.

126. _____ Place all sterile items inside the 1-inch margin of the sterile field.

127. _____ Do not turn your back on a sterile field.

128. _____ Prevent drafts by closing the door and avoiding extra movements.

129. _____ Avoid spilling and splashing when pouring sterile fluids into sterile containers.

130. _____ If you cannot see an item, it is contaminated.

131. _____ You know when you contaminated an item or a field. Report it to the nurse.

132. _____ Hold wet items down.

A. A sterile item can touch only another sterile item.
B. A sterile field or sterile items are always kept within your vision and above your waist.
C. Airborne microbes can contaminate sterile items or a sterile field.
D. Fluids flow downward, in the direction of gravity.
E. The sterile field is kept dry unless the area below it is sterile.
F. The edges of a sterile field are contaminated.
G. Honesty is essential to sterile technique.

LABELING

133. The illustration shows how to remove gloves. List the steps of the procedure shown in each drawing

    A. (1) _____

        (2) _____

B. (1) _____

C. (1) _____

   (2) _____

D. (1) _____

134. In this figure, color the part of the sterile field that would not be sterile.
How wide is this space? _____

[ ]

OPTIONAL LEARNING EXERCISES

135. Compare medical asepsis to surgical asepsis.

136. Medical asepsis is _____
_____. Surgical asepsis is
_____.

137. Why are hands and forearms kept lower than elbows in hand washing? _____
_____
_____

138. What is the least time you should wash hands? ___
_____

139. Why is lotion applied after hand washing? _____
_____

140. Gloves are worn in Standard Precautions when contact is likely with

  A. _____

  B. _____

  C. _____

  D. _____

  E. _____

141. Masks, goggles, and face shields are worn for procedures and tasks that are likely to cause _____
_____
_____.

142. What information does the nursing assistant need from the nurse or care plan when the person requires isolation precautions?

  A. _____

  B. _____

  C. _____

143. If a person has measles and you are susceptible, what should you do? _____

144. If a person in airborne precautions must leave the room, the person must wear _____.

145. How is preventing the spread of infection an important part of your job? _____

146. How does wearing gloves protect you and the person? It protects you _____.

    It protects the person _____.

147. Why is a gown turned inside out as you remove it? _____

148. If you are wearing gloves, gown, eyewear, and mask, in what order are they donned? _____

149. When you remove gloves, gown, eyewear, and mask, in what order are they taken off? _____

150. Why is a moist mask or gown changed? _____

151. What basic needs may not be met when a person is in isolation? _____

152. In addition to blood, what are other potentially infectious materials (OPIM)?

    A. _____
    B. _____
    C. _____

153. What information is included in training about bloodborne pathogens?

    A. _____
    B. _____
    C. _____
    D. _____
    E. _____
    F. _____
    G. _____
    H. _____
    I. _____
    J. _____

154. How are containers used for contaminated sharps identified? _____

155. OSHA requires these measures for safely handling and using personal protective equipment.

    A. _____
    B. _____
    C. _____
    D. _____
    E. _____
    F. _____
    G. _____
    H. _____

156. If you are asked to assist with a sterile procedure, what information do you need before beginning?

    A. _____
    B. _____
    C. _____
    D. _____
    E. _____
    F. _____

INDEPENDENT LEARNING ACTIVITIES

- Hand-washing practices are important to use whenever you are to prevent the spread of infection. Use this exercise to make yourself aware of your own habits.
  - Make a list of when you washed your hands for 1 day.
  - How did you wash your hands? Did you use the method taught in this chapter?
  - How many times did you wash your hands at work? At home?
  - How many times did you realize you had forgotten to wash your hands? What were the reasons you forgot?
  - How can you improve your hand-washing practices? What will you change after studying this chapter?

- How would you feel if you could not have visitors in a care center where you resided as a result of a pandemic, such as COVID-19? If you were a nursing assistant at a care center, how could you help residents stay in touch with family and friends?

CROSSWORD

Fill in the crossword by choosing words from this list.

Asepsis   Germicide
Biohazard   HAI
Carrier   HBV
Contamination   HIV
Latex   PPE
Microbe   Reservoir
MSRA   Virus
OPIM   VRE

Across

1. Small living plant or animal
4. Abbreviation for personal protective equipment—gloves, mask, gown, and goggles or face shield worn to protect yourself
6. Abbreviation for methicillin-resistant *Staphylococcus aureus*—a bacterium that can cause serious wound infections and pneumonia
9. Abbreviation for infection acquired in a health care agency
10. One type of microbe; it grows in living cells
11. Abbreviation for human immunodeficiency virus
12. A rubber product used to make some gloves; some people are allergic to this
13. Abbreviation for vancomycin-resistant *Enterococcus*—a bacterium that can cause urinary tract, wound, pelvic, and other infections
14. Human body fluids, any tissue or organ, and HIV-containing cells that may cause infections
15. Humans and animals where a pathogen can grow and multiply

Down

2. The process of becoming unclean
3. Disinfectant applied to the skin, tissue, and non-living objects
5. Symbol placed on contaminated linens or contaminated items before removing them from a person's room
7. A reservoir that does not have signs or symptoms of infection but can pass the infection to others
8. Being free of disease-producing microbes
9. Hepatitis B virus

15 Body Mechanics and Safe Resident Handling, Positioning, and Transfers

FILL IN THE BLANKS: KEY TERMS

Base of support
Body alignment
Body mechanics
Dorsal recumbent position
Ergonomics
Fowler position

Friction
Lateral position
Left semiprone position
Logrolling
Posture
Prone position

Shearing
Side-lying position
Supine position
Transfer

1. _____ is another name for lateral position.

2. _____ or posture is the way the head, trunk, arms, and legs are aligned with one another.

3. When the skin sticks to a surface while muscles slide in the direction the body is moving, it is called _____ _____.

4. The _____ is the same as the back-lying or supine position.

5. The area on which an object rests is the _____ _____.

6. _____ is a left side-lying position in which the upper leg is sharply flexed so that it is not on the lower leg and the lower arm is behind the person.

7. A semi-sitting position with the head of the bed elevated 45–90 degrees is _____.

8. Lying on the abdomen with the head turned to one side is _____.

9. _____ is using the body in an efficient and careful way.

10. The back-lying or dorsal recumbent position is also called the _____.

11. _____ is another name for body alignment.

12. _____ is turning the person as a unit, in alignment, with one motion.

13. _____ is the science of designing the job to fit the worker.

14. When the person lies on one side or the other, it is the side-lying or _____ position.

15. Moving the person from one place to another is to _____.

16. _____ is the rubbing of one surface against another.

CIRCLE THE BEST ANSWER

17. Using good body mechanics will
    A. Prevent good posture
    B. Cause back injuries
    C. Reduce the risk of injury to you and the person you care for
    D. Cause muscle injury

18. For a wider base of support
    A. Keep your feet close together
    B. The head, trunk, arms, and legs are aligned with one another
    C. Stand with your feet apart
    D. Make sure you are in good physical condition

19. When you bend your knees and squat to lift a heavy object, you are
    A. Using good body alignment
    B. In danger of injury
    C. Likely to strain your back
    D. Using good body mechanics

20. If you need to move a heavy object
    A. Push, slide, or pull the object
    B. Always work alone
    C. Bend at the waist to lift from the floor
    D. Keep feet close together

21. The risk of work-related musculoskeletal disorders (MSDs) increases
    A. When the worker does not exercise regularly
    B. When the worker is small and weak
    C. When a task involves repeating an action to move persons
    D. Only when the staff member is using poor body mechanics

71

22. If you have pain when standing or rising from a seated position, you
    A. May have a back injury
    B. Are using poor body mechanics
    C. Have worked too many hours
    D. Should exercise more
23. Which of these nursing tasks is known to be a high risk for musculoskeletal disorders (MSDs)?
    A. Using good body mechanics when transferring a person
    B. Getting help when lifting or moving heavy objects
    C. Picking up a person from the floor to the bed
    D. Lifting with forceful movement
24. Which of these activities will help prevent back injury?
    A. Reach across the bed to give care
    B. Bend at the waist to pick up an object from the floor
    C. Lift an object above your shoulder
    D. Get help from a coworker to move heavy objects
25. When caring for a person, regular position changes and good alignment
    A. Cause pressure ulcers and contractures
    B. Promote comfort and well-being
    C. Interrupt rest and sleep
    D. Decrease circulation
26. A resident who depends on the nursing team for position changes needs to be positioned
    A. At least every 2 hours
    B. Once an hour
    C. Every 15 minutes
    D. Once a shift
27. Linens need to be clean, dry, and wrinkle-free to help prevent
    A. Pressure injuries
    B. Contractures
    C. Breathing problems
    D. Frequent repositioning
28. Most older persons have limited range of motion in their necks and so do not tolerate
    A. Lateral position
    B. Chair position
    C. Fowler position
    D. Prone position
29. When positioning a person in the supine position, the nurse may ask you to place a pillow under the person's lower legs to
    A. Improve the circulation
    B. Assist the person to breathe easier
    C. Lift the heels off of the bed
    D. Prevent swelling of the legs and feet
30. A small pillow is positioned against the person's back in the
    A. Lateral position
    B. Prone position
    C. Supine position
    D. Semi-Fowler position
31. In the chair position, a pillow is not used
    A. To position paralyzed arms
    B. To support the feet
    C. Under the upper arm and hand
    D. Behind the back if restraints are used
32. To prevent injuries when moving older persons
    A. Move the person without help
    B. Grab the person under the arms
    C. Allow the person to move himself or herself
    D. Move the person carefully to prevent injury or pain
33. To prevent work-related injuries, OSHA recommends that
    A. Manual lifting be minimized or eliminated when possible
    B. Manual lifting be used at all times
    C. You never lift any person or object alone
    D. You always use mechanical lifts for any lifting
34. When moving residents, it is best if you move the person
    A. By yourself
    B. With 2–3 staff members
    C. Always using a mechanical lift
    D. Only with staff members that you like
35. When moving a person up in bed, prevent hitting the headboard with the head by
    A. Keeping the person in good body alignment
    B. Placing the pillow upright against the headboard
    C. Placing your hand on the person's head
    D. Asking the person to bend his or her neck forward
36. Which of these would be correct when you are using manual lifting?
    A. Reach across the bed to grasp the person
    B. Stand with good posture and keep your back straight
    C. Keep the bed in the lowest position
    D. Do not ask coworkers for help
37. If a person with dementia resists being moved, you should
    A. Move the person by yourself
    B. Proceed slowly and use a calm, pleasant voice
    C. Leave the person alone and do not re-position him or her
    D. Tell the person firmly that he or she must cooperate with being moved
38. When you are delegated to move a person in bed, you need to know
    A. Whether the person has eaten recently
    B. Whether the person is awake
    C. How many workers are needed to move the person safely
    D. Whether the person wishes to be moved at this time
39. When the person can bear some weight, can sit up with help, and may be able to pivot to transfer, you know that the person's level of dependence is
    A. Code 4
    B. Code 3
    C. Code 2
    D. Code 1

72

40. When turning a person, it is important to
    A. Place the person in the prone position
    B. Make sure the person's face, nose, and mouth are not obstructed by a pillow
    C. Always turn the person toward you
    D. Only use logrolling
41. Why are beds raised to move persons in bed?
    A. It prevents the person from falling out of bed
    B. It reduces friction and shearing
    C. It prevents pulling on drainage tubes
    D. This reduces bending and reaching
42. How can you reduce friction and shearing?
    A. Raise the head of the bed to a sitting position before moving the person
    B. Roll the person to re-position him or her
    C. Pull the person up in bed by grasping under the arms
    D. Massage the skin
43. When raising a person's head and shoulders
    A. It is best to have help with an older person to prevent pain and injury
    B. A mechanical lift should be used
    C. You can always do this alone
    D. A transfer belt will be needed
44. In order to correctly raise the head and shoulders
    A. Both of your hands are placed under the person's back
    B. The person puts his near arm under your near arm and behind your shoulder
    C. Use a lift sheet to raise the person up
    D. Your free arm rests on the edge of the bed
45. You may move a person up in bed alone if the
    A. Person can assist and use a trapeze
    B. Rest of the staff is busy and cannot help
    C. Nurse tells you to use a lift sheet or slide sheet
    D. Nurse tells you have to move the person alone
46. What is the position of the bed when you are moving a person up in bed?
    A. Fowler
    B. Flat
    C. As flat as possible for the person's condition
    D. Semi-Fowler
47. The person is moved
    A. On the "count of 3"
    B. On the "count of 2"
    C. When the person says he or she is ready
    D. As soon as all workers are in position
48. An assist device such as a lift sheet is used
    A. For most residents
    B. Only for a person with a dependence level of Code 1
    C. Only for a person with a dependence level of Code 4
    D. For a person with dementia
49. Where is the lift sheet positioned?
    A. Under the head and shoulders
    B. Under the buttocks
    C. From the head to above the knees or lower
    D. From the hips to below the knees

50. When using a lift sheet as an assist device, the workers should
    A. Roll the sheet up close to the person
    B. Grasp the sheet at the edges
    C. Move one side of the sheet at a time
    D. Grasp the sheet only at the top edge
51. A person is moved to the side of the bed before turning because
    A. It makes it easier to turn the person
    B. It prevents injury to the person
    C. Otherwise, after turning, the person lies on the side of the bed and not in the middle
    D. It prevents friction and shearing
52. When you move a person in segments, you should
    A. Begin by first moving the hips and legs
    B. First place your arms under the person's neck and shoulders and grasp the far shoulder
    C. Move the center part of the body by placing one arm under the waist and one arm under the legs
    D. First move the legs and feet
53. When using a drawsheet to move a person to the side of the bed, support the
    A. Back
    B. Knees
    C. Head
    D. Hips
54. After the person is turned
    A. Give the person good personal care
    B. Position him or her in good body alignment
    C. Elevate the head of the bed
    D. Elevate the bed to its highest position
55. When delegated to turn a person, you get the information you need
    A. From the doctor's orders
    B. By asking your coworkers
    C. From the nurse and care plan
    D. By asking the person how he or she wants to be turned
56. When a person is turned, musculoskeletal injuries, skin breakdown, and pressure ulcers could occur if a person is not in
    A. A special bed
    B. Good body alignment
    C. Good body mechanics
    D. The middle of the bed
57. How do you decide whether to turn the person toward you or away from you?
    A. Check the doctor's order
    B. It depends on the person's condition and the situation
    C. Use the method you like best
    D. Ask the person which way is best
58. Why do you need 2 or 3 staff members to logroll a person?
    A. A person who is being logrolled is usually in pain
    B. It is important to keep the spine straight and in alignment
    C. The person probably has a Code 4 level of dependence and needs extra help
    D. No assist devices are used when you logroll

73

59. When preparing to logroll a person, place a pillow
    A. At the head of the bed
    B. Between the knees
    C. Under the head
    D. Under the shoulders
60. What information do you need before dangling a person?
    A. The person's diagnosis
    B. When the person ate last
    C. The person's dependence level
    D. Whether the person likes to dangle
61. What should you do if a person who is dangling becomes faint or dizzy?
    A. Lay the person down
    B. Go and report this to the nurse
    C. Tell the person to take deep breaths
    D. Have the person move his or her legs back and forth in circles
62. When preparing to dangle a person, the head of the bed should be
    A. Flat
    B. Slightly raised
    C. In a sitting position
    D. At a comfortable height for the person
63. When preparing to transfer a person, you should
    A. Arrange the room so there is enough space for a safe transfer
    B. Keep furniture in the position the resident likes
    C. Remove all furniture from the room
    D. Ask the person how to arrange the furniture
64. The person being transferred should wear non-skid footwear to
    A. Protect the person from falls
    B. Allow the person to bend the feet more easily
    C. Promote comfort for the person
    D. Keep the feet warm
65. Lock the bed, wheelchair, or assist device wheels when transferring to
    A. Help the staff use good body mechanics
    B. Prevent damage to the equipment being used
    C. Prevent the bed and the device from moving during the transfer
    D. Make sure the person is kept in good body alignment
66. When a person is transferring from a chair or wheelchair, help the person out of bed on
    A. The right side of the bed
    B. His or her strong side
    C. His or her weak side
    D. The side of the bed that is most convenient for the staff
67. Which of these is the preferred method for chair or wheelchair transfers?
    A. Use a gait/transfer belt
    B. Have the person put his or her arms around your neck
    C. Put your arms around the person and the grasp the shoulder blades
    D. Always use a mechanical lift
68. When a person is seated in a wheelchair, you can increase the person's comfort by
    A. Placing pillows around the person
    B. Making sure nothing covers the vinyl seat and back
    C. Covering the back and seat with a folded bath blanket
    D. Removing any cushions or positioning devices
69. When you transfer a person, the nurse may ask you to take and report what before and after the transfer?
    A. Blood pressure
    B. Pulse rate
    C. Respiration
    D. Temperature
70. When using a transfer belt, you can prevent the person from sliding or falling by
    A. Moving the person quickly from the bed to the wheelchair
    B. Blocking the person's weak leg with your legs or knees
    C. Straddling your legs around the person's strong leg
    D. Planning the transfer so the person moves his or her weak side first
71. When you are transferring a person back to bed from a chair or wheelchair, the person should be positioned
    A. With the weak side near the bed
    B. With the strong side near the bed
    C. With the chair in the same position as it was when the person got out of bed
    D. Where you have the most space to work
72. A mechanical lift is used
    A. For all persons regardless of the level of dependence
    B. For persons who are too heavy for the staff to transfer
    C. When staff members prefer to use it instead of lifting manually
    D. Only when ordered by the doctor
73. When you are delegated to use a mechanical lift, you need to know
    A. Whether the doctor has ordered using the mechanical lift
    B. What sling the person prefers
    C. How many staff members are needed to perform the task safely
    D. When the mechanical device was used last
74. As a person is lifted in the sling of the mechanical lift, he or she
    A. May hold the swivel bar
    B. May hold the straps or chains
    C. Should keep the arms crossed over the chest
    D. Should keep the legs outstretched
75. When transferring a person from a wheelchair to the toilet
    A. The toilet should have a raised seat
    B. The toilet seat should be removed
    C. Always position the wheelchair next to the toilet
    D. Unlock the wheelchair to allow movement during the transfer

76. A slide board may be used to transfer a person from a wheelchair to a toilet if
    A. The person can stand and pivot
    B. There is enough room to position the wheelchair next to the toilet
    C. The staff member does not want to use a transfer belt
    D. The person has lower body strength
77. When moving a person who weighs more than 200 pounds to a stretcher, OSHA recommends
    A. Using a lateral sliding aid and 2 staff members
    B. Using a lateral sliding aid and 3 staff members
    C. Using a lateral sliding aid or a friction-reducing device and 2 staff members
    D. Using a drawsheet, turning pad, or large incontinence underpad
78. During transport on the stretcher, the person is moved feet first so
    A. The staff member at the feet can clear the pathway
    B. The staff member at the head can watch the person's breathing and color
    C. The person can see where he or she is going
    D. The person does not become disoriented

FILL IN THE BLANKS

Write out the meaning of each abbreviation.

79. ID _____

80. OSHA _____

81. MSD _____

82. Where are strong, large muscles that are used to lift and move heavy objects located?
    A. _____
    B. _____
    C. _____
    D. _____

83. Back injuries are a major risk when lifting. For good body mechanics, you should
    A. _____
    B. _____

84. Describe these risk factors for musculoskeletal disorders (MSDs) in nursing centers.
    A. Force _____
    _____
    B. Repeating action _____
    _____
    C. Awkward postures _____
    _____
    D. Heavy lifting _____
    _____

85. Early signs and symptoms of MSDs are
    A. _____
    B. _____
    C. _____

86. What nursing tasks are known to be high risk for MSDs?
    A. _____
    B. _____
    C. _____
    D. _____
    E. _____
    F. _____
    G. _____
    H. _____
    I. _____
    J. _____
    K. _____
    L. _____
    M. _____
    N. _____
    O. _____
    P. _____

87. Instructions to re-position a person are received from the _____ and the _____.

88. If you are delegated the task to position the person, what information do you need?
    A. _____
    B. _____
    C. _____
    D. _____
    E. _____
    F. _____
    G. _____
    H. _____
    I. _____
    J. _____
    K. _____

89. What measures are needed for good alignment when the person is in Fowler position?

A. _____

B. _____

C. _____

90. In supine position?

A. _____

B. _____

C. _____

91. In prone position?

A. _____

B. _____

C. _____

92. In lateral position?

A. _____

B. _____

C. _____

D. _____

E. _____

F. _____

93. In left semiprone position?

A. _____

B. _____

C. _____

D. _____

94. In chair position?

A. _____

B. _____

C. _____

95. To prevent injuries in older persons with fragile bones and joints, what safety measures must be used?

A. _____

B. _____

C. _____

D. _____

E. _____

F. _____

G. _____

96. To promote mental comfort when handling, moving, or transferring the person, you should

A. _____

B. _____

97. To promote physical comfort when handling, moving, or transferring the person, you should

A. _____

B. _____

C. _____

D. _____

98. When lifting manually, you use good body mechanics when you

A. _____

B. _____

C. _____

D. _____

E. _____

99. Explain how a person is lifted and transferred for each level of dependence.

A. Code 4: Total Dependence _____

_____

B. Code 3: Extensive Assistance _____

_____

C. Code 2: Limited Assistance _____

_____

D. Code 1: Supervision _____

_____

E. Code 0: Independent _____

_____

100. When you move a person in bed, report and record

A. _____

B. _____

C. _____

D. _____

E. _____

101. Friction and shearing can be reduced when moving a person in bed by

A. _____

B. _____

102. You can sometimes move a person up in bed alone if the person can use a _____.

103. When moving a person up in bed and the person can assist

A. Flex _____

B. Ask the person to grasp the _____

_____

C. Tell the person to move _____

_____

104. An assist device is used to move persons

    A. Who are recovering from _____

    _____

    B. Older _____

    _____

105. What assist devices, other than mechanical lifts, are used to move persons to the side of the bed?_____
_____

106. Before turning and repositioning a person, what information do you need from the nurse and the care plan?

    A. _____

    B. _____

    C. _____

    D. _____

    E. _____

    F. _____

    G. _____

    H. _____

107. What observations are reported and recorded after turning a person?

    A. _____

    B. _____

    C. _____

    D. _____

    E. _____

108. After turning and repositioning a person, it is common to place pillows

    A. _____

    B. _____

    C. _____

    D. _____

109. When a person is logrolled, the spine must be _____.

110. Logrolling is used to turn these persons:

    A. _____

    B. _____

    C. _____

    D. _____

111. When a person is dangling, the circulation can be stimulated by having the person move _____
_____.

112. What observations should be reported and recorded after dangling a person?

    A. _____

    B. _____

    C. _____

    D. _____

    E. _____

    F. _____

    G. _____

113. While a person is dangling, check the person's condition by

    A. Asking _____

    B. Checking _____

    C. Checking _____

    D. Noting _____

114. A person can transfer from the bed to the chair with a stand and pivot transfer if

    A. _____

    B. _____

    C. _____

115. During a chair or wheelchair transfer, the person must not put his or her arms around your neck because _____
_____.

116. Locked wheelchairs may be considered restraints if the person _____

117. When using a transfer belt to transfer a person to a chair or wheelchair, grasp the belt at _____
_____ and grasp _____
_____ the belt.

118. If you transfer a person to a chair without a transfer belt, place your hands _____ and around the person's _____.

119. For what reasons would you use the slings listed?

A. Standard full sling _____

_____

B. Extended length sling _____

_____

C. Bathing sling _____

_____

D. Toileting sling _____

_____

E. Amputee sling _____

_____

120. What information do you need when you are delegated to use a mechanical lift?

A. _____

B. _____

C. _____

D. _____

E. _____

F. _____

LABELING

_____

124. Identify the positions in each of the illustrations.

121. To promote mental comfort when using a mechanical lift, you should explain and show the person

_____.

122. A slide board can be used when transferring a person to and from a toilet if

A. _____

B. _____

C. _____

D. _____

123. If a person weighs more than 200 pounds and is being moved to a stretcher, OSHA recommends the use of one of the following.

A. _____

B. _____

C. _____

A. _____

B. _____

C. _____

D. _____

E. _____

F. _____

Chapter **15** **Body Mechanics and Safe Resident Handling, Positioning, and Transfers**

OPTIONAL LEARNING EXERCISES

125. According to OSHA, certain activities can lead to back injuries. Read the examples below and state the factor that could cause a back injury in each activity. (Factors listed in textbook)

   A. The nursing assistant does not raise the level of the bed when changing linens. _____
   _____

   B. While you are walking with Mr. Smith, he slips and starts to fall. _____
   _____

   C. Mrs. Tippett slides down in bed and looks uncomfortable. _____
   _____

   D. You assist Mrs. Miller to use the toilet in her small bathroom. _____
   _____

   E. Water is spilled on the hallway floor. _____
   _____

   F. You lean across the bed to hold the person in position while the nurse changes a dressing. ___
   _____
   _____

126. When caring for a person, regular position changes and good alignment promote

   A. _____
   B. _____
   C. _____
   D. _____

   Position changes and good alignment prevent

   E. _____
   F._____

127. If you need to move a person with dementia, the person may resist because he or she may not _____
   _____

   What measures in the care plan will help you give safe care?

   A. _____
   B. _____
   C. _____

128. What type of pad is not strong enough to be used during a lift? _____

129. For a safe lift, the underpad must

   A. _____

   B. _____

   C. _____

130. When you turn a person and re-position him or her, what must be done to the level of the bed before you leave the room? _____
   _____

131. When two staff members are logrolling a person without a turning sheet, where does each person stand?

   A. First worker stands near _____
   _____

   B. Coworker stands near _____
   _____

132. What should you do if the mechanical lift available is different than ones you have used before? _____
   _____
   _____

INDEPENDENT LEARNING ACTIVITIES

- After learning about using good body mechanics in this chapter, think about how well you practice good body mechanics in your daily life and answer these questions.
  - How much do the books you carry with you each day weigh? How do you carry them? When carrying them, where is your base of support? Is your body in good alignment?
  - Do you have small children you pick up? How do you lift them? What methods listed in the chapter do you use?
  - When carrying groceries into the house, do you carry them held close to the body? How well are you using good body mechanics?
  - At the end of the day, how do you feel? How could using good body mechanics help you avoid any discomfort?
- Work with classmates and practice the following activities. Each of you should take a turn as the resident.
  - Practice moving a person up in bed with and without assist devices. Answer the following questions after you have completed this exercise.
  - Which method was easier for the worker? For the person being moved?
  - How did you feel when you were being moved? Did anyone explain what was being done?

- Practice transferring a person who is weak on one side to a chair from the bed and then return the person to the bed. Answer the following questions after you complete the exercise.
  - As the worker: How did you position the chair? How did the chair position change when you returned the person to bed?
  - As the person: How safe did you feel during the transfer? What could the worker have done to help you feel safe? What else could the staff have done to make you more comfortable?
- Practice logrolling a person with and without a turning sheet. Answer the following questions after you have completed the exercise.
  - As the worker: How many workers were used to logroll the person? Which method was easier—with or without the turning sheet? How well do you think the workers did with the turns? Did the spine stay straight?
  - As the person: How did you feel? Did you understand what was being done? Was the turn smooth or did you feel as if your spine twisted?
- Overall, how will these practices help you as you move residents? What would you do differently now that you have practiced these exercises?

Chapter **15 Body Mechanics and Safe Resident Handling, Positioning, and Transfers**

16 The Resident's Unit

FILL IN THE BLANKS: KEY TERMS

Fowler position
Full visual privacy
High-Fowler position

Resident unit
Reverse Trendelenburg position

Semi-Fowler position
Trendelenburg position

1. The personal space, furniture, and equipment provided for the individual by the nursing center is the _____.

2. In _____, the head of the bed is raised 30 degrees; or the head of the bed is raised 30 degrees and the knee portion is raised 15 degrees.

3. _____ is a semi-sitting position; the head of the bed is raised 45 to 60 degrees.

4. The head of the bed is raised and the foot of the bed is lowered in _____.

5. In _____, the head of the bed is lowered and the foot of the bed is raised.

6. The person has the means to be completely free from public view while in bed when they have _____.

7. The bed is in a semi-sitting position; the head of the bed is raised between 60 and 90 degrees in _____ _____.

CIRCLE THE BEST ANSWER

8. When residents share a room
   A. You may rearrange items and furniture in the room as needed
   B. Each person has a private area of the room
   C. They may use each other's belongings
   D. They generally share furniture such as a dresser

9. OBRA requires that nursing centers maintain a temperature range of
   A. 68°F to 74°F
   B. 61°F to 71°F
   C. 71°F to 81°F
   D. 78°F to 85°F

10. Persons who are older and those who are ill
    A. May need cooler room temperatures
    B. May need higher temperatures for comfort
    C. Are insensitive to room temperature changes
    D. Will need a warmer room at night

11. Which of these factors that affect comfort cannot be controlled by the nursing staff?
    A. Illness
    B. Temperature
    C. Noise
    D. Odors

12. If an older person complains of a draft
    A. Have the person go to bed
    B. Give the person a hot shower
    C. Offer a lap robe or a warm sweater to wear
    D. Pull the privacy curtain around the person

13. If unpleasant odors occur, these may be controlled when you
    A. Use spray deodorizers around all residents
    B. Provide good hygiene to prevent body and breath odors
    C. Make sure incontinent persons are taken to the toilet once an hour
    D. Empty laundry hampers once a shift

14. A person with dementia may react to loud noises, especially
    A. At night
    B. When the room is well lighted
    C. During meal time
    D. When he or she is in an area with others present

15. Which of these measures will reduce noises in a nursing center?
    A. Have drapes in rooms
    B. Use only metal equipment
    C. Wait for the nurse to answer the telephone
    D. Talk loudly in halls so others can hear you clearly

16. Soft, non-glare lighting is used with dementia residents because it
    A. Helps residents to relax
    B. Increases agitation in residents
    C. Improves orientation in residents with dementia
    D. Helps residents to see more clearly

17. Cranks on manual beds are kept down when not in use to
    A. Prevent residents from operating the bed
    B. Prevent anyone walking past the crank from bumping into it
    C. Keep the bed in the correct position
    D. Make sure they are ready to use at all times

18. How can the staff prevent a person from adjusting an electric bed into unsafe positions?
    A. Lock the bed into a position
    B. Unplug the bed
    C. Put the person in a bed that cannot be repositioned
    D. Keep reminding the person not to change the position
19. What bed position may adjust the head of the bed and the knee portion to prevent sliding down in bed?
    A. Fowler
    B. Semi-Fowler
    C. Trendelenburg
    D. Reverse Trendelenburg
20. If a person becomes trapped in the hospital bed system, you should
    A. Call for the nurse at once
    B. Call 911
    C. Make sure the person is comfortable
    D. Lower the bed rails
21. If a person becomes trapped between the end of the bed rail and the side edge of the headboard, the area is called
    A. Zone 1
    B. Zone 2
    C. Zone 6
    D. Zone 7
22. Which of these items can be placed on the overbed table?
    A. Urinals
    B. Personal care items
    C. Soiled linens
    D. Bedpans
23. Where are the bedpan and urinal kept in the bedside table?
    A. Wherever the person wants
    B. The top shelf or drawer
    C. The bottom shelf or drawer
    D. The middle shelf or drawer
24. OBRA requires that the resident unit always has
    A. Two chairs
    B. A straight-back chair
    C. A reclining chair
    D. At least one chair for personal and visitor use
25. Privacy curtains
    A. Are sometimes used in rooms with more than one bed
    B. Are always pulled completely around the bed when care is given
    C. Can block sounds and conversations
    D. May be open when giving personal care
26. Personal care items
    A. Are often supplied by the nursing center
    B. Must be provided by the resident
    C. Must be ordered by the doctor
    D. Are required by OBRA

27. When the resident is weak on the left side, the call light
    A. Is placed on the left side
    B. Is removed from the room
    C. Is placed on the right side
    D. Is replaced by an intercom
28. If a confused person cannot use a call light
    A. Explain often how to use the call light
    B. Use an intercom instead
    C. Remove the call light
    D. Check the person often
29. Elevated toilet seats
    A. Help residents with joint problems
    B. Make wheelchair transfers more difficult
    C. Are required by OBRA
    D. Are used on all toilets in a nursing center
30. When a person uses a bathroom call light
    A. It flashes above the room door and at the nurses' station
    B. It makes the same sound as the room call light
    C. It activates the intercom
    D. The signal sounds and flashes only above the bathroom door
31. Closet and drawer space
    A. Are shared by persons in a room with more than one person
    B. Can be opened and searched by a staff member at any time
    C. Cannot be searched without the resident's permission
    D. Are not required in a nursing center
32. What equipment may be in rehabilitation centers but usually is not found in long-term care centers?
    A. Televisions
    B. Commode chairs
    C. Blood pressure equipment or wall outlets for oxygen and suctioning
    D. Electric beds
33. Residents can bring some furniture and personal items to use in the room as long as the items
    A. Do not interfere with the rights of others
    B. Match the color and decoration in the room
    C. Can be cared for by the resident or the family
    D. Do not need to be attached to the wall

FILL IN THE BLANKS

34. What are three factors that affect comfort and that usually cannot be controlled?

    A. _____

    B. _____

    C. _____

35. What factors that affect comfort can be controlled?

A. _____

B. _____

C. _____

D. _____

E. _____

36. Describe the entrapment zones that can occur in a hospital bed system.

A. Zone 1 _____

B. Zone 2 _____

C. Zone 3 _____

D. Zone 4 _____

E. Zone 5 _____

F. Zone 6 _____

G. Zone 7 _____

37. The resident is allowed to bring personal items to make his space as homelike as possible. The health team must make sure the resident's choices

A. _____

B. _____

C. _____

LABELING

38. In this figure

A. What is the bed position called? _____
_____

B. What is the angle of the head of the bed?
_____

39. In this figure

A. What is the bed position called? _____
_____

B. What is the angle of the head of the bed? _____
_____

40. In this figure

A. What is the bed position called? _____
_____

B. What is the angle of the head of the bed? _____
_____

C. What is the angle of the knee portion of the bed?
_____

D. Raising the knee portion of the bed can _____
_____

41. In this figure

    A. What is the bed position called? _____
    _____

    B. What is the position of the head of the bed and the foot of the bed? _____

    C. This position requires a _____
    _____

42. In this figure

    A. What is the bed position called? _____
    _____

    B. What is the position of the head of the bed and the foot of the bed? _____

    C. This position requires a _____
    _____

43. In these situations, how would you help protect a resident from drafts?

    A. The person is dressing for the day. _____
    _____

    B. The person is sitting in a wheelchair. _____
    _____

    C. You are assisting a resident who is going to bed for the night. _____

    D. You are giving personal care to the resident. ____
    _____

44. How can you help eliminate odors in these situations?

    A. You are caring for a person who is frequently incontinent. _____

    B. The person is vomiting and has wound drainage.
    _____

    C. The person uses the bathroom by herself. _____
    _____

    D. The person keeps a urinal at his bedside and uses it himself during the day. _____

45. When the staff talk loudly and laugh in the hallways, some persons may think that _____
_____
_____.

46. Why do persons with dementia react more to loud noises at night? _____
_____

47. How can the staff reduce noises and increase resident comfort?

    A. Control _____
    _____

    B. Handle _____
    _____

    C. Keep _____
    _____

    D. Answer _____
    _____

48. What are two situations when bright lights are helpful for a resident with poor vision? _____
_____ and
_____.

49. In dementia units, how does adjusting lighting help the residents?

    A. Soft, non-glare _____
    _____.

    B. Brighter _____
    _____.

85

50. The bed in the flat position is used for

    A. _____

    B. _____

51. Semi-Fowler position has two definitions. They are

    A. _____

    B. _____

52. How do you position the bed when semi-Fowler position is ordered? _____
    _____

53. In order to raise the foot of the bed with Trendelenburg position, you may put _____
    _____.

54. When the nursing team uses the overbed table as a work area, what are the only items that can be placed on it? _____
    _____

55. What are your responsibilities in these situations regarding the call light?

    A. The resident is sitting in a chair next to the bed.
    _____

    B. The person is weak on the right side. _____
    _____

    C. The person calls out instead of using the call light.
    _____

    D. The resident is embarrassed because she soiled the bed after signaling for assistance. _____
    _____

    E. The bathroom light in a room rings while you are busy in another room. _____
    _____

56. List the OBRA requirement that relates to each of these items in the resident unit.

    A. Number of residents in a room _____
    _____
    _____

    B. Windows _____
    _____

    C. Closets _____
    _____

    D. Call system _____
    _____

    E. Odors, noise, and lighting _____
    _____

    F. Handrails _____
    _____

INDEPENDENT LEARNING ACTIVITIES

- When you are in the health care center as a student, find an empty resident room and practice using the equipment. Answer the following questions about the equipment.
  - Where are the controls for the bed?
    - How do you operate the head of the bed?
    - How do you operate the knee control of the bed?
    - How do you adjust the height of the bed?
  - Where is the call light located?
  - Where are the controls for the television and radio?
  - Does the center have an intercom system? How is it used?
- Ask the staff the following questions about the call lights.
  - How does the staff know when a resident turns on the call light?
  - When a resident uses a bathroom call light, how does the staff know the difference?
  - Does the health care center use wireless call buttons or pendant call buttons? If so, what are the advantages?
- Think about what temperature is comfortable for you and answer the following questions. This exercise will help you understand the importance of individual preferences for residents in the health care center.
  - What is the usual temperature of your home?
  - Who decides what the temperature will be in your home? Partner, spouse, roommate, or children?
  - Would the temperature you prefer be comfortable for an infant? An older person? Why or why not?
- Think about the noises in your home and how they affect you. This exercise will help you understand why noise levels in the nursing center can affect the residents.
  - When you study, do you turn on the TV or radio? Listen to music? Prefer complete silence?
  - What noises do you like when going to sleep? TV? Radio? Soft music?
  - Does everyone in your household agree on how loud or soft to play a radio or TV? How are conflicts about noise levels resolved?
  - If you are in noisy surroundings, how do you react? How does it affect your ability to think? To rest? To study? How does it affect your relationship with others?

17 Bedmaking

FILL IN THE BLANKS: KEY TERMS

Cotton drawsheet
Drawsheet
Waterproof drawsheet

1. A drawsheet made of plastic, rubber, or absorbent material used to protect the mattress and bottom linens from dampness and soiling is a _____
_____.

2. A _____ is a small sheet placed over the middle of the bottom sheet.

3. A drawsheet made of cotton that helps keep the mattress and bottom linens clean and dry is a _____
_____.

CIRCLE THE BEST ANSWER

4. In nursing centers, bed linens are changed
   A. Only if the person asks for a change
   B. Every day
   C. On the person's bath or shower day
   D. Once a week on a scheduled day
5. Follow Standard Precautions and the Bloodborne Pathogen Standard when you
   A. Handle any bed linens
   B. Make the bed every morning
   C. May have contact with wet, soiled, or damp linens
   D. Place clean linens on the bed
6. When handling linens and making beds, you should
   A. Put the dirty linens on the floor
   B. Hold the linens away from your body and uniform
   C. Shake linens in the air to straighten them
   D. Use any extra linens for another resident
7. A closed bed
   A. Is made with the person in the bed
   B. Has the top linens fan-folded back so the person can get into bed
   C. Is made for residents who are up for most or all of the day
   D. Has the linens fan-folded lengthwise to the side of the bed
8. When making a bed, you use good body mechanics when you
   A. Bend from the waist when removing and replacing the linens
   B. Stretch across the bed to smooth the linens
   C. Raise the bed to a comfortable height
   D. Lock the wheels

9. If extra clean linens are brought to a person's room, you should
   A. Return the unused linens to the linen room
   B. Store the extra linens in the person's closet
   C. Put the unused linens in the dirty laundry
   D. Use the linens for a person in the next room
10. An open bed
    A. Is made with the person in it
    B. Lets the person get into the bed with ease
    C. Is not in use until bedtime; the top linens are not folded back
    D. Is made to transfer a person from a stretcher to the bed
11. Which of these linens will be collected first?
    A. Bath towel
    B. Bath blanket
    C. Mattress pad
    D. Top sheet
12. When you remove dirty linens, it is correct to
    A. Gather all the linens in one large roll
    B. Roll each piece of dirty linen away from you
    C. Place disposable pads in the laundry hamper with the dirty linens
    D. Replace all linens with clean linens every day
13. A waterproof drawsheet
    A. Can cause discomfort and skin breakdown
    B. Is used to keep linens tight and wrinkle-free
    C. Is used for all residents
    D. Is disposable and can be placed in the trash when soiled
14. When you are delegated to make a bed, why do you need to know the person's schedule for treatments, therapies, and activities?
    A. You need to make sure the bed is flat.
    B. It is best to change linens after the treatment or when the person is out of the room.
    C. You need to unlock beds that have been locked in a certain position.
    D. You will then know what type of bed to make.
15. When assigned to make a bed, what information do you need from the nurse or care plan?
    A. How the person wants the bed made
    B. Whether the person is confused
    C. When the bed was changed last
    D. How to position the person and the positioning devices needed

16. When a person is discharged from a hospital or nursing center, what is done in addition to changing the bed?
    A. New pillows are placed on the bed.
    B. The bed frame and mattress are cleaned and disinfected.
    C. The bed is sterilized.
    D. The bedspread and blanket may be reused.
17. When making a bed with a flat sheet, position the bottom sheet with
    A. The lower edge even with the top of the mattress
    B. The hemstitching facing downward, away from the person
    C. The large hem at the bottom and the small hem at the top
    D. The center crease across the bed
18. When the top sheet, blanket, and bedspread are in place on the bed
    A. Each one is tucked under the mattress separately
    B. The sheet and blanket are tucked together and the bedspread is allowed to hang loose over them
    C. All three are tucked together under the foot of the bed and the corners are mitered
    D. All three are allowed to hang loose over the foot of the bed
19. The pillow is placed on the bed so
    A. The open end of the pillowcase is away from the door
    B. The seam of the pillowcase is toward the foot of the bed
    C. It is leaning against the head of the bed
    D. The open end of the pillowcase is toward the door
20. If you are making an occupied bed for a person who is comatose, it is important to
    A. Keep the bed in the low position
    B. Unlock the wheels
    C. Use special linens
    D. Explain each step of the procedure to the person before it is done
21. A bath blanket is used when making an occupied bed to
    A. Protect the person from injury
    B. Provide warmth and privacy for the person
    C. Protect the bed linens
    D. Protect the person from dirty linens
22. To provide safety when making an occupied bed for a person who does not use bed rails, you should
    A. Have a coworker work on the opposite side of the bed
    B. Push the bed against the wall
    C. Always keep one hand on the person while you are making the bed
    D. Only change linens when the person is out of the bed for tests or therapies

23. When making an occupied bed, privacy is provided when you
    A. Close the door and pull curtains around the bed
    B. Ask the roommate to leave the room
    C. Work alone so there is only one worker in the room
    D. Lock the door so no one can enter the room
24. Which of these steps is done when making a surgical bed?
    A. Fan-fold linens lengthwise to the side of the bed farthest from the door.
    B. Remove all linens from the bed if the person is arriving from the hospital.
    C. Remove the mattress pad, as it is never used on a surgical bed.
    D. Cover the person with a bath blanket.
25. You allow the person the right of personal choice when you
    A. Allow the person to use bed linens from home
    B. Decide which linens will look best in the room
    C. Tell the person you will make the bed at 9 AM
    D. Choose the pillows and blanket the person needs for comfort

FILL IN THE BLANKS

26. Number the following list from 1 to 13 in the order you would collect the linens to make a bed.

    _____ Pillowcase(s)

    _____ Top sheet

    _____ Gown or pajamas

    _____ Bottom sheet (flat or fitted)

    _____ Mattress pad

    _____ Bedspread

    _____ Waterproof drawsheet

    _____ Bath blanket

    _____ Hand towel

    _____ Cotton drawsheet

    _____ Bath towel(s)

    _____ Blanket

    _____ Washcloth

OPTIONAL LEARNING EXERCISES

27. When is a complete linen change made in a nursing center? _____

28. Clean, dry, and wrinkle-free linens are important to promote _____ and to prevent _____ .

29. What should you do to keep beds neat and clean?

    A. _____

    B. _____

    C. _____

    D. _____

    E. _____

    F. _____

30. When handling linens, practice medical asepsis. Explain why each of the following actions would be poor medical asepsis.
    A. Holding the linens close to your body and uniform _____
    B. Shaking the linens to straighten them _____
    _____
    C. Placing the dirty linens on the floor _____
    _____

31. Family and visitors may question the quality _____ _____ and the quality _____ _____ if the bed is unmade, messy, or dirty.

INDEPENDENT LEARNING ACTIVITIES

- When you make beds at home this week, practice the methods you learned in this chapter.
  ○ What linens did you collect? In what order did you collect the linens?
  ○ Did you remember to make as much of one side of the bed as possible before moving to the other side?
  ○ What step could *not* be carried out at home that would have helped you to use good body mechanics?
  ○ Think about the methods you used to change your bed before reading this chapter. How will you change your bedmaking practices now that you have studied this chapter?
- How is a surgical bed different from an open bed?
- A new resident is arriving at the center by ambulance. She will be brought to the room by a stretcher. What is the best way to make the bed?
- Practice with a classmate and take turns as a resident who must have an occupied bed made. Ask the following questions about your feelings.
  ○ In what ways was your privacy protected?
  ○ Did the caregiver offer you any choices before making your bed? What were these choices?
  ○ Did you feel safe at all times? If not, what made you feel unsafe?
  ○ What was uncomfortable during the bed change?
  ○ How were you positioned after the bed was made?
- It is sometimes difficult for a new nursing assistant to remember the order in which to collect linens. Make a list in a pocket notebook or on a 3×5-inch index card so you can carry it with you when you are working.

18 Hygiene

FILL IN THE BLANKS: KEY TERMS

AM care
Aspiration
Denture
Early morning care
Evening care

HS care
Morning care
Oral hygiene
Pericare
Perineal care

Plaque
PM care
Tartar

1. Another name for PM care is _____ _____.

2. _____ is cleansing the genital and anal areas; it is sometimes called pericare.

3. Sometimes evening care is called _____ _____.

4. Routine care performed before breakfast or early morning care is called _____.

5. _____ is mouth care or measures that keep the mouth and teeth clean.

6. Hardened plaque on teeth is _____ _____.

7. _____ occurs when breathing fluid, food, vomitus, or an object into the lungs.

8. Care given after breakfast when hygiene measures are more thorough is called _____.

9. Another name for perineal care is _____ _____.

10. _____ is a thin film that sticks to the teeth. It contains saliva, microbes, and other substances.

11. Another name for AM care is _____ _____.

12. An artificial tooth or a set of artificial teeth is a _____.

13. Another name for evening care is _____ _____.

CIRCLE THE BEST ANSWER

14. If a person needs help with personal hygiene, you can find out what needs they have by
    A. Following the nurse's directions and the care plan
    B. Asking the family
    C. Asking other staff members
    D. Making your own decisions

15. You should assist a person with personal hygiene
    A. Only when the person asks
    B. Only in the morning
    C. Whenever help is needed
    D. Only when it is your assignment

16. When giving personal hygiene, you need to remember to protect the person's right to
    A. Privacy and personal choice
    B. Care and security of personal possessions
    C. Activities
    D. Environment

17. When giving routine care before breakfast, you should
    A. Assist with activity by ambulating the person
    B. Give a complete bath
    C. Change wet or soiled linens and garments
    D. Change all of the bed linens for every person

18. Which of these is done every time you assist with hygiene measures throughout the day?
    A. Assisting with dressing and hair care
    B. Face and hand washing
    C. Assisting with ambulation
    D. Helping the person change into sleepwear

19. If good oral hygiene is not done regularly, the person may develop tartar, which will lead to
    A. A dry mouth
    B. Periodontal disease
    C. A bad taste in the mouth
    D. Plaque

20. The nurse may be assisted in assessing the person's need for mouth care by the
    A. Nursing assistant
    B. Physical therapist
    C. Doctor
    D. Dietitian

21. Teeth are flossed
    A. When brushing the teeth is not possible
    B. When the person is in a coma
    C. When you do not have time to give complete oral hygiene
    D. To remove food from between the teeth

22. Which of these steps is correct when flossing the teeth?
    A. Floss dentures in the same way you floss natural teeth
    B. Use a new piece of floss for each section of the mouth
    C. Move the floss gently up and down between the teeth
    D. Move to a new section of floss when moving from the upper to lower teeth
23. Sponge swabs are used for
    A. Persons who are unconscious
    B. Cleaning dentures
    C. Oral care on children
    D. Oral care on all residents
24. You follow Standard Precautions and the Bloodborne Pathogen Standard when giving oral hygiene because
    A. You will not spread bacteria to the person
    B. It will help you avoid bad breath odors from the person
    C. Gums may bleed during mouth care
    D. You will avoid any loose teeth or rough dentures
25. When the person is able to perform oral hygiene in bed, you arrange the items on
    A. The overbed table
    B. The bedside table
    C. The sink counter
    D. The bed
26. When you are brushing the person's teeth, you should
    A. Let the person rinse the mouth with water
    B. Use only a sponge swab to clean the teeth
    C. Have the person floss his or her teeth
    D. Wear gloves only if bleeding occurs
27. When providing mouth care for an unconscious person, position the person on one side with the head turned well to the side to
    A. Make it easier to brush the teeth
    B. Make the person more comfortable
    C. Prevent the risk of aspiration
    D. Make it easier for the person to breathe
28. When giving oral hygiene to an unconscious person who wears dentures, you should
    A. Remove the dentures, clean them, and replace them in the mouth
    B. Know that dentures are not worn when the person is unconscious
    C. Clean the dentures in the mouth without removing them
    D. Insert your fingers to keep the mouth open
29. Mouth care is given to an unconscious person
    A. After each meal
    B. When AM and PM care is given
    C. At least every 2 hours
    D. Once a day
30. A padded tongue blade is used when giving oral hygiene to an unconscious person to
    A. Keep the mouth open
    B. Clean the teeth
    C. Clean the tongue
    D. Prevent aspiration
31. When cleaning dentures at a sink, line the sink with a towel to
    A. Prevent infections
    B. Prevent the dentures from falling on a hard surface
    C. Dry the dentures
    D. Clean the dentures
32. If dentures are not worn after cleaning, store them in
    A. Cool water or a denture soaking solution
    B. Hot water
    C. A soft towel
    D. Soft tissues or a napkin
33. If the person cannot remove the dentures, you can use which of these to get a good grip on the slippery dentures?
    A. Gloves
    B. Washcloth
    C. Gauze squares
    D. Bare hands
34. Older persons usually need a complete bath or shower twice a week because
    A. They are less active
    B. They are often ill
    C. They have increased perspiration
    D. Dry skin often occurs with aging
35. If a person has dry skin, which of these will help keep it soft?
    A. Soaps
    B. Lotions and oils
    C. Frequent baths or showers
    D. Deodorants and antiperspirants
36. If a person with dementia resists bathing, you should
    A. Hurry through the bath
    B. Speak firmly in a loud voice
    C. Try giving a partial bath or try giving the bath later
    D. Use restraints so the person will not harm you
37. When choosing skin care products for bathing, you should use
    A. Soap
    B. Products the person prefers or those listed in the care plan
    C. Bath oils
    D. Creams and lotions
38. The water temperature for a complete bed bath is usually between 110°F and 115°F (43.3°C and 46.1°C) for adults. For older persons, the temperature
    A. Should be between 110°F and 115°F (43.3°C and 46.1°C)
    B. May need to be lower
    C. Should be whatever you feel is comfortable
    D. May need to be warmer

39. When applying powder
    A. Shake or sprinkle the powder directly on the person
    B. Sprinkle a small amount of powder on your hands or a cloth
    C. Apply a thick layer of powder
    D. You should never use powder on any older person
40. A complete bed bath is given to
    A. Those who cannot bathe themselves
    B. Persons with dementia or confusion
    C. All residents who need help with hygiene
    D. A person who walks independently
41. When you are giving a complete bed bath, the bed linens are changed
    A. Only if needed
    B. Before the bath begins
    C. After the bath
    D. After the person gets out of bed
42. The person is offered the bedpan, urinal, or commode or is taken to the bathroom
    A. Before the bath begins
    B. After the bath ends
    C. During the bath, before perineal care is done
    D. Only if this step is part of the care plan
43. During the bed bath, the bath blanket is placed
    A. Over the top linens
    B. Under the top linens
    C. Over the person as the top linens are removed
    D. Under the person
44. Do not use soap when washing
    A. The face, ears, and neck
    B. Around the eyes
    C. The abdomen
    D. The perineal area
45. How do you avoid exposing the person when washing the chest?
    A. Keep the bath blanket over the area
    B. Keep the top linens over the chest
    C. Place a bath towel over the chest crosswise
    D. Make sure the curtains are closed
46. Bath water is changed during a bed bath
    A. Every 5 minutes
    B. Only if the person asks you to change it
    C. Before giving perineal care
    D. After washing the face, ears, and neck
47. Which of these persons may respond well to a towel bath?
    A. Person with dementia
    B. Person who has been incontinent
    C. Person with breaks in the skin
    D. Person who needs a partial bath
48. A partial bath involves bathing
    A. Areas the person cannot reach
    B. The face, hands, axillae (underarms), back, buttocks, and perineal area
    C. The arms, legs, and feet
    D. The chest, abdomen, and underarms

49. When giving any type of bath, you should
    A. Wash from the dirtiest to cleanest areas
    B. Allow the skin to air-dry to avoid rubbing
    C. Provide for privacy
    D. Decide what is best for the person
50. A tub bath should not last longer than
    A. 10 minutes
    B. 15 minutes
    C. 20 minutes
    D. 30 minutes
51. If a person is weak or unsteady, which of these should be used when the person showers?
    A. Shower chair
    B. Transfer belt
    C. Wheelchair
    D. Stretcher
52. Which of these would be good time management when giving a tub bath or shower?
    A. Take the person to the shower room and then collect your equipment
    B. Ask a coworker to give the shower for you
    C. Ask a coworker to make the person's bed while you give the bath
    D. Clean and disinfect the tub or shower before returning the person to his or her room
53. When assisting with a tub bath or shower, which of these steps is done first?
    A. Help the person undress and remove footwear
    B. Assist or transport the person to the tub or shower room
    C. Put the OCCUPIED sign on the door
    D. Place a rubber bath mat in the tub or on the shower floor
54. The best position for a back massage is
    A. Prone position
    B. Supine position
    C. Side-lying position
    D. Semi-Fowler position
55. Back massages are dangerous for persons
    A. Who are bedridden
    B. With heart and kidney diseases
    C. Who have arthritis
    D. Who have intact skin
56. When giving a back massage, the strokes
    A. Start at the shoulders and go down to the buttocks
    B. Should be light and gentle
    C. Start at the buttocks and go up to the shoulders
    D. Are continued for at least 10 minutes
57. When cleaning the perineal area
    A. You do not need to wear gloves
    B. Work from the anal area to the urethral area
    C. Work from the urethral area to the anal area
    D. Work from the dirtiest area to the cleanest area
58. When gathering equipment for perineal care, you will need
    A. One washcloth
    B. Two washcloths
    C. At least three washcloths
    D. At least four washcloths

59. When giving perineal care to a male, you
    A. Retract the foreskin if he is uncircumcised
    B. Wash from the scrotum to the tip of the penis
    C. Use one washcloth for the entire procedure
    D. Leave the foreskin retracted after finishing the care

60. If a family member or friend offers to help provide hygiene to a person
    A. You should check the center policy
    B. The person must consent to this
    C. Accept the offer and allow him or her to give the care
    D. Tell the family member or friend that this is not allowed

MATCHING

Match the skin care product with the benefits or the problem that may occur if you use the product. (Use Table 18-1 to answer.)

61. _____ Absorbs moisture and prevents friction

62. _____ Makes showers and tubs slippery

63. _____ Protects skin from the drying effect of air and evaporation

64. _____ Excessive amounts can cause caking and crusts that can irritate the skin

65. _____ Masks and controls body odors

66. _____ Tends to dry and irritate skin

67. _____ Keeps skin soft and prevents drying of skin

68. _____ Removes dirt, dead skin, skin oil, some microbes, and perspiration

A. Soaps
B. Bath oils
C. Creams and lotions
D. Powders
E. Deodorants and antiperspirants

FILL IN THE BLANKS

69. C is an abbreviation for _____.

70. F is an abbreviation for _____.

71. ID is an abbreviation for _____.

72. The _____ and _____ must be intact to prevent microbes from entering the body and causing an _____.

73. When is oral hygiene given to a person? _____ _____

74. When you are delegated to give oral hygiene, what observations should you report?
    A. _____
    B. _____
    C. _____
    D. _____
    E. _____
    F. _____

75. If flossing is done only once a day, the best time to floss is at _____.

76. When giving oral care to an unconscious person, explain what you are doing because you always assume _____.

77. When following the rules for bathing in Box 18-1, you protect the skin by these actions:
    A. Rinse _____
    _____
    B. Pat _____
    _____
    C. Dry _____
    _____

78. What methods can be used to measure the water temperature when giving a bed bath?
    A. _____
    B. _____

79. When you place a person's hands in the basin during the bed bath, you may have the person _____ _____ the hands and fingers.

80. When assisting a person to take a partial bath, you know that most people need help washing the _____ _____.

81. When a person has been on bedrest, safety is a concern because the bath can make the person feel _____ _____ or _____.

82. When the shower room has more than one stall or cabinet, you must protect the person's right. What can you do to protect this right for privacy?

A. _____

B. _____

C. _____

83. When giving a tub bath or shower, you use safety measures to protect the person from _____ _____, _____, and _____.

84. When giving a back massage and the person does not want the buttocks exposed, you should _____ _____.

85. When you are delegated to give a back massage, what observations should you report and record?

A. _____

B. _____

C. _____

D. _____

86. When you are assisting a person with perineal care, what terms can you use to help the person understand what you are going to do? _____ _____

LABELING

87. Look at the figure and answer the following questions.

A. Why is the person positioned on his side? _____ _____

B. What is the purpose of the padded tongue blade? _____

88. In this figure, what is the staff member using to remove the upper denture? _____ _____

Why? _____ _____

89. In this figure, explain what the staff member is doing. _____

Why is the towel positioned vertically on the person? _____

OPTIONAL LEARNING EXERCISES

90. Hygiene promotes comfort, safety, and health. Answer the following questions about hygiene.

A. Why is intact skin important? _____ _____.

B. What other areas must be clean to maintain intact skin? _____

C. Besides cleansing, what are the other benefits of good hygiene? _____

D. What are two other reasons that hygiene is important? _____

91. What factors cause mouth dryness in an unconscious person?

    A. _____

    B. _____

    C. _____

92. The factors listed above cause crusting on the _____ and _____.

93. Oral hygiene keeps the mouth and teeth _____ _____. It also prevents _____ and _____.

94. What are the benefits of bathing?

    A. Cleans _____

    B. Also cleans _____

    C. Removes _____

    D. Bath is _____ and

    _____

    E. Stimulates _____

    F. Exercises _____

    G. You can make _____

    H. You have time _____

95. When you are bathing a person with dementia, what measures are important to help the person through the bath?

    A. _____

    B. _____

    C. _____

    D. _____

    E. _____

    F. _____

    G. _____

    H. _____

    I. _____

    J. _____

    K. _____

    L. _____

    M. _____

    N. _____

    O. _____

    P. _____

96. You are delegated to give Mrs. Johnson a bath. Before beginning, what information do you need?

    A. _____

    B. _____

    C. _____

    D. _____

    E. _____

    F. _____

    G. _____

    H. _____

97. As you are bathing Mrs. Johnson, what observations should you make to report and record?

    A. _____

    B. _____

    C. _____

    D. _____

    E. _____

    F. _____

    G. _____

    H. _____

    I. _____

    J. _____

    K. _____

98. When you are preparing to give perineal care to Mrs. Johnson, how many washcloths should you gather? Why? _____ _____

INDEPENDENT LEARNING ACTIVITIES

- Have you ever been comforted by a warm towel or blanket that just came out of the dryer? Can you see how this warmth would also be pleasing to a resident after a bath or shower?
- Have you ever spent time in a whirlpool tub or hot tub? Perhaps you found this relaxing. Can you see how this might be frightening, however, for a person with dementia?

95

19 Grooming

FILL IN THE BLANKS: KEY TERMS

Alopecia
Anticoagulant
Bed bugs
Dandruff

Hirsutism
Lice
Mite
Pediculosis

Pediculosis capitis
Pediculosis corporis
Pediculosis pubis

1. A very small spider-like organism is a _____ _____.

2. An infestation with lice is _____.

3. _____ is an excessive amount of dry, white flakes from the scalp.

4. The infestation of the body with lice is _____ _____.

5. Hair loss is _____.

6. _____ is the infestation of the pubic hair with lice.

7. Excessive body hair in women and children is _____.

8. The infestation of the scalp with wingless insects is _____.

9. A medication that prevents or slows blood-clotting time is an _____.

10. Another name for pediculosis is _____ _____.

11. Small, flat insects that feed on the blood of sleeping people and animals are _____.

CIRCLE THE BEST ANSWER

12. Hair care, shaving, and nail and foot care are important to residents because they also affect the need for
    A. Safety and security
    B. Love and belonging and self-esteem
    C. Basic physical needs
    D. Self-actualization

13. If you see any signs of lice, you should report them to the nurse because
    A. Lice bites can cause severe infections
    B. Lice are easily spread to other persons through clothing, furniture, bed linens, and sexual contact
    C. Lice can cause the person's hair to fall out
    D. Lice will cause the hair to mat and tangle

14. The nurse tells you that a person you are caring for has scabies. When giving care, you observe
    A. Dry, white flakes on the scalp
    B. A rash in the underarm area, on the thighs, and in the genital area
    C. White or yellow oval nits on the hair
    D. Tan to grayish-white objects the size of sesame seeds in the pubic hair

15. Who chooses how you will brush, comb, and style a person's hair?
    A. The person
    B. You
    C. The nurse
    D. The care plan

16. If long hair becomes matted or tangled, you should
    A. Braid the hair
    B. Cut the hair to remove the tangles and matting
    C. Talk to the nurse and ask for directions
    D. Get the family's permission to change the hairstyle

17. When caring for a person with hair that is curly, coarse, and dry, which of these would you do?
    A. Braid or cut the hair
    B. Use a wide-toothed comb
    C. Start at the ends and work toward the scalp
    D. Use a fine-tooth comb

18. If a woman's hair is done by the beautician
    A. Wash her hair only once a week
    B. Shampoo her hair on the day she goes to the beautician
    C. Make sure she wears a shower cap during the tub bath or shower
    D. Wash her hair each time she gets a shower or tub bath

19. If a person has limited range of motion in the neck, he or she is not shampooed
    A. At the sink or on a stretcher
    B. In the tub or shower with the head tipped forward
    C. During a tub bath
    D. In bed

20. What observation is made and reported when shampooing?
    A. The hair color
    B. The presence of nits or lice
    C. The texture of the hair
    D. The hairstyle

21. If a person receives anticoagulants and needs shaving
    A. An electric razor is used
    B. Use disposable safety razors
    C. It must be done by the nurse or barber
    D. It should be done only during the shower or bath
22. When using safety razors (blade razors)
    A. The same razor can be used for several persons until it becomes dull
    B. Use the resident's own razor several times
    C. Discard the razor blade or disposable razor in the sharps container
    D. Be careful when shaving a person who takes anticoagulants
23. Why is an electric razor used when shaving a person with dementia?
    A. They usually bleed easily
    B. The person may resist care and move suddenly
    C. It is faster than using a safety razor
    D. The person's skin is tender and sensitive
24. When shaving a person with a safety razor, wear gloves
    A. To protect the person from infections
    B. To prevent contact with blood
    C. When applying shaving cream
    D. To maintain sterile technique
25. When caring for a mustache and beard, you should
    A. Wash and comb the mustache or beard daily
    B. Allow only the barber to groom the mustache or beard
    C. Wash with shampoo and conditioner
    D. Trim a mustache or beard when needed
26. Nursing assistants can trim nails
    A. Whenever they have time
    B. On all persons
    C. Only if center policy allows them to do so
    D. If the person agrees to the care
27. When caring for the fingernails, you should
    A. Cut the nails with small scissors
    B. Shape the nails with an emery board or nail file
    C. Round the nails at the corners with nail clippers
    D. Soak the hands for 15 to 20 minutes
28. When changing clothing, remove the clothing from
    A. The weak side first
    B. The lower limbs first
    C. The right side last
    D. The strong or "good" side first
29. When you are undressing a person, it is usually done
    A. In the bed in the supine position
    B. With the person sitting in a chair
    C. With the person standing at the bedside
    D. In the bathroom
30. When you are changing the person's clothes, you use good body mechanics by
    A. Having a good base of support
    B. Holding objects close to your body
    C. Raising the bed to a good working level
    D. Lifting with the large muscles

31. To provide warmth and privacy when changing clothes, you
    A. Keep the top sheets in place
    B. Cover the person with a bath blanket
    C. Close the curtains
    D. Close the door
32. When changing the hospital gown of a person with an IV
    A. Turn off the IV
    B. Lay the IV bag on the bed and remove the gown
    C. Use a gown with shoulder snaps, if available
    D. Disconnect the IV
33. When you have finished changing the gown of a person with an IV, always
    A. Restart the pump
    B. Reconnect the IV
    C. Ask the nurse to check the flow rate
    D. Check the flow rate

FILL IN THE BLANKS

34. Write the meaning of the following abbreviations

    A. C_____

    B. F_____

    C. ID_____

    D. IV_____

35. When you are giving care, report these signs and symptoms of lice to the nurse at once:

    A. _____

    B. _____

    C. _____

    D. _____

    E. _____

36. When you brush and comb the hair, you should report and record

    A. _____

    B. _____

    C. _____

    D. _____

    E. _____

    F. _____

    G. _____

    H. _____

37. If you give hair care to a person in bed after a linen change, collect falling hair by _____ _____.

38. Brush and comb matted hair by starting at the _____ and working up to the _____.

39. You can protect the person's eyes during shampooing by asking the person to hold a _____ _____.

40. What delegation guidelines do you need when shaving a person?

A. _____

B. _____

C. _____

D. _____

E. _____

F. _____

G. _____

H. _____

41. What should be reported at once when you are shaving a person?

A. _____

B. _____

C. _____

42. When you are shaving the face and underarms with a safety razor, shave in the direction of the _____ _____.

43. When shaving legs with a safety razor, shave _____ _____.

44. When using an electric shaver, shave _____ _____.

45. When you are delegated to give nail and foot care, report and record

A. _____

B. _____

C. _____

D. _____

E. _____

46. Foot care for persons with diabetes or poor circulation is provided by _____ or _____ _____.

47. When undressing the person who cannot raise the head and shoulders

A. _____

B. _____

C. _____

D. _____

E. _____

48. When dressing the person who cannot raise the hips and buttocks

A. _____

B. _____

C. _____

D. _____

E. _____

49. Before changing the hospital gown of a person with an IV, what information do you need from the nurse and the care plan?

A. _____

B. _____

50. When using a shampoo cap

A. _____

B. _____

C. _____

D. _____

E. _____

OPTIONAL LEARNING EXERCISES

51. You are caring for a person who is receiving cancer treatments. What effect could this treatment have on the person's hair? _____ _____

52. Dandruff not only occurs on the scalp, but it may involve the _____.

53. How are each of these problems treated?
A. Lice _____
B. Scabies _____
C. Bed bugs _____

54. Brushing the hair increases _____ to the scalp. It also brings _____ along the hair shaft.

55. Why do older persons usually have dry hair? _____ _____

56. What water temperature is usually used when shampooing the hair? _____

57. How can the beard be softened before shaving?

_____

58. After shaving, why do some people apply aftershave or lotion?

A. Lotion _____

B. Aftershave _____

59. Injuries to the feet of a person with poor circulation are serious because poor circulation _____
_____.

60. When changing clothing or hospital gowns, what rules should be followed?

A. _____

B. _____

C. _____

D. _____

E. _____

F. _____

61. How does grooming improve the quality of life?

A. Promotes _____
_____

B. Helps the person's _____
_____ and _____
_____

C. Whenever possible, it allows for _____
_____

D. Treats person's property with _____
and _____

INDEPENDENT LEARNING ACTIVITIES

- Role-play this situation with a classmate. Take turns being the resident and the nursing assistant. Remember to keep your left arm and leg limp when you are the resident.

SITUATION: *Mr. Olsen is a 58-year-old resident who has weakness on the left side. You are assigned to take off his sleepwear and dress him for the day. You need to remove his pajamas and dress him in a shirt, a pullover sweater, slacks, socks, and shoes.*

- ○ How did you provide privacy?
- ○ How was Mr. Olsen positioned for the clothing change?
- ○ What difficulties did you have when you removed his pajamas?
- ○ Which arm did you re-dress first? What difficulty did you have getting his arms into the shirt?
- ○ How did you put on the sweater? What was most difficult about this?
- ○ What was the most difficult part of putting on the slacks?
- ○ How did you put on the socks and shoes?
- ○ What did you learn from this role-play situation? Did you follow the procedure in the chapter to assist you?
- ○ Discuss with each other how it felt to have someone dress you when you were "Mr. Olsen."

20 Nutrition and Fluids

Anorexia   Dehydration   Intake
Aspiration   Dysphagia   Nutrient
Calorie   Edema   Nutrition
Daily Value (DV)   Graduate   Output

1. _____ is the amount of fluid taken in.

2. The _____ is how a serving fits into the daily diet. It is expressed in a percentage based on a daily diet of 2000 calories.

3. The loss of appetite is _____ __.

4. The amount of fluid lost is _____ _____.

5. A substance that is ingested, digested, absorbed, and used by the body is a _____.

6. _____ is difficulty swallowing.

7. The breathing of fluid, food, vomitus, or an object into the lungs is _____.

8. The process involved in the ingestion, digestion, absorption, and use of food and fluids by the body is _____.

9. The fuel or energy value of food is a _____.

10. A decrease in the amount of water in body tissues is _____.

11. A _____ is a measuring container for fluid.

12. _____ is the swelling of body tissues with water.

CIRCLE THE BEST ANSWER

13. When a person has a poor diet and poor eating habits, he or she is likely to have
    A. Decreased risk for infection
    B. Improved wound healing
    C. Increased risk for accidents and injuries
    D. Decreased risk of acute and chronic diseases

14. Body fuel for energy is found in
    A. Vitamins
    B. Minerals
    C. Fats, proteins, and carbohydrates
    D. Water

15. The *Dietary Guidelines for Americans, 2020–2025* help people
    A. Recover from chronic illnesses
    B. Promote overall health
    C. Develop a vegetarian diet
    D. Aim to include 2500 mg of sodium in their diet each day

16. The *Dietary Guidelines for Americans, 2020–2025* recommends
    A. Eating a diet with more than 300 mg of cholesterol
    B. Including raw fish or shellfish in the diet
    C. Reducing daily sodium intake to less than 2300 mg for healthy people
    D. Eating plenty of refined grain foods, especially those that contain solid fats

17. What type of fat should be kept as low as possible in the diet, according to the *Dietary Guidelines for Americans, 2020–2025*?
    A. Trans fatty acids
    B. Saturated fatty acids
    C. Monosaturated fatty acids
    D. Polyunsaturated fatty acids

18. According to the *Dietary Guidelines for Americans, 2020–2025*, persons over 51 years of age and those with certain chronic diseases should reduce sodium intake to
    A. Less than 1000 mg a day
    B. No more than 3500 mg a day
    C. No more than 1500 mg a day
    D. No more than 5000 mg a day

19. In the *Dietary Guidelines for Americans, 2020–2025*, building healthy eating patterns includes
    A. Eating the same foods every day
    B. Eating only fruits and vegetables
    C. Selecting an eating pattern that meets nutrient needs over time
    D. Taking a multivitamin to supplement the diet

20. The MyPlate plan recommends increasing
    A. The size of portions eaten
    B. Fruits and vegetables to half of your plate
    C. Sodium intake
    D. Intake of sugary drinks

21. Which of these is an example of moderate physical activity?
    A. Playing singles tennis
    B. Walking at about 2 miles per hour
    C. Participating in water aerobics
    D. Swimming freestyle laps
22. Dairy products in the MyPlate plan should
    A. Supply more than half of the calories in the diet
    B. Be a very small amount of the calories in the diet
    C. Be mostly fat-free or low-fat products
    D. Be mostly high-fat products
23. Vegetables in the MyPlate plan should be
    A. High in cholesterol
    B. Served only uncooked
    C. Always dark green in color
    D. Fresh, frozen, or canned
24. Oils are
    A. One of the food groups in the MyPlate plan
    B. Low in calories
    C. Liquid at room temperatures
    D. Solid at room temperature
25. Which nutrient is needed for tissue growth and repair?
    A. Carbohydrates
    B. Fats
    C. Vitamins
    D. Protein
26. Which vitamin is needed for the formation of substances that hold tissue together?
    A. Vitamin K
    B. Vitamin C
    C. Vitamin A
    D. Vitamin B_{12}
27. Food labels are important because they help people
    A. Determine the cost of the food
    B. Know all of the vitamins and minerals in the food
    C. Know the total amount of fat and the amount of saturated and trans fats
    D. Determine the flavor of the food
28. What health benefits do vegetables have?
    A. Contain high cholesterol
    B. Protect against certain cancers
    C. Promote development of kidney stones
    D. Help lower calorie intake, but only when cut up and mashed
29. People with limited incomes often buy
    A. More protein foods
    B. Foods high in carbohydrates
    C. Foods high in vitamins and minerals
    D. Fatty foods
30. When people buy cheaper foods, the diet may lack
    A. Fats
    B. Starchy foods
    C. Protein and certain vitamins and minerals
    D. Sugars
31. Appetite can be stimulated by
    A. Illness and medications
    B. Decreased senses of taste and smell
    C. Aromas and thoughts of food
    D. Anxiety, pain, and depression

32. During illness
    A. Appetite increases
    B. Fewer nutrients are needed
    C. Nutritional needs increase to fight infection and heal tissue
    D. The person will prefer protein foods
33. As a person ages, changes in the GI system can cause
    A. Increases in taste and smell
    B. Increases in secretion of digestive juices
    C. Difficulty swallowing
    D. A decrease in the appetite
34. Requirements for food served in long-term care centers are made by
    A. MyPlate
    B. OBRA and CMS
    C. The nursing center
    D. The public health department
35. A requirement for food served in long-term care centers is
    A. All food served must be cut up or ground
    B. The person's diet is well-balanced, nourishing, and tastes good
    C. All food is served at room temperature
    D. No salt or sugar is added to the food
36. A general diet
    A. Is ordered for the person with difficulty swallowing
    B. Has no dietary limits or restrictions
    C. May have restricted amounts of sodium
    D. Increases the amount of sugar in the diet
37. The body needs no more than which amount of sodium each day?
    A. 2400 mg
    B. 3000 mg
    C. 5000 mg
    D. 1000 mg
38. When the body tissues swell with water, what organ has to work harder?
    A. Kidneys
    B. Liver
    C. Heart
    D. Lungs
39. When you are caring for a person with diabetes, you should
    A. Serve the person's meals and snacks when the person requests food
    B. Give the person extra salt or sugar as requested
    C. Give the person extra food and snacks whenever requested
    D. Serve meals and snacks at regular times
40. When a person has swallowing difficulties, he or she will be given foods that
    A. Are thickened to meet the person's needs
    B. Are easy to chew
    C. Have been pureed and are very liquid
    D. Can be given through a feeding tube

101

41. A person may be given a mechanical soft diet because
    A. Nausea and vomiting have occurred
    B. The person has chewing difficulties
    C. The person has been advanced from a clear-liquid diet
    D. The person has constipation
42. If you are serving a meal to a person on a fiber- and residue-restricted diet, the meal would *not* include
    A. Raw fruits and vegetables
    B. Strained fruit juices
    C. Canned or cooked fruit without skin or seeds
    D. Plain pasta
43. A person who has serious burns would receive a
    A. Sodium-controlled diet
    B. Fat-controlled diet
    C. High-calorie diet
    D. High-protein diet
44. When a person has dysphagia, the thickness of the food served is chosen by the
    A. Person
    B. Nursing assistant
    C. Family
    D. Speech-language pathologist, dietitian, and doctor or nurse
45. A thickened liquid on a dysphagia diet is served
    A. From a cup
    B. In a bowl
    C. By stirring immediately before serving
    D. According to the care plan
46. When assisting a person with dysphagia, you can help prevent aspiration while the person is eating by placing him or her in
    A. Semi-Fowler position
    B. Fowler position or upright in a chair
    C. The side-lying position
    D. The supine position
47. If fluid intake exceeds fluid output, the person may
    A. Have edema in the tissues
    B. Be dehydrated
    C. Have vomiting and diarrhea
    D. Have increased urinary output
48. How much fluid is needed every day for normal fluid balance?
    A. 1500 mL
    B. 1000–1500 mL
    C. 2000–2500 mL
    D. 3000–4000 mL
49. If the person you are caring for has an order for restricted fluids, which of these should you do?
    A. Offer a variety of liquids
    B. Thicken all fluids
    C. Remove the water pitcher from the room
    D. Do not allow the person to swallow any liquids during oral hygiene

50. When you are keeping I&O records, you should measure all of these except
    A. Milk, water, coffee, and tea
    B. Mashed potatoes and creamed vegetables
    C. Gelatin and popsicles
    D. Ice cream, custard, and pudding
51. When you are measuring I&O, you need to know that 1 ounce equals
    A. 10 mL
    B. 500 mL
    C. 100 mL
    D. 30 mL
52. When you are using the graduate to measure output, you read the amount by
    A. Holding the graduate at waist level and reading the amount
    B. Looking at the graduate while it is held above eye level
    C. Keeping the container at eye level
    D. Setting the graduate on the floor and reading it
53. When I&O is ordered, which of the following is measured as output?
    A. Perspiration
    B. Solid stool
    C. Drainage from wound suction
    D. Solid foods
54. A quietly confused person may sometimes be served meals in a _____ dining program.
    A. Social
    B. Family
    C. Low-stimulation
    D. Restaurant-style
55. Which of the following needs to be done before the person is served a meal?
    A. Give complete personal care
    B. Change all linens
    C. Make sure the person is clean and dry
    D. Make sure the person has been shaved or has make-up applied
56. What should you do if a food tray has not been served within 15 minutes?
    A. Re-check the food temperatures
    B. Serve the tray immediately
    C. Throw the food away
    D. Serve only the cold items on the tray
57. How can you make sure the food tray is complete?
    A. Ask the person being served
    B. Ask the nurse
    C. Call the dietary department
    D. Check items on the tray with the dietary card
58. If you become impatient while feeding a resident with dementia, you should
    A. Refuse to continue caring for the person
    B. Return the person to his or her room
    C. Talk to the nurse
    D. Make the person eat his or her food

59. When you are feeding a person, you should
    A. Not allow the person to assist
    B. Give the person a fork and knife to assist with cutting the food
    C. Feed the person in a private area to maintain confidentiality
    D. Use a spoon because it is less likely to cause injury
60. When feeding a person, liquids are given
    A. Only at the start of feeding
    B. During the meal, alternating with solid foods
    C. At the end of the meal when all solids have been eaten
    D. Only if the person has difficulty swallowing
61. When providing fresh water to residents, you would
    A. Give fresh water once each shift
    B. Put ice in all pitchers
    C. Practice the rules of medical asepsis to prevent the spread of microbes
    D. Give each person one glass of water at a time
62. When you keep track of calorie intake, you include
    A. What time the person ate
    B. Only the liquids that the person drinks
    C. All of the food that was served to the person
    D. What the person ate and how much
63. When residents are included in deciding what foods they eat, which of their rights is being met?
    A. Personal choice
    B. Privacy
    C. Confidentiality
    D. Good nutrition

FILL IN THE BLANKS

64. Write out the meaning of each abbreviation.
    A. CMS _____
    B. DV _____
    C. F _____
    D. FDA _____
    E. GI _____
    F. ID _____
    G. IDDSI _____
    H. I&O _____
    I. mg _____
    J. mL _____
    K. NDD _____
    L. NPO _____
    M. OBRA _____
    N. oz _____
    O. USDA _____

65. How many calories are in each of these?
    A. 1 gram of fat _____
    B. 1 gram of protein _____
    C. 1 gram of carbohydrate _____

Questions 66 to 70 relate to the Dietary Guidelines for Americans, 2020–2025.

66. The Dietary Guidelines help people
    A. _____
    B. _____
    C. _____

67. Which foods or food components should be reduced in the diet?
    A. _____ to less than 2300 mg
    B. Consume less than 10% of calories from _____
    _____
    C. Consume less than 300 mg of _____
    _____
    D. Keep _____ consumption as low as possible

68. What foods and nutrients should be increased?
    A. A variety of _____, especially
    _____
    B. Half of all grains should be _____
    _____
    C. Fat-free or low-fat _____
    _____
    D. _____ should be chosen in place of meat and poultry

69. What recommendations are made to manage weight?
    A. _____
    B. _____
    C. _____
    D. _____

70. What guidelines are given to build healthy eating patterns?
    A. _____
    B. _____
    C. _____

Questions 71 to 76 relate to MyPlate.

71. What are the five food groups included in MyPlate?
    A. _____
    B. _____
    C. _____
    D. _____
    E. _____

103

72. _____are also included in food patterns but are not a food group.

73. What foods contain the entire grain kernel?

    A. _____

    B. _____

    C. _____

    D. _____

    E. _____

74. What are five vegetable subgroups?

    A. _____

    B. _____

    C. _____

    D. _____

    E. _____

75. What are the health benefits of milk and milk products?

    A. _____

    B. _____

    C. _____

76. What nutrients are provided in protein foods?

    A. _____

    B. _____

    C. _____

77. If dietary fat is not needed by the body, it is stored as _____.

78. What is the function of each of these nutrients?

    A. Protein _____

    B. Carbohydrates _____

    C. Fats _____

    D. Vitamins _____

    E. Minerals _____

    F. Water _____

79. Which vitamins can be stored by the body? _____
    _____

80. Which vitamins must be ingested daily? _____
    _____

81. What vitamin is important for these functions? *Formation of substances that hold tissues together; healthy blood vessels, skin, gums, bones, and teeth; wound healing; prevention of bleeding; resistance to infection* _____

82. Milk and milk products, liver, green leafy vegetables, eggs, breads, and cereals are good sources of which vitamin? _____
    _____

83. What mineral allows red blood cells to carry oxygen? _____

84. When the diet does not have enough _____ _____, it may affect nerve function, muscle contraction, and heart function.

85. Calcium is needed for _____
    _____.

86. What information is found on food labels?

    A. _____

    B. _____

    C. _____

87. What are the health benefits of grains?
    _____.

88. Nutritional needs increase during illness when the body must _____.

89. Why do the diets of people with limited income sometimes lack protein? _____
    _____
    _____

90. What OBRA requirement relates to the temperature of foods served in long-term care centers? _____
    _____
    _____

91. What foods are included in a clear-liquid diet? ____
    _____

92. When the person receives a full-liquid diet, it will include all of the foods on the clear-liquid diet as well as these foods: _____
    _____.

93. If a person has poorly fitted dentures and has chewing difficulties, the doctor may order a _____ _____ diet.

94. A person who is constipated and has other GI disorders may receive a _____ diet. The foods in this diet increase the amount of _____ to stimulate _____.

95. If a person is receiving a high-calorie diet, the calorie intake is increased to _____ calories.

96. What vegetable juices are high in sodium? _____
    _____

97. When a person is receiving a diabetic diet, the same amount of _____ are eaten each day.

98. If you are feeding a person a dysphagia diet, what observations should be reported to the nurse immediately?

    A. _____, _____, or _____ during or after meal

    B. _____ or _____

99. Why is it important to offer water often to older persons? _____

100. When you give oral hygiene to a person who is receiving nothing by mouth, the person must not _____.

101. List the amount of millimeters in the following:

    A. 1 ounce equals _____ mL.

    B. 1 pint equals about _____ mL.

    C. 1 quart equals about _____ mL.

102. What information do you need when you are delegated to measure intake and output?

    A. _____

    B. _____

    C. _____

    D. _____

    E. _____

103. What type of dining programs may be used with persons who are oriented or are quietly confused? _____ _____

104. What can be done to promote comfort when preparing residents for meals?

    A. _____

    B. _____

    C. _____

    D. _____

    E. _____

    F. _____

105. If a food tray is not served within 15 minutes, what should be checked? _____ _____

106. When you are delegated to serve meal trays, what information do you need from the nurse or the care plan?

    A. _____

    B. _____

    C. _____

    D. _____

    E. _____

    F. _____

107. When you are serving meal trays, you make sure the right person gets the right tray by checking _____ _____.

108. When you are feeding a person, the spoon should be filled _____.

109. Why is it important to sit facing the person when you feed him or her?

    A. _____

    B. _____

    C. _____

110. What should be reported after you have fed a person?

    A. _____

    B. _____

    C. _____

    D. _____

111. What are safety tips from the USDA to keep food safe to eat?

    A. Clean _____

    B. Separate _____

    C. Cook _____

    D. Chill _____

Chapter **20** **Nutrition and Fluids**

112. Enter this information on the intake and output record. Total amounts are for the 8-hour and 24-hour periods. Amounts in ( ) indicate how much a person ate or drank. Use 2400–0800, 0800–1600, and 1600–2400 as 8-hour periods.

0200	Voided 300 mL	1530	Vomited 50 mL
0600	Voided 500 mL	1545	1 can of soda (whole can)
0730	Breakfast	1730	Dinner
	Orange juice (whole glass)		Soup (whole bowl)
	Milk (1/2 carton)		Tea (1 cup)
	Coffee (1 cup)		Juice (whole glass)
0700	Voided 300 mL		Ice cream (all)
1000	Water pitcher filled	1730	Voided 250 mL
1130	Lunch	1830	Vomited 100 mL
	Soup (whole bowl)	1915	Voided 500 mL
	Milk (1/2 carton)	2000	Milk (1 carton)
	Tea (1 cup)	2015	Voided 300 mL
	Jell-O (1 serving)	2330	Voided 200 mL
1330	Voided 450 mL		
1430	Water pitcher 500 mL (refilled)		

(Modified from OSF St. Joseph Medical Center, Bloomington, IL.)

113. Label the plate with numbers so that you can describe the location of food to a blind person. How would you tell a visually impaired person who asks you where to find the food items on the plate?

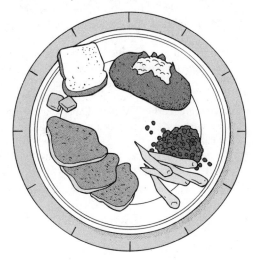

A. Bread _____

B. Baked potato _____

C. Vegetables _____

D. Meat _____

OPTIONAL LEARNING EXERCISES

114. John is 40 years old. The following is his food intake for one day. List the foods in the correct food group from MyPlate and list the number of servings in each group.

BREAKFAST
6 oz orange juice
1 cup oatmeal
½ cup milk
2 slices toast with 1 tablespoon butter
1 cup black coffee

LUNCH
1 cup tomato soup
Grilled cheese sandwich (with 1 oz natural cheese and 2 slices bread)
12 oz diet soda

DINNER
2 pork chops (4 oz each)
4 oz baked potato with 2 tablespoons butter
¼ cup green beans
4 oz pudding
1 cup black coffee
SNACKS
1 apple
2 oz peanuts
1 can regular soda
½ cup ice cream

A. Grains _____
_____ servings

B. Vegetables _____
_____ servings

C. Fruits _____
_____ servings

D. Dairy _____
_____ servings

E. Protein _____
_____ servings

F. Other, including oils _____
_____ servings

115. How many servings of each food group should John have? How many did he actually consume?

	Daily Servings	Consumed Servings
A. Grains	_____	_____
B. Vegetables	_____	_____
C. Fruits	_____	_____
D. Dairy	_____	_____
E. Protein	_____	_____

INDEPENDENT LEARNING ACTIVITIES

- Now that you have learned about good nutrition, use this exercise to find out whether you eat a nutritious diet. List your intake for 1 day. Be sure to include the amount of each item—remember, the portion size is important.

  Group the foods and liquids you eat according to the parts of MyPlate. If you wish, you may go to www.ChooseMyPlate.gov and follow the directions there to group the foods. Answer the following questions.
  - How many servings of grains did you eat? How many of these servings were whole grain?
  - How many servings of fruit did you eat? How many were fresh fruit? Canned fruit? Fruit juice? Had added sugars?
  - How many servings of vegetable did you eat? How many were raw? Cooked? How much sodium was contained in prepared vegetables?
  - How many servings of dairy products did you eat? How many were low-fat or fat-free?
  - How many servings of protein foods did you eat? How many were high in fat? Low in fat? High in sodium?
  - How many foods did you eat that count as oils?
  - In which food groups are you meeting your daily needs?
  - In which groups do you need to increase your intake? Decrease your intake?

- How much physical activity did you include in your daily plan?
- After completing this exercise, what changes in your diet and activity level will you consider?

- Role-play with a classmate and take turns feeding each other as you would a resident. You may choose any spoon-fed foods you wish. (Pudding, gelatin, and soup are suggestions.) You should also give a beverage to the person.

  After you have fed each other, answer the following questions.

  - How were your physical needs met before you were fed? (toileting, hand washing, oral hygiene)
  - Where were you fed? (bed, chair, at a table) Who made the decision about your location?
  - Was a clothing protector applied? How did this make you feel?
  - Which food was offered first? Who made the choice of how food was offered? Were you offered a variety of foods?
  - When was a beverage offered? Between food items? Only at the end of feeding? How did the person feeding you decide the order of foods and beverages? The temperature of these items?
  - When you were being fed, how was the nursing assistant positioned? Sitting? Standing? How did the person's position make you feel?
  - What kind of conversation was carried on while you were eating? What chances were offered to rest while you were eating? Did you feel relaxed or rushed?
  - After this exercise, what will you do differently when you feed a resident?

21 Nutritional Support and IV Therapy

FILL IN THE BLANKS: KEY TERMS

Aspiration   Intravenous (IV) therapy   Parenteral nutrition
Enteral nutrition   Jejunostomy tube   Percutaneous endoscopic gastros-
Flow rate   Nasoenteral tube   tomy (PEG) tube
Gastrostomy tube   Nasogastric (NG) tube   Regurgitation
Gavage

1. Giving nutrients into the gastrointestinal (GI) tract through a feeding tube is _____.

2. A _____ is a tube inserted through a surgically created opening in the stomach.

3. A feeding tube inserted through the nose into small bowel is a _____.

4. _____ is the backward flow of stomach contents into the mouth.

5. A _____ is a feeding tube inserted into a surgically created opening in the jejunum of the small intestine.

6. The process of giving a tube feeding is called _____

7. The _____ is the number of drops per minute.

8. _____ is breathing fluid or an object into the lungs.

9. Giving nutrients through a catheter inserted into a vein is _____.

10. _____ is giving fluids through a needle or catheter inserted into a vein.

11. A feeding tube inserted through the nose into the stomach is a _____.

12. A _____ is a feeding tube inserted into the stomach through a small incision made through the skin.

CIRCLE THE BEST ANSWER

13. The doctor may order nutritional support for a person who
    A. Cannot eat enough to meet his or her nutritional needs
    B. Is underweight
    C. Does not like the food served
    D. Is overweight

14. Which of these tubes are used for short-term nutritional support?
    A. Nasogastric (NG) tubes
    B. Gastrostomy tubes
    C. Jejunostomy tubes
    D. PEG tubes

15. Opened formula for a gavage feeding can remain at room temperature for
    A. 1 hour
    B. About 8 hours
    C. About 2 hours
    D. Overnight

16. If a person is receiving intermittent (scheduled) feedings, the nurse will
    A. Attach the feeding to a pump
    B. Give feeding four or more times each day
    C. Give the feedings over a 24-hour period
    D. Give the feeding directly from the refrigerator

17. A major risk with tube feedings is
    A. Nausea
    B. Complaints of flatulence
    C. Aspiration
    D. Elevated temperature

18. If a person is receiving a gavage feeding, you should report at once if
    A. The blood pressure is elevated
    B. The person has signs and symptoms of respiratory distress
    C. The pulse rate is within normal range
    D. The person is sleeping

19. You can help prevent regurgitation when a person is receiving gavage by
    A. Positioning the person in a left side-lying position
    B. Maintaining Fowler or semi-Fowler position after the feeding
    C. Positioning the person in a supine position
    D. Positioning the person in prone position

20. When a person is receiving nutrition through a tube, frequent mouth care is needed because
    A. It stimulates peristalsis to aid digestion
    B. It prevents discomfort from dry mouth, dry lips, and sore throat
    C. It provides additional fluid intake
    D. It provides additional nutrition
21. Which of these is never done by nursing assistants?
    A. Inserting a feeding tube
    B. Removing a feeding tube
    C. Giving tube feedings
    D. Cleaning area around a feeding tube
22. When a person is receiving TPN, the nursing assistant would assist by
    A. Removing the tube
    B. Inserting the tube
    C. Providing frequent oral hygiene and other basic needs
    D. Giving the feedings
23. When caring for a person receiving IV therapy, the nursing assistant should
    A. Adjust the flow rate if it is too fast or too slow
    B. Report to the nurse if no fluid is dripping
    C. Disconnect the IV to give basic care
    D. Change the IV bag when it is empty
24. You may change a dressing on a peripheral IV if
    A. The nurse asks you to do this
    B. You observe that it is loose and soiled
    C. Your state allows nursing assistants to perform the procedure
    D. You think you know how to do this procedure

FILL IN THE BLANKS

25. Write out the meaning of each abbreviation.

    A. GI _____

    B. gtt _____

    C. gtt/min _____

    D. IV _____

    E. mL _____

    F. NG _____

    G. NPO _____

    H. oz _____

    I. PEG _____

    J. PICC _____

    K. TPN _____

26. Nasogastric and nasointestinal tubes are in place for short-term nutritional support, usually for less than _____.

27. Gastrostomy, jejunostomy, and PEG tubes are used for long-term support, usually longer than _____ _____.

28. Formula is given through a feeding tube at room temperature because cold fluids cause _____.

29. Coughing, vomiting, suctioning, and poor positioning can move a tube out of place and are common causes of _____.

30. What can the nursing assistant do to assist the nurse in preventing regurgitation and aspiration?

    A. _____

    B. _____

    C. _____

31. What comfort measures will help a person with a feeding tube who has a dry mouth?

    A. _____

    B. _____

    C. _____

32. The nose and nostrils are cleaned every 4 to 8 hours because a feeding tube can _____ and _____.

33. If your state and job description allow you to be delegated the task of giving a tube feeding, what should the nurse identify and check first?

    A. _____

    B. _____

34. How much flushing solution is used before giving a tube feeding to an adult? _____ _____

35. When a person is receiving TPN, what signs and symptoms should be reported to the nurse at once?

    A. _____

    B. _____

    C. _____

    D. _____

    E. _____

    F. _____

    G. _____

    H. _____

    I. _____

    J. _____

    K. _____

    L. _____

    M. _____

    N. _____

36. When caring for a person receiving IV therapy, what complications at the IV site would you observe and report?

A. _____

B. _____

C. _____

D. _____

E. _____

OPTIONAL LEARNING EXERCISES

37. What type of feeding tube would each of these persons probably have in place?

A. The nurse tells you Mr. S. is expected to have a feeding tube to his stomach for 2 to 3 weeks

_____

B. Mrs. G. has had a feeding tube to her stomach for 9 months. _____, _____, or _____ _____

C. The nurse tells you to observe Mr. H. for irritation of his nose and nostril when you give care. _____ or _____ _____

D. The nurse tells you that Mrs. K. is at great risk for regurgitation from her feeding tube. _____ _____ or _____

38. Why is formula warmed to room temperature when it has been refrigerated? _____ _____

39. Why are older persons more at risk for regurgitation and aspiration?

A. _____

B. _____

40. What would you do if a person with a feeding tube asks you for something to eat or drink? _____ _____ _____

He or she may be allowed to have_____ _____

41. Mrs. H. has a feeding tube in her nose. Answer these questions about caring for her nose and nostrils.

A. How often should the nose and nostrils be cleaned? _____

B. How is the tube secured to the nose? _____ _____

C. Why is the tube secured to the person's garment at the shoulder? _____

D. What are two ways the tube can be secured at the shoulder?

1. _____

2. _____

42. When giving tube feedings, what answers would you likely get if you asked the nurse these questions?

A. What feeding methods are used? _____ _____

B. What size syringe is used? _____ _____

C. How is the person positioned for the feeding? ___ _____

D. How is the person positioned after the feeding? _____

E. How high is the syringe raised or the feeding bag hung? _____

F. How much fluid is used to flush the tubing? _____ _____

G. How fast is the feeding given if using a syringe? _____

43. If a person is receiving TPN, how will you assist the nurse?

A. _____

B. _____

C. _____

44. How can you check the flow rate of an IV? _____ _____

45. What would you tell the RN at once when you check the flow rate?

A. _____

B. _____

C. _____

46. When you assist the person with an IV in turning and repositioning, how should the IV bag be handled?

A. _____

B. _____

47. Mrs. H. is receiving intermittent IV administration.

A. This is also called _____ _____

B. This allows her to be _____ _____

INDEPENDENT LEARNING ACTIVITIES

- Have you or anyone you know ever needed enteral nutrition? Either answer these questions yourself or ask the person you know to answer them.
  - How long was the tube in place? What type of tube was used?
  - What discomfort or pain was felt?
  - How did having a feeding tube affect your activity? Your personal care and grooming?
- Have you ever had an IV? Answer these questions about the experience.
  - What type of IV did you have? Where was it inserted?
  - How long was the IV in place?
  - How did the IV interfere with your care, grooming, or activity?
- You may care for a person who is not receiving any nutritional support or IV therapy. Answer these questions about how you handle this situation.
  - How would you feel about caring for a person who is not receiving any nutritional support?
  - How would your religious or cultural values affect you in this situation?
- If the situation made you uncomfortable, what would you do?

CROSSWORD

Fill in the crossword by choosing words from this list.

Aspiration	gtt	nasoenteral	oz
Gastrostomy	IV	nasogastric	regurgitation
Gavage	Jejunostomy	NPO	TPN
GI	mL	PEG	

Across
7. Feeding tube inserted through the nose into the small intestine
9. Tube inserted through surgically created opening in the stomach
10. Abbreviation for giving fluids through a needle or catheter inserted into a vein
11. Backward flow of stomach contents into the mouth
13. Abbreviation for total parenteral nutrition
14. Abbreviation for drop
15. Abbreviation for gastrointestinal

Down
1. Process of giving a tube feeding
2. Feeding tube inserted through the nose into the stomach
3. Abbreviation for feeding tube inserted into the stomach through a small incision made through the skin
4. Feeding tube inserted in a surgically created opening in the jejunum or the small intestine
5. Abbreviation for milliliter
6. Abbreviation for nothing by mouth
8. Breathing fluid, food, vomitus, or an object into the lungs
12. Abbreviation for ounce

22 Urinary Elimination

FILL IN THE BLANKS: KEY TERMS

Catheter
Catheterization
Dysuria
External catheter
Foley catheter
Functional incontinence
Hematuria
Incontinence
Indwelling catheter

Micturition
Mixed incontinence
Nocturia
Oliguria
Overflow incontinence
Polyuria
Reflex incontinence
Retention catheter
Straight catheter

Stress incontinence
Transient incontinence
Urge incontinence
Urinary frequency
Urinary incontinence
Urinary urgency
Urination
Voiding

1. Abnormally large amounts of urine are called _____.

2. _____ is the combination of stress incontinence and urge incontinence.

3. A Foley or indwelling catheter is also called a _____.

4. The process of inserting a catheter is _____.

5. _____ is the involuntary loss or leakage of urine.

6. Frequent urination at night is _____.

7. A catheter left in the bladder so urine drains constantly into a drainage bag is called a retention, Foley, or _____.

8. _____ is temporary or occasional incontinence that is reversed when the cause is treated.

9. The loss of small amounts of urine from a full bladder is _____.

10. Another word for urination is _____.

11. _____ occurs when the person has bladder control but cannot use the toilet in time.

12. Another name for micturition or voiding; the process of emptying urine from the bladder is _____.

13. A _____ is a tube used to drain or inject fluid through a body opening.

14. Blood in the urine is _____.

15. A catheter that drains the bladder and then is removed is a _____.

16. Voiding at frequent intervals is _____.

17. An indwelling or retention catheter is also called a _____.

18. When urine leaks during exercise and certain movements that cause pressure on the bladder, it is called _____.

19. Another word for urination or micturition is _____.

20. _____ is the need to void at once.

21. The loss of urine in response to a sudden, urgent need to void is _____.

22. Painful or difficult urination is _____.

23. The loss of urine at predictable intervals when the bladder is full is _____.

24. A scant amount of urine, usually less than 500 mL in 24 hours, is _____.

25. The inability to control urination or defecation is _____.

26. A catheter placed on the outside of the body (male or female) and drains urine to a collection container is called a(n) _____.

CIRCLE THE BEST ANSWER

27. Solid wastes are removed from the body by the
    A. Digestive system
    B. Urinary system
    C. Blood
    D. Integumentary system

113

28. A healthy adult produces about _____ of urine a day.
    A. 500 mL
    B. 1000 mL
    C. 1500 mL
    D. 2000 mL
29. You can provide privacy when the person is voiding by
    A. Warming the bedpan
    B. Staying in the room
    C. Pulling the curtain around the bed
    D. Asking the roommate to leave the room
30. If the person has difficulty starting the urine stream, you can
    A. Play music on the TV
    B. Provide perineal care
    C. Use a stainless steel bedpan
    D. Run water in a nearby sink
31. The urine may be bright yellow if the person eats
    A. Asparagus
    B. Carrots and sweet potatoes
    C. Beets and blackberries
    D. Rhubarb
32. When using a metal bedpan you should
    A. Keep the pan in the utility room
    B. Warm the pan with water and dry it before use
    C. Sterilize the pan after each use
    D. Cool the pan with water and dry it before use
33. When you are getting ready to give a person the bedpan, you should
    A. Raise the head of the bed slightly
    B. Position the person in Fowler position
    C. Wash the person's hands
    D. Place the bed in a flat position
34. Urinals are usually placed at the bedside on
    A. Bed rails
    B. Overbed tables
    C. Bedside stands
    D. The floor
35. If a man is unable to place a urinal to void, you should
    A. Tell the nurse
    B. Ask a male coworker to help the man
    C. Place the penis in the urinal
    D. Pad the bed with incontinence pads
36. A commode chair is used when
    A. The person is unable to walk to the bathroom
    B. You need to obtain a urine specimen
    C. The person does not want to use the toilet
    D. The bathroom is occupied by another person
37. When you place a commode over the toilet
    A. Restrain the person
    B. Stay in the room with the person
    C. Lock the wheels
    D. Make sure the container is in place

38. Dribbling of urine that occurs with laughing, sneezing, coughing, lifting, or other activities means the person has
    A. Urge incontinence
    B. Stress incontinence
    C. Overflow incontinence
    D. Functional incontinence
39. When you do not answer lights quickly or do not position the call light within the person's reach, it can cause
    A. Overflow incontinence
    B. Mixed incontinence
    C. Reflex incontinence
    D. Functional incontinence
40. When a person with dementia is incontinent, you can provide safe care by
    A. Telling the person it is wrong to be incontinent
    B. Changing the person's wet clothing once every 2 hours to establish a schedule
    C. Reassuring the person if he or she becomes upset when incontinent
    D. Wait for the person to tell you when he or she needs to void
41. It will help prevent urinary tract infections if you
    A. Avoid having the person wear underwear
    B. Decrease fluid intake
    C. Encourage the person to wear cotton underpants
    D. Keep side rails of the bed up
42. When providing perineal care for an incontinent person, you should
    A. Provide perineal care once a day
    B. Dry the perineal area and buttocks after cleaning the area
    C. Remove wet incontinence products, garments, and linens once every 2 hours
    D. Wipe the area with tissue paper or dry washcloths
43. A catheter that is inserted and then removed is
    A. An indwelling catheter
    B. A straight catheter
    C. A condom catheter
    D. A Foley catheter
44. A person may have an indwelling catheter when
    A. He or she is incontinent
    B. A urine specimen is needed
    C. He or she has a bladder infection
    D. He or she has wounds and pressure injuries from contact with urine
45. A last resort for incontinence is
    A. Bladder training
    B. Answering call lights promptly
    C. An indwelling catheter
    D. Adequate fluid intake
46. When cleaning a catheter, you should
    A. Wipe 4 inches up the catheter to the meatus
    B. Disconnect the tubing from the drainage bag
    C. Clean the catheter from the meatus down the catheter about 4 inches
    D. Wash and rinse the catheter by washing up and down the tubing

47. The drainage bag from a catheter should not hang from the
    A. Bed frame
    B. Chair
    C. Wheelchair
    D. Bedrail
48. If a catheter is accidentally disconnected from the drainage bag, you should tell the nurse at once and then
    A. Quickly reconnect the drainage system
    B. Clamp the catheter to prevent leakage
    C. Wipe the end of the tube and end of the catheter with antiseptic wipes and reconnect
    D. Discard the drainage bag and get a new bag
49. If a person uses a leg drainage bag, it
    A. Is changed to a drainage bag when the person is in bed
    B. Is attached to the clothing with tape or safety pins
    C. Is attached to the bed rail when the person is in bed
    D. Can be worn 24 hours a day
50. A leg bag needs to be emptied more often than a drainage bag because
    A. It holds less than 1000 mL and the drainage bag holds about 2000 mL
    B. It is more likely to leak than the drainage bag
    C. It holds about 250 mL and the drainage bag holds 1000 mL
    D. It interferes with walking if it is full
51. When you empty a drainage bag, you
    A. Disconnect the bag from the tubing
    B. Clamp the catheter to prevent leakage
    C. Open the clamp on the drain and drain into a graduate
    D. Take the bag into the bathroom to empty it
52. When applying a condom catheter
    A. Apply elastic tape in a spiral around the penis
    B. Make sure the catheter tip is touching the head of the penis
    C. Apply adhesive tape securely in a circle entirely around the penis
    D. Remove and reapply every shift
53. The goal of bladder training is
    A. To keep the person dry and clean
    B. Control of urination
    C. Prevention of skin breakdown
    D. Prevention of infection
54. When you are assisting the person with habit training for bladder rehabilitation,
    A. Help the person to the bathroom every 15 or 20 minutes
    B. The voiding is scheduled at regular times to match the person's voiding habits
    C. Clamp the catheter for 1 hour
    D. Tell the person he or she can void only once a shift
55. When you assist with bladder training for a person with an indwelling catheter,
    A. Empty the drainage bag every hour
    B. At first, clamp the catheter for 1 hour
    C. At first, clamp the catheter for 3 to 4 hours
    D. Give the person 15 to 20 minutes to start voiding

FILL IN THE BLANKS

56. What do the following abbreviations mean?

    A. CMS _____

    B. IV _____

    C. mL _____

    D. UTI _____

57. What substances increase urine production?

    A. _____

    B. _____

    C. _____

    D. _____

58. A normal position for voiding for women is _____ _____. For men, a normal position is _____.

59. What can you do to mask urination sounds?

    A. _____

    B. _____

    C. _____

60. Fracture pans are used for persons

    A. _____

    B. _____

    C. _____

    D. _____

    E. _____

    F. _____

61. When a person voids in a bedpan or urinal, what observations about the urine are important?

    A. _____

    B. _____

    C. _____

    D. _____

    E. _____

    F. _____

62. When you are handling bedpans, urinals, and commodes and their contents, you should follow _____ _____ and _____.

63. When you are delegated to provide a urinal, what guidelines should you follow?

A. _____

B. _____

C. _____

D. _____

E. _____

F. _____

G. _____

H. _____

64. When you transfer a person to a commode from bed, you must practice safe transfer practices and use a _____ and _____ .

65. Name five causes of urge incontinence.

A. _____

B. _____

C. _____

D. _____

E. _____

66. Stress incontinence is common in women because the pelvic muscles weaken from _____ _____and with _____ _____ .

67. Overflow incontinence may occur in men because of a _____ .

68. _____ incontinence occurs with nervous system disorders and injuries.

69. When a catheter is inserted after a person voids, it is measuring how _____ .

70. The female external catheter is placed _____ _____ .

71. When you provide perineal care after a person is incontinent, remember to

A. _____

B. _____

C. _____

D. _____

E. _____

F. _____

72. A catheter is secured to the inner thigh or the man's abdomen to prevent _____ _____ .

73. When a person has a catheter, what observations should you report and record?

A. _____

B. _____

C. _____

D. _____

E. _____

F. _____

G. _____

H. _____

74. When you give catheter care, clean the catheter about _____ inches. Clean _____ and _____ from the meatus with _____ stroke.

75. Is the urinary system sterile or nonsterile? _____

76. What happens if a drainage bag is higher than the bladder? _____ This can cause ___ _____ _____ .

77. If a drainage system is disconnected accidentally, what should you do?

A. Tell _____

B. Do not _____

C. Practice _____

D. Wipe _____

E. Wipe _____

F. Do not _____

G. Connect _____

H. Discard _____

I. Remove _____

78. Before applying a condom catheter, you should

A. Provide_____ _____

B. Observe the penis for_____ _____

79. The catheter is clamped for 1 hour at first and eventually for 3 to 4 hours when _____ being done.

LABELING

80. Mark the places you would secure the catheter. Explain why the catheter is secured this way.

81. Mark the places you would secure the catheter. Explain why the catheter is secured this way.

CROSSWORD

Fill in the crossword by answering the clues with words from this list.

Dysuria   Nocturia
Frequency   Oliguria
Hematuria   Polyuria
Incontinence   Urgency

Across

6. Scant amount of urine, usually less than 500 mL in 24 hours
8. Inability to control loss of urine from bladder

Down

1. Production of abnormally large amounts of urine
2. Painful or difficult urination
3. Blood in the urine
4. Voiding at frequent intervals
5. Frequent urination at night
7. Need to void immediately

82. When a person eats a diet high in salt, it causes the body to _____. When this happens, how does it affect urine output _____ _____?

83. You would ask the nurse to observe urine that looks or _____. You would also report complaints of _____ _____.

84. A fracture pan can be used with older persons who have _____ or _____ _____.

85. Covering the lap and legs of a person using a commode provides _____ and promotes _____.

86. If you are caring for an incontinent person and you become short-tempered and impatient, you should _____.

What right are you protecting when you do this? _____

87. Even though catheters are a last resort for incontinent persons, they may be used with weak, disabled, or dying persons to

A. Promote_____

B. Prevent_____

C. Protect _____ and _____ _____

D. Allow_____

88. Catheters may have diagnostic reasons for use, such as
   A. _____
   B. _____

89. What can happen if microbes enter a closed drainage system? _____.

90. What type of tape is used to apply a condom catheter? _____ Why? _____ _____ What can happen if you use the wrong tape? _____ _____

INDEPENDENT LEARNING ACTIVITIES

- Role-play the following situation with a classmate. Take turns playing the person using the bedpan and the nursing assistant. Answer the questions about the activity.

SITUATION: Mrs. Donnelly is a 70 year old resident who must use the bedpan. She finds it difficult to move easily and usually does not have enough strength to raise her hips to get on the bedpan. She tells you she will try to help as much as she can.

As Mrs. Donnelly:
- When you tried to assist, how easy was it to raise your hips? How did the nursing assistant help you get on the pan?
- When you were rolled onto the bedpan, how did it feel? How well was the pan positioned under you?
- How did you feel about sitting on the pan in bed? Did you feel as if this would be an easy or difficult way to void? Explain your feelings.
- How could the nursing assistant have made this procedure better?

As the nursing assistant:
- How did you position the bedpan to get ready to slide it under Mrs. Donnelly? Did this method work? How could you improve this?
- When you rolled Mrs. Donnelly onto the pan, how well positioned was she? What adjustments were necessary?
- When you rolled her off the pan, what happened? If urine had been in the pan, what would have occurred?
- How could you change some of your steps to make this procedure better?

23 Bowel Elimination

Colostomy
Constipation
Defecation
Dehydration
Diarrhea
Enema

Fecal impaction
Fecal incontinence
Feces
Flatulence
Flatus
Ileostomy

Melena
Ostomy
Peristalsis
Stoma
Stool
Suppository

1. A surgically created opening for the elimination of body wastes is a _____.

2. The process of excreting feces from the rectum through the anus is a bowel movement or _____.

3. The excessive formation of gas in the stomach and intestines is _____.

4. A _____ is a cone-shaped solid drug that is inserted into a body opening.

5. The frequent passage of liquid stools is _____.

6. _____ is the prolonged retention and buildup of feces in the rectum.

7. _____ is the excessive loss of water from tissues.

8. Gas or air passed through the anus is _____ _____.

9. The introduction of fluid into the rectum and lower colon is an _____.

10. Excreted feces is _____.

11. An artificial opening between the colon and the abdominal wall is a _____.

12. _____ is the alternating contraction and relaxation of intestinal muscles.

13. The passage of a hard, dry stool is _____ _____.

14. _____ is the inability to control the passage of feces and gas through the anus.

15. An opening that can be seen on the abdominal wall is a _____.

16. The semi-solid mass of waste products in the colon is _____.

17. A surgically created opening between the ileum and the abdominal wall is an _____ _____.

18. _____ are black and tarry stools caused by GI bleeding.

CIRCLE THE BEST ANSWER

19. People usually have a bowel movement
    A. After every meal
    B. When they have consumed large amounts of fluids
    C. At a regular time and pattern that is normal for the person
    D. Once a week

20. Bleeding in the stomach and small intestines causes stool to be
    A. Brown
    B. Black
    C. Red
    D. Clay-colored

21. The characteristic odor of stool is caused by
    A. Poor personal hygiene
    B. Poor nutrition
    C. Bacterial action in the intestines
    D. Adequate fluid intake

22. When you observe stool that is abnormal
    A. Ask the nurse to observe the stool
    B. Report your observations and discard the stool
    C. Ask the person if the stool is normal for him or her
    D. Record your observations when you finish giving care

23. Which of these could interfere with defecation?
    A. Being able to relax by reading a book or newspaper
    B. Eating a diet with high-fiber foods
    C. Using a bedpan, commode, or bathroom when others are present
    D. Drinking 6 to 8 glasses of water daily

119

24. A person who must stay in bed most of the time may have irregular elimination and constipation because of
    A. Poor diet
    B. Poor fluid intake
    C. Lack of activity
    D. Lack of privacy
25. Which of these would provide safety for a person during bowel elimination?
    A. Make sure the bedpan is warm
    B. Place the call light and toilet tissue within the person's reach
    C. Provide perineal care
    D. Allow enough time for defecation
26. Constipation can be relieved by
    A. Giving the person a low-fiber diet
    B. Increasing activity
    C. Decreasing fluids
    D. Ignoring the urge to defecate
27. A person tries several times to have a bowel movement and cannot. Liquid feces seep from the anus. This probably means the person has
    A. Diarrhea
    B. Constipation
    C. A fecal impaction
    D. Fecal incontinence
28. When the nurse finds a fecal impaction is present, he or she sometimes tries to relieve it by
    A. Changing the person's diet
    B. Telling the nursing assistant to give more fluids
    C. Removing the fecal mass with a gloved finger
    D. Increasing the activity of the person
29. Good skin care is important when a person has diarrhea because
    A. This prevents odors
    B. Skin breakdown and pressure injuries are risks
    C. It prevents the spread of microbes
    D. It prevents fluid loss
30. Diarrhea can be very serious in older persons, especially because it
    A. Causes skin breakdown
    B. Causes odors
    C. Can cause dehydration
    D. Increases activity
31. When caring for a person with *Clostridium difficile* (*C. difficile*), you practice good hand hygiene by
    A. Washing your hands in alcohol
    B. Washing your hands with soap and water
    C. Using alcohol-based hand rubs
    D. Wearing sterile gloves
32. When a person has fecal incontinence, it is important to
    A. Increase fluid intake
    B. Help the person with elimination once a shift
    C. Help the person with elimination after meals and every 2 to 3 hours
    D. Tell the person to turn on the call light in time for help to arrive

33. If flatus is not expelled, the person may complain of
    A. Abdominal cramping or pain
    B. Diarrhea
    C. Fecal incontinence
    D. Nausea
34. What is a goal of bowel training?
    A. To give laxatives daily to maintain regular bowel movements
    B. To gain control of bowel movements
    C. To make sure the person has at least one bowel movement each day
    D. To prevent abdominal cramping
35. When bowel training is planned, which of these is included in the care plan?
    A. The amount of stool the person expels
    B. How many bowel movements the person has each day
    C. The usual time of day the person has a bowel movement
    D. The foods that cause flatus
36. When the nurse delegates preparing a soapsuds enema for an adult to you, mix
    A. 2 teaspoons of salt in 1000 mL of tap water
    B. 3 to 5 mL of castile soap in 500 to 1000 mL of tap water
    C. 2 mL of castile soap in 500 mL of tap water
    D. Mineral oil with sterile water
37. When you give an enema of 750 to 1000 mL, it should be given to the person
    A. Within 5 minutes
    B. Over about 30 minutes
    C. Over about 10 to 15 minutes
    D. Over about 20 minutes
38. The person receiving an enema is usually placed in a
    A. Supine position
    B. Prone position
    C. Semi-Fowler position
    D. Left side-lying position
39. When the doctor orders enemas until clear
    A. Give one enema
    B. Give as many enemas as necessary to return a clear fluid
    C. Ask the nurse how many times to repeat the enema
    D. Give only tap water enemas
40. If you are giving an enema and the person complains of cramping
    A. Tell the person it is normal and continue to give the enema
    B. Clamp the tube until the cramping subsides
    C. Discontinue the enema immediately and tell the nurse
    D. Lower the bag below the level of the bed
41. When giving a small-volume enema, do not release pressure on the bottle because
    A. It will cause cramping if pressure is released
    B. The fluid will leak from the rectum
    C. Solution will be drawn back into the bottle
    D. It will cause flatulence

42. When giving a small-volume enema
   A. Place the person in the prone position
   B. Insert the enema tip 2 inches into the rectum
   C. Heat the solution to 105°F
   D. Clamp the tubing if cramping occurs

43. An oil-retention enema is given to
   A. Cleanse the bowel to prepare for surgery
   B. Regulate the person who is receiving bowel training
   C. Relieve flatulence
   D. Soften the feces and lubricate the rectum

44. If you feel resistance when you are giving a cleansing enema
   A. Lubricate the tube more thoroughly
   B. Push more firmly to insert the tube
   C. Stop and report this to the nurse
   D. Ask the person to take a deep breath and relax

45. When you are caring for a person with any type of ostomy, you know
   A. All of the stools are solid and formed
   B. A stoma does not have sensation and is not painful
   C. An ostomy is always temporary and is reconnected after healing
   D. A pouch is worn to protect the stoma

46. Which of these statements is true about an ileostomy?
   A. The stool is solid and formed
   B. The stoma is an opening into the colon
   C. The pouch is changed daily
   D. The skin around the ileostomy can be irritated by the digestive juices in the stool

47. When caring for a person with a stoma, the pouch is
   A. Changed daily
   B. Changed every 3 to 7 days and when it leaks
   C. Worn only when the person thinks he or she will have a bowel movement
   D. Changed every time the person has a bowel movement

48. The best time to change the ostomy bag is after sleep because
   A. The stoma is less likely to expel stool at this time
   B. The person has more time in the morning
   C. It should be changed before morning care
   D. The person tolerates the procedure better before eating

49. When cleaning the skin around the stoma, you use
   A. Sterile water and sterile gauze squares
   B. Alcohol and sterile cotton
   C. Soap and other cleansing agents as directed by the nurse
   D. Adhesive remover and sterile cotton balls

50. You give the person with an ostomy the right of personal choice when you
   A. Allow the person to manage the care when able
   B. Choose the time when care is done
   C. Choose the care measures and equipment used
   D. Ask the nurse to determine the care to be done

FILL IN THE BLANKS

51. What do these abbreviations mean?
   A. BM _____
   B. GI _____
   C. oz _____
   D. SSE _____
   E. TWE _____

52. When observing stool, what should be reported to the nurse?
   A. _____
   B. _____
   C. _____
   D. _____
   E. _____
   F. _____
   G. _____
   H. _____

53. What three food groups are high in fiber?
   A. _____
   B. _____
   C. _____

54. Name six gas-forming foods.
   A. _____
   B. _____
   C. _____
   D. _____
   E. _____
   F. _____

55. Drinking warm fluids such as coffee, tea, hot cider, and warm water will increase _____.

56. How will dehydration affect these?
   A. Skin is _____
   B. Urine is _____
   C. Blood pressure _____
   D. Pulse and respirations _____

57. Persons at risk for developing a *Clostridium difficile* infection are those who are
   A. _____
   B. _____
   C. _____

58. The *Clostridium difficile* microbe is found in the
    _____.

59. Flatulence may be caused when the person _____
    _____ while eating and drinking.

60. When a nurse inserts a suppository for bowel train-
    ing, how soon would you expect the person to defe-
    cate? _____

    _____

61. Before giving an enema, make sure that

    A. _____

    B. _____

    C. _____

    D. _____

    E. _____

62. After giving an enema, what should be reported and
    recorded?

    A. _____

    B. _____

    C. _____

    D. _____

    E. _____

    F. _____

    G. _____

63. Because it is likely you will come in contact with
    stool while giving an enema, you should follow
    _____ and
    _____.

64. How can cramping be prevented during an enema?

    A. _____

    B. _____

65. How long does it usually take for a tap water, saline, or
    soapsuds enema to take effect? _____

66. A small-volume enema contains _____
    of solution.

67. A person should retain a small-volume enema for
    _____.

68. When you start to insert the tube to give an enema,
    ask the person to _____.

69. What can you place in the ostomy pouch to prevent
    odors? _____

70. Showers and baths are delayed 1 or 2 hours after apply-
    ing a new pouch to allow _____.

LABELING

*Answer Questions 71 through 74 using the illustrations
of colostomies.*

71. Name the four types of colostomies shown

    A. _____

    B. _____

    C. _____

    D. _____

72. Which colostomy will have the most solid and
    formed stool? _____

73. Which colostomy will have the most liquid stool?

    _____

74. Which colostomy is a temporary colostomy?

    _____

75. What type of ostomy is shown? _____
_____

Stoma ———

   A. What part of the bowel has been removed? _____
   _____

   B. Will the stool from the ostomy be liquid or formed? _____

OPTIONAL LEARNING EXERCISES

76. You are caring for Mr. Evans, who is in a semi-private room. His roommate has a large family and many visitors. Mr. Evans has not had a bowel movement in 3 days, even though he is eating well and taking medications to assist elimination. What could be a reason he has not had a bowel movement? _____
_____
_____

77. Mrs. Weller usually has a bowel movement after breakfast. What are some activities that may assist her to defecate more easily? _____
_____

78. Mrs. Shaffer tells you she cannot digest fruits and vegetables and she refuses to eat them. What may be added to her cereal and prune juice to provide fiber? _____

79. You offer Mr. Murphy _____ of water each day to promote normal bowel elimination.

80. Mr. Hernandez has been taking an antibiotic, which is a drug to treat his pneumonia, and he has developed diarrhea. You think he may have diarrhea because _____.

81. Mr. Hernandez has continued to have diarrhea and the nurse tells you he has *Clostridium difficile*. His signs and symptoms are

   A. _____

   B. _____

   C. _____

   D. _____

   E. _____

82. When you care for Mr. Hernandez, you can spread the microbes if your contaminated hands or gloves

   A. _____

   B. _____

83. You are caring for 83-year-old Mrs. Chen. You helped her to the bathroom 30 minutes ago, where she had a bowel movement. When you enter her room to make her bed, she tells you she needs to use the bathroom for a bowel movement. You know that older people
_____
_____

84. The two goals of bowel training are _____
_____ and _____.

85. Why can tap water enemas be dangerous? _____
_____

86. How many tap water enemas can be given? _____
Why? _____

87. Compare small-volume enemas and oil-retention enemas.
   A. Small-volume enemas are given to _____
   _____.

   Oil-retention enemas are given to _____
   _____.

   B. Small-volume enemas take effect in about _____ minutes.

   Oil-retention enemas should be retained for at least _____ minutes.

   C. An oil-retention enema may be retained for _____ hours.

123

INDEPENDENT LEARNING ACTIVITIES

- Think about times when you have had a problem with bowel irregularity. Answer these questions about how you handled the problems.
  - What causes you to have irregularity? Foods? Illness? Stress? Inactivity?
  - What methods have you used to treat irregularity? Diet? Medication?
  - How does irregularity affect you physically? Your appetite? Energy level? Sleep and rest?
  - How does irregularity affect your mood? Your daily activities?
- Interview a person who has a colostomy or an ileostomy. You may know someone who has an ostomy. Or you may care for someone who has one. Your community may have an ostomy support group that you can contact. Talk to the person and ask the following questions.
  - How long has the person had the ostomy? Is it permanent or temporary?
  - What was the hardest part of learning to live with an ostomy? What was the easiest part?
  - How has living with an ostomy affected the person's life? Has the person's work been affected? Were leisure activities affected?
  - How has the ostomy affected the person's family? What changes have occurred?
  - What equipment works best for the person? How expensive is the equipment? How much time is required each day to care for the ostomy?

24 Exercise and Activity

FILL IN THE BLANKS: KEY TERMS

Abduction
Adduction
Ambulation
Atrophy
Contracture
Deconditioning
Dorsiflexion

Extension
External rotation
Flexion
Footdrop
Hyperextension
Internal rotation
Orthostatic hypotension

Plantar flexion
Postural hypotension
Pronation
Range of motion (ROM)
Rotation
Supination
Syncope

1. If _____ is present, the foot is bent down at the ankle.

2. A brief loss of consciousness or fainting is _____.

3. Bending a body part is _____ _____.

4. Moving a body part away from the midline of the body is _____.

5. _____ is the movement of a joint to the extent possible without causing pain.

6. Turning the joint outward is _____ _____.

7. A drop in blood pressure when the person stands is postural hypotension or _____.

8. _____ occurs when moving a body part toward the midline of the body.

9. Turning the joint upward is called _____ _____.

10. Bending the toes and foot up at the ankle is _____.

11. Excessive straightening of a body part is _____ _____.

12. A decrease in size or a wasting away of tissue is _____.

13. Turning the joint is _____.

14. _____ is the straightening of a body part.

15. _____ is another name for orthostatic hypotension.

16. _____ is permanent plantar flexion; the foot falls down at the ankle.

17. The act of walking is _____ _____.

18. _____ is turning the joint downward.

19. The loss of muscle strength from inactivity is _____.

20. _____ is turning the joint inward.

21. The lack of joint mobility caused by abnormal shortening of a muscle is a _____.

CIRCLE THE BEST ANSWER

22. If a person is on bedrest, he or she
    A. May be allowed to do some activities of daily living (ADL)
    B. Can use the bedside commode for elimination needs
    C. May not perform any activities of daily living
    D. Can use the bathroom for elimination needs

23. Complications of bedrest include
    A. Contractures in fingers, wrists, knees, and hips
    B. Increased muscle strength
    C. Increased appetite and improved muscle strength
    D. Normal blood pressure when getting out of bed

24. If a contracture develops
    A. It will require extra range of motion exercises to correct it
    B. You need to position the person in good body alignment
    C. The person is permanently deformed and disabled
    D. It will be relieved as soon as the person is able to walk and exercise

25. When you are caring for a person who has orthostatic hypotension, you should
    A. Raise the head of the bed slowly to Fowler position
    B. Have the person get out of bed quickly to prevent weakness
    C. Keep the bed flat when getting the person out of bed
    D. Have the person walk around to decrease weakness and dizziness
26. Nursing care that helps prevent complications from bedrest will include
    A. Positioning frequently in good body alignment
    B. Doing all ADL for the person
    C. Changing position once a shift
    D. Allowing the person to sleep as much as possible
27. If a person sitting on the edge of the bed complains of weakness, dizziness, or spots before the eyes, you should
    A. Assist the person to stand
    B. Help the person to sit in a chair or walk around
    C. Help the person to return to Fowler position
    D. Tell the person it is a normal response and continue to get the person up
28. Bedboards are used to
    A. Keep the person in alignment by preventing the mattress from sagging
    B. Prevent plantar flexion that can lead to footdrop
    C. Keep the hips abducted
    D. Keep the weight of top linens off the feet
29. Plantar flexion must be prevented to
    A. Keep the feet from bending down at the ankle (footdrop)
    B. Keep the hips from rotating outward
    C. Keep the wrist, thumb, and fingers in normal position
    D. Maintain good body alignment
30. To prevent the hips and legs from turning outward, you can use
    A. Bed cradles
    B. Hip abduction wedges
    C. Trochanter rolls
    D. Splints
31. When a trapeze bar is used for exercise, it will strengthen the
    A. Trunk and hips
    B. Shoulders
    C. Legs and hips
    D. Arms
32. When you move a person's joints through range of motion exercises, it is called
    A. Active range of motion
    B. Activities of daily living
    C. Active-assistive range of motion
    D. Passive range of motion
33. A nursing assistant can perform range of motion exercises on the _____ only if allowed by center policy.
    A. Shoulder
    B. Neck
    C. Hip
    D. Knee
34. When exercising the wrist, which of these exercises turns the hand toward the thumb?
    A. Abduction
    B. Hyperextension
    C. Radial flexion
    D. Extension
35. Which of these joints is adducted and abducted?
    A. Neck
    B. Hip
    C. Elbow
    D. Knee
36. When you help a person to walk, you should
    A. Apply a gait (transfer) belt
    B. Help the person lean on furniture to walk around the room
    C. Put soft socks on the feet without shoes
    D. Let the person walk without any help
37. When the person is walking with crutches, the person should wear
    A. Soft slippers on the feet
    B. Clothes that fit well
    C. Clothes that are loose
    D. A gait belt
38. When walking with a cane, it is held
    A. On the strong side of the body
    B. On the weak side of the body
    C. In the right hand
    D. On the left side of the body
39. When a person is using a walker, it is
    A. Picked up and moved 3 to 4 inches in front of the person
    B. Moved forward with a rocking motion
    C. Moved first on the left side and then on the right
    D. Picked up and moved about 10 inches in front of the person
40. When you are caring for a person who wears a brace, it is important to report at once
    A. How far the person walks
    B. What care the person can do alone
    C. The amount of mobility in joints when doing range of motion exercises
    D. Any redness or signs of skin breakdown when you remove a brace
41. Recreational activity is important because
    A. It forces the person to find new interests
    B. It prevents boredom
    C. Circulation is stimulated and joints and muscles are exercised
    D. It forces the person to do things that do not interest him or her

FILL IN THE BLANKS

42. Write out the meaning of each abbreviation.

    A. ADL_____

    B. PT_____

    C. ROM_____

43. To prevent deconditioning, is it important to promote _____ and _____
    in all persons to the extent possible.

44. Bedrest is ordered to

    A. _____

    B. _____

    C. _____

    D. _____

    E. _____

45. The nurse tells you the resident is on bedrest but can use the bathroom for elimination. This means the resident is ordered _____
    _____.

46. When a person has a contracture, the person is _____ deformed and disabled.

47. When a person is suddenly moved from lying or sitting to a standing position, the blood pressure may _____. This is called _____
    _____.

48. Supportive devices such as bedboards, footboards, and trochanter rolls are used to _____
    and _____ the person in a certain position.

49. When you use a footboard, the soles of the feet are against it to prevent _____.

50. A trochanter roll is placed along the body to prevent the hips and legs from _____.

51. Hand rolls or grips prevent _____
    of the thumb, fingers, and wrists.

52. A device used to keep the wrist, thumb, and fingers in normal position is a _____.

53. Bed cradles are used because the weight of top linens can cause _____ and
    _____.

54. A trapeze bar allows the person to lift the _____
    _____ off the bed. It also allows the person to _____ and _____
    _____ in bed.

55. When a person does exercises with some help, he or she is doing _____ range of motion exercises.

56. When range of motion exercises are done, what should be reported and recorded?
    A. _____

    B. _____

    C. _____

    D. _____

    E. _____

57. When performing range of motion exercises, each movement should be repeated _____ times or the
    _____.

58. When performing range of motion exercises, you should

    A. _____

    B. _____

    C. _____

    D. _____

    E. _____

    F. _____

    G. _____

    H. _____

    I. _____

59. When you help a person to walk, you should walk to the _____ and
    _____ the person. Provide support with the _____ or have one arm _____ and the other
    _____.

60. Many people prefer a walker because it gives more support than a _____.

61. When many recreational activities are offered, it protects the person's right to _____
    _____.

LABELING

62. ROM exercises for the _____ joint are shown in these drawings. Name the movements shown in each drawing.

A. _____

B. _____

C. _____

63. ROM exercises for the _____ are shown in these drawings. Name the movements shown in each drawing.

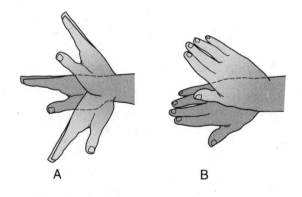

A. _____

B. _____

64. ROM exercises for the _____ are shown in these drawings. Name the movements shown in each drawing.

A. _____

B. _____

C. _____

D. _____

CROSSWORD

Fill in the crossword by choosing words from the following list.

Abduction
Adduction
ADL
Ambulation
Atrophy
Contracture
Deconditioning
Dorsiflexion
Extension
Flexion
Footdrop
Hyperextension
Pronation
PT
ROM
Rotation
Supination
Syncope

Across

4. Loss of muscle strength from inactivity
8. Abbreviation for range of motion
10. Bending a body part
12. Decrease in size or wasting away of tissue
13. Abbreviation for physical therapy
14. Moving a body part away from the midline of the body
15. Straightening a body part
16. Brief loss of consciousness; fainting
17. Bending the toes and foot up at the ankle
18. Moving a body part toward the midline of the body

Down

1. Foot falls down at the ankle; permanent plantar flexion
2. Abbreviation for activities of daily living
3. Turning a joint
5. Lack of joint mobility caused by abnormal shortening of a muscle
6. Act of walking
7. Excessive straightening of body part
9. Turning the joint downward
11. Turning the joint upward

65. What kind of range of motion would be used with each of these residents?

A. The resident needs complete care for bathing, grooming, and feeding. _____

B. The resident takes part in many activities in the center. She walks to most activities independently. _____

C. The resident has weakness on his left side. He is able to feed himself but needs help with bathing and dressing. _____

66. As you plan to help a person out of bed, you are concerned about orthostatic hypotension. In order to make sure the person is able to stand and get up safely, you plan to take the blood pressure and pulse several times. When would you take the blood pressure and pulse?

A. _____

B. _____

C. _____

D. _____

E. _____

67. When doing range of motion exercises, you should ask the person if he or she has _____ or _____

68. When performing range of motion exercises, you do not

A. _____

B. _____

69. When you ambulate a person, what observations are reported and recorded?

A. _____

B. _____

C. _____

D. _____

E. _____

70. Why does the nurse assess the skin under braces every shift? _____

- Role-play with a classmate and take turns acting as the nursing assistant and a person with left-sided weakness. Perform range of motion exercises on the person. Answer the following questions about how you felt after this activity.
  ◦ What did the nursing assistant explain to you before performing the exercises?
  ◦ How were you positioned for exercising? What did the nursing assistant ask about your comfort and personal wishes in the position used?
  ◦ How was your privacy maintained? Was there anything that made you feel exposed or embarrassed?
  ◦ How were your joints supported during the exercises? Did you feel any discomfort or pain during the exercises?
  ◦ What exercises were you encouraged to carry out independently? With some assistance?
  ◦ Which exercises were done first? Were the exercises carried out in an organized pattern? How did you know what exercise would be done next?
  ◦ After this activity, what will you do differently when giving range of motion exercises to a person?
- With a classmate, role-play assisting a weak, older person to ambulate. Take turns acting as the person and the nursing assistant. Answer the following questions about how you felt and what you learned.
  ◦ What did the nursing assistant tell you before preparing to walk with you? What choices were offered about the time you were to ambulate, what clothing to wear, and where you were going to walk?
  ◦ What safety devices were used? What did the nursing assistant tell you about the devices or equipment used?
  ◦ What assessments were made before you sat up? When you dangled? After walking?
  ◦ How did the nursing assistant make you feel secure during ambulation? How did the nursing assistant hold you?
  ◦ What did you learn from this activity that will help you when you ambulate a person?

25 Comfort, Rest, and Sleep

FILL IN THE BLANKS: KEY TERMS

Acute pain
Chronic pain
Circadian rhythm
Comfort
Discomfort
Distraction

Enuresis
Guided imagery
Insomnia
NREM sleep
Pain
Persistent pain

Phantom pain
Radiating pain
Relaxation
REM sleep
Rest
Sleep

1. Another name for discomfort is _____ _____.

2. _____ is pain that is felt suddenly from injury, disease, trauma, or surgery; it generally lasts less than 6 months.

3. _____ is a way to change a person's center of attention.

4. A state of unconsciousness, reduced voluntary muscle activity, and lowered metabolism is _____.

5. Pain lasting longer than 6 months is _____. It may be constant or occur off and on.

6. _____ is to be free from mental or physical stress.

7. _____ is a state of well-being. The person has no physical or emotional pain and is calm and at peace.

8. To be calm, at ease, and relaxed is to _____. The person is free of anxiety and stress.

9. Creating and focusing on an image is _____.

10. The stage of sleep when there is rapid eye movement is _____.

11. _____ is a chronic condition in which the person cannot sleep or stay asleep throughout the night.

12. The "day-night" cycle or body rhythm is also called _____. This daily rhythm is based on a 24-hour cycle.

13. _____ is pain felt at the site of tissue damage and in nearby areas.

14. To ache, hurt, or be sore is _____. It is also called pain.

15. _____ is the phase of deep sleep when there is no rapid eye movement.

16. Pain felt in a body part that is no longer there is _____.

17. Urinary incontinence in bed at night is _____.

18. Another name for chronic pain is _____.

CIRCLE THE BEST ANSWER

19. Rest and sleep are needed to
    A. Restore energy and well-being
    B. Decrease energy needed for daily functions
    C. Increase muscle strength
    D. Increase the appetite

20. OBRA requirements related to comfort, rest, and sleep include
    A. Only two people in a room
    B. Bright lighting in all areas
    C. Room temperature between 65°F and 71°F
    D. Adequate ventilation and room humidity

21. When a person complains of pain or discomfort
    A. The person has pain or discomfort
    B. It must be measured carefully to see if the person really has pain or discomfort
    C. You can easily measure to find out how much pain is present
    D. You can tell if the person really has pain or discomfort by the way he or she acts

22. When a person complains of pain that is at the site of tissue damage and in nearby areas, this is _____ pain.
    A. Acute
    B. Chronic
    C. Radiating
    D. Phantom

131

23. If pain is ignored or denied, it may be because the person thinks pain is a sign of weakness. Which factor that affects pain would this be?
    A. Attention
    B. Past experience
    C. Value or meaning of pain
    D. Support from others
24. A person from some cultures may be very stoic when experiencing pain. You would expect the person to
    A. Show a strong emotional response
    B. Show no reaction to the pain
    C. Accept pain quietly
    D. View it as the will of God
25. When a person has anxiety, the person
    A. May feel increased pain
    B. Will usually feel less pain
    C. May deny having pain
    D. May be stoic and show no reaction to pain
26. When you ask a person "Where is the pain?," you are asking the person to
    A. Describe the pain
    B. Explain the intensity of the pain
    C. Tell you the onset and duration of the pain
    D. Tell you the location of the pain
27. When a person tells you he has pain when coughing or deep breathing, this is
    A. A factor causing pain
    B. A measurement of the onset of pain
    C. Words used to describe the pain
    D. The location of the pain
28. A distraction measure to promote comfort and relieve pain may be
    A. Asking the person to focus on an image
    B. Learning to breathe deeply and slowly
    C. Listening to music or playing games
    D. Contracting and relaxing muscle groups
29. If the nurse has given a person pain medication, it is best if you
    A. Give the person a bath
    B. Walk the person according to the care plan
    C. Wait 30 minutes before giving care
    D. Give care before the medication makes the person sleepy
30. You may help to promote comfort and relieve pain when you
    A. Tell family members and friends to leave the person alone
    B. Keep the room brightly lit and play loud music
    C. Provide blankets for warmth and to prevent chilling
    D. Avoid touching the person to give care or back massages
31. You can help to promote rest when you
    A. Meet physical needs such as thirst, hunger, and elimination needs
    B. Check the person every 10 minutes to ask if he or she is resting
    C. Provide snacks that include caffeine drinks
    D. Give care at a time most convenient to you

32. When caring for an ill or injured person, you know the person may need more rest. You can help the person to get rest by making sure you
    A. Provide plenty of exercise to prevent weakness
    B. Provide rest periods during or after a procedure
    C. Give complete hygiene and grooming measures quickly
    D. Spend time talking with the person to distract him or her
33. During sleep
    A. The person is aware of the environment
    B. Metabolism is increased
    C. Vital signs (blood pressure, temperature, pulse, and respirations) increase
    D. There are no voluntary arm or leg movements
34. Some people function better in the morning because of
    A. The circadian rhythm
    B. Getting enough sleep
    C. Interference with the body rhythm
    D. Changes in the work schedule
35. During REM sleep, the person
    A. Is hard to arouse
    B. Has a gradual fall in vital signs
    C. Is easily aroused
    D. Has tension in voluntary muscles
36. Which stage of sleep is usually not repeated during the cycles of sleep?
    A. REM
    B. Stage 1: NREM
    C. Stage 2: NREM
    D. Stage 3: NREM
37. Which age group requires less sleep than middle-aged adults?
    A. Toddlers
    B. Young adults
    C. Adolescents
    D. Older adults
38. Which of these factors increases the need for sleep?
    A. Illness
    B. Weight loss
    C. Emotional problems
    D. Medications and other substances
39. When a person takes sleeping pills, sleep may not restore the person mentally because
    A. Caffeine prevents sleep
    B. Some have difficulty falling asleep
    C. The length of REM sleep is reduced
    D. It upsets the usual sleep routines
40. Exercise should be avoided for 2 hours before sleep because
    A. It requires energy
    B. People usually feel good after exercise
    C. It causes the release of substances in the bloodstream that stimulate the body
    D. The person tires after exercise

41. Persons who are ill, in pain, or hospitalized may experience
    A. Sleep deprivation
    B. Sleepwalking
    C. Insomnia
    D. Increased sleep times
42. If a person has decreased reasoning, red, puffy eyes, and coordination problems, report this to the nurse because the person
    A. Is having a reaction to sleeping medications
    B. Has signs and symptoms of sleep disorders
    C. Needs more exercise before bedtime
    D. May need an increase in sleeping pills
43. Which of these measures would help to promote sleep?
    A. Turn on several lights in the room
    B. Have the person void or make sure that incontinent persons are clean and dry
    C. Encourage the person to take part in an exercise class shortly before bedtime
    D. Offer the person a cup of coffee or tea at bedtime

FILL IN THE BLANKS

44. Write out the meaning of each abbreviation

    A. CPAP _____

    B. HS _____

    C. NREM _____

    D. REM _____

    E. TENS _____

45. OBRA has requirements about the person's room. List the requirements that relate to each of these.

    A. Suspended curtain _____

    B. Linens _____

    C. Bed _____

    D. Room temperature _____

    E. Persons in room _____

46. Name the type of pain described.

    A. A person with an amputated leg may still sense leg pain. _____

    B. There is tissue damage. The pain decreases with healing. _____

    C. Pain from a heart attack is often felt in the left chest, left jaw, left shoulder, and left arm. _____

    D. The pain remains long after healing. Common causes are arthritis and cancer. _____

47. Older persons may ignore or deny new pain because

    A. _____

    B. _____

48. Persons with dementia may signal pain by changes _____.

49. When gathering information about a person in pain, you can use a scale of 1 to 10. Which end of the scale is the most severe pain? _____

50. What happens to vital signs when the person has acute pain? _____

51. When the person uses words such as aching, knife-like, or sore to describe pain, what do you report to the nurse? _____

52. What body responses may be objective signs or symptoms (signs you can measure or see) that the person has acute pain?

    A. _____

    B. _____

    C. _____

    D. _____

53. What changes in these behaviors may be symptoms of pain?

    A. Speech _____
    _____

    B. Affected body part _____
    _____

    C. Positioning _____
    _____

54. List nursing measures to promote comfort and relieve pain related to these clues.

    A. Position of the person _____
    _____

    B. Linens _____
    _____

    C. Blankets _____
    _____

    D. Pain medications _____
    _____

    E. Family members _____
    _____

133

55. If a person is receiving strong pain medication or sedatives, what safety measures are important?

A. _____

B. _____

C. _____

D. _____

56. When you explain the procedure before performing it, you may help a person to rest better because you met the need for _____.

57. A clean, neat, and uncluttered room can promote rest by meeting _____ needs.

58. The mind and body rest, the body saves energy, and body functions slow during _____.

59. Mental restoration occurs during a phase of sleep called _____.

60. The deepest stage of sleep occurs during _____ _____.

61. If work hours change, it can affect the normal _____ cycle or _____ rhythm.

62. Alcohol tends to cause drowsiness and sleep but it interferes with _____.

63. Insomnia may be caused by

A. Fear of _____

B. Fear of not _____

C. Fear of not being able _____

D. Physical and emotional _____

64. When a person has dementia and wanders at night, the best approach for some persons is to allow _____ _____

OPTIONAL LEARNING EXERCISES

65. You are caring for two residents who both have arthritis. Mr. Forman tells you this is the first time he has had any health problems. Mrs. Wegman tells you she has had several surgeries and has had three children. Which of these two persons is likely to be more anxious about the pain and to be unable to handle the pain well? Why? _____ _____

66. Mr. Forman tells you his pain seems much worse at night. What could be the reason for this reaction? _____ _____

67. You are caring for Mrs. Reynolds. She tells you she misses her children, who have moved to another state. Today, Mrs. Reynolds is complaining of pain in her abdomen. In spite of providing nursing comfort measures, she still rates her pain at a 7. What is a possible reason Mrs. Reynolds is not getting relief from her pain? _____ _____

68. When a person is ill, how do these affect sleep?

A. Treatments and therapies _____ _____

B. Care devices such as traction or a cast _____ _____

C. Motions _____ _____

69. Certain foods affect sleep. Tell how these foods affect sleep and list foods that contain the substances.

A. Caffeine _____ sleep. It is found in _____.

B. Tryptophan _____ sleep. It is found in _____.

INDEPENDENT LEARNING ACTIVITIES

- Form a group with several classmates and share your personal experiences with pain. Discuss the following questions to understand the different ways you respond to pain and treat the pain.
  - What experiences have you had with pain? Accidents? Illnesses? Childbirth? Surgery?
  - What type of pain have you had? Acute? Chronic? Other types?
  - How would you rate your pain on a scale of 1 to 10? How long did it last?
  - How did your family and friends respond to your pain? How much support did you receive from them? How did the support (or lack of it) affect the pain?
  - What measures were used to treat the pain? What was the most effective? The least effective?
  - What did you learn from this discussion with others about their pain? How will this help you as you care for others with pain?
- Form a group with several classmates to talk about differences in sleep habits. Answer these questions to understand differences in personal practices concerning rest and sleep.
  - How many hours do you sleep each day? How many hours of sleep do you think you *should* get each day?
  - If you did not have to follow a schedule (work, school, etc.), when would you go to bed and wake up?
  - What rituals do you perform before going to bed? How is your sleep affected if you cannot perform these rituals?

28. Respirations that are slow, shallow, and sometimes irregular are _____.

29. A _____ is a surgically created opening into the trachea.

CIRCLE THE BEST ANSWER

30. Oxygen (O₂) is carried to cells by the
    A. Alveoli
    B. Red blood cells
    C. Bone marrow
    D. White blood cells

31. Oxygen needs increase when
    A. The person is aging
    B. Medications are taken
    C. The person has fever or pain
    D. The person is well-nourished

32. Respiratory depression can occur when
    A. The person exercises
    B. Allergies are present
    C. Narcotics are taken in large doses
    D. The person smokes

33. Restlessness is an early sign of
    A. Hypoxia
    B. Apnea
    C. Hyperventilation
    D. Bradypnea

34. Signs of hypoxia may be
    A. Disorientation and confusion
    B. Decrease in pulse rate and respirations
    C. Being relaxed and calm
    D. The skin, mucous membranes, and nail beds are pink

35. When you prepare a person for a bronchoscopy, you
    A. Make sure the person does not eat for 6 to 8 hours before the test
    B. Help the person remove all clothing and jewelry from the waist to the neck
    C. Place the person in a sitting position
    D. Keep the person on bedrest for at least 1 hour before the x-ray

36. If you are caring for a person who just had a pulmonary function test, you would expect the person to
    A. Tell you he or she has chest pain
    B. Be very tired
    C. Have hemoptysis
    D. Complain of nausea and vomiting

37. If a pulse oximeter is being used on a person with tremors or poor circulation, which of these sites would be best to use?
    A. A toe on a foot that is swollen
    B. A finger that has nail polish on the nail
    C. A toe with an open wound
    D. An earlobe

38. When you are delegated to place a pulse oximeter on a person, report to the nurse if
    A. The person is sleeping
    B. The person's pulse rate goes above or below the alarm limit
    C. You remove nail polish on the nail before attaching the pulse oximeter
    D. You tape the oximeter in place

39. When a person has breathing difficulties, it is usually easier for the person to breath
    A. In the supine position
    B. Lying on one side for long periods
    C. In the semi-Fowler or Fowler position
    D. In the prone position

40. Deep-breathing and coughing exercises
    A. Help prevent pneumonia and atelectasis
    B. Decrease pain after surgery or injury
    C. Are done once a day
    D. Cause mucus to form in the lungs

41. When assisting with coughing and deep breathing, you tell the person to
    A. Inhale through the mouth
    B. Hold the breath for 30 seconds
    C. Exhale slowly through pursed lips
    D. Repeat the exercise 1 or 2 times

42. When a person uses an incentive spirometer, it allows the person to
    A. Take shallow breaths
    B. See air movement when inhaling
    C. See air movement with exhaling
    D. Exhale quickly

43. If a person is receiving oxygen, you may
    A. Set the flowmeter rate
    B. Apply the oxygen device to the person
    C. Set up the system
    D. Turn on the oxygen

44. If a person receives oxygen through a nasal cannula, it is important to look for irritation
    A. On the nose, ears, and cheekbones
    B. Under the mask
    C. In the throat
    D. In the oral cavity

45. If you are near a person receiving oxygen, which of these should you report?
    A. The humidifier is bubbling
    B. The humidifier has enough water
    C. The humidifier is not bubbling
    D. The person is in a semi-Fowler position

46. If a person uses an inhaler, it is important to
    A. Make sure they use the inhaler frequently
    B. Notify the nurse quickly if the person cannot catch his or her breath
    C. Make sure the inhaler is bubbling
    D. Store it safely with the nurse

47. When caring for a person with an artificial airway, you should tell the nurse at once if
    A. The vital signs remain stable
    B. Frequent oral hygiene is done
    C. The airway comes out or is dislodged
    D. The person feels as if he or she is gagging
48. Because a person with an endotracheal tube (ET) cannot speak, it is important to
    A. Never ask questions
    B. Avoid talking to the person
    C. Always keep the call light within reach
    D. Avoid explaining what you are going to do
49. The person with an ET can communicate by
    A. Whispering or speaking softly
    B. Using paper and pencil, Magic Slates, or communication boards
    C. Having a family member ask and answer questions
    D. Covering the tube opening
50. If you are caring for a person with an artificial airway, your care should always include
    A. Removing the device to clean it
    B. Comforting and reassuring the person that the airway helps breathing
    C. Suctioning to maintain the airway
    D. Making sure the person never takes a tub bath
51. The stoma or tube must be
    A. Covered when the person is shaving
    B. Covered with plastic when the person is outdoors
    C. Covered with a loose gauze dressing when the person is bathing
    D. Uncovered when the person is outdoors
52. When suctioning is done, the nurse
    A. Follows Standard Precautions and the Bloodborne Pathogen Standard
    B. Makes sure a suction cycle is not more than 20 to 30 seconds
    C. Waits about 5 seconds between each suction cycle
    D. Suctions as many times as needed to clear the airway
53. If you are caring for a person who needs suctioning, you know that suctioning is done
    A. On a regular schedule
    B. As needed when signs and symptoms of respiratory distress are observed
    C. When the nurse directs you to do the suctioning
    D. When the person asks for suctioning
54. When the alarm sounds on a machine used for mechanical ventilation, you should first
    A. Report it to the nurse at once
    B. Reset the alarms
    C. Reassure the person that the alarm is normal
    D. Check to see if the person's tube is attached to the ventilator
55. Petrolatum gauze is kept at the bedside of a person with chest tubes to
    A. Cover the insertion site if the chest tube comes out
    B. Lubricate the site of the chest tube
    C. Cleanse the skin around the chest tube
    D. Cover the site of the chest tube insertion to prevent drainage

FILL IN THE BLANKS

56. Write out the meaning of each abbreviation.
    A. CO_2 _____
    B. ET _____
    C. L/min _____
    D. O_2 _____
    E. RBC _____
    F. SpO_2 _____

57. As a person ages, several factors affect the person's oxygen needs. List what happens in each of the areas listed below.
    A. Respiratory muscles _____
    _____
    B. Lung tissue _____
    _____
    C. Strength for coughing _____
    _____
    D. Risk for respiratory _____
    _____

58. Three diseases are caused by or are risk factors related to smoking. They are
    A. _____
    B. _____
    C. _____

59. How does alcohol increase the risk of aspiration? It depresses the _____, reduces the _____, and increases _____
    _____.

60. How many respirations per minute occur with
    A. Normal respirations _____
    B. Tachypnea _____
    C. Bradypnea _____

61. What signs and symptoms can be used to describe sputum when reporting and recording these areas of observation?
    A. Color _____
    _____
    B. Odor _____
    _____
    C. Consistency _____
    _____
    D. Hemoptysis _____
    _____

62. If a person has difficulty breathing, he or she may prefer a position in which the person is sitting _____. This position is called _____.

63. If a person has a productive cough, what respiratory hygiene and cough etiquette should be taught?

   A. _____

   B. _____

   C. _____

   D. _____

64. If a person is using an incentive spirometer, how long is the breath held to keep the balls floating? _____ _____

65. What observations should be reported after a person uses an incentive spirometer?

   A. _____

   B. _____

   C. _____

   D. _____

66. When a person wears a mask to receive oxygen, what should you do when the person needs to eat? _____ _____ How will the person receive oxygen during the meal? _____ _____

67. Oxygen is humidified because it will _____ _____.

68. When caring for a person with an artificial airway, you may be delegated to

   A. Check _____ often

   B. Observe for _____ _____

   C. Give frequent _____ _____

   D. Report to the nurse at once if _____ _____

69. What are the three parts of a tracheostomy tube?

   A. _____

   B. _____

   C. _____

Questions 70 to 77 relate to caring for a tracheostomy and assisting the nurse during suctioning. You must know whether your state laws or job description allows you to assist with these procedures.

70. Which part of the tracheostomy tube is removed for cleaning and mucus removal? _____

71. Which part of the tracheostomy tube is not removed? _____

72. If a person with a tracheostomy is outdoors, what is used to cover the tracheostomy? _____ _____

73. A suction cycle takes no more than _____ seconds. The cycle involves

   A. _____

   B. _____

   C. _____

74. Before, during, and after suctioning, what is checked and observed?

   A. _____

   B. _____

   C. _____

   D. _____

75. When you are observing a person when suctioning is being done, what should be reported to the nurse at once?

   A. _____

   B. _____

   C. _____

   D. _____

   E. _____

76. When a person has mechanical ventilation, what should you say when you enter the room? _____ _____ _____ When you leave the room? _____

77. If chest tubes are in place, what should be reported to the nurse?

   A. Signs and symptoms of _____ and _____

   B. Complaints of _____ or ___ _____

CROSSWORD

Fill in the crossword by choosing words from the following list.

Apnea   Hyperventilation
Biot   Hypoventilation
Bradypnea   Kussmaul
"Cheyne-Stokes"   Orthopnea
Dyspnea   Tachypnea

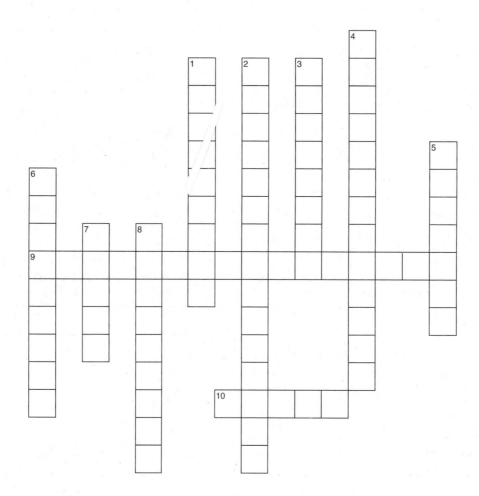

Across

9. Respirations are rapid and deep
10. Rapid and deep respirations followed by 10 or 20 seconds of apnea; occur with nervous disorders

Down

1. Respirations are 24 or more per minute
2. Respirations are slow, shallow, and sometimes irregular
3. Very deep and rapid respirations; signal diabetic coma
4. Respirations gradually increase in rate and depth; common when death is near
5. Difficult, labored, or painful breathing
6. Breathing deeply and comfortably only when sitting
7. Lack or absence of breathing
8. Respirations are fewer than 12 per minute

OPTIONAL LEARNING EXERCISES

Situation: *You are caring for Mr. R., age 84, who has chronic obstructive pulmonary disease.*

78. What position would make it easier for Mr. R. to breathe when he is in bed? _____
_____

79. How can you increase his comfort when he is sitting up? _____What is this position called? _____

Situation: *Mrs. F. is receiving oxygen through a nasal cannula at 2 L/min. Her respirations are unlabored at 16 per minute unless she is walking about or doing personal care. Then her respirations are 28 per minute and dyspneic.*

80. Where should you check for signs of irritation from the cannula? _____

81. You should make sure there are _____ in the tubing and that Mrs. F. does not _____ of the tubing.

82. What are the abnormal respirations that Mrs. F. has with activity called? _____

83. If you are caring for a person with a tracheostomy, why is the tracheostomy covered when the person is outdoors? _____
_____

84. What is done to protect the stoma in the following situations?
    A. Tub baths or showers _____
    _____
    B. Shaving _____
    _____
    C. Shampooing _____
    _____

85. The stoma is never covered with _____
    _____
    Why? _____

86. What do you need to check before you use an Ambu bag attached to oxygen? _____
    Why? _____

87. If a person has mechanical ventilation, where do you find a plan for communication? _____
_____

Why is it important for everyone to use the same signals for communication? _____
_____

88. If a person has chest tubes, why is it important to prevent kinks in the tubing? _____
_____

INDEPENDENT LEARNING ACTIVITIES

- Work with a classmate and carry out these exercises. They will help you understand how it feels to be a person with breathing problems.
  - Have your partner count your respirations while you are at rest. Then exercise by running or jogging in place for at least 2 minutes. Now have your partner check your respirations again. How have they changed? Rate? Rhythm or pattern? Easy or labored?
  - While you exercise, try first to breathe only through your nose. Then try breathing through your mouth. Which way makes you feel you are getting enough air?
  - Place a drinking straw in your mouth and close your lips tightly around it. Now breathe only through the straw while at rest and during exercise. When you are at rest, how comfortable does this feel? Are you getting enough air? How is your air supply during exercise?
  - Take a drinking straw and place small pieces of paper in one end so that it is fairly tight. Now try breathing through the straw at rest and during exercise. What is the difference between the open and blocked straw? Imagine that every breath you take feels like it does with the blocked straw. This is how many people with breathing problems feel all the time.
- Try to find a person who has had a type of artificial ventilation discussed in this chapter. Ask the person the following questions.
  - What was the worst part of the experience?
  - How did the person communicate his or her needs with others?
  - What did the staff do that helped make the person comfortable?
  - What would have helped to make the experience better?

27 Measuring Vital Signs

FILL IN THE BLANKS: KEY TERMS

"Apical-radial pulse"
Blood pressure (BP)
Body temperature
Bradycardia
Diastole
Diastolic pressure
Fever

Hypertension
Hypotension
Pulse
Pulse deficit
Pulse rate
Respiration

Sphygmomanometer
Stethoscope
Systole
Systolic pressure
Tachycardia
Vital signs

1. A rapid heart rate is _____. The heart rate is over 100 beats per minute.

2. The _____ is taking the apical and radial pulse at the same time.

3. An instrument used to listen to the sounds produced by the heart, lungs, and other body organs is a _____.

4. A condition in which the systolic blood pressure is below 90 mm Hg and the diastolic pressure is below 60 mm Hg is _____ _____.

5. The _____ is the number of heartbeats or pulses felt in 1 minute.

6. The amount of heat in the body that is a balance between the amount of heat produced and amount lost by the body is the _____.

7. _____ is the period of heart muscle contraction.

8. _____ is persistent blood pressure measurements above the normal systolic (140 mm Hg) or diastolic (90 mm Hg) pressures.

9. The instrument used to measure blood pressure is a _____.

10. The beat of the heart felt at an artery as a wave of blood passes through the artery is the _____.

11. Temperature, pulse, respirations, and blood pressure are _____.

12. _____ is a slow heart rate; the rate is less than 60 beats per minute.

13. The amount of force it takes to pump blood out of the heart into the arterial circulation is the _____ _____.

14. The period of heart muscle relaxation is _____.

15. The difference between the apical and radial pulse rates is the _____.

16. _____ is the amount of force exerted against the walls of an artery by the blood.

17. The act of breathing air into and out of the lungs is _____.

18. _____ is the pressure in the arteries when the heart is at rest.

19. Elevated body temperature is _____ _____.

CIRCLE THE BEST ANSWER

20. Vital signs are
    A. Temperature, pulse, respirations, and blood pressure
    B. Temperature, pulse, and respirations
    C. Blood pressure and pulse oximeter reading of oxygen level
    D. Tachycardia, bradypnea, and bradycardia

21. Unless otherwise ordered, take vital signs when the person
    A. Is lying or sitting
    B. Has been walking or exercising
    C. Has just finished eating
    D. Is getting ready to take a shower or tub bath

22. Body temperature is lower in the
    A. Afternoon
    B. Morning
    C. Evening
    D. Night

23. If you are taking vital signs on a person with dementia, it may be better if
    A. You have 2 or 3 coworkers restrain the person
    B. The vital signs are taken when the person is asleep
    C. You take the pulse and respirations at one time and the temperature and blood pressure at another time
    D. You ask the nurse to take the vital signs

24. What should you do if a resident asks his or her vital sign measurements?
    A. You can tell the person the measurements if center policy allows
    B. Tell the nurse that the person wants to know the measurements
    C. Tell the person you cannot tell him or her this information
    D. This information is private and cannot be shared

25. If you take a rectal temperature, the normal range of the temperature would be
    A. 96.6 °F to 98.6 °F (35.9 °C to 37.0 °C)
    B. 97.6 °F to 99.6 °F (36.5 °C to 37.5 °C)
    C. 98.6 °F to 100.6 °F (37.0 °C to 38.1 °C)
    D. 98.6 °F (37 °C)

26. If you are taking the temperature of an older person, you would expect the temperature to be
    A. Lower than the normal range
    B. Higher than the normal range
    C. About in the middle of the normal range
    D. The same as a younger adult

27. When recording an axillary temperature of 97.6 °F, it is written
    A. 97.6°
    B. 97.6° R
    C. 97.6° Ax
    D. 97.6° axillary

28. When using an electronic thermometer, you can prevent the spread of infection by
    A. Discarding the thermometer after each use
    B. Discarding the probe cover after each use
    C. Keeping a thermometer for each person at the bedside
    D. Sterilizing the thermometer after each use

29. When taking a temperature on a resident with dementia, the best choice is to
    A. Take a rectal temperature
    B. Take an oral temperature
    C. Take an axillary temperature
    D. Use a tympanic membrane, temporal artery thermometer, or infrared thermometer

30. Which pulse is most commonly used?
    A. Carotid
    B. Brachial
    C. Radial
    D. Popliteal

31. A _____ pulse is taken during cardiopulmonary resuscitation (CPR).
    A. Carotid
    B. Temporal
    C. Femoral
    D. Radial

32. When using a stethoscope, you can help to prevent infection by
    A. Warming the diaphragm in your hand
    B. Wiping the earpieces and diaphragm with antiseptic wipes before and after use
    C. Placing the diaphragm over the artery
    D. Placing the earpieces in your ears so the bend of the tips point forward

33. When a pulse rate is 120 beats per minute, you
    A. Report that the person has bradycardia
    B. Know that this is a normal pulse rate
    C. Report that the person has tachycardia
    D. Report that the pulse is irregular

34. The pulse rate is the number of heartbeats or pulses felt in
    A. 30 seconds
    B. 15 seconds
    C. 1 minute
    D. 5 minutes

35. Electronic blood pressure equipment will not give you information about
    A. Pulse force
    B. Pulse rate
    C. Tachycardia
    D. Bradycardia

36. When taking the radial pulse, place
    A. The thumb over the pulse site
    B. 2 or 3 fingers on the middle of the wrist
    C. 2 or 3 fingers on the thumb side of the wrist
    D. The stethoscope on the chest wall

37. The apical pulse is counted for
    A. 30 seconds
    B. 15 seconds
    C. 1 full minute
    D. The amount of time directed by the nurse

38. An apical pulse of 72 is recorded as
    A. Pulse 72
    B. 72 – Apical pulse
    C. 72Ap
    D. P 72

39. An "apical-radial" pulse is taken by
    A. Taking the radial pulse for 1 minute and then taking the apical pulse for 1 minute
    B. Subtracting the apical pulse from the radial pulse
    C. Having one staff member take the radial pulse at the same time that another staff member takes the apical pulse
    D. Having two persons take the apical pulse at the same time

40. When counting respirations, the best way is to
    A. Stand quietly next to the person and watch the chest rise and fall
    B. Keep your fingers or stethoscope over the pulse site so the person thinks you are still counting the pulse
    C. Tell the person to breathe normally so you can count the respirations
    D. Use the stethoscope to hear the respirations clearly and count for 1 full minute

143

41. Each respiration involves
    A. One inhalation
    B. One exhalation
    C. One inhalation (chest rises) and one exhalation (chest falls)
    D. Counting for 15 seconds and multiplying by four
42. The blood pressure should not be taken on an arm
    A. If the person has had breast surgery on that side
    B. If the arm was used for a blood draw earlier in the day
    C. If it is the dominant arm used for eating and writing
    D. If the person has arthritis in the hand
43. You will find out the size of blood pressure cuff needed
    A. By asking the nurse
    B. By measuring the person's arm
    C. By reading the doctor's orders
    D. By asking the person
44. When taking the blood pressure, you place the stethoscope diaphragm
    A. Over the radial artery on the thumb side of the wrist
    B. Over the brachial artery at the inner aspect of the elbow
    C. Lightly against the skin
    D. Over the apical pulse site
45. When getting ready to take the blood pressure, position the person's arm
    A. Above the level of the heart
    B. Level with the heart
    C. Below the level of the heart
    D. Abducted from the body
46. The blood pressure cuff is inflated between
    A. 100 mm Hg and 120 mm Hg
    B. 2 to 4 mm per second
    C. 160 mm Hg and 180 mm Hg
    D. 180 mm Hg and 200 mm Hg
47. When taking a resident's temperature with an infrared thermometer,
    A. Always use a new probe cover
    B. Have the resident close their eyes when using thermometer near their forehead
    C. The thermometer sensing area should be held perpendicular to the forehead
    D. Ask that the resident not eat or drink at least 15–20 minutes prior to the measurement

FILL IN THE BLANKS

48. Write out the meaning of each abbreviation.
    A. BP _____
    B. C _____
    C. F _____
    D. Hg _____
    E. mm _____
    F. mm Hg _____
    G. TPR _____
49. Vital signs are taken when medications are taken that affect _____.
50. When taking vital signs, report to the nurse at once if
    A. _____
    B. _____
    C. _____
51. Sites for measuring temperature are the
    A. _____
    B. _____
    C. _____
    D. _____
    E. _____
52. Which site has the highest baseline temperature?
    _____
53. Which site has the lowest baseline temperature?
    _____
54. When taking an axillary temperature, the axilla must be _____.
55. Tympanic membrane and temporal artery thermometers are used for confused persons because they are _____.
56. When using an electronic thermometer, what does the color of the probe mean?
    A. Blue _____
    B. Red _____
57. When you take a rectal temperature, you apply _____ to the tip of the thermometer or the end of the covered probe.
58. When taking a tympanic membrane temperature, pull up and back on the adult's ear to _____ _____.
59. The pulse rate for a person 12 years or older is between _____ and _____ per minute.
60. List words used to describe the following:
    A. Forceful pulse _____
    _____
    B. Hard-to-feel pulse _____
    _____
61. If a pulse is irregular, count the pulse for _____.

62. When you take a pulse, what observations should be reported and recorded?

A. _____

B. _____

C. _____

D. _____

E. _____

F. _____

G. _____

63. Do not use your thumb to take a pulse because _____.

64. When taking an apical pulse, each lub-dub sound is counted as _____.

65. The radial pulse rate is never greater than the _____ pulse.

66. A healthy adult has _____ respirations per minute.

67. What observations should be reported and recorded when counting respirations?

A. _____

B. _____

C. _____

D. _____

E. _____

F. _____

G. _____

H. _____

68. Each respiration involves one _____ and one _____.

69. Respirations are counted for _____ if they are abnormal or irregular.

70. Blood pressure is controlled by

A. _____

B. _____

C. _____

71. Normal ranges for blood pressures are

A. Systolic less than _____

B. Diastolic less than _____

72. If a person has been exercising, let the person rest for _____ before taking the blood pressure.

73. The blood pressure is normally taken when the person is _____ or _____. The doctor may also order the blood pressure to be taken when the person is _____.

74. When listening to the blood pressure, the first sound you hear is the _____ pressure and the point where the sound disappears is the _____ pressure.

LABELING

75. Name the pulse sites shown.

A. _____

B. _____

C. _____

D. _____

E. _____

F. _____

G. _____

H. _____

I. Which pulse is used during cardiopulmonary resuscitation (CPR)? _____

J. Which pulse is most commonly taken? _____ _____

K. Which pulse is used when taking the blood pressure? _____

L. Which pulse is found with a stethoscope? _____ _____

76. Fill in the drawings so the dials show the correct blood pressures.

    A. 168/102

    B. 104/68

OPTIONAL LEARNING EXERCISES

Taking Temperatures

77. How would you record these temperature readings?

A. An oral temperature of 97.4 °F, 36.5 °C

_____

B. A rectal temperature of 99.8 °F, 38.1 °C

_____

C. An axillary temperature of 96.2 °F, 36.1 °C

_____

Taking Pulses and Respirations

78. You are assigned to take Mrs. Sanchez's pulse and respirations. You note that the pulse rate and respirations are regular, so you take each one for

_____

When you complete counting the pulse and are ready to count respirations, you keep your _____. This is done so that Mrs. Sanchez will _____

79. When you finish counting Mrs. Sanchez's pulse and respirations for 30 seconds, your numbers are pulse 36 and respirations 9. What numbers should be recorded? Pulse _____ Respirations _____ Why? _____

80. The nurse tells you to take an "apical-radial" pulse on Mrs. Hellman. Why do you ask a coworker to help you? _____
_____

81. How long is an "apical-radial" pulse counted? _____
_____

After you have taken the "apical-radial" pulse, how do you find the pulse deficit? _____
_____
_____

Taking Blood Pressures

82. You are assigned to take Mr. Hardaway's blood pressure. You know that he goes for dialysis three times a week. What do you need to know before you take his blood pressure? _____ Why?
_____

83. When inflating the cuff, how high is the cuff inflated? _____ When deflating the cuff, you should deflate the cuff at an even rate of _____ per second.

INDEPENDENT LEARNING ACTIVITIES

- Take turns measuring vital signs on 3 or 4 classmates. If possible, use electronic, tympanic, infrared, and temporal thermometers for each person to see if they give similar results. Use the following table to record the results.

Person	Temperature	Pulse	Respiration	Blood Pressure
#1	Electronic Tympanic Temporal Infrared	Radial Apical	Rate Rhythm Depth	
#2	Electronic Tympanic Temporal Infrared	Radial Apical	Rate Rhythm Depth	
#3	Electronic Tympanic Temporal Infrared	Radial Apical	Rate Rhythm Depth	
#4	Electronic Tympanic Temporal Infrared	Radial Apical	Rate Rhythm Depth	

Answer the following questions about this exercise.

○ If you used different thermometers, how did the results compare?

○ What differences were there in finding the radial pulses among your classmates?

○ What differences did you find in the rates and rhythms?

○ How were you able to measure respirations so the person did not know you were watching?

○ What differences in rhythm and depth of respirations did you find among your classmates?

○ What differences did you find in locating the brachial artery in different people?

○ How did the sounds of the blood pressure differ among your classmates?

○ What difficulties did you have with any of the measurements taken?

○ What will you change about measuring vital signs on a resident after this practice?

• Practice taking an "apical-radial" pulse with classmates. Take turns acting as the staff members and the person having the pulse taken. Answer the following questions after the exercise is completed.

○ How was privacy maintained for the person having the pulse measured?

○ How did the "staff members" decide who would begin and end the count?

○ What problems did you have in counting for 1 minute?

○ How did the apical and radial counts compare?

○ What will you change about measuring the "apical-radial" pulses on a resident after this experience?

28 Assisting with the Physical Examination

FILL IN THE BLANKS: KEY TERMS

Dorsal recumbent position
Genupectoral position
Horizontal recumbent position
Knee-chest position

Laryngeal mirror
Lithotomy position
Nasal speculum
Ophthalmoscope

Otoscope
Percussion hammer
Tuning fork
Vaginal speculum

1. An instrument vibrated to test hearing is a _____.

2. In the _____, the person lies on the back with the hips at the edge of the exam table; the knees are flexed, the hips are externally rotated, and the feet are in stirrups.

3. The supine position with the legs together is called the _____.

4. An _____ is a lighted instrument used to examine the external ear and the eardrum (tympanic membrane).

5. A _____ is an instrument used to open the vagina so it and the cervix can be examined.

6. When a person kneels and rests the body on the knees and chest, so that the head is turned to one side, the arms are above the head or flexed at the elbows, the back is straight, and the body is flexed about 90 degrees at the hip, the person is in the _____.

7. A _____ is an instrument used to tap body parts to test reflexes.

8. An instrument used to examine the mouth, teeth, and throat is called a _____.

9. An instrument used to examine the inside of the nose is a _____.

10. The dorsal recumbent position is also called the _____.

11. An _____ is a lighted instrument used to examine the internal structures of the eye.

12. Another name for the knee-chest position is _____.

CIRCLE THE BEST ANSWER

13. When weighing a person, have him or her
    A. Wear only socks and shoes and a bathrobe
    B. Remove regular clothes and wear a gown or pajamas
    C. Wear regular street clothes
    D. Remove any clothing worn after being weighed and then weigh the clothes

14. Chair, bed, lift, and wheelchair scales are used when
    A. A person can transfer from a wheelchair to the scale
    B. A person cannot stand
    C. A person can stand and walk independently
    D. A person is in the supine position

15. When a person cannot stand on the scale to have the height measured
    A. Ask the person or the family the person's height
    B. Have the person sit in a chair and use a measuring tape to measure the person from head to toe
    C. Position the person in a supine position in bed and measure with a measuring tape
    D. Estimate the height of the person by observing him or her

16. In nursing centers, residents have a physical examination
    A. Only when the person is admitted
    B. Once a month
    C. At least once a year
    D. Only when the person is ill

17. If a resident is having a physical examination, you may be asked to assist by
    A. Measuring vital signs, height, and weight
    B. Having the person remove all clothing and cover with a sheet
    C. Explaining why the examination is being done and what to expect
    D. Leaving the person alone after you have taken the vital signs and positioned the person

18. When the doctor is examining the person's mouth, teeth, and throat, you may be asked to hand him or her the
    A. Ophthalmoscope
    B. Percussion hammer
    C. Tuning fork
    D. Laryngeal mirror
19. The right to personal choice for a person having a physical examination is protected during a physical exam when you
    A. Have the person urinate before the examination begins
    B. Tell the person who will do the exam and when it will be done
    C. Keep the person screened and the room door closed
    D. Allow a family member to be present if the person requests it
20. The right to privacy is protected by
    A. Removing all clothes for a complete examination
    B. Explaining the reasons for the examination
    C. Exposing only the body part being examined
    D. Explaining the exam results with a family member present
21. Before the exam begins, you should
    A. Make sure the person has a bowel movement
    B. Have the person void so the bladder is empty
    C. Give the person an enema to empty the colon
    D. Have the person drink a large glass of water
22. After you have taken the person to the exam room and placed the person in position, you should
    A. Put the call light on for the nurse or examiner
    B. Leave the room
    C. Go to the nurse or examiner to report that the person is ready
    D. Open the door so the nurse or examiner knows you are ready
23. When the abdomen, chest, and breasts are to be examined, you will place the person in the
    A. Lithotomy position
    B. Lateral position
    C. Dorsal recumbent (horizontal recumbent) position
    D. Knee-chest position
24. If a person is asked to stand on the floor during an exam, you should
    A. Assist the person to put on shoes or slippers
    B. Place paper or paper towels on the floor
    C. Place a sheet on the floor
    D. Wipe the floor carefully with an antiseptic cleaner before the person stands on it

FILL IN THE BLANKS

25. List the equipment you need to collect when the ears are being examined.
    A. _____
    B. _____
26. List the items needed to examine the eyes.
    A. _____
    B. _____
27. When the nose, mouth, and throat are being examined, you should collect
    A. _____
    B. _____
    C. _____
    D. _____
28. What is done to the balance scale before having the person step on it?
    A. _____
    B. _____
    C. _____
29. When measuring a person in the supine position, the ruler is placed _____.
30. What are common fears the person may have when a physical examination is done?
    A. _____
    B. _____
    C. _____
    D. _____
    E. _____
    F. _____
    G. _____
    H. _____
31. To maintain the person's right to privacy, who are the only persons who have a right to see the person's body during the exam? _____ _____
32. Who are the staff members who need to know the reason for the exam and its results? _____ _____ _____

LABELING

Look at the instruments and answer questions 33 to 37.

33. Name the instruments.

A. _____

B. _____

C. _____

D. _____

E. _____

F. _____

G. _____

34. Which instrument is used to examine the nose? _____

35. When the eye is examined, the examiner uses the ___ _____.

36. If a person has a sore throat, the examiner will look at the throat with the _____.

37. The reflexes are examined by using the _____ _____.

Look at the positions and answer questions 38 to 41.

38. Name the positions.

A. _____

B. _____

C. _____

D. _____

39. Which positions may be used when a rectal examination is done?

A. _____

B. _____

40. When the abdomen, chest, and breasts are examined, the person is placed in _____.

41. The _____ is used for a vaginal exam.

Chapter **28** **Assisting with the Physical Examination**

OPTIONAL LEARNING EXERCISES

42. When you are delegated the job of preparing a person for an exam, why do you need the following information?

   A. What time is the examination? _____
   _____

   B. What are two reasons it would be helpful to know which examinations will be done? _____
   _____
   _____

   C. What equipment will you need if you are assigned to take vital signs? _____

43. You are a female nursing assistant assisting a male examiner with an examination of a female resident. The nurse tells you to stay in the exam room during the entire procedure. Why is this important to the examiner and to the woman? _____
   _____

INDEPENDENT LEARNING ACTIVITIES

• You probably have had a physical examination at some time. Perhaps you needed one to be a student in this class. Answer the following questions about your experience when you had the physical done to you.
   ◦ Who explained what to expect during the exam? What were you told about any discomfort?
   ◦ What steps were taken to give you privacy? While you changed clothes? During the exam?
   ◦ Who was present during the exam? Were you given a choice of having another person in the room with you and the examiner? How did you feel about having (or not having) another person in the room?
   ◦ How did you know what was being done? How much information were you given about procedures? Positions? Tests?
   ◦ What positions were used during the exam? Which positions shown in this chapter were used? How comfortable did you feel? How did the examiner and assistant help make you more comfortable with the positions?
   ◦ What questions did you have during the exam? Who was able to answer these? How well were they answered to make you understand what was being done?
   ◦ How comfortable did you feel about the exam? What could have been done to make you more comfortable physically and psychologically?
   ◦ How did this experience help you understand the feelings of persons you may assist during an exam?

29 Collecting and Testing Specimens

FILL IN THE BLANKS: KEY TERMS

Acetone
Glucosuria
Glycosuria
Hematoma

Hematuria
Hemoptysis
Ketone

Ketone body
Melena
Sputum

1. Bloody sputum is _____.

2. A ketone is also called _____.

3. A black, tarry stool is _____.

4. _____ is glucosuria, or sugar in the urine.

5. _____ is mucus from the respiratory system that is expectorated through the mouth.

6. Acetone is called _____ or ketone body.

7. A substance that appears in urine from the rapid breakdown of fat for energy is _____.

8. Sugar in the urine is called glycosuria or _____.

9. _____ is blood in the urine.

10. A swelling that contains blood is a _____.

CIRCLE THE BEST ANSWER

11. Specimens are collected and tested to
    A. Measure the specimen
    B. Measure output
    C. Detect diseases
    D. Assist the person with personal care
12. When you are collecting a specimen, you should
    A. Use a sterile container for each specimen
    B. Follow the rules of medical asepsis
    C. Label the specimen after taking it to the clean utility room
    D. Carry the specimen to the lab wrapped in a clean paper towel
13. A urine specimen may be placed in a paper bag to
    A. Prevent embarrassing the person
    B. Protect the specimen from light
    C. Follow Standard Precautions
    D. Keep the specimen sterile

14. A random urine specimen is collected
    A. First thing in the morning
    B. After meals
    C. At any time
    D. At bedtime
15. When a person is collecting a random urine specimen, ask the person to put the toilet tissue in
    A. The wastebasket or toilet
    B. The specimen container
    C. The specimen pan
    D. A BIOHAZARD bag
16. When obtaining a midstream specimen, the perineal area is cleaned to
    A. Remove all microbes from the area
    B. Reduce the number of microbes in the urethral area
    C. Follow Standard Precautions and the Bloodborne Pathogen Standard
    D. Reduce infection during the specimen collection
17. When collecting a midstream specimen, which of these is correct?
    A. Collect the entire amount of urine voided
    B. Collect about 4 oz (120 mL) of urine
    C. Have the person void and then pass the receptacle into the stream of urine
    D. Collect several specimens and mix them together
18. When collecting a 24-hour urine specimen, the urine is kept
    A. Chilled on ice or refrigerated during the 24-hour period
    B. At room temperature
    C. In a sterile container at the nurses' station
    D. In a drainage collection bag at the bedside
19. A 24-hour urine specimen collection is started
    A. At the beginning of a shift
    B. After a meal
    C. At night
    D. After the person voids and that urine is discarded
20. At the end of 24-hour specimen collection
    A. The person voids and that urine is saved
    B. Write down any missed or spilled urine
    C. Record the amount of urine collected
    D. The person voids and that urine is discarded

153

21. When you test urine with reagent strips (dipsticks), it is important that you
    A. Follow the manufacturer's instructions
    B. Use a sterile urine specimen
    C. Wear sterile gloves
    D. Make sure the urine is cold

22. When you are assigned to strain a person's urine, you
    A. Have the person void directly into the strainer
    B. Send all urine to the lab
    C. Have the person void into the receptacle and then pour the urine through the strainer
    D. Discard the strainer if it contains any stones

23. If a warm stool specimen is required, it is
    A. Placed it in an insulated container
    B. Taken to the laboratory at once
    C. Tested at once on the nursing unit
    D. Taken at once to the storage area for transport to the laboratory

24. When collecting a stool specimen, ask the person to
    A. Void and have a bowel movement in a bedpan
    B. Use only a bedpan or commode to collect the specimen
    C. Urinate into the toilet and collect the stool in the specimen pan
    D. Place the toilet tissue in the bedpan, commode, or specimen pan with the stool

25. When collecting the stool specimen
    A. Pour it into the specimen container
    B. Use your gloved hand to obtain a specimen to place in the container
    C. Use a tongue blade to take about two tablespoons of stool from the middle of the formed stool
    D. Use a tongue blade to place the entire stool specimen in the container

26. When you test a stool specimen for blood
    A. It must be sent to the laboratory
    B. The specimen must be sterile
    C. You will need to test the entire stool specimen
    D. Use separate tongue blades to obtain a small amount of stool from two different areas

27. A sputum specimen is more easily collected
    A. Upon awakening
    B. After eating
    C. At bedtime
    D. After activity

28. Before obtaining a sputum specimen, ask the person to
    A. Rinse the mouth with water
    B. Brush the teeth and use mouthwash
    C. Cough and discard the first sputum expectorated
    D. Sit in an upright position to loosen secretions

29. Postural drainage is used when collecting a sputum specimen to
    A. Collect sterile specimens
    B. Make the sputum specimen more liquid
    C. Stimulate coughing
    D. Help secretions drain by gravity

30. When choosing a site for blood glucose testing, the best choice is
    A. The thumb
    B. The fleshy part of the middle finger
    C. The side toward the tip of the middle or ring finger
    D. The index finger

31. To increase the blood flow in the fingers before a blood glucose test
    A. Apply a warm washcloth or wash the hands in warm water
    B. Massage the fingers vigorously
    C. Apply cool compresses to the fingers and hands
    D. Have the person hang the hand over the edge of the bed for several minutes

FILL IN THE BLANKS

32. Write out the meaning of each abbreviation
    A. BM _____
    B. ID _____
    C. I&O _____
    D. mL _____
    E. oz _____

33. When collecting urine specimens, what observations are reported and recorded?
    A. _____
    B. _____
    C. _____
    D. _____
    E. _____

34. How much urine is collected for a random urine specimen? _____

35. When collecting a midstream urine specimen, the person starts to void and then stops. After the specimen container is positioned, the person _____ _____.

36. When you are obtaining a midstream specimen from a female, spread the labia with the thumb and index finger of your _____ hand.

37. When cleaning the female perineum for a midstream specimen, clean from _____.

38. When cleaning the male perineum for a midstream specimen, clean the penis starting _____ _____.

39. When you make labels for a 24-hour urine collection to place in the room and bathroom, what information is marked? _____ _____

40. Urine pH measures if the urine is _____ _____ or _____.

41. When you use reagent strips, you read the strip by comparing it to the _____.

42. When you strain urine, you are looking for stones that can develop in the

    A. _____

    B. _____

    C. _____

43. The strainer or gauze is placed in the specimen container if any _____ appear.

44. Stool specimens are studied and checked for

    A. _____

    B. _____

    C. _____

    D. _____

    E. _____

45. After collecting a stool specimen, place the container in a _____.

46. When you are delegated to collect a stool specimen, what observations are reported and recorded?

    A. _____

    B. _____

    C. _____

    D. _____

    E. _____

47. When stools are black and tarry, there is bleeding in the _____.

48. Blood in the stool that is hidden is called _____.

49. Mouthwash is not used before a sputum specimen is collected because it _____.

50. When you are delegated to collect a sputum specimen, report and record

    A. _____

    B. _____

    C. _____

    D. _____

    E. _____

    F. _____

    G. _____

    H. _____

    I. _____

51. When you are assisting a person to collect a sputum specimen, ask the person to take 2 or 3 _____ and _____ the sputum.

52. When preparing to carry out a blood glucose test, how will you make sure

    A. The glucose meter was tested for accuracy? ____

    _____

    B. You have the correct reagent strips for the meter you are using? _____

    C. The strips are not too old to use? _____

    _____

OPTIONAL LEARNING EXERCISES

53. If you are collecting a midstream specimen, what should you do if it is hard for the person to stop the stream of urine? _____

    _____

54. You are caring for a person who is having a 24-hour urine specimen test. He tells you he forgot to save a specimen 1 hour ago. What should you do and why?

    _____

55. What is normal pH for urine? _____

    _____

    What can cause changes in the normal pH? _____

    _____

56. When the body cannot use sugar for energy, it uses fat. When this happens, _____ appear in the urine.

57. Why is privacy important when collecting a sputum specimen? _____

INDEPENDENT LEARNING ACTIVITIES

- Answer the following questions about collecting specimens.
  - What specimens may be collected by nursing assistants in your state?
  - What special training is given to make sure that nursing assistants understand how to collect specimens?
  - Ask permission to look at specimen containers used at your clinical site. Are any directions included with the containers?
  - Where is information about collecting specimens kept at the clinical site?

Chapter **29** **Collecting and Testing Specimens**

CROSSWORD

Fill in the crossword by choosing words from this list.

Calculi	Labia	Postural	Specimens
Dysuria	Midstream	Random	Suctioning
Expectorated	Occult		

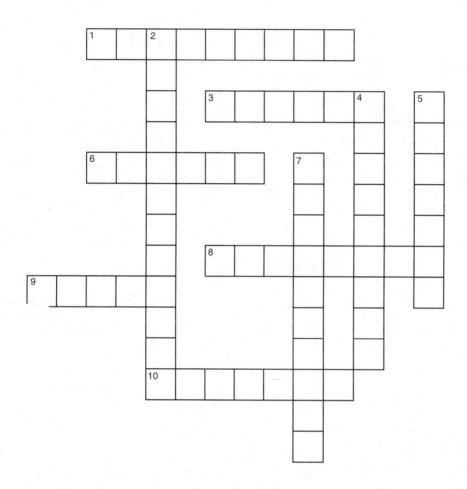

Across

1. Samples
3. Urine specimen that can be collected at any time
6. Hidden, as in blood in the stool
8. Position with head lower than body used to cause fluid to flow down
10. Pain when urinating

Down

2. Expelled, as in sputum, through the mouth
4. Urine specimen that is collected after the person starts to void
5. Stones that develop in the kidneys, ureters, or bladder
7. Removal of sputum from the trachea with a machine

30 Admissions, Transfers, and Discharges

Admission
Discharge
Transfer

1. _____ is moving a person from one room or nursing unit to another.

2. The official entry of a person into a nursing center is _____.

3. _____ occurs with the official departure of a person from a nursing center.

CIRCLE THE BEST ANSWER

4. Usually, _____ to a home setting is a happy time.
   A. Admission
   B. Discharge
   C. Transfer
   D. Home care

5. What staff member starts the admissions process?
   A. The doctor
   B. The nurse
   C. The admission coordinator
   D. The activities director

6. When a person with dementia is admitted to a nursing center, the person
   A. Is usually depressed
   B. May have an increase in confusion
   C. May have a decrease in confusion
   D. Usually feels safer in the new setting

7. Persons admitted to a rehabilitation unit from the hospital
   A. Are always admitted by the RN
   B. Are always admitted by the nursing assistant
   C. May be admitted by the nursing assistant after the nurse determines that the person's condition is stable and the person has no discomfort or distress
   D. Are never admitted by the nursing assistant

8. If a person being admitted is arriving by stretcher, you should
   A. Raise the bed to its highest level
   B. Leave the bed closed
   C. Raise the head of the bed to Fowler position
   D. Lower the bed to its lowest level

9. During admission, you can help the person feel more comfortable by
   A. Taking the person to his or her room and leaving the person alone
   B. Telling family members they must leave
   C. Talking quickly and answering questions with short answers
   D. Assisting the person to hang up pictures or display photos

10. When a person is being moved to a new room, who is notified?
    A. The doctor
    B. The social worker
    C. The family and business office
    D. The person's roommate

11. When you are transferring a person, you should
    A. Identify the person by checking the ID bracelet against the transfer slip
    B. Explain the reasons for the transfer
    C. Call the person's family to let them know about the transfer
    D. Wear gloves when gathering the person's belongings

12. If a person wishes to leave the center without the doctor's permission, you should
    A. Tell the person this is not allowed
    B. Prevent the person from leaving
    C. Tell the nurse at once
    D. Try to convince the person to stay

13. When you are assisting a person who is being discharged, you should
    A. Strip the bed and disinfect the equipment in the room while the person is packing
    B. Check off items on the clothing list and personal belongings list
    C. Call the family to ask them to assist the person in getting ready to go home
    D. Give the person prescriptions written by the doctor

14. OBRA has standards for transfers and discharges. List the ways these standards affect the person's rights.

    A. Reasons for _____ and are part of the person's _____.

    B. The _____ and _____ _____ are told of transfer or discharge plans.

    C. A procedure is followed if the person _____.

    D. An _____ often works with the person and family to ensure that _____.

15. When you are delegated to assist with admissions, transfers, or discharges, what information do you need from the nurse?

    A. _____
    B. _____
    C. _____
    D. _____
    E. _____
    F. _____
    G. _____
    H. _____
    I. _____
    J. _____

16. When a person is being admitted, what identifying information is obtained?

    A. _____
    B. _____
    C. _____
    D. _____
    E. _____

17. During admission, why does the person have a photo taken or receive an ID bracelet? _____ _____

18. When you are asked to admit a person, what can you do to make a good first impression?

    A. _____
    B. _____
    C. _____
    D. _____
    E. _____

19. What are reasons a person is moved to a new room?

    A. _____
    B. _____
    C. _____
    D. _____
    E. _____

20. According to OBRA and the CMS, reasons for a transfer or discharge are

    A. _____
    B. _____
    C. _____
    D. _____
    E. _____

21. When you transfer a person to a new unit, use good communication skills by

    A. _____
    B. _____
    C. _____
    D. _____

22. When a person is transferred or discharged, the nurse will tell you when to start and when the person is ___ _____.

23. When you assist with a discharge, you should report and record

    A. _____
    B. _____
    C. _____
    D. _____
    E. _____
    F. _____

24. During admission, transfer, or discharge, you can help the person and his or her family experience quality of life by

    A. Being_____
    B. Being_____
    C. Handling_____
    D. Treating_____

Situation: *Rosa Romirez, age 65, had a stroke (CVA) last week and is being admitted to a rehabilitation unit in the nursing care center where you work.*

Answer the following questions about Mrs. Romirez.

25. Because you know Mrs. Romirez is arriving by wheelchair, you leave the bed

    A. _____

    B. _____

26. The nurse instructs you to collect the equipment needed to admit a new person. You collect

    A. _____

    B. _____

    C. _____

    D. _____

    E. _____

    F. _____

    G. _____

    H. _____

    I. _____

    J. _____

27. When Mrs. Romirez arrives with her husband, it may help them feel more comfortable if you offer them

    _____

    _____.

28. You greet Mrs. Romirez by name and ask if she prefers a certain _____.

When you arrive at work one day, you are told Mrs. Romirez is being transferred to another room and you are asked to assist. Answer the following questions about transferring her.

29. When you transport Mrs. Romirez in a wheelchair, she is covered with a _____.

30. What items are taken with Mrs. Romirez to the new unit? _____

31. What information is recorded and reported about the transfer?

    A. _____

    B. _____

    C. _____

    D. _____

    E. _____

    F. _____

    G. _____

Several weeks later, you are assigned to care for Mrs. Romirez and find she is going home. Answer the following questions about her discharge.

32. What information and teaching should Mrs. Romirez receive from the health team before discharge?

    A. _____

    and _____

    B. Teaching about _____ and

    _____

    C. Arrangements for

    (1) _____

    (2) _____

    (3) _____

    D. Appointment with _____

    _____

33. Good communication skills should be used when assisting with the discharge. When Mrs. Romirez and her family leave, you should wish

    _____

INDEPENDENT LEARNING ACTIVITIES

- Have a discussion with 3 or 4 classmates to share experiences you have had with admissions to care facilities. You may have had personal experience or you may have observed a friend or family member being admitted. If you have not had this experience, perhaps you can relate the feelings you have had when admitted to a hospital or visiting a doctor's office. Answer the following questions during the discussion.

  ○ Who was the first person you met when you arrived to be admitted? How were you greeted? Did you feel welcome?

  ○ How did you arrive at your room? Were you escorted or did you have to find your way?

  ○ How long did you wait in the room before a staff member came to admit you? How did this affect your feelings about the place?

  ○ How were you addressed? First name? Last name? Did anyone ask you what you preferred?

  ○ What information were you given to make you feel more comfortable? What printed information was provided?

  ○ Overall, how did the admission procedure affect your feelings about the facility? Negative? Positive?

  ○ How will your personal experience and the experiences of others in this group affect your approach to new persons in a care facility?

31 Wound Care

FILL IN THE BLANKS: KEY TERMS

Abrasion
Arterial ulcer
Chronic wound
Clean wound
Clean-contaminated wound
Closed wound
Compress
Constrict
Contaminated wound
Contusion
Dehiscence
Diabetic foot ulcer
Dilate
Dirty wound
Edema

Embolus
Evisceration
Full-thickness wound
Gangrene
Hyperthermia
Hypothermia
Incision
Infected wound
Intentional wound
Laceration
Open wound
Pack
Partial-thickness wound
Penetrating wound
Phlebitis

Puncture wound
Purulent drainage
Sanguineous drainage
Serosanguineous drainage
Serous drainage
Skin tear
Stasis ulcer
Thrombus
Trauma
Ulcer
Unintentional wound
Vascular ulcer
Venous ulcer
Wound

1. A _____ is a break or rip in the skin that separates the epidermis from underlying skin.

2. A cut produced surgically by a sharp instrument is a(n) _____.

3. A shallow or deep crater-like sore of the skin or mucous membrane is an _____.

4. When tissues are injured but the skin is not broken, it is a _____.

5. _____ is thick green, yellow, or brown drainage.

6. When the dermis and epidermis of the skin are broken, it is called a _____.

7. A _____ is a break in the skin or mucous membrane.

8. A wound that is not infected is a _____.

9. A(n) _____ is a partial-thickness wound caused by the scraping away or rubbing of the skin.

10. A _____ is an open wound on the foot caused by complications from diabetes.

11. Thin, watery drainage that is blood-tinged is called _____.

12. A(n) _____ is a wound containing large amounts of microbes that shows signs of infection.

13. Another name for a blood clot is a _____.

14. _____ is an inflammation of a vein.

15. A wound with a high risk of infection is a _____.

16. A condition in which there is death of tissue is _____.

17. A body temperature that is much higher than the person's normal range is _____.

18. A _____ is an open wound with torn tissues and jagged edges.

19. A wound resulting from trauma is an _____.

20. A(n) _____ is an open wound on the lower legs or feet caused by poor arterial blood flow.

21. Clear, watery fluid is _____.

22. A blood clot that travels through the vascular system until it lodges in a distant vessel is called an _____.

23. Another name for an infected wound is _____.

24. A _____ is a wound that does not heal easily.

25. An open sore on the lower legs or feet caused by poor blood flow through the veins is a _____.

26. An open wound made by a sharp object is a _____ _____.

27. A wound created for therapy is a(n) _____ _____.

28. A _____ is an open wound that breaks the skin and enters a body area, organ, or cavity.

29. _____ is the separation of wound layers.

30. Swelling that is caused by fluid collecting in tissues is _____.

31. A _____ occurs when the dermis, epidermis, and subcutaneous tissue are penetrated. Muscle and bone may be involved.

32. An accident or violent act that injures the skin, mucous membranes, bones, and internal organs is called _____.

33. The separation of the wound along with the protrusion of abdominal organs is _____.

34. A _____ is another name for a venous ulcer.

35. Bloody drainage is called _____ _____.

36. A closed wound caused by a blow to the body is a _____.

37. A(n) _____ occurs when the skin or mucous membrane is broken.

38. A soft pad applied over a body part is a _____ _____.

39. A _____ is a wet or dry application wrapping a body part.

40. To expand or open wider is to _____ _____.

41. A very low body temperature is _____ _____.

42. _____ means to narrow.

43. A wound that occurs from the surgical entry of the reproductive, urinary, respiratory, or gastrointestinal system is a _____.

44. A _____ is an open sore on the lower legs or feet caused by decreased blood flow through the arteries or veins.

CIRCLE THE BEST ANSWER

45. When you inspect a resident's elbow, you find some of the skin is rubbed away. You would report this to the nurse as a(n)
    A. Laceration
    B. Abrasion
    C. Contusion
    D. Incision

46. When you look at a resident's arm that caught on the wheelchair, the tissue is torn with jagged edges. You know this is a
    A. Puncture wound
    B. Abrasion
    C. Penetrating wound
    D. Laceration

47. Which of these would place a person at risk for skin tears?
    A. The person is obese
    B. The person is able to walk to the dining room
    C. The person is very thin
    D. The person is alert and oriented

48. Applying lotion will help prevent skin breakdown or skin tears because it may
    A. Prevent loss of fatty layer under the skin
    B. Increase general thinning of the skin
    C. Keep the skin moisturized
    D. Prevent moisture in areas of the body where perspiration occurs

49. Venous ulcers of the feet and legs are caused by
    A. Poorly fitted shoes
    B. Poor venous blood flow
    C. Increased activity
    D. Increased fluid intake

50. A measure to promote circulation to prevent venous (stasis) ulcers is to
    A. Use elastic or rubber band–type garters to hold the person's socks in place
    B. Keep the person's feet flat on the floor while sitting in a chair
    C. Apply compression stockings or elastic wraps to legs
    D. Massage the legs and feet

51. Compression stockings
    A. Are usually removed every 8 hours for 30 minutes
    B. Are applied after the person has been out of bed for 30 minutes or more
    C. Normally cause the person to complain of tingling or numbness in the feet
    D. Are removed only at bedtime or for a bath or shower

52. When applying compression stockings, it is correct to
    A. Position the person in the chair
    B. Turn the stocking inside out down to the heel
    C. Make sure the stocking is large enough to fit loosely
    D. Fold over the top of the stocking if it is too long

53. Compression stockings and elastic bandages are
    A. Applied loosely to prevent discomfort
    B. Applied starting at the knee
    C. Used with persons at risk for developing a thrombus
    D. Used with all older persons

54. When applying elastic bandages, you should
 A. Apply the bandage so it completely covers the fingers or toes
 B. First apply the bandage to the lowest (distal) part of the wrist, foot, ankle, or knee
 C. Secure the bandage at the back of the leg with a safety pin
 D. Remove the bandage only when it becomes loose or falls off the extremity
55. Common causes of arterial ulcers are
 A. Poor blood flow through the veins
 B. Leg or foot surgery
 C. Smoking, high blood pressure, and diabetes
 D. Surgery on bones and joints
56. When caring for a person at risk for vascular ulcers, you should
 A. Remind the person not to sit with the legs crossed
 B. Assist the person to apply garters to hold up socks or hose
 C. Massage pressure points
 D. Encourage the person to use elastic garters to hold stockings in place
57. When caring for a person with diabetes, it is important to
 A. Massage the feet and ankles frequently
 B. Ask the person if the feet are too cold or too hot
 C. Check the person's feet every day
 D. Tell the person not to wear any shoes
58. During wound healing, what phase is happening when the wound is about 1 year old?
 A. Initial phase
 B. Inflammatory phase
 C. Maturation phase
 D. Proliferative phase
59. The nurse tells you to make sure Mrs. Reyn supports her abdominal wound when she gns. The nurse wants this done to protect agai
 A. Secondary intention healing
 B. Infection
 C. Scarring
 D. Dehiscence
60. When you are caring for Mrs. Reynolds, you notice thin, watery drainage that is blood-tinged. When you report your observations, you tell the nurse that the wound has _____ drainage.
 A. Purulent
 B. Serosanguineous
 C. Serous
 D. Sanguineous
61. Which of these methods used in wound care will prevent microbes from entering a wound when large amounts of drainage are expected?
 A. Wet-to-dry dressings
 B. Closed drainage system attached to suction
 C. Penrose drain
 D. Nonadherent gauze

62. Transparent adhesive film applied to a wound
 A. Absorbs dead tissue, which is removed when dressings are dry
 B. Allows drainage to be absorbed
 C. Allows air to reach the wound but does not allow fluids and bacteria to reach it
 D. Can be lifted to observe the wound
63. Plastic and paper tape may be used to secure a dressing
 A. Because they allow movement of the body part
 B. When the dressing must be changed frequently
 C. If the person is allergic to adhesive tape
 D. Because they stick well to the skin
64. A wet-to-wet dressing
 A. Is allowed to dry before being removed
 B. Is kept wet at all times
 C. Provides pressure to support the wound
 D. Prevents microbes from entering the wound
65. If you are assigned to change a dressing, which of these is important information to have?
 A. What kind of medication the person receives
 B. The person's diagnosis
 C. When pain medication was given and when it will take effect
 D. The person's age
66. You can make the person more comfortable when changing a dressing by
 A. Changing the dressing immediately after pain medication is given
 B. voiding body language that indicates the wound is unpleasant
 C. Encouraging the person to look at the wound
 D. Removing the dressing quickly by pulling the tape and dressing off all at once
67. When you are assigned to change dressings, you should
 A. Follow Standard Precautions and the Bloodborne Pathogen Standard
 B. Use sterile technique
 C. Wear gloves only to remove old dressings
 D. Use one pair of gloves throughout the dressing change
68. Binders promote healing because they
 A. Prevent infection
 B. Prevent drainage
 C. Support wounds and hold dressings in place
 D. Prevent bleeding
69. A binder should be applied
 A. With firm, even pressure over the area
 B. With safety pins positioned where they are easy to reach
 C. Very loosely to prevent interfering with movement
 D. Only once a day and be removed only during AM care
70. When heat is first applied to the skin
 A. Blood vessels in the area dilate
 B. Tissues receive less oxygen
 C. Blood flow decreases
 D. Blood vessels constrict

71. When heat is applied for too long, a complication that occurs is
    A. Blood vessels dilate
    B. Blood flow increases
    C. Blood vessels constrict
    D. More nutrients reach the area
72. Moist heat applications have lower temperatures than dry heat applications because
    A. Dry heat penetrates more deeply
    B. Dry heat cannot cause burns
    C. Moist heat has greater and faster effects than dry heat
    D. Moist heat has a slower effect than dry heat
73. Heat and cold applications are applied for no longer than
    A. 1 hour
    B. 30 minutes
    C. 15 to 20 minutes
    D. 4 hours
74. When a warm or cold application is in place, you should check the area
    A. Every 15 to 20 minutes
    B. Every 5 minutes
    C. About every 30 minutes
    D. Once an hour
75. When giving a sitz bath
    A. Give the person privacy for the entire time
    B. Observe for signs of weakness, faintness, or fatigue
    C. Observe for signs of swelling in the perineal area
    D. Check the person every 15 minutes
76. When warm or cold applications are in place, you should report if
    A. The skin is warm and red with a heat application
    B. The person tells you the cold application has relieved some of the pain
    C. The skin appears pale, white, gray, or bluish in color
    D. The person is slightly chilled and asks for an extra blanket
77. When a person has hyperthermia, ice packs are applied to
    A. The abdomen
    B. The extremities
    C. The head, neck, underarms, and groin
    D. The back

FILL IN THE BLANKS

78. Write out the meaning of each abbreviation.

    A. C _____

    B. F _____

    C. GI _____

    D. ID _____

    E. PPE _____

79. What are common causes of wounds?
    A. _____
    B. _____
    C. _____
    D. _____
    E. _____

80. You can cause a skin tear when moving, repositioning, and transferring by holding on to a person's arm or leg _____.

81. List ways to prevent skin tears:

    A. Improve hydration by offering the person _____ _____.

    B. What kind of clothing would be helpful? _____ _____.

    C. Nail care of the person _____ _____.

    D. Lift and turn the person with an _____ _____.

    E. Support the arms and legs with _____ _____.

    F. Pad _____.

    G. Keep your fingernails _____ and _____. Do not wear rings with _____.

82. Skin tears are portals _____ _____.

83. When the person has vascular ulcers, report any _____.

84. You are caring for a person with a disease that affects venous circulation. You notice her toenails are long and sharp. You should tell _____ because _____.

85. Compression (anti-embolism, AE, or TED) stockings help prevent the development of thrombi because they _____.

86. When you are delegated to apply compression (AE, TED) stockings, what observations should you report and record?
    A. _____
    B. _____
    C. _____
    D. _____
    E. _____
    F. _____
    G. _____
    H. _____
    I. _____

87. When you apply elastic bandages, the fingers or toes are exposed to allow _____.

88. After applying elastic bandages, you should check the fingers or toes for _____.

Also ask about _____
_____.

If any of these are noted, you should _____
_____.

89. What two diseases are common causes of arterial ulcers? _____

90. When a person has diabetes, what complications can occur with the following?

A. Nerves—Person may not feel _____.
Can develop _____.

B. Blood vessels—Blood flow_____.
What can occur? _____

91. Explain what can happen if a person with diabetes has the following foot problems.

A. Corns and calluses _____

_____

B. Ingrown toenails _____

_____

C. Hammer toes _____

_____

D. Dry and cracked skin _____

_____

92. With primary intention healing, the wound edges are held together with _____.

93. Secondary intention healing is used for _____ wounds. Because healing takes longer, the threat of _____ is great.

94. What should you do if you find a person's wound has dehiscence or evisceration? _____
_____

95. What observations would you make about wound appearance?

A. _____
B. _____
C. _____
D. _____
E. _____

96. When you are delegated to change a dressing, what may the nurse tell you to do if the old dressings stick to the wound? _____
_____

97. If the person has drainage from a wound, how is it measured?

A. _____
B. _____

98. What are purposes of a transparent adhesive film dressing?

A. _____
B. _____
C. _____
D. _____

99. What is the difference between wet-to-dry dressings and wet-to-wet dressings? _____
_____

100. When taping a dressing in place, the tape should not encircle the entire body part because _____
_____.

101. When delegated to apply dressings, what observations should be reported and recorded?

A. _____
B. _____
C. _____
D. _____
E. _____
F. _____
G. _____
H. _____
I. _____
J. _____
K. _____
L. _____
M. _____

102. What are the uses of warm applications?

A. _____
B. _____
C. _____
D. _____
E. _____

103. When you are caring for a confused person and heat or cold is applied, how can you know if the person is in pain? _____

_____

104. When you prepare an ice bag, collar, or glove, remove the excess air by _____.

105. When heat or cold applications are in place, you can help promote comfort and safety and maintain quality of life by

A. _____

B. _____

C. _____

D. _____

OPTIONAL LEARNING EXERCISES

You are assigned to care for Mrs. Stevens. She is 87 years old and has diabetes and high blood pressure. She walks with difficulty and spends most of her day sitting in her chair. She is somewhat overweight and tells you she had a knee replacement 5 years ago and had phlebitis after surgery. The nurse tells you to watch carefully for signs of vascular ulcers.

106. What risk factors does Mrs. Stevens have that may make her develop vascular ulcers?

A. _____

B. _____

C. _____

D. _____

E. _____

107. If arterial ulcers develop, they are usually found _____.

Mr. Hawkins, age 74, was in an automobile accident and has a wound on his leg that is large and open. It has become infected and he is being treated with antibiotics. When you are talking with him, he tells you he has smoked for 55 years and has poor circulation in his legs. He lives alone and generally eats takeout foods or cereal when he is at home.

108. Why is he receiving antibiotics? _____

_____

109. What side effect of the antibiotics can cause a problem that could interfere with healing? _____

_____

_____

110. What factors would increase Mr. Hawkins's risk for complications?

A. _____

B. _____

C. _____

D. _____

111. What is missing in Mr. Hawkins's diet that is needed to help in healing the wound? _____

_____

The nurse instructs you to apply a cold pack to Mrs. Wilson, a resident who has twisted her ankle. Use the information you learned in this chapter to answer the following questions.

112. What is the purpose of the cold application for this injury? _____

113. What can you use to make a cold pack if no commercial cold packs are available? _____

_____

_____

114. How will you protect Mrs. Wilson's skin? _____

_____

115. How often should you check the area under the cold pack? _____

116. How long should the cold pack remain in place?

_____

117. Mrs. Wilson tells you the cold pack is helping reduce the pain. She asks you to leave it in place when you start to remove it. What should you tell her? _____

INDEPENDENT LEARNING ACTIVITIES

- Role-play this situation with a classmate. One of you should act as the person and the other should act as the nursing assistant. Work together to answer the questions for each role.

  Situation: *Mr. Chavez is 45 years old and has a reddened area on his left calf. The doctor has ordered moist warm compresses to the area and the nurse has delegated this task to you.*

  - As the nursing assistant:
    - What questions would you ask the nurse before you applied the compresses?
    - How will you check the temperature of the compresses?
    - How will you keep the compresses at the correct temperature?
    - How often will you check the compresses? What will you observe when you check the area?
  - As Mr. Chavez:
    - How was the treatment explained to you?
    - How were you positioned? What did the nursing assistant do to make sure you were comfortable?
    - How did the compresses feel? Was the temperature maintained? How?
    - How often were the compresses checked?

Fill in the crossword by choosing words from this list.

Abrasion	Dilate	Gangrene	Thrombus
Compress	Edema	Hypothermia	Trauma
Constrict	Embolus	Incision	Ulcer
Contusion	Evisceration	Phlebitis	Wound
Dehiscence			

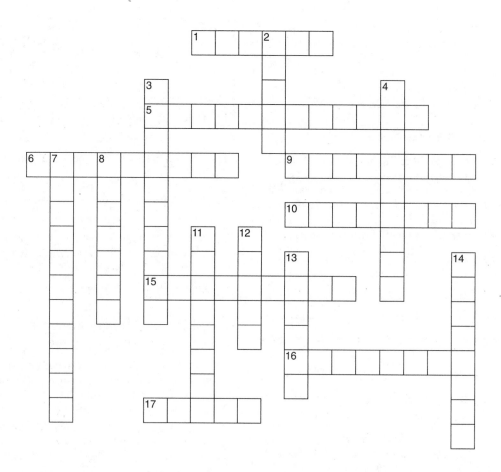

Across

1. Accident or violent act that injures the skin, mucous membranes, bones, and organs
5. Separation of the wound along with the protrusion of abdominal organs
6. Inflammation of a vein
9. Partial-thickness wound caused by scraping away or rubbing of the skin
10. Soft pad applied over a body area
15. Closed wound caused by a blow to the body
16. Blood clot
17. Swelling caused by fluid collecting in tissues

Down

2. Shallow or deep crater-like sore of the skin or mucous membranes
3. Separation of wound layers
4. To narrow
7. Very low body temperature
8. Blood clot that travels through the vascular system until it lodges in a distant vessel
11. Condition where there is death of tissue
12. Break in the skin or mucous membrane
13. To expand or open wider
14. Cut produced surgically by a sharp instrument

32 Pressure Injuries

Avoidable pressure injury   Colonized   Pressure injury
Bedfast   Eschar   Shear
Bony prominence   Friction   Slough
Chairfast   Intact skin   Unavoidable pressure injury

1. _____ is the presence of bacteria on the wound surface or in wound tissue; the person does not have signs and symptoms of an infection.

2. Dead tissue that is shed from the skin is _____ _____.

3. A pressure injury that develops from the improper use of the nursing process is an _____ _____.

4. A _____ is an area where the bone sticks out or projects from the flat surface of the body.

5. Thick, leathery dead tissue that may be loose or adhered to the skin is _____.

6. _____ occurs when layers of the skin rub against each other, or when the skin remains in place and underlying tissues move and stretch and tear underlying capillaries and blood vessels, causing tissue damage.

7. _____ means confined to bed.

8. The rubbing of one surface against another is _____ _____.

9. An _____ is a pressure injury that occurs despite efforts to prevent one through proper use of the nursing process.

10. A localized injury to the skin and/or underlying tissue, usually over a bony prominence, that results from pressure or pressure in combination with shear, is a _____.

11. _____ means confined to a chair.

12. _____ is normal skin without opening or damage.

CIRCLE THE BEST ANSWER

13. A pressure injury occurs because
    A. The person repositions himself or herself in the bed or chair
    B. The person drinks too many fluids
    C. Skin and underlying tissue is damaged by unrelieved pressure
    D. The person is repositioned too frequently

14. Older and disabled persons are at great risk for pressure injuries because of
    A. Acute illnesses
    B. Increased activity
    C. Age-related skin changes
    D. Good nutrition

15. The first sign of a pressure injury in an area would be
    A. Skin color over a bony area is reddened or a different color than surrounding tissue
    B. Swelling in the area
    C. A break in the skin
    D. Exposed tissue and some drainage from the area

16. Mrs. Greene keeps sliding down in bed. The nurse tells you to raise the head of the bed no more than 30 degrees. This position will prevent tissue damage caused by
    A. Pressure over hard surfaces
    B. Shearing
    C. Poor body mechanics
    D. Poor fluid balance

17. According to the CMS, the most common site of pressure injuries is
    A. The ears
    B. Underneath the breasts
    C. Between abdominal folds
    D. The sacrum

18. A Stage 3 pressure injury would have
    A. Intact skin with redness or different skin coloring over a bony prominence
    B. Exposed subcutaneous fat and slough
    C. Full-thickness tissue loss with muscle, tendon, and bone exposure
    D. A blister or shallow injury

19. When there is a purple or maroon localized area of discolored intact skin or a blood-filled blister, this is
    A. A Stage 2 pressure injury
    B. A suspected deep tissue injury
    C. An unstageable pressure injury
    D. A Stage 4 pressure injury
20. When following a repositioning schedule, a bedfast person should be repositioned
    A. According to the schedule in the person's care plan
    B. Three times a day
    C. Every 15 minutes
    D. As often as you have time
21. One way to prevent friction in the bed is to
    A. Use soap when cleansing the skin
    B. Rub or massage reddened areas
    C. Use pillows and blankets to prevent skin from being in contact with skin
    D. Powder sheets lightly
22. Bed cradles are used to
    A. Position the person in good body alignment
    B. Prevent pressure on the legs, feet, and toes
    C. Keep the heels off the bed
    D. Distribute body weight evenly

FILL IN THE BLANKS

23. Name the stage of pressure injury described in each of the following.

    A. The skin is gone and subcutaneous fat may be exposed. _____

    B. Full-thickness tissue loss occurs and the injury is covered by slough and/or eschar. _____ _____

    C. The skin is red with light skin or red, blue, or purple with dark skin. The color does not return to normal when the skin is relieved of pressure. _____

    D. Muscle, tendon, and bone are exposed and damaged. Eschar may be present. _____

    E. Usually this pressure injury is due to damage of underlying soft tissue from pressure and/or shear. _____

    F. The wound may involve an abrasion, blister, or shallow crater. _____

24. You can help prevent shearing by raising the head of the bed only _____. The care plan tells you

    A. _____

    B. _____

    C. _____

25. Explain how the following conditions place a person at risk for pressure injuries.

    A. Urinary or fecal incontinence _____ _____

    B. Poor nutrition _____ _____

    C. Poor fluid balance _____ _____

    D. Lowered mental awareness _____ _____

    E. Circulatory problems _____ _____

    F. Older person _____ _____

26. Explain how these protective devices help prevent pressure injuries.

    A. Bed cradle prevents pressure on _____ _____.

    B. Heel and elbow protectors prevent _____ _____ and _____.

    C. Heel and foot elevators raise _____ _____.

    D. Gel or fluid-filled pads and cushions _____ _____.

    E. Alternating air mattress overlays distribute _____ _____.

    F. Special beds distribute _____ _____. There is little pressure on _____.

27. List six examples of medical device-related pressure injuries (MDRPI)

    A. _____
    B. _____
    C. _____
    D. _____
    E. _____
    F. _____

OPTIONAL LEARNING EXERCISES

28. After admission to a nursing center, many pressure injuries develop with the first _____ after admission.

29. A person at risk can develop a pressure injury within _____ after the onset of pressure.

30. When handling, moving, and positioning a person, it is important to follow the _____ in the person's care plan.

   A. How often should a bedfast person be repositioned? _____

   B. How often should a chairfast person be repositioned? _____

   C. Remind a person sitting in a chair to shift their position every_____.

31. What are two ways pressure injuries can occur on the ears?

   A. _____

   B. _____

32. If you are interviewed by the CMS staff about pressure injuries, what questions may be asked?

   A. _____

   B. _____

   C. _____

   D. _____

   E. _____

INDEPENDENT LEARNING ACTIVITIES

- Take turns with a classmate and carry out these exercises. They will help you understand how a person who cannot move without assistance feels when pressure is unrelieved. NOTE: These exercises work best if the person wears thin clothing so the discomfort is more noticeable.
  - Place a pencil or similar hard object on the seat of a chair and have a classmate sit on the object for 10 minutes. Keep time and remind the person not to move, to make it more uncomfortable. Remember, persons at risk for pressure injuries often are unable to change position without assistance.
  - Position a classmate in bed, making sure the bed linens are wrinkled to form lumps under bony pressure points. (For example, place a wrinkle under the sacrum in the supine position or under the hip or shoulder in the lateral position.)
- Answer the following questions about the exercises done.
  - How long did it feel like when you were waiting for 10 minutes to pass?
  - How many times did you begin to reposition yourself without thinking about it?
  - How did the pressure areas feel when you completed the 10 minutes? What color was the area?
  - How will this exercise affect your care of persons who cannot move?

33 Hearing, Speech, and Vision Problems

FILL IN THE BLANKS: KEY TERMS

Aphasia
Blindness
Braille
Broca's aphasia
Cerumen
Deafness

Expressive aphasia
Expressive-receptive aphasia
Global aphasia
Hearing loss
Low vision
Mixed aphasia

Motor aphasia
Receptive aphasia
Tinnitus
Vertigo
Wernicke aphasia

1. _____ is a touch reading and writing system that uses raised dots for each letter of the alphabet.

2. Another name for receptive aphasia is _____ _____.

3. Another name for earwax is _____ _____.

4. _____is dizziness.

5. A ringing, roaring, hissing, or buzzing sound in the ears is _____.

6. The total or partial loss of the ability to use or understand language; a language disorder resulting from damage to parts of the brain responsible for language is _____.

7. _____ is not being able to hear the normal range of sounds associated with normal hearing.

8. _____is difficulty expressing or sending out thoughts.

9. Eyesight that cannot be corrected with eyeglasses, contact lenses, medicine, or surgery is _____ _____.

10. _____ is also called expressive aphasia or Broca's aphasia.

11. A hearing loss in which it is impossible for the person to understand speech through hearing alone is _____.

12. Another name for expressive aphasia or motor aphasia is _____.

13. _____ is also called expressive-receptive aphasia or mixed aphasia.

14. The absence of sight is _____ _____.

15. Difficulty expressing or sending out thoughts and difficulty understanding language is _____ _____.

16. Another name for expressive-receptive aphasia or global aphasia is _____.

17. Difficulty understanding language is _____ _____; also called Wernicke aphasia.

CIRCLE THE BEST ANSWER

18. If a person has chronic otitis media, the person may develop
    A. Vertigo
    B. Permanent hearing loss
    C. Diarrhea
    D. Nausea and vomiting

19. How would you know a person with dementia has otitis media?
    A. The person would tell you he or she has pain
    B. The person would not be able to hear you
    C. You might notice the person tugging or pulling at one or both ears
    D. The person would have tinnitus

20. If you are caring for a person who has Meniere's disease, it is important to
    A. Prevent falls
    B. Assist the person to move quickly
    C. Keep the lights in the room very bright
    D. Encourage the person to be active

21. Which of these is a preventable cause of hearing loss?
    A. Aging
    B. Heredity
    C. Exposure to very loud music
    D. Birth defects

22. When you are caring for a person with a hearing loss, which of these would help communication?
    A. Gain the person's attention by lightly touching the person's arm
    B. Speak as loudly as possible
    C. Make sure the radio or TV is playing in the room
    D. Sit next to the person out of his or her line of sight
23. When you are caring for a person with a hearing aid, follow the nurse's directions and the manufacturer's instructions before
    A. Turning the hearing aid off at night
    B. Inserting a new battery if needed
    C. Cleaning the hearing aid
    D. Removing the battery at night
24. If a person has expressive aphasia, he or she
    A. Would not understand simple language
    B. Would speak in complete sentences
    C. Would have difficulty hearing what was said
    D. Might speak in single words or put words in the wrong order
25. When a person is speech-impaired, he or she
    A. Speaks rapidly in long sentences
    B. Often becomes angry and depressed
    C. Usually does not understand what is being said
    D. Needs to have his or her speech corrected
26. An effective measure to use when caring for a speech-impaired person is to
    A. Speak in a child-like way
    B. Ask the person questions to which you know the answer
    C. Use long, involved sentences
    D. Make sure the TV and radio are loud
27. When a person has glaucoma, he or she may have difficulty seeing objects
    A. That are far away
    B. To the right or left of him or her
    C. Directly in front of him or her
    D. That are bright colors
28. A risk factor for glaucoma is
    A. Everyone over 40 years of age
    B. Caucasian and Asians over 40 years of age
    C. Those with a family history of glaucoma
    D. Those who have poor nutrition
29. Cataracts most commonly are caused by
    A. Aging
    B. Injury
    C. Increased pressure in the eye
    D. Surgery
30. When a person has had eye surgery for cataracts, the care includes
    A. Removing the eye shield or patch for naps and at night
    B. Explaining the location of food on the food tray
    C. Reminding the person not to rub or press the affected eye
    D. Placing the overbed table on the operative side

31. After cataract surgery, report to the nurse if
    A. The person complains of eye pain or has eye drainage
    B. Glasses need to be cleaned
    C. The person needs help with his or her food tray
    D. The person asks for help with basic needs
32. If a person has dry age-related macular degeneration (AMD)
    A. It can be treated with surgery
    B. The person will need to use eye drops for the rest of his or her life
    C. The person will eventually be blind
    D. The person will need to wear corrective glasses to see clearly
33. Which of these measures can reduce the risk of AMD?
    A. Exposing the eyes to sunlight
    B. Eating a healthy diet high in green leafy vegetables and fish
    C. Eating a diet high in red meats
    D. Decreasing the amount of exercise
34. Diabetic retinopathy is the result of
    A. High blood pressure
    B. Tiny blood vessels in the retina being damaged as a complication of diabetes
    C. Pressure increasing in the eye
    D. The lens becoming cloudy
35. A person with low vision
    A. Can be fitted with glasses that will improve vision to normal
    B. Can have corrective surgery to improve the vision
    C. Learns to use one or more visual and adaptive devices
    D. Is unable to see anything
36. A person who is legally blind
    A. Sees at 20 feet what a person with normal vision sees at 20 feet
    B. Is always totally blind
    C. Is usually blind from birth
    D. Sees at 20 feet what a person with normal vision sees at 200 feet
37. When you enter the room of a blind person, you should first
    A. Touch the person to let him or her know you are there
    B. Speak loudly to make sure the person knows you are there
    C. Make sure the lights are bright
    D. Identify yourself by giving your name, title, and reason for being there
38. When a person is blind, you should avoid
    A. Rearranging furniture and equipment
    B. Using words such as "see," "look," or "read"
    C. Letting the person move about
    D. Letting the person perform self-care

171

39. When you offer to assist a blind person to walk, it is best if you
    A. Walk slightly behind the person
    B. Walk one step ahead of the person
    C. Grasp the person's arm firmly to guide him or her
    D. Walk very slowly to allow the person to take small steps
40. If a blind person uses a cane, you can assist by
    A. Grasping the person by the arm holding the cane
    B. Coming up behind the person and grasping his or her elbow
    C. Giving the person verbal cues to avoid objects in the way
    D. Asking if you can assist before trying to help
41. If a blind person uses a guide dog, you
    A. Take the person by the arm on the side opposite the dog
    B. May pet, feed, or distract the dog
    C. May give the dog commands to avoid danger
    D. Understand that the dog sees for the person and is trained to keep the person safe
42. Eyeglasses should be cleaned with
    A. Cleaning solution or warm water
    B. Boiling water
    C. Detergent
    D. Dry cleansing tissues
43. When cleaning an ocular prosthesis (artificial eye), you should
    A. Wash the prosthesis with strong soap and hot water
    B. Wash the eyelid and eyelashes using sterile water and sterile wipes
    C. Use a small brush to remove any debris from the artificial eye
    D. Rinse the eye with sterile water before the person inserts the eye

FILL IN THE BLANKS

44. Write out the meaning of each abbreviation.

    A. AFB _____

    B. AMD _____

    C. ASL _____

    D. HOH _____

45. Otitis media often begins with _____
    _____.

46. If a person has chronic otitis media, it can cause permanent _____.

47. When a person has Meniere's disease, symptoms or attacks can occur _____ or just _____
    _____.

48. With Meniere's disease, the person should not walk alone in case _____.

49. What are examples of noises that can cause hearing loss?

    A. _____

    B. _____

    C. _____

    D. _____

50. When persons are 75 years of age or older, about _____ have a hearing loss.

51. Symptoms of hearing loss include

    A. _____

    B. _____

    C. _____

    D. _____

    E. _____

    F. _____

    G. _____

    H. _____

    I. _____

    J. _____

    K. _____

52. If a woman is speaking to a hearing-impaired person, why should she adjust the pitch of her voice? _____
    _____
    _____

53. Why is it important for a person with a hearing loss to see your face when you are speaking to him or her? _____
    _____

54. What are common causes of speech disorders?

    A. _____

    B. _____

    C. _____

55. If a person has apraxia, the brain _____
    _____.

56. Measures you can use to communicate with a speech-impaired person include:

    A. Listen and give _____

    B. Repeat _____

    C. Write down _____

    D. Allow the person _____

    E. Watch _____

57. When a person has expressive aphasia, the person knows what _____.

Thinking is _____.

58. When a person has receptive aphasia, the person may speak in _____ that have no _____.

59. Symptoms of glaucoma include:

A. Peripheral vision is _____ and the person sees through a _____.

B. Blurred

C. Halos

60. Medications and surgery are used with glaucoma to _____ and _____.

61. Most cataracts are caused by _____. Other risk factors are

A. _____

B. _____

C. _____

D. _____

E. _____

62. When you are caring for a person after cataract surgery, an eye shield is worn as directed and is worn for _____.

63. When assisting a blind or visually impaired person, what can be done to provide a consistent meal time setting?

A. _____

B. _____

C. _____

D. _____

E. _____

F. _____

64. A person with age-related macular degeneration (AMD) would develop a blind spot _____.

65. Everyone with diabetes is at risk for _____.

66. How can a person with low vision use a computer as an adaptive device?

A. _____

B. _____

67. When you orient a person with low or no vision to the room, why do you let the person move about the room? _____

OPTIONAL LEARNING EXERCISES

Mr. Herman is an 85-year-old man with hearing loss that has developed as he has become older. Answer the following questions about his care.

68. Two nursing assistants are caring for Mr. Herman—a male and a female. They notice that he answers questions asked by the male nursing assistant more quickly. What is the likely reason for this? _____

69. The nursing assistants have found that Mr. Herman is alert and oriented. They are surprised when Joan, another nursing assistant, tells them he is "senile." Why would Joan make this statement? _____

70. Mr. Herman says he is too tired to go to the game room for a party. He says no one likes him. What are some reasons for his actions and statements?

A. Tired because _____

B. No one likes him because _____

71. When giving care, the nursing assistant turns off the TV and radio in Mr. Herman's room. Why is this done? _____

You are caring for Mrs. Sanchez, who is legally blind because of glaucoma. Answer the following questions about her care.

72. When you enter the room, you notice that Mrs. Sanchez is looking at her mail with a magnifying glass. How is this possible, since you thought she was blind? _____

73. When you enter the room, Mrs. Sanchez asks you to adjust the blinds. Why? _____

74. When you are helping Mrs. Sanchez to move about the room, you allow her to touch the furniture and equipment. Why? _____

173

INDEPENDENT LEARNING ACTIVITIES

- Cover your ears so you cannot hear clearly. Use one of these methods or one that you devise:
    - Commercial earplugs
    - Cotton plugs in ears
    - Cover ears with earmuffs or similar devices
- Keep your ears covered and your hearing muffled for at least 1 hour as you go about your daily activities. A wise student will not wear earplugs during class time! Answer the following questions about the experience.
    - How did you find yourself compensating for the hearing loss? Turning up the TV or radio? Asking others to write out information? Staying away from others? Getting angry or frustrated?
    - When you could not understand someone, what did you do? Ask them to repeat? Ask them to speak louder? Answer even if you were unsure of what was said? Not respond at all?
    - If you answered when unsure, what was your response? Did you tend to agree or disagree with the speaker? Why?
    - What methods listed in the chapter were helpful? What other methods did you use to understand what was being said? Watching the speaker? Cupping a hand around an ear?
    - How will this experience assist you when you care for a person with a hearing loss?
- Cover your eyes with a blindfold so you cannot see. Keep the blindfold on for at least 1 hour as you go about your normal activities. Have someone act as a guide during this time. In addition to your normal activities, include the activities listed.
    - Go outside with your guide and cross a street.
    - Visit a store or restaurant with your guide.
    - Eat a simple snack or meal.
    - Go to the toilet, wash your hands, and comb your hair.
    - Have your guide take you to a public area, place you in a chair or on a bench, and leave you alone for 5 to 10 minutes.

NOTE: You may wish to carry out this exercise using the blindfold and using this alternate method. If you wear glasses, cover the center of the lens with a coating of petroleum jelly. This will simulate the vision experienced by a person with cataracts. Answer the following questions for either or both experiences.

- How did you feel when you were unable to see what was going on around you? What noises or other sensory stimulants did you notice?
- When you were crossing the street, how did you feel? Safe? Frightened?
- When you were in a public area, what did you notice? How did you feel? How did others respond to you?
- How comfortable did you feel about eating when you could not see the food? How were you able to locate the food? What problems did you have?
- How did you manage in the bathroom? Were you able to find the equipment you needed? How competent did you feel about carrying out hand washing and grooming without being able to see?
- What were your feelings when left alone in a public area for 5 to 10 minutes? How long did it *seem* to be before your guide returned? What concerns did you have? Safety? Fear of injury? Desertion?
- How will this experience assist you when caring for a person with a vision loss?

Have a group discussion with your classmates after they have all carried out the exercises to simulate vision and hearing problems. Answer the following questions.

- Which disability did you find the most difficult to tolerate? Why?
- If you had to live with one of these disabilities, which one would you choose? Why?
- What happened during these exercises that surprised you about being unable to see or hear? How does this discovery change your attitude about the disabilities?

34 Cancer, Immune System, and Skin Disorders

FILL IN THE BLANKS: KEY TERMS

Autoimmune disorder   Malignant tumor   Stem cells
Benign tumor   Metastasis   Stomatitis
Cancer   Port   Tumor

1. A _____ is a tumor that invades and destroys nearby tissue and can spread to other body parts.

2. Inflammation of the mouth is _____
   _____.

3. A tumor that does not spread to other body parts is a _____.

4. A new growth of abnormal cells that may be benign or malignant is a _____.

5. The spread of cancer to other body parts is _____
   _____.

6. Another name for a malignant tumor is _____
   _____.

7. An implanted device in the body that allows medications or fluids to be given into a vein is a _____
   _____.

8. An _____ is a condition where the body attacks itself.

9. Cells with the potential to develop into many different types of cells in the body are _____
   _____.

CIRCLE THE BEST ANSWER

10. Benign tumors
    A. Do not spread to other body parts
    B. Invade healthy tissue
    C. Are always very small
    D. Divide in an orderly and controlled way

11. A factor that increases the risk of cancer is
    A. Limiting exposure to sun
    B. Smoking and drinking alcohol
    C. A diet high in fresh fruits and vegetables
    D. Taking multivitamins and minerals

12. When surgery is done to treat cancer
    A. It always cures the cancer
    B. It may relieve pain from advanced cancer
    C. The person will continue to have pain
    D. The person loses body hair

13. When you care for a person receiving radiation therapy, you might expect the person to
    A. Need physical therapy
    B. Need special skin care measures
    C. Have dressings over the site
    D. Have weight gain

14. Chemotherapy involves
    A. X-ray beams aimed at the tumor
    B. Giving medications that prevent the production of certain hormones
    C. Therapy to help the immune system
    D. Giving medications that kill cells

15. While caring for a person receiving chemotherapy, she tells you she is upset because her hair is falling out. You know that
    A. The hair often falls out when a person receives chemotherapy
    B. This is symptom of her disease
    C. You should report this to the nurse at once
    D. You should change the subject so she will not be so upset

16. When hormone therapy is used to treat cancer, a woman may experience
    A. Stomatitis
    B. Flu-like symptoms
    C. Weight gain, hot flashes, and fluid retention
    D. Burns and skin breakdown

17. A person with cancer may complain of constipation because of
    A. The side effects of pain-relief medication
    B. Pain
    C. The side effects from cancer treatments
    D. Fluid and nutrition intake

18. When a person has cancer and expresses anger, fear, and depression, you can help most by
    A. Telling the person not to worry or get upset
    B. Giving the person privacy and time alone
    C. Being there when needed and listening to the person
    D. Changing the subject to distract the person

175

19. Treatment for autoimmune disorders is aimed at
    A. Curing the illness
    B. Controlling the autoimmune response
    C. Removing the affected organs
    D. Preventing metastasis
20. HIV is *not* spread by
    A. Blood
    B. Semen
    C. Sneezing or coughing
    D. Breast milk
21. To protect yourself from HIV and AIDS, you should
    A. Avoid all body fluids when giving care
    B. Refuse to give care to persons diagnosed with these diseases
    C. Follow Standard Precautions and the Bloodborne Pathogen Standard when giving care
    D. Always use sterile technique when giving any care
22. Shingles is caused by the same virus that causes
    A. HIV
    B. Measles
    C. Chicken pox
    D. Mumps

FILL IN THE BLANKS

23. Write out the abbreviations.
    A. AIDS _____
    B. HIV _____
    C. IV _____
24. Cancer is the _____ most common cause of death in the United States.
25. The goals of cancer treatment are
    A. _____
    B. _____
    C. _____
26. Some signs and symptoms of cancer are
    A. _____
    B. _____
    C. _____
    D. _____
    E. _____
    F. _____
    G. _____
    H. _____
    I. _____
    J. _____

27. With radiation therapy, skin care measures are needed at the treatment site because _____ and _____ can occur.
28. When chemotherapy is used, it affects _____ _____ cells and _____ cells.
29. When a person is receiving chemotherapy, what side effects might occur?
    A. _____
    B. _____
    C. _____
30. When a person has an autoimmune disorder, it means the _____ system can cause disease by attacking _____ _____.
31. Acquired immunodeficiency syndrome (AIDS) is caused by a _____ that attacks the _____.
32. How does the human immunodeficiency virus (HIV) enter the bloodstream? _____ _____
33. When caring for a person with HIV, the main threat to health care workers is from _____ _____.
34. Those at risk for developing shingles are
    A. _____
    B. _____
    C. _____
35. Treatment for eczema includes:
    A. _____
    B. _____
    C. _____
    D. _____
    E. _____
    F. _____

Mrs. Myers is a 62-year-old woman who is having chemotherapy to treat cancer. She has not been eating well and complains of feeling very tired. When you assist her with personal care, you notice a large amount of hair on her pillow. Answer the following questions about Mrs. Myers and her care.

36. Mrs. Myers may not be eating well because the chemotherapy _____ the gastrointestinal tract and causes _____, _____, and _____ _____.

37. She may also have _____, which is called stomatitis. You can help relieve the discomfort from this side effect when you provide _____.

38. What is causing Mrs. Myers to lose her hair? _____ _____

    This condition is called _____ _____.

Answer this question about HIV.

39. What are reasons that many older persons do not consider themselves at risk for HIV?

    A. _____

    B. _____

    C. _____

- Interview a person who has been treated for cancer and ask the following questions.
  - How was the person told about the diagnosis of cancer? What kind of reaction did the person have? Was he or she frightened, angry, depressed, etc.?
  - What treatment was used to treat the cancer? What side effects did the person have? Did any of the treatments affect body image? Did the treatment leave any permanent disfigurement?
  - How did the cancer and the treatment affect the person's life? How able was the person to carry on normal activities, such as caring for family members or working?
  - How long ago did this occur? How is the person feeling now? What long-term effects have the cancer and treatments had on the person?

- If you have cared for a person with HIV/AIDS, answer the following questions about the experience. If you have not, think about how you might feel in that situation.
  - How did you react when you knew the person had HIV? What questions did you ask the nurse? The person?
  - What special precautions did you take when you were caring for the person?
  - How would you feel if you found out a person you had been caring for was diagnosed with HIV? How would this diagnosis affect the care you give?
  - When you use Standard Precautions and the Bloodborne Pathogen Standard for *all* persons you care for, how does that affect your reaction to an HIV patient?

35 Nervous System and Musculoskeletal Disorders

FILL IN THE BLANKS: KEY TERMS

Amputation
Arthritis
Arthroplasty
Closed fracture
Compound fracture

Fracture
Gangrene
Hemiplegia
Open fracture
Paralysis

Paraplegia
Quadriplegia
Simple fracture
Tetraplegia

1. An open fracture is also called a _____ _____.

2. Another name for quadriplegia is _____ _____.

3. The removal of all or part of an extremity is _____.

4. A _____ is when the bone is broken but the skin is intact.

5. _____ is paralysis and loss of sensory function in the arms, legs, and trunk. It can also be called tetraplegia.

6. Paralysis on one side of the body is _____.

7. Joint inflammation is _____ _____.

8. A closed fracture can also be called _____ _____.

9. A _____ is a broken bone.

10. An _____ occurs when the broken bone has come through the skin. It is also called a compound fracture.

11. An _____ is the surgical replacement of a joint.

12. Paralysis and loss of sensory function in the legs is _____.

13. A condition in which there is death of tissue is _____.

14. _____ is loss of motor function, loss of sensation, or both.

CIRCLE THE BEST ANSWER

15. The leading cause of disability in adults in the United States is
    A. Heart disease
    B. Cancer
    C. Stroke
    D. Diabetes

16. If a person has symptoms of a stroke that last a few minutes, it means that
    A. The person has had a transient ischemic attack (TIA)
    B. It is not a dangerous situation because it was temporary
    C. The person needs to lie down at once
    D. No further treatment is needed

17. Which of these persons has the most risk factors for stroke?
    A. A 70-year-old White man with hypertension and diabetes
    B. A 50-year-old White woman who smokes and is slightly overweight
    C. A 70-year-old African-American man who has hypertension and diabetes
    D. A 75-year-old Asian woman who is inactive and has normal blood pressure and diabetes

18. If a person who has had a stroke ignores and forgets about the weaker side of the body, it is called
    A. Paralysis
    B. Incontinence
    C. Aphasia
    D. Neglect

19. When you are caring for a person who has had a stroke, the call light and other objects
    A. Should be removed from the room
    B. Are placed on the weak side of the body
    C. Are placed on the strong side of the body
    D. Are given to a family member to use for the person

20. Safety measures are needed for a person with Parkinson's disease to prevent
    A. Problems with communication
    B. Elimination difficulties
    C. Falls and injury
    D. Emotional changes
21. Multiple sclerosis (MS) is a disease that
    A. Is an acute illness from which the person recovers completely
    B. Always follows the same course with the same symptoms
    C. May have long periods without symptoms before a flare-up occurs
    D. Is easily treated with medications
22. When a person has secondary-progressive MS
    A. The symptoms gradually disappear with partial or complete recovery
    B. The person has no remissions
    C. More symptoms appear with each flare-up and the person's condition declines
    D. This stage follows relapsing-remitting MS
23. A person with amyotrophic lateral sclerosis (ALS) would be
    A. Confused and disoriented
    B. Able to walk with assistance even as the disease progresses
    C. Incontinent of bladder and bowel functions
    D. Unable to move the arms, legs, and body
24. If a person is in a persistent vegetative state after a traumatic brain injury, he or she
    A. Is unconscious and unaware and cannot be aroused
    B. Is unconscious and has sleep-wake cycles and alert periods
    C. Is unresponsive but can be aroused briefly
    D. Is unconscious and has sleep-wake cycles and alert periods. These symptoms last longer than 1 month
25. A person who has a spinal cord injury in the lumbar region will likely have
    A. Quadriplegia
    B. Paraplegia
    C. Hemiplegia
    D. Tetraplegia
26. When caring for a person with paralysis, it is important to
    A. Turn and reposition the person at least every 4 hours
    B. Check bath water, heat applications, and food for proper temperature
    C. Encourage the person to do as much as he or she can to maintain mobility
    D. Encourage deep-breathing and coughing exercises to prevent pneumonia
27. Autonomic dysreflexia occurs in a person who has paralysis
    A. Of any kind
    B. Above the mid-thoracic level
    C. In the lumbar region
    D. That is incomplete

28. If you are caring for a person with autonomic dysreflexia, report to the nurse at once if
    A. The person has sweating above the level of the injury
    B. The blood pressure is low
    C. The person complains of pain below the level of the injury
    D. The person has sweating below the level of the injury
29. If a person is at risk for autonomic dysreflexia, it is best if only the nurse
    A. Gives basic care
    B. Makes sure the catheter is draining properly
    C. Checks for fecal impactions or gives an enema
    D. Repositions the person at least every 2 hours
30. Osteoarthritis differs from rheumatoid arthritis because osteoarthritis
    A. Is an inflammatory disease
    B. Occurs with aging
    C. Means that the person does not feel well
    D. Occurs on both sides of the body
31. When you are caring for a person with osteoarthritis, which of these would be most helpful to the person?
    A. Allow the person to stay in bed as much as desired
    B. Keep the room cool, as osteoarthritis improves with cold temperatures
    C. Help the person use good body mechanics and good posture and get regular rest
    D. Tell the person not to exercise, as the exercise will prevent healing
32. If you are caring for a person who has rheumatoid arthritis and the person has a flare-up of the disease, you should
    A. Make sure the person exercises more often
    B. Position the person in good alignment
    C. Encourage the person to rest in bed as much as possible
    D. Instruct the person to avoid any type of exercise that affects the joints
33. When caring for a person who has had a total hip replacement, it is correct to
    A. Have a high, firm chair with arms for the person to use when out of bed
    B. Remove the abductor splint or pillow when turning the person in bed
    C. Remind the person to cross his or her legs when sitting in a chair
    D. Instruct the person that he or she should only use a bedpan for elimination
34. Which of these will help strengthen bones in a person at risk for osteoporosis?
    A. Bedrest
    B. Decreased calcium intake
    C. Exercise of weight-bearing joints
    D. Increased alcohol and caffeine intake

179

35. When a closed reduction and external fixation is done following a fracture
    A. The bone is moved back into place and is not exposed
    B. Surgery is used to expose the bone and move it into alignment
    C. Pins, screws, or wires are attached to keep the bones in place
    D. A cast is applied without moving the bone ends into alignment
36. When a person has a newly applied plaster cast, it will dry in
    A. 2 to 4 hours
    B. 3 to 4 days
    C. 24 to 48 hours
    D. 12 to 24 hours
37. You can prevent flat spots on a cast by
    A. Positioning the cast on a hard, flat surface
    B. Supporting the entire cast with pillows
    C. Using your fingertips to lift the cast
    D. Covering the cast with a blanket
38. If a person complains of numbness in a part that is in a cast, you should
    A. Tell the person to move the limb a little to relieve the numbness
    B. Reposition the person to help the numbness
    C. Gently rub the exposed toes or fingers
    D. Tell the nurse at once
39. When giving care to a person in traction, you should
    A. Put bottom linens on the bed from the top down
    B. Remove the weights while you are giving care
    C. Turn the person from side to side to change the bed and to give care
    D. Assist the person to use the commode chair when needed
40. When caring for a person who has had surgery to repair a hip fracture, the operated leg should be
    A. Abducted at all times
    B. Adducted at all times
    C. Exercised with range of motion exercises every 4 hours
    D. Positioned to keep the leg in external rotation
41. When you assist a person to get up in a chair after hip surgery
    A. Place the chair on the affected side
    B. Place the chair on the unaffected side
    C. Have a low, soft chair for the person to use
    D. Remind the person to cross the legs
42. If a person complains of pain in the amputated part
    A. Report this to the nurse at once
    B. Assume that the person is confused or disoriented
    C. Reassure the person that this is a normal reaction
    D. Tell the person that this a temporary sensation that will go away shortly

FILL IN THE BLANKS

43. Write out the meaning of each abbreviation.
    A. ADL _____
    B. AKA _____
    C. ALS _____
    D. BKA _____
    E. CVA _____
    F. EMS _____
    G. FAST _____
    H. MS _____
    I. RA _____
    J. ROM _____
    K. TBI _____
    L. TIA _____
44. What risk factors for stroke cannot be controlled?
    A. _____
    B. _____
    C. _____
    D. _____
45. What are the warning signs of stroke?
    A. _____
    B. _____
    C. _____
    D. _____
    E. _____
46. What are signs and symptoms of Parkinson's disease?
    A. _____
    B. _____
    C. _____
    D. _____
    E. _____
47. Which type of multiple sclerosis causes the person's condition to gradually decline with more and more symptoms and no remissions? _____
    _____

48. What effect does amyotrophic lateral sclerosis have on

A. Mind, intelligence, and memory _____
_____

B. Senses _____
_____

C. Bowel and bladder functions _____
_____

D. Motor nerve cells _____
_____

49. If a person survives traumatic brain injury, some permanent _____. Disabilities depend on the _____ and _____ of the injury.

50. When caring for a person with paralysis, you must check the person often if he or she is unable to use _____.

51. Range of motion exercises are important when caring for a person with paralysis because they will maintain _____ and prevent _____.

52. Raising the head of the bed 45 degrees or more for a person with a spinal cord injury may relieve signs and symptoms of _____.

53. If you are caring for a person with osteoarthritis, exercise is important because it

A. Decreases _____

B. Increases _____

C. Improves _____

D. Also helps with _____
and promotes _____

54. Rest and joint care are also used to treat osteoarthritis. Explain how these treatments help.

A. Regular rest _____

B. Canes and walkers _____
_____

C. Splints _____

55. Which type of arthritis generally develops between the ages of 20 and 50? _____

56. What are the treatment goals for rheumatoid arthritis?

A. _____

B. _____

C. _____

D. _____

57. When caring for a person who has had a hip replacement, what measures are used to protect the hip?

A. _____

B. _____

C. _____

D. _____

E. _____

F. _____

G. _____

H. _____

58. List how these risk factors affect developing osteoporosis.

A. Women's risk increases after _____
_____

B. Family _____

C. Weight _____
_____

59. Calcium is lost from bone if it does not _____. What happens to the bone when calcium is lost? _____
_____

60. What joints are exercised to help prevent osteoporosis? What exercises are often used on these joints? _____

61. When a person has a cast on a fracture, what do these symptoms mean?

A. Pain _____

B. Odor _____

C. Numbness _____

D. Cool skin _____

E. Hot skin _____

62. When caring for a person in traction, what would you do in these situations?

A. Weights are touching the floor _____
_____

B. Rope is frayed _____
_____

C. Perform ROM exercises on _____
_____

D. Usual position allowed _____
_____

E. Redness, drainage, and odor noted at pin site _____
_____

F. Person complains of numbness _____
_____

Chapter **35 Nervous System and Musculoskeletal Disorders**

63. After hip surgery, what positions of the hip are avoided?

A. _____

B. _____

C. _____

D. _____

64. When turning and positioning a person after hip surgery, usually the person is not positioned on _____ _____.

65. If the person has an internal fixation device, the operative leg is not elevated when sitting in a chair because _____ _____.

66. _____ is a common cause of vascular changes that can lead to an amputation.

OPTIONAL LEARNING EXERCISES

You are caring for Mrs. Huber, who has had a stroke. Questions 67 to 71 relate to Mrs. Huber and her care. Explain the reasons why the care plan gives each of the following instructions.

67. Position Mrs. Huber in a side-lying position. _____ _____

68. Approach Mrs. Huber from the unaffected side. _____

69. Give Mrs. Huber a dysphagia diet. _____ _____

70. Apply elastic stockings as part of her care. _____ _____

71. Perform range of motion exercises. _____ _____

72. List the ages when the following diseases are most likely to occur.
A. Parkinson's disease_____ _____
B. Multiple sclerosis _____
C. Amyotrophic lateral sclerosis _____ _____

You are caring for two persons who have arthritis. Read the information about each of them and answer Questions 73 to 75 about these two persons.

- *Mr. Miller is 78 years old. He worked in construction for many years and did heavy physical work. He complains about pain in his hips and right knee. His fingers are deformed by arthritis and interfere with good range of motion.*
- *Mrs. Haxton is 40 years old. She has swelling, warmth, and tenderness in her wrists, several finger joints on both hands and both knees. She tells you that she has had arthritis for about 10 years and it "comes and goes." At present, Mrs. Haxton has a temperature of 100.2°F and she states that she is tired and does not feel well.*

73. Which type of arthritis does Mr. Miller probably have? _____ At what time of day is he likely to have more joint stiffness? _____

74. Mrs. Haxton most likely has _____ arthritis. She complains of not feeling well because the arthritis affects _____ as well as the joints.

75. It is cold and raining today. Which of these persons is more likely to be affected by the weather? _____ _____

INDEPENDENT LEARNING EXERCISES

- Many people have had a fracture at some time. If you have had a broken bone, answer these questions about your experience.
  - When did you know the bone was broken? Immediately? Several hours or days later? How did you find out?
  - What signs and symptoms did you have? Describe these signs and symptoms.
  - What treatment was done? Cast? Surgery? Pins, plates, screws, or traction? Describe the treatment and how you felt about it.
  - How did the fracture affect your day-to-day life? Work? School? Leisure activities?
  - What changes were needed for you to carry out ADL? How much help did you need from others? How did the need for help make you feel?
  - How was your mobility affected? Walking? Getting out of bed or out of a chair? Driving?
  - What discomfort did you have during the healing process? With the cast or surgical site?
  - What permanent or long-term problems happened? Periodic pain? Limited mobility?
- Try this experiment to have a "fractured leg." It will help you understand how a fracture interferes with normal activities. Make an immobilizer for your leg. Use one of the methods suggested or devise one of your own.
  - Find four pieces of sturdy cardboard that are long enough to reach from the ankle to mid-thigh. Place them on the front, back, and sides of the leg and secure them with elastic bandages or cloth strips. You should not be able to bend the knee.
  - Use several layers of newspaper or magazines and wrap them around the leg from the ankle to above the knee. Secure them with elastic bandages or cloth strips. You should not be able to bend the knee.

- After the "cast" is in place, leave it on for 1 to 2 hours and go about your normal routine. Answer these questions about the experience.
  - How much did the cast interfere with your routine?
  - How did the cast affect ADL? Driving? Walking?
  - What other problems did you have with the cast?
  - How did you feel when you were in the cast? Awkward? Embarrassed?
  - How do you think this short experience may help you when you care for a person with a cast?
- Try this experiment to understand how osteoporosis affects bone.
  - Fold a piece of standard 8½ × 11-inch paper in half length-wise three times (it will now be about 1 inch × 11 inches). Try to tear it in half along the fold and along the 1-inch edge.
  - What happens? Unfold the paper once (it will be 2 inches × 11 inches) and cut pieces out along all of the edges. This step will make the paper porous, much like the bone becomes with osteoporosis.
  - Refold the paper to the 1 × 11-inch size and try to tear it again. What happens now?
- Role-play with a partner. One person is experiencing a CVA (stroke). The other partner will implement FAST to try to determine if their partner might be having a stroke. Using the acronym ask the person questions (can you smile, etc).

36 Cardiovascular and Respiratory Disorders

Hypertension stage 1   Hypertension stage 2   Hypertensive crisis

1. When the systolic pressure is 140 mm Hg or higher or the diastolic pressure is 90 mm Hg or higher, it is _____.

2. _____ is when the systolic pressure is higher than 180 mm Hg and/or the diastolic pressure is higher than 120 mm Hg.

3. _____ is when the systolic pressure is between 130 and 139 mm Hg or the diastolic pressure is between 80 and 89 mm Hg.

CIRCLE THE BEST ANSWER

4. The leading cause of death in the United States is
   A. Cardiovascular and respiratory disorders
   B. Cancer
   C. Strokes
   D. Accidents
5. Elevated blood pressure would be indicated by a reading of
   A. 120/70 mm Hg
   B. 100/60 mm Hg
   C. 140/90 mm Hg
   D. 130/60 mm Hg
6. A risk factor for hypertension that a person cannot change is
   A. Stress
   B. Being overweight
   C. Age
   D. Lack of exercise
7. The most common cause of coronary artery disease is
   A. Lack of exercise
   B. Atherosclerosis
   C. Family history
   D. Stress
8. When a person has angina pectoris, the chest pain occurs when
   A. Oxygen does not reach the lungs
   B. The heart needs more oxygen
   C. The blood pressure is too high
   D. Heart muscle dies

9. If a person has angina pain, it usually will be relieved by
   A. Resting for 3 to 15 minutes
   B. Taking narcotic medications
   C. Using oxygen therapy
   D. Getting up and walking for exercise
10. If a person takes a nitroglycerin tablet for angina, you should
    A. Give them a large glass of water to swallow the pill
    B. Take the pills back to the nurses' station
    C. Make sure the person tells the nurse that a pill was taken
    D. Encourage the person to walk around the room
11. When a myocardial infarction occurs, it means that
    A. A part of the heart muscle dies
    B. The heart muscle is not receiving enough oxygen
    C. Pain can be relieved by rest
    D. Blood backs up into the lungs
12. If a person complains of pain or numbness in the back, neck, jaw, or stomach, you should tell the nurse at once because the person
    A. Is having an angina attack
    B. May be having a stroke
    C. May be having a myocardial infarction
    D. Has symptoms of COPD
13. When heart failure occurs, you may assist in the person's care by
    A. Encouraging increased exercise
    B. Promoting a diet high in sodium
    C. Assisting with self-care activities
    D. Giving the person plenty of fluids
14. An older person with heart failure is at risk for
    A. Contractures
    B. Skin breakdown
    C. Fractures
    D. Urinary tract infections
15. The most common risk factor for chronic obstructive pulmonary disease (COPD) is
    A. Family history
    B. Respiratory infections
    C. Cigarette smoking
    D. Exercise

16. When caring for a person who has COPD, you should
    A. Make sure the person has increased activity
    B. Encourage the person to sleep or rest in the supine position
    C. Encourage the person to stop smoking and to avoid secondhand smoke
    D. Complete all ADL for the person
17. If a person has chronic bronchitis, one of the first symptoms is
    A. Wheezing and tightening in the chest
    B. Shortness of breath on exertion
    C. A smoker's cough in the morning
    D. A high temperature for several days
18. When a person has an asthma attack, it is treated with
    A. Medications, including inhalers
    B. Oxygen therapy
    C. Cold air
    D. Increased fluid intake
19. If an older person has influenza, he or she may
    A. Have a very high body temperature
    B. Have an increased appetite
    C. Feel more energy than usual
    D. Not have signs and symptoms usually seen in influenza
20. Which of these symptoms is more likely to be from a cold rather than the flu?
    A. Sinus congestion (stuffy nose)
    B. High fever (100°F to 102°F)
    C. Fatigue for 2 to 3 weeks
    D. Bronchitis or pneumonia
21. When a person has pneumonia, fluid intake is increased because of fever and to
    A. Decrease the amount of bacteria in the lungs
    B. Dilute medication given to treat the disease
    C. Thin secretions
    D. Decrease inflammation of the breathing passages
22. Breathing is easier for a person with pneumonia when the person is positioned in
    A. Semi-Fowler position
    B. Side-lying position
    C. Supine position
    D. A soft chair
23. When you care for a person with tuberculosis (TB), you should
    A. Use Standard Precautions and isolation precautions when caring for the person
    B. Avoid the person when possible
    C. Ask the facility to provide you with medication to prevent contracting TB
    D. Increase the person's fluid intake

FILL IN THE BLANKS

24. Write out the meaning of each abbreviation.

    A. AHA _____

    B. CAD _____

    C. CDC _____

    D. CO_2 _____

    E. COPD _____

    F. COVID-19 _____

    G. MI _____

    H. mm Hg _____

    I. O_2 _____

    J. TB _____

25. What risk factors that you cannot change increase blood pressure?

    A. _____

    B. _____

    C. _____

    D. _____

26. The most common cause of coronary artery disease (CAD) is _____. When this occurs, _____collects on the _____.

27. What activities or other factors can cause angina?

    A. _____

    B. _____

    C. _____

    D. _____

    E. _____

    F. _____

28. Where is nitroglycerin (tablets or spray) kept? _____
    _____

29. Signs and symptoms of a myocardial infarction may be chest pain that is

    A. _____

    B. _____

    C. _____

    D. _____

30. The goals of cardiac rehabilitation after a myocardial infarction are

    A. _____

    B. _____

    C. _____

31. When left-sided heart failure occurs, blood backs up into _____. What effect does this have on these areas and features of the body?

A. Brain _____

B. Kidneys _____

C. Skin _____

D. Blood pressure _____

32. When the person has right-sided heart failure, blood backs up into the _____. What happens to these areas?

A. Feet and ankles _____

B. Liver _____

C. Abdomen _____

33. Older persons with heart failure are at risk for skin breakdown because of

A. _____

B. _____

C. _____

34. How can you help prevent skin breakdown in older persons with heart failure? _____

35. What changes occur in the lungs when a person has chronic obstructive pulmonary disease (COPD)?

A. _____

B. _____

C. _____

D. _____

36. If a person has chronic bronchitis, the person must stop _____.

37. A common complication of influenza is _____ _____.

38. If an older person has influenza, they may not have typical signs and symptoms. They may instead have these symptoms:

A. _____

B. _____

C. _____

D. _____

E. _____

39. What signs and symptoms may be present if a person has active tuberculosis (TB)?

A. _____

B. _____

C. _____

D. _____

E. _____

F. _____

G. _____

H. _____

40. Why does TB sometimes become active as a person ages? _____

41. Besides COVID-19, what are two other coronaviruses?

A. _____

B. _____

MATCHING

Match the symptom listed with disorders of coronary artery disease.

42. _____ Chest pain occurs with exertion

43. _____ Blood flow to the heart is suddenly blocked

44. _____ Blood backs up into the venous system

45. _____ Fluid occurs in the lungs

46. _____ Rest and nitroglycerin often relieve the symptoms

47. _____ Pain is described as crushing, stabbing, or squeezing

A. Angina
B. Myocardial infarction
C. Heart failure

Match the form of chronic obstructive pulmonary disorder (COPD) with the related symptom.

48. _____ Person develops a barrel chest

49. _____ Mucus and inflamed breathing passages obstruct airflow

50. _____ Alveoli become less elastic

51. _____ Air passages narrow

52. _____ First symptom is often a smoker's cough in the morning

53. _____ Normal O_2 and CO_2 exchange cannot occur in affected alveoli

54. _____ Allergies and air pollutants are common triggers

A. Chronic bronchitis
B. Emphysema
C. Asthma

OPTIONAL LEARNING EXERCISES

55. Why is hypertension called "the silent killer?"
_____

56. When a person has CAD, what lifestyle changes are needed?

A. Quit _____

B. Increase regular_____

C. Reduce _____

D. Healthy diet to reduce _____,
_____, and _____
_____

E. If overweight, _____
_____

INDEPENDENT LEARNING ACTIVITIES

- If possible, visit a cardiac rehabilitation center. Observe and ask the staff the following questions.
  - What exercises are included for a person recovering from an MI? Cardiac surgery?
  - How is the person monitored while exercising?
  - How long does the person need to continue the program?
  - How often does the person come to the rehabilitation center? How much time is spent on each visit?
- Get permission from the staff to ask the following questions of one of the persons exercising.
  - What condition do you have that made you need this program?
  - When did your rehabilitation begin after your diagnosis?
  - How long will you need to continue the rehabilitation program?
  - What benefits do you feel you are getting from the program?
  - What exercise will you continue after the rehabilitation program is completed?
  - What other lifestyle changes have you made?

37 Digestive and Endocrine Disorders

FILL IN THE BLANKS: KEY TERMS

Emesis	Hyperglycemia	Jaundice
Heartburn	Hypoglycemia	Vomitus

1. High sugar in the blood is _____ _____.

2. _____ is when food and fluids are expelled from the stomach through the mouth.

3. Low sugar in the blood is _____ _____.

4. Another word for vomitus is _____ _____.

5. _____ is yellowish color of the skin or whites of the eyes.

6. A burning sensation in the chest and sometimes the throat is _____.

CIRCLE THE BEST ANSWER

7. A risk factor for gastroesophageal reflux disease (GERD) is
   A. Eating small, frequent meals
   B. Eating spicy or tomato-based foods
   C. Maintaining normal weight
   D. Respiratory illnesses

8. If you are caring for a person with GERD, the person may be
   A. Encouraged to eat large meals 2 or 3 times a day
   B. Instructed not to lay down for 3 hours after eating
   C. Told to sleep in a bed with no pillow
   D. Told to drink a glass of wine at bedtime

9. Vomiting can be life-threatening when it
   A. Is caused by an infection
   B. Is aspirated and obstructs an airway
   C. Contains undigested food
   D. Has a bitter taste

10. If vomitus looks like coffee grounds, you should report this to the nurse at once because
    A. It signals bleeding
    B. The person may need a diet change
    C. This indicates an infection
    D. The person may need pain medication

11. Diverticular disease may occur because of
    A. A high-fiber diet
    B. Regular bowel movements
    C. Aging
    D. Infections

12. Gallstones are
    A. Needed for digestion of fats
    B. Formed in the small intestine
    C. Formed when bile hardens into stone-like pieces
    D. Passed easily through the kidneys

13. A symptom of gallstones is
    A. Pain radiating down one or both arms
    B. Diarrhea
    C. Constipation
    D. Pain located between the shoulder blades

14. When hepatitis is contracted by eating or drinking food or water contaminated by feces, it is
    A. Hepatitis A
    B. Hepatitis B
    C. Hepatitis C
    D. Hepatitis D

15. Cirrhosis is often caused by
    A. Eating a high fat diet
    B. Eating food or drinking water contaminated with feces
    C. Chronic alcohol abuse
    D. Gallstones

16. When caring for a person with cirrhosis, itching may be decreased by
    A. Using very hot water when bathing
    B. Using warm water and baking soda for bathing
    C. Reminding the person not to scratch the skin
    D. Increasing fluid intake

17. An obese 50-year-old woman with hypertension is diagnosed with diabetes. She most likely has
    A. Type 1
    B. Type 2
    C. Gestational
    D. None of the above

18. A diabetic complains of thirst and frequent urination. You notice the person has a flushed face and slow, deep respirations. You know these are signs and symptoms of
   A. Hyperglycemia
   B. Hypoglycemia
   C. Diabetic coma
   D. An infection

MATCHING

Match the type of hepatitis with the correct statement.

19. _____ Occurs in persons infected with hepatitis B

20. _____ Occurs in international travelers (especially to developing countries)

21. _____ Caused by HBV

22. _____ Ingested when eating food or water contaminated with feces

23. _____ Person may have virus but no symptoms

24. _____ Serious liver damage shows up years later

A. Hepatitis A
B. Hepatitis B
C. Hepatitis C
D. Hepatitis D

Match the symptom with either hypoglycemia or hyperglycemia.

25. _____ Trembling, shakiness

26. _____ Sweet breath odor

27. _____ Tingling around the mouth

28. _____ Cold, clammy skin

29. _____ Slow, deep, and labored respirations

30. _____ Headache

31. _____ Flushed face

32. _____ Frequent urination

A. Hypoglycemia
B. Hyperglycemia

FILL IN THE BLANKS

33. Write out the meaning of each abbreviation.
   A. GERD _____
   B. HBV _____
   C. IBD _____
   D. I&O _____
   E. IV

34. What lifestyle changes may be needed for a person with GERD?
   A. _____
   B. _____
   C. _____

D. _____

E. _____

F. _____

G. _____

35. What measures will help the person who is vomiting?
   A. Turn _____
   B. Place _____
   C. Move _____
   D. Provide _____
   E. Eliminate _____

36. The following are risk factors for diverticular disease. What is the specific risk for each of these related to the disease?

A. Age _____

B. Diet _____

C. Bowel function _____

37. If a person with gallstones has jaundice, the skin and whites of the eyes will appear _____.

38. A gallbladder attack often follows a _____ _____.

39. List the characteristics of the types of hepatitis.

A. Hepatitis A is spread by the _____ _____ route.

B. Hepatitis B is present in the _____ _____ of infected persons.

C. Hepatitis C can be transmitted even when the person has _____.

D. Hepatitis D occurs only in people with _____.

E. Hepatitis E is not common in _____ _____.

40. Cirrhosis is caused by

A. Chronic _____ abuse

B. Chronic _____ and _____ _____ __ __

C. _____ is becoming a common cause.

41. A person with _____ _____ diabetes will be treated with healthy eating, exercise, and sometimes oral medications.

42. A person with_____ diabetes will be treated with daily insulin therapy as well as healthy diet and exercise.

OPTIONAL LEARNING EXERCISES

You are caring for several persons with diabetes. Answer Questions 43–48 about these persons.

- *Mr. Jones, a 75-year-old African-American man*
- *Ms. Miller, a 45-year-old White, overweight woman*
- *Mrs. Thorpe, a 32-year-old pregnant woman*
- *Ms. Hernandez, a 60-year-old Hispanic woman with hypertension*

43. Three of these persons are most likely to have type 2 diabetes. They are

A. _____

B. _____

C. _____

44. Mrs. Thorpe probably has _____ diabetes. She is at risk for developing _____ later in life.

45. Which type of diabetes develops rapidly? _____ _____

46. Mrs. Hernandez has an open wound on her ankle. Why is this wound a concern? _____ _____

47. Why is Ms. Miller instructed to decrease her food intake? _____

48. Mr. Jones tells you he feels shaky and dizzy and has a headache when he misses a meal.

He probably is experiencing _____ _____.

Edward P. has been diagnosed with cirrhosis. Answer the following questions about his disease and care.

49. Abdominal pain and bloating occur with cirrhosis when _____.

50. What skin changes may be observed?

A. _____

B. _____

51. Edward P. is likely to have dietary restrictions. These will include

A. Healthy diet limited in _____ _____

B. Diet to reduce edema and ascites _____ _____

INDEPENDENT LEARNING ACTIVITIES

- Talk with a person who has gastroesophageal reflux disease (GERD) and ask the following questions.
  - What symptoms does the person have related to GERD?
  - What risk factors does the person have that may have caused the GERD?
  - What lifestyle changes has the person made since the diagnosis?
- Talk with a person who has had gallstones and ask the following questions.
  - What risk factors does the person have related to gallstone formation?
  - What signs and symptoms did the person have that helped the doctor diagnose gallstones?

- What treatment did the person have to relieve the symptoms?
- After treatment, what signs or symptoms have changed?
- Talk with a person with diabetes and ask the following questions.
  - What type of diabetes does the person have: type 1 or type 2?
  - How old was the person when diabetes was diagnosed?
  - What lifestyle changes have been made to treat the diabetes?
- What complications of diabetes have occurred?
- Ask your instructor to help you arrange to attend a diabetic education class, if these are available at your agency. After attending, answer the following questions.
  - What are the ages of the members of the class? Are family members included in the class?
  - What information is given to the class about diet?
  - What exercise programs are recommended to the class?
  - What information is given about medications used to treat diabetes?

38 Urinary and Reproductive Disorders

FILL IN THE BLANKS: KEY TERMS

Cystocele
Dialysis
Diuresis
Dysuria

Hematuria
Oliguria
Pyuria
Rectocele

Suprapubic
Urinary diversion
Urostomy
Uterine prolapse

1. Scant urine is _____
_____.

2. Difficult or painful urination is _____
_____.

3. A _____ is a surgically
created opening between the ureter and the abdomen.

4. _____ is the process of pass-
ing urine; large amounts of urine are produced—1000
to 5000 mL a day.

5. A new pathway for urine to exit the body is a
_____.

6. Blood in the urine is _____
_____.

7. _____
is pus in the urine.

8. _____ is the process of
removing waste products from the blood.

9. An area above the pubic bone is
_____.

10. _____ occurs when the
bladder drops down.

11. When the uterus shifts downward into the vaginal
canal, it is called _____.

12. A _____ occurs when the
rectum shifts downward.

CIRCLE THE BEST ANSWER

13. Women have a higher risk of urinary tract infections
because of
A. Hormone levels in the body
B. The short female urethra
C. Bacteria
D. Prostate gland secretions

14. If a person has cystitis, the care plan will include
A. Restricting fluid intake
B. Assisting the person to ambulate frequently
C. Straining the urine
D. Encouraging the person to drink 2000 mL of fluid
a day

15. If a man has benign prostatic hyperplasia (BPH), he
will probably
A. Be incontinent of urine
B. Have frequent voiding at night
C. Have increased urine output
D. Have renal failure

16. After surgery to correct BPH, the care plan may
include
A. A balanced diet to prevent constipation
B. Increased activity with an exercise plan
C. Restricted fluid intake
D. Care of the surgical incision

17. When caring for a person with a urinary diversion,
the pouch is changed
A. Each time the person voids
B. Anytime it leaks
C. Only once a week
D. When the pouch is full

18. When caring for a person with a stoma, the nursing
assistant knows
A. The stoma does not have sensation
B. Sterile technique is used when cleaning the area
C. Pain medication is given before caring for the
stoma
D. The person is never allowed to help with the care

19. If you are caring for a person with renal calculi (kid-
ney stones), your care will include
A. Restricting fluids
B. Keeping the person on strict bedrest
C. Straining all urine
D. Maintaining a strict diet

20. When you care for a person with acute renal failure,
the care plan will include
A. Increasing fluid intake to 2000 to 3000 mL per day
B. Measuring and recording urine output every hour
C. Making sure the person does not drink any fluids
D. Measuring weight weekly

21. Chronic renal failure
    A. Occurs suddenly
    B. Generally improves and kidney function returns to normal within 1 year
    C. Occurs when nephrons of the kidney are destroyed over many years
    D. Has very little effect on the person's overall health
22. If a person has chronic renal failure, which of these would be included in the care plan?
    A. A diet high in protein, potassium, and sodium
    B. Plenty of exercise
    C. Measures to prevent itching
    D. Frequent bathing with soap
23. When a person is receiving hemodialysis, you will
    A. Make sure the person drinks about 2000 mL each day
    B. Never take the blood pressure on the arm with the fistula

C. Assist the person to ambulate several times a day
D. Allow the person to eat whatever he or she wants to maintain weight

24. A woman with pelvic organ prolapse may be encouraged to
    A. Drink plenty of fluids
    B. Perform Kegel exercises several times a day
    C. Exercise vigorously each day
    D. Remain on complete bedrest
25. A woman who complains about frothy, thick, foul-smelling vaginal discharge most likely has
    A. Gonorrhea
    B. Genital warts
    C. Syphilis
    D. Trichomoniasis

MATCHING

Match the sexually transmitted disease with the correct statement.

26. _____ Surgical removal if ointment is not effective

27. _____ Sores may have a watery discharge

28. _____ No symptoms in men, only in women

29. _____ May have vaginal bleeding

30. _____ Urinary urgency and frequency is present

31. _____ Treated with antiviral medications

32. _____ Painless sores appear on genitals 10 to 90 days after exposure

33. _____ May not show symptoms

A. Herpes
B. Genital warts
C. Gonorrhea
D. Chlamydia
E. Syphilis
F. Trichomoniasis

FILL IN THE BLANKS

34. Write out the meaning of the abbreviations.
    A. AIDS _____
    B. BPH _____
    C. HIV _____
    D. mL _____
    E. STI _____
    F. UTI _____

35. Why are older persons at high risk for urinary tract infections?
    A. _____
    B. _____
    C. _____
    D. _____

36. After a transurethral resection of the prostate (TURP), the person's care plan may include
    A. _____
    B. _____
    C. _____
    D. _____
    E. _____

37. When you care for a person with a urinary diversion, you should follow _____ _____ for safety.

38. What are the risk factors for developing renal calculi?
    A. Age, race, sex _____
    B. _____
    C. _____
    D. _____

39. A person with renal calculi needs to drink 2000 to 3000 mL of fluid a day to help _____ _____.

40. When acute renal failure occurs, there are two phases. Name and explain each phase.

    A. At first, _____ occurs.

    Urine output is _____.

    This phase lasts _____ _____.

    B. Then _____ occurs.

    Urine output is _____.

    This phase lasts _____ _____.

41. When caring for a person with acute renal failure, report to the nurse at once if the person has _____ _____.

42. Signs and symptoms of chronic renal failure appear when _____ is lost.

43. You may need to assist a person in chronic renal failure with nutritional needs. List what the care plan is likely to include for the following.

    A. Diet _____

    B. Fluids _____

44. Sexually transmitted infections are transmitted by _____.

45. Using _____ can help prevent the spread of STIs.

46. When caring for a person with an STI, you should follow _____ and _____ _____.

OPTIONAL LEARNING EXERCISES

You give home care to Mrs. Eunice Weber twice a week. She is 92 years old and lives alone. She has severe osteoporosis and uses a walker to move about in her home. She receives Meals on Wheels and spends most of the day sitting on the sofa. She has periods of incontinence or dribbling because of poor bladder control. When you arrive to care for her, she tells you she is not feeling well. She tells you it burns when she urinates, and when she needs to urinate, the urge comes on suddenly and she often does not get to the toilet in time. Answer the following questions about Mrs. Weber.

47. You should tell the _____ because these symptoms may mean Mrs. Weber has _____ _____.

48. What is the urge to void called? _____ _____.

49. How does Mrs. Weber's immobility affect the following?
    A. Fluid intake_____
    B. Perineal care_____

50. The doctor will probably order _____ to treat the condition.

51. The care plan will probably include "Encourage fluids to _____ per day."

Two weeks later you notice that Mrs. Weber has chills. When you take her temperature, it is 102°F. She tells you she has been vomiting since yesterday. You observe her urine and see that it is very cloudy.

52. You report these symptoms to the nurse because it can indicate that Mrs. Weber now has _____ _____. This means the infection has moved from the _____ to the _____ _____.

INDEPENDENT LEARNING ACTIVITIES

- Talk with someone who has had urinary tract infections (UTIs). If you have had a UTI, answer these questions about your own experience.
    ○ What signs and symptoms were present?
    ○ How many UTIs have occurred?
    ○ What risk factors may have placed the person (or you) at risk for developing UTIs?
    ○ What treatment was used to treat the UTI?
    ○ What lifestyle changes were recommended to prevent a recurrence of the UTI?
- Talk with someone who has had renal calculi and ask the following questions.
    ○ What signs and symptoms were present?
    ○ How was the problem treated?
    ○ What dietary changes have been prescribed to prevent future attacks?

39 Mental Health Disorders

FILL IN THE BLANKS: KEY TERMS

Affect	Hallucination	Psychiatric disorder
Anxiety	Mental	Psychosis
Compulsion	Mental disorder	Stigma
Defense mechanism	Mental health	Stress
Delusion	Mental illness	Stressor
Delusion of grandeur	Obsession	Suicide
Delusion of persecution	Panic	Suicide contagion
Emotional illness	Paranoia	Withdrawal syndrome
Flashback	Phobia	

1. Exposure to suicide or suicidal behaviors within one's family, one's peer group, or media reports of suicide is _____.

2. _____ is reliving a trauma in thoughts during the day and in nightmares during sleep.

3. When a person has an exaggerated belief about one's own importance, wealth, power, or talents, it is called _____.

4. A mental disorder, emotional disorder, or psychiatric disorder is also called a _____.

5. A _____ is any emotional, physical, social, or economic factor that causes stress.

6. The person's physical and mental response after stopping or severely reducing the intake of a substance that was used regularly is _____ _____.

7. _____ means relating to the mind. It is something that exists in the mind or is performed by the mind.

8. A feeling of shame or judgment from someone else is a _____.

9. The response or change in the body caused by any emotional, physical, social, or economic factor is _____.

10. _____ is a vague, uneasy feeling that occurs in response to stress.

11. _____ is another name for mental illness, mental disorder, or psychiatric disorder.

12. A _____ is an intense fear.

13. A false belief is a _____ _____.

14. _____ is a disturbance in the ability to cope or adjust to stress; behavior and functioning are impaired. This condition is also called a mental disorder, emotional illness, or psychiatric disorder.

15. A state of severe mental impairment is _____ _____.

16. A _____ is seeing, hearing, or feeling something that is not real.

17. _____ is a disorder of the mind. The person has false beliefs and suspicion about a person or situation.

18. Repeating an act over and over again is a _____.

19. _____ is when the person copes with and adjusts to the stresses of everyday living in ways accepted by society.

20. _____ is a false belief that one is being mistreated, abused, or harassed.

21. An intense and sudden feeling of fear, anxiety, terror, or dread is _____.

22. _____ is another name for mental illness, mental disorder, or emotional disorder.

23. A _____ is an unconscious reaction that blocks unpleasant or threatening feelings.

195

24. To kill oneself is _____ _____.

25. Feelings and emotions are _____ _____.

26. An _____ is a recurrent, unwanted thought, idea, or image.

CIRCLE THE BEST ANSWER

27. Which of these statements about anxiety is *true*?
    A. Anxiety often occurs when needs are not met.
    B. Anxiety is always abnormal.
    C. The body does not respond to anxiety with physical symptoms.
    D. The level of anxiety is the same regardless of the cause.
28. An unhealthy coping mechanism would be
    A. Talking about the problem
    B. Playing music
    C. Smoking
    D. Exercising
29. Panic is
    A. The highest level of anxiety
    B. A disorder that occurs gradually
    C. A psychosis
    D. Vague, normal response to stress
30. When a person with obsessive-compulsive disorder is unable to perform his or her ritual (compulsion), the person
    A. Will become less anxious
    B. Will gradually forget about performing the ritual
    C. Will have more anxiety
    D. Will learn to use good coping mechanisms
31. Flashbacks occur in persons with
    A. Panic attacks
    B. Post-traumatic stress disorder (PTSD)
    C. Schizophrenia
    D. Depression
32. A person you are caring for tells you he is the president of the United States. He has a delusion of grandeur, which is a part of
    A. Obsessive-compulsive disorder
    B. Phobias
    C. Bipolar disorders
    D. Schizophrenia
33. During a manic phase, a person with bipolar disorder may
    A. Be sad, anxious, or have an empty mood
    B. Complain of chronic pain not caused by physical illness or injury
    C. Have an unrealistic belief in his or her abilities and powers
    D. Startle easily
34. A major risk of a depressive episode is that the person
    A. Is very sad
    B. May attempt suicide

C. Has depressed body functions
D. Cannot concentrate
35. If an older person is depressed, it may be wrongly diagnosed as a
    A. Cognitive disorder
    B. Physical problem
    C. Hormonal change
    D. Side effect of medications
36. A person with an antisocial personality disorder may
    A. Be suspicious and distrust others
    B. Have violent behavior
    C. See, hear, or feel something that is not real
    D. Blame others for actions and behaviors
37. An adult is considered an alcoholic if the person
    A. Enjoys a glass of wine with dinner
    B. Becomes "high" or drunk after 1 or 2 drinks
    C. Cannot stop drinking once drinking has begun
    D. Drinks only liquor with a high alcohol content
38. Alcohol can be more dangerous for an older person because
    A. The person has been drinking for a long period of time
    B. The person eats a poor diet
    C. Older people tend to take more medications that may be harmful when taken with alcohol
    D. The person is more likely to lie about alcohol intake than a young person
39. When a person is addicted to medications or drugs, he or she
    A. Takes the medication only as prescribed
    B. Takes smaller and smaller amounts to get the same effect
    C. Is only taking illegal drugs
    D. Continues to use the substance even when he or she knows it makes a situation worse
40. If a resident you are caring for tells you he has thoughts of suicide, you should
    A. Promise him you will not tell anyone
    B. Ignore him, as he often says this and nothing has happened before
    C. Tell the nurse at once
    D. Report this conversation when you give a report at the end of the shift

FILL IN THE BLANKS

41. Write out the meaning of each abbreviation.
    A. BPD _____
    B. NIAAA _____
    C. NIMH _____
    D. OCD _____
    E. PTSD _____
    F. NAMI _____
    G. SUD _____

42. What are causes of mental health disorders?

A. _____

B. _____

C. _____

D. _____

E. _____

F. _____

G. _____

43. Name the defense mechanism being used in the following situations.

A. A girl fails a test. She blames another girl for not helping her study. _____

B. A man does not like his boss. He buys the boss an expensive Christmas present. _____

_____

C. A girl complains of a stomach ache so she will not have to read aloud. _____

D. A child is angry with his teacher. He hits his brother. _____

E. A woman misses work frequently and is often late. She gets a bad job evaluation. She says that the boss does not like her. _____

_____

44. When a person is having a panic attack, what changes would you expect to find when assessing the vital signs?

A. Pulse _____

B. Respirations _____

C. Blood pressure _____

45. If a person has an intense fear of being in an open, crowded, or public place, this is called _____

_____

46. After a terrifying ordeal, a person may develop _____. Signs and symptoms of this disorder usually develop about _____ after the harmful event.

47. Below are examples of problems that occur with schizophrenia. Name each one.

A. A man believes his neighbor is poisoning his water. _____

B. A woman says that voices told her to set fire to her apartment. _____

C. A man believes he can fly like a bird. _____

_____

D. A woman tells you she owns 3 BMW cars and is the president of McDonald's. _____

_____

48. What disorders of movement may occur when a person has schizophrenia?

A. _____

B. _____

C. _____

D. _____

E. _____

49. The following are signs and symptoms of bipolar disorder. Name the episode (mania or depression) for each sign or symptom listed.

A. Extreme irritability _____

B. Thoughts of death or suicide _____

_____

C. Denial that anything is wrong _____

_____

D. Loss of interest in sex _____

_____

E. Jumping from one idea to another _____

_____

F. Feelings of guilt, worthlessness, or helplessness

_____

G. Unrealistic beliefs in one's abilities or powers

_____

50. What losses in older persons may cause depression?

A. _____

B. _____

C. _____

D. _____

51. A person with antisocial personality disorder will display thinking and behaviors that show no regard for _____.

52. A person who greatly admires and loves family members and friends but suddenly shifts to intense anger and dislike may have a _____.

53. Describe the following symptoms of alcoholism.

A. Craving _____

_____

B. Loss of control _____

_____

C. Physical dependence _____

_____

_____

D. Tolerance _____

_____

54. According to the NIAAA, a person needs help for alcohol abuse if he or she has the following problems:

A. _____

B. _____

C. _____

D. _____

E. _____

F. _____

G. _____

H. _____

I. _____

J. _____

55. What signs and symptoms occur with withdrawal syndrome when the person is in withdrawal from an addictive substance?

A. _____

B. _____

C. _____

D. _____   _____

E. _____   _____

F. _____

56. It is important to identify depression in elderly men because the highest rate of suicide is among _____ _____.

57. When interacting with persons with mental disorders, you should

A. _____

B. _____

C. _____

D. _____

E. _____

F. _____

58. When a person has mental health disorders, quality of life must be met. Which right is being protected in each of these examples?

A. All harmful items are removed from the person's setting. _____

B. When the person says or does something, you share it only with the nurse. _____

C. The person is given very simple choices so that he or she still feels in control. _____ _____

D. You report bruises or other signs that the person is not well cared for. _____ _____

59. The three digit code to call for suicide or mental health related crisis support is _____ _____

OPTIONAL LEARNING EXERCISES

60. Mr. Johnson is very worried about his surgery tomorrow. You notice that he is talking very fast and is sweating. You give him directions to collect a urine specimen. Five minutes later, he turns on his call light to ask you to repeat the directions. He tells you he is using the toilet "all the time" because he has diarrhea and frequent urination. The nurse tells you that all of these are signs and symptoms of _____ _____.

61. You are assigned to care for Mrs. Grand, a new resident. She is getting ready to go to the dining room. You assist her to get dressed and she tells you she wants to wash her hands before going to the dining room. She goes to the bathroom and washes her hands for several minutes. As she leaves the room, she stops to turn off the light. Then she tells you she must wash her hands again. She repeats washing her hands and turning the lights on and off 4 or 5 times. You report this to the nurse, who tells you Mrs. Grand has _____.

INDEPENDENT LEARNING ACTIVITIES

• Try this experiment with a group of classmates. Make labels with various roles for "staff members" and "mentally ill persons." A list is provided but you may add or subtract according to the size of your group. Make sure the group includes a mix of people with mental health diseases and staff or visitors.

Doctor
A person with bipolar disorder
Nurse
A person with delusions of grandeur
Visitor
A person with obsessive-compulsive disorder
Nursing assistant
A person with schizophrenia with paranoia
Recreational therapist
A person with hallucinations
Dietitian
A person with anorexia nervosa

- Attach a label to each person so that he or she cannot read it. (It may be placed on the back or the forehead.) Have everyone move about the group and talk to each other based on how the person thinks he or she should approach the person with a certain "label." Continue the experiment for about 15 minutes and then use the following questions to guide a group discussion.
  - How did you feel talking to a person with a mental health disorder?
  - How were the people with a mental health disorder approached? How quickly were the "mentally ill persons" able to sense that this was their label? What cues did they receive from others?
  - How quickly did "staff members" recognize the label they had? What cues did they receive from others?
  - In what ways did the approach of others cause people to respond in a way that was expected? Did the people with mental health disorders show signs of the illness based on the reaction of others?
  - What did the group learn about approaching a person with a mental health disorder?
- Consider this situation and answer the following questions concerning how you would feel about caring for a person with a mental health disorder.

Situation: Marion Cross, age 65, is a patient in an acute care hospital with a diagnosis of pneumonia. The nurse tells you Mrs. Cross has a history of schizophrenia. You are assigned to provide AM care for Mrs. Cross.
- How would you approach Mrs. Cross when you enter her room? How would your knowledge about her mental health disorder affect your initial contact with her?
- What would you do if Mrs. Cross told you she sees an elephant in the room? What would you say to her?
- How would you react if Mrs. Cross told you that she owns Disney World and goes there free anytime she wants? How would you respond?
- How would you provide good oral hygiene if Mrs. Cross refuses to cooperate because she is sure the staff is trying to poison her? What could you try that might be helpful?
- What would you do if Mrs. Cross curls up in a tight ball and refuses to talk or cooperate during AM care? What could you do to maintain her hygiene?
- How would you feel about caring for a person with abnormal behavior? Why?

40 Confusion and Dementia

FILL IN THE BLANKS: KEY TERMS

Cognitive function   Dementia   Paranoia
Delirium   Elopement   Pseudodementia
Delusion   Hallucination   Sundowning

1. When the person has false beliefs and suspicions about a person or situation, it is called _____ _____.

2. A false belief is a _____ _____.

3. Seeing, hearing, or feeling something that is not real is _____.

4. Increased signs, symptoms, and behaviors of AD during hours of darkness is _____.

5. _____ is a state of temporary but acute mental confusion that comes on suddenly.

6. The loss of cognitive function and social function caused by changes in the brain is _____ _____.

7. _____ is a false disorder of the mind.

8. _____ involves memory, thinking, reasoning, ability to understand, judgment, and behavior.

9. When a person leaves the center without staff knowledge, it is _____.

CIRCLE THE BEST ANSWER

10. Confusion caused by physical changes
    A. Occurs suddenly
    B. Cannot be cured
    C. Is cured by aiming treatment at the cause
    D. Is usually temporary
11. When a person is confused, it is helpful if you
    A. Repeat the date and time as often as needed
    B. Change the routine each day to stimulate the person
    C. Keep the drapes pulled during the day
    D. Give complex answers to questions
12. Hearing and vision decrease with confusion, so you should
    A. Speak in a loud voice
    B. Write out directions for the person
    C. Face the person and speak clearly
    D. Keep the lighting dim in the room
13. Dementia
    A. Is a normal part of aging
    B. Causes the person to have difficulty with routine personal, social, and occupational activities
    C. Is always temporary and can be cured
    D. Affects most older people
14. The most common type of permanent dementia is
    A. Alzheimer disease
    B. Dementia
    C. Depression
    D. Delirium
15. The classic sign of Alzheimer disease (AD) is
    A. Forgetting simple tasks
    B. Gradual loss of short-term memory
    C. Acute confusion and delirium
    D. Wandering and sundowning
16. In stage 1 of AD (mild), the person may
    A. Walk slowly with a shuffling gait
    B. Be totally incontinent
    C. Blame others for mistakes
    D. Become agitated and may be violent
17. In stage 2 of AD (moderate), the person may
    A. Have difficulty performing everyday tasks
    B. Need help with activities of daily living
    C. Be disoriented to time and place
    D. Have seizures
18. In stage 3 of AD (severe), the person may
    A. Forget recent events
    B. Lose impulse control and use foul language or have poor table manners
    C. Be less interested in things or be less outgoing
    D. Be disoriented to person, time, and place
19. When a person wanders, the major concern is
    A. The person's comfort
    B. The person is at risk for life-threatening accidents
    C. Inconvenience for the family or facility
    D. Making sure the person gets enough rest and sleep

20. When sundowning occurs, it may be related to
    A. Being tired or hungry
    B. Having poor judgment
    C. Impaired vision or hearing
    D. The person looking for something or someone
21. When you are caring for a person with paranoia and the person accuses you of stealing an item, you should
    A. Argue with the person and say you are not a thief
    B. Help the person search for the item and talk about what is found
    C. Leave the room immediately and report to the nurse
    D. Refuse to care for the person as long as the item is missing
22. Too much stimuli from being asked too many questions at once can overwhelm a person and cause
    A. Delusions
    B. Catastrophic reactions
    C. Hallucinations
    D. Sundowning
23. A caregiver may cause agitation and restlessness by
    A. Calling the person by name
    B. Selecting tasks and activities specific to the person's cognitive abilities and interests
    C. Encouraging activity early in the day
    D. Making the person hurry in order to complete care quickly
24. When you are caring for a person with AD, it is helpful if you
    A. Give simple, step-by-step instructions
    B. Play loud, familiar TV programs during meals and care activities
    C. Encourage late afternoon or early evening exercise and activity
    D. Restrain a person who insists on going outside
25. If a person with AD displays sexual behaviors, the nurse may tell you to
    A. Tell the person this behavior is not acceptable
    B. Make sure the person has good hygiene to prevent itching
    C. Avoid caring for the person
    D. Ignore the behavior because the disease causes it
26. What should you do when a person repeats the same motions or repeats the same words over and over?
    A. Remind the person to stop the repeating behavior
    B. Report this to the nurse immediately
    C. Take the person for a walk or distract the person with music or picture books
    D. Isolate the person in his or her room until the repeating behavior stops
27. A person with AD is encouraged to take part in therapies and activities that
    A. Increase the level of confusion
    B. Help the person to feel useful, worthwhile, and active
    C. Will prevent aggressive behaviors
    D. Improve physical problems such as incontinence and contractures

28. How do AD special care units differ from other areas of a care facility?
    A. Complete care is provided.
    B. Entrances and exits are locked.
    C. Meals are served in the person's room.
    D. No activities are provided.
29. A person with AD no longer stays in a secured unit when
    A. The condition improves
    B. The family requests a move to another unit
    C. The person cannot sit or walk
    D. Aggressive behaviors disrupt the unit
30. A family that cares for a person with dementia at home
    A. Usually does not need any help
    B. Cannot afford to have the person cared for in a nursing facility
    C. Needs assistance from others to cope with the person
    D. Must have special training to care for the person

FILL IN THE BLANKS

31. Write out the meaning of each abbreviation.

    A. AD _____

    B. ADL _____

    C. GDS _____

    D. MCI _____

    E. NIA _____

32. Cognitive function involves

    A. _____

    B. _____

    C. _____

    D. _____

    E. _____

    F. _____

33. When caring for a confused person, how can you help the person know the date and time?

    A. _____

    B. _____

34. How can you help the confused person maintain the day-night cycle?

    A. _____

    B. _____

    C. _____

35. What senses decrease with changes in the nervous system from aging? _____ _____

36. Give examples of how early warning signs of dementia may be seen in these areas.

    A. Memory _____

    _____

    B. Doing tasks _____

    _____

    C. Language _____

    _____

    D. Judgment _____

    _____

37. What substances can cause dementia? _____ _____

38. Pseudodementia can occur with _____ and _____.

39. The most common mental health disorder in older persons is _____.

40. A person with mild cognitive impairment has problems with

    A. _____

    B. _____

    C. Other mental functions _____

    _____

    D. These problems do not interfere with _____ _____.

41. Alzheimer disease (AD) damages brain cells that control these functions.

    A. _____

    B. _____

    C. _____

    D. _____

    E. _____

    F. _____

    G. _____

    H. _____

42. Which of the seven stages of AD are described in the following examples?

    A. The person cannot walk without help. _____

    B. The person may need help choosing correct clothes to wear. _____

C. The person shows no signs of memory problems. _____

D. Family, friends, and others notice problems. _____

E. The person has problems with shopping, paying bills, and managing money. _____ _____

F. The person may forget names but recognizes faces. _____

G. The person does not know where to find keys, eyeglasses, or other objects. _____ _____

43. The *MedicAlert + Safe Return* program will help an AD person who has the behavior of _____ _____.

44. Which behavior of AD is described in the following examples?

    A. Confusion and restlessness increase after dark. _____

    B. Too much stimulation may trigger this behavior. _____

    C. The person may use this behavior to communicate as the disease progresses. _____ _____

    D. The person may walk into traffic or go out not properly dressed for the weather. _____ _____

    E. The person repeats the same words or motions over and over. _____ _____

    F. The person may have false beliefs about who he or she is or who the caregiver may be. _____ _____ _____

    G. The person may pace, hit, or yell. _____ _____

    H. The person touches himself or others in a sexual way that is inappropriate. _____

    I. The person complains of feeling bugs crawling or seeing animals that are not there. _____ _____ _____

    J. The person hits, pinches, grabs, bites, or swears at others. _____

    K. The person hides her dentures in a wastebasket. _____

45. When a person has dementia or AD, what is the reason the following items may be part of the care plan?

A. Approach the person from the front. _____
_____

B. Provide plastic eating and drinking utensils. ____
_____

C. Respond to door alarms at once. _____
_____

D. Do not argue with a person who wants to leave.
_____

E. Do not ask a person to tell you what is bothering him or her. _____

F. Turn off TV or movies when violent or disturbing programs are on. _____

G. Use nightlights so the person can see. _____
_____

H. Promote exercise and activity during the day. ___
_____

I. Have equipment ready for any procedure. _____
_____

46. Validation therapy is based on these principles.

A. _____
B. _____
C. _____
D. _____
E. _____
F. _____

OPTIONAL LEARNING EXERCISES

You are caring for Mr. Harris, a 78-year-old who is confused. You know there are ways to help a person to be more oriented. Answer the following questions about ways to help a confused person.

47. How can you help orient Mr. Harris to who he is every time you are in contact with him? _____
_____

48. How can you avoid startling Mr. Harris? _____
_____

49. When helping Mr. Harris with basic needs, what can you do to prevent these problems?

A. Wandering and sundowning _____
_____

B. Restlessness, confusion, and agitation _____
_____

C. Fear of bathing _____

You are caring for Mrs. Matthews, an 82-year-old resident. The nurse tells you she lived with her daughter for the last 2 years but the family is now concerned for her safety. She left home when the temperature was 35°F and was found 2 miles away wearing a light sweater. On another occasion, she turned on the gas stove and could not remember how to turn it off. Sometimes, she did not recognize her daughter and resisted getting a bath or changing her clothes. Since admission to the care facility, she tells everyone she must leave to go to her birthday party. Answer these questions about Mrs. Matthews and her care.

50. Why would Mrs. Matthews most likely be in a special care unit in the nursing facility? _____
_____
_____

51. What disease is it likely that Mrs. Matthew has? ___
_____

52. Mrs. Matthews is probably in stage _____ of the disease. What activities would indicate she is in this stage?

A. _____
B. _____
C. _____
D. _____

53. How often will the health team review Mrs. Matthews's need to stay on this unit? _____
Why is this done? _____
_____

54. The nurse may encourage Mrs. Matthews's daughter to join a _____ group.
How can this be helpful to the daughter? _____
_____

INDEPENDENT LEARNING ACTIVITIES

• Consider the situation and answer the following questions about how you would feel.

Situation: *Imagine you are in a strange country where people talk to you but you do not understand what they are saying. They use strange tools to eat and you cannot figure out how to use them. They try to feed you food you do not recognize. Sometimes these people seem friendly and caring but at other times they become angry because you are not doing what they ask you to do. You become frightened when they try to remove your clothes and take you in a room to shower you. You become frightened and upset because you do not know what will happen next. At times other strangers come to your room and bring gifts. They talk kindly to you but you do not know them. They seem upset when you do not respond to their gifts and gestures. The doors*

203

and windows in this country are all locked and you cannot find a way out so you can go home.

- How does this situation relate to the information in this chapter?
- How would you react if you were the person in this situation? Why?
- What methods might you use to try to communicate with the person in this situation?
  - Why would the person want to go home? What does "home" mean to him or her?
  - How will this exercise help you when you care for a person who is confused?
- Consider the situation and answer the following questions about how you would care for a person who has dementia.

Situation: *You are assigned to care for Ronald Myers, age 85, who has Alzheimer disease. He often wanders from room to room and tries to open the outside doors. He frequently becomes agitated and restless, especially in the evenings. Most of the time Mr. Myers is unable to feed himself and he is often incontinent. He keeps repeating all day: "Help me, help me."*

- How do you feel about caring for a person like this? Frightened? Angry? Impatient? How do you deal with your feelings so you can give care to the person?
- At what stage of Alzheimer disease is Mr. Myers? What signs and symptoms support your answer?
- Why would it be ineffective to remind Mr. Myers of the date and time during your shift? Why is this a good technique with some confused persons and not with others?
- Why does Mr. Myers become more agitated toward evening? What is this called?
- What methods could you use to make sure Mr. Myers receives the care needed to maintain good personal hygiene? How could you get him to cooperate or participate in his care?
- What parts of Mr. Myers' behavior would be most difficult for you to tolerate? What would you do if you found yourself becoming irritated and angry with Mr. Myers?
- What information in this chapter has helped you understand persons like Mr. Myers better? How will this information help you give better care to these persons and maintain their quality of life?

41 Intellectual and Developmental Disabilities

Birth defect   Disability   Spastic
Developmental disability   Inherited
Diplegia   Intellectual disability

1. _____ involves severe limits in intellectual function and adaptive behavior occurring before age 18.

2. An abnormality present at birth that can involve a body structure or function is a _____.

3. When similar body parts are affected on both sides of the body, it is called _____.

4. _____ is the uncontrolled contractions of skeletal muscles.

5. A disability that occurs before 22 years of age is _____.

6. A _____ is any lost, absent, or impaired physical or mental function.

7. That which is passed down from parents to children is _____.

CIRCLE THE BEST ANSWER

8. A developmental disability (DD)
   A. Always occurs at birth
   B. Is usually temporary
   C. Limits function in three or more life skills
   D. Is present before the age of 12

9. Developmentally disabled adults
   A. Need lifelong assistance, support, and special services
   B. Usually can live independently after they become adults
   C. Always need to be in long-term care in special centers
   D. Generally outgrow the problems as they mature

10. A person with intellectual disabilities would not usually have
    A. An IQ score about 70 or below
    B. Difficulty with interpersonal skills
    C. Limited skills needed to live, work, and play
    D. Mental health disorders

11. The Arc of the United States is a national organization
    A. Related to Alzheimer disease
    B. That deals with intellectual and related developmental disabilities
    C. That provides care for people with physical disabilities
    D. For persons with cerebral palsy

12. The Arc beliefs about sexuality for those with DD include
    A. The right to have control over their own bodies
    B. Encouraging persons with DD to be sterilized
    C. Preventing persons with DD from learning about sex, marriage, and family
    D. Denying interaction with members of the opposite sex

13. Down syndrome (DS) is caused by
    A. An extra 21st chromosome
    B. Head injury during birth
    C. Diseases of the mother during pregnancy
    D. Lack of oxygen to the brain

14. A person with Down syndrome is at risk for
    A. Cerebral palsy
    B. Diplegia
    C. Leukemia
    D. Poor nutrition

15. Fragile X syndrome (FXS) occurs because of
    A. An extra 21st chromosome
    B. An inherited intellectual disability
    C. Lack of oxygen to the brain during birth
    D. A traumatic brain injury

16. Cerebral palsy is a group of disorders involving
    A. Intellectual disabilities
    B. Muscle weakness or poor muscle control
    C. Abnormal genes from one or both parents
    D. An increased risk of developing leukemia

17. When a person has spastic cerebral palsy, the symptoms include
    A. Constant slow weaving or writhing motions
    B. Uncontrolled contractions of skeletal muscles
    C. Using little or no eye contact
    D. A strong attachment to a single item, idea, activity, or person

18. A person with autism may
    A. Dislike being held or cuddled
    B. Have bladder and bowel control problems
    C. Have generalized seizures
    D. Have diplegia or hemiplegia

205

19. A person with autism
    A. Needs to develop social and work skills
    B. Will outgrow the condition
    C. Will always live in group homes or residential care centers
    D. Will have severe physical problems
20. Spina bifida occurs
    A. At birth due to injury during delivery
    B. Because of traumatic injury in childhood
    C. During the first month of pregnancy
    D. As a result of child abuse
21. Which of these types of spina bifida causes the person to have leg paralysis and lack of bowel and bladder control?
    A. Spina bifida cystica
    B. Myelomeningocele
    C. Spina bifida occulta
    D. Meningocele
22. A shunt placed in the brain of a child with hydrocephalus will
    A. Increase pressure on the brain
    B. Drain fluid from the brain to the abdomen or heart chamber
    C. Cause intellectual disabilities or neurological damage
    D. Cure the hydrocephalus
23. A person with a developmental disability will
    A. Always need to live with family or in a nursing care center
    B. Have his or her rights protected by the Americans with Disabilities Act of 1990 and the Developmental Disabilities Assistance and Bill of Rights Act of 2000
    C. Not be admitted to a nursing facility until he or she is past 60 years of age
    D. Outgrow the disability as he or she ages

FILL IN THE BLANKS

24. Write out the meaning of each abbreviation.
    A. ADA _____
    B. ASD _____
    C. CP _____
    D. DS _____
    E. FXS _____
    F. IDD _____
    G. IQ _____
    H. SB _____
25. A developmental disability is present when function is limited in three or more of these life skills.
    A. _____
    B. _____

C. _____
D. _____
E. _____
F. _____
G. _____

26. What genetic conditions can cause intellectual disabilities?
    A. _____
    B. _____
    C. _____
    D. _____
    E. _____
27. Intellectual disabilities may be caused after birth by childhood diseases such as
    A. _____
    B. _____
    C. _____
    D. _____
    E. _____
    F. _____
28. Intellectual disabilities involve the condition being present before _____.
29. The Arc belief about sexuality for persons with intellectual disabilities includes the right to
    A. _____
    B. _____
    C. _____
    D. _____
    E. _____
    F. _____
    G. _____
    H. _____
    I. _____
    J. _____
    K. _____
30. If a child has Down syndrome (DS), what features are present in the following areas?
    A. Head _____
    B. Eyes _____
    C. Tongue _____

D. Nose _____

E. Hands and fingers _____
_____

31. Persons with Down syndrome need therapy in these areas.

A. _____

B. _____

C. _____

D. _____

32. What problems will boys with Fragile X syndrome have in the areas listed?

A. Social and emotional _____
_____

B. Speech and language _____
_____

33. The usual cause of cerebral palsy is a lack of _____
_____.

34. Which type of cerebral palsy is described in each example?

A. Arm and leg on one side are paralyzed. _____
_____

B. Muscles contract or shorten. They are stiff and cannot relax. _____

C. Both arms and both legs are paralyzed. _____
_____

D. Person has constant, slow, weaving, or writhing motions. _____

E. Both arms *or* both legs are paralyzed. _____
_____

35. The goal for a person with cerebral palsy is to be ____
_____.

36. A person with autism spectrum disorder (ASD) has

A. _____

B. _____

C. _____

37. Spina bifida is a defect of the _____
_____.

38. Children with spina bifida may have learning problems in these areas:

A. _____

B. _____

C. _____

D. _____

39. Which type of spina bifida would cause the problems in each of the examples given?

A. The person has leg paralysis and a lack of bowel and bladder control. _____

B. The person may have no symptoms. _____
_____

C. Nerve damage usually does not occur and surgery corrects the defect. _____

40. If hydrocephalus is not treated, pressure increases in the head and causes _____
and _____.

OPTIONAL LEARNING EXERCISES

Mr. Murphy is one of the residents you care for. He has Down syndrome. Answer Questions 41 to 43, which relate to this person.

41. Mr. Murphy is 40 years old. What disease may appear in adults with Down syndrome? _____
_____.

42. Mr. Murphy is encouraged to eat a well-balanced diet and to attend regular exercise classes. Including these in the care plan will help prevent the problems of _____ and
_____.

43. What two therapies may help Mr. Murphy to communicate more clearly? _____
and _____.

You care for Mary Reynolds, who has cerebral palsy. Answer Questions 44 and 45 about Ms. Reynolds.

44. It is difficult to feed Ms. Reynolds because she drools, grimaces, and moves her head constantly. You know that she does this because she has a type of cerebral palsy called _____
_____.

45. Because Ms. Reynolds remains in bed or a special chair all the time, she is at special risk for _____ because of immobility. She needs to be repositioned at least every _____
_____.

Chapter **41** **Intellectual and Developmental Disabilities**

INDEPENDENT LEARNING ACTIVITIES

- Many communities have services available for families with children and adults who are developmentally disabled. Some communities have sheltered workshops, day care, sheltered living centers, or physical and occupational therapy programs available. If your community has these services, ask permission to visit them and observe the persons being served there. Answer the following questions when you observe in the agency.
    - What age groups are served in this program?
    - What activities are available to the group?
    - What training is required for the people who work there?
    - How do the persons in the program act? Happy? Bored? Withdrawn? Other reactions?
    - What other services are available to these individuals in the agency? In the community?
    - Where do the persons in this program live? With family? Group homes? Other?
- Do you know a family who has a developmentally disabled family member? Ask the family if they will answer the following questions about living with this person.
    - How old is the developmentally disabled person? Where does the person live?
    - What abilities does the person have? What disabilities interfere with the activities of daily living for the person?
    - What therapies are being done to help the person reach his or her highest level of function?
    - What community programs have been helpful for the person?
    - How does this person's disability affect the family? Physical? Emotional? Financial? Day-to-day activities?

42 Rehabilitation and Restorative Care

FILL IN THE BLANKS: KEY TERMS

Activities of daily living   Prosthesis   Restorative aide
Disability   Rehabilitation   Restorative nursing care

1. A nursing assistant with special training in restorative nursing and rehabilitation skills is a _____
_____.

2. _____ are activities usually done during a normal day in a person's life.

3. An artificial replacement for a missing body part is a _____.

4. Care that helps persons regain their health, strength, and independence is _____.

5. A _____ is any lost, absent, or impaired physical or mental function.

6. The process of restoring the disabled person to the highest possible level of physical, psychological, social, and economic functioning is _____
_____.

CIRCLE THE BEST ANSWER

7. The focus of rehabilitation is on
   A. Improving abilities
   B. Restoring function to normal
   C. Helping the person regain health and strength
   D. Preventing injury
8. Restorative nursing will
   A. Cure the problem
   B. Allow the person to be independent
   C. Maintain the highest level of function
   D. Teach family members to care for the person
9. If you are a restorative aide, it means you have
   A. Special training in restorative nursing and rehabilitation skills
   B. Taken required classes for restorative aides
   C. Passed a special test to show you can perform these duties
   D. The most seniority at the facility

10. When assisting with rehabilitation and restorative care, it is important to
    A. Give complete care to prevent exertion by the person
    B. Make sure you do everything for the person
    C. Encourage the person to perform ADL to the extent possible
    D. Complete care quickly
11. Which of these would be most helpful for a person receiving rehabilitative care?
    A. Give the person pity or sympathy when tasks are difficult
    B. Remind the person not to try new skills or those that are difficult
    C. Give praise when even a little progress is made
    D. Encourage the person to perform ADL quickly
12. Complications can be prevented by
    A. Doing all ADL for the person
    B. Allowing the person to decide if he or she wants to move or exercise
    C. Making sure the person is in good alignment, is turned and repositioned, and performs range of motions exercises
    D. Making sure rehabilitation is fast-paced
13. Rehabilitation begins
    A. After the person has recovered
    B. When the person first seeks health care
    C. When the person asks for help
    D. When a discharge date has been set
14. Self-help devices help meet the goal of
    A. Recovery of all normal abilities
    B. Self-care
    C. Living alone
    D. Dependence on others
15. When dysphagia occurs after a stroke, a person
    A. May learn exercises to improve swallowing
    B. Must be fed by the staff
    C. Will always need enteral nutrition
    D. Will be given a clear liquid diet to prevent choking
16. Rehabilitation stresses plans that address
    A. Only physical care needs
    B. Only ambulation needs
    C. Physical, psychological, social, and economic needs
    D. Only psychological and social needs

209

17. The rehabilitation team meets to evaluate the person's progress
    A. Every 90 days
    B. Often, to change the plan as needed
    C. Every week
    D. Only when requested by the family or person
18. OBRA requires that nursing centers
    A. Have a full-time physical therapist
    B. Provide rehabilitation services
    C. Provide physical care only
    D. Employ full-time occupational and speech therapists

FILL IN THE BLANKS

19. Write out the meaning of the abbreviations.

    A. ADL _____

    B. OBRA _____

    C. OT _____

    D. PT _____

    E. ROM _____

    F. SNF _____

20. Restorative nursing programs do the following:

    A. _____

    B. _____

21. A person in rehabilitation needs help to restore or adjust in these areas:

    A. _____

    B. _____

    C. _____

    D. _____

22. Rehabilitation takes longer in which age group?
    _____

    What are the reasons for this?

    A. Changes affect _____

    _____

    B. Chronic _____

    _____

    C. Risk for _____

    _____

23. What are some self-help devices that will assist in self-feeding?

    A. _____

    B. _____

    C. _____

24. The goal for a prosthesis is to have the device _____
    _____.

25. When you are assisting with rehabilitation and restorative nursing care, why is it helpful to listen to how the nurse or therapist guides and directs the person? _____
    _____

26. When assisting with rehabilitation and restorative nursing care, what complications can be prevented if you report early signs and symptoms? _____
    _____

27. What can you do to promote the person's quality of life?

    A. _____

    B. _____

    C. _____

    D. _____

    E. _____

    F. _____

    G. _____

OPTIONAL LEARNING EXERCISES

Mrs. Mercer is 82 years old. She is a resident in a rehabilitation unit because she had a stroke that has caused weakness on her left side. Although she is right-handed, she needs to learn to use several self-help devices as she relearns ways to carry out ADL. She often becomes angry or depressed. Answer Questions 28 to 33 about Mrs. Mercer and her care. (You will need to use information learned in previous chapters for some of the answers.)

28. Mrs. Mercer is having difficulty with controlling urinary and bowel elimination. What would be the goal of her care for these problems? _____
    _____

    Her plan of care would include programs for _____
    _____.

29. What should you do to prepare Mrs. Mercer's food at mealtime so she can feed herself? _____
    _____

30. Mrs. Mercer can brush her teeth but needs help getting prepared. What should you do to get her ready to brush her teeth? _____
    _____

31. Why does she need help at mealtime and to brush her teeth? _____

32. Mrs. Mercer needs help to get in and out of bed. When helping her to transfer, you remember to position the chair on her _____ side.

33. When Mrs. Mercer becomes discouraged because progress is slow, how can you help her? You can stress _____ and focus on _____.

INDEPENDENT LEARNING ACTIVITIES

- Role-play the following situation with a classmate. Answer the questions about how you felt when you played Mrs. Leeds to understand how a person with a disability feels. Use your nondominant hand to attempt the activities Mrs. Leeds must do.

  Situation: Mary Leeds is 62 years old and had a stroke last month. She has weakness on her dominant side and has been admitted to a rehabilitation unit to relearn activities of daily living (ADL). She is practicing eating by using a spoon to place fluids and food in her mouth. She is also learning to button clothing.

  - How well could you hold the spoon with your nondominant hand?
  - What problems did you have controlling the spoon?
  - How rapidly could you eat? What type of food was easier to eat?
  - How well were you able to button your clothing? What techniques did you find that made you more successful?

  - How did this experience make you feel? How will it affect the way you interact with persons who have similar disabilities?

- With your instructor's permission, borrow a wheelchair from your school to use for 1 to 2 hours. Have a classmate push you around in the chair in a grocery store, mall, or your school. *Stay in the chair for the entire time to experience the feelings of a person who must use a wheelchair.* Use a handicap-equipped bathroom during this experience.

  - How comfortable was the wheelchair? Did you use any special padding or cushion in the seat?
  - What difficulties were encountered while moving about? Doorways? Steps? Aisles? Crowds? How did you deal with any difficulties?
  - How accessible was the handicap-equipped bathroom? How much room was available for you to transfer from the wheelchair to the toilet?
  - How did other people treat you? How many spoke to you? How many talked to your classmate and avoided you?
  - How did this experience make you feel? How will it affect the way you interact with a person in a wheelchair?

43 Assisted Living

FILL IN THE BLANKS: KEY TERMS

Assisted living   Medication reminder   Service plan

1. A _____ is reminding the person to take medications, observing that they were taken as prescribed, and charting that they were taken.

2. A written plan that lists the services needed by the person and who provides them is a _____ _____.

3. _____ provides housing, support services, and health care to persons needing help with activities of daily living.

CIRCLE THE BEST ANSWER

4. Which of these persons *would not* be living in an ALR?
   A. Someone who needs help taking medications at certain times
   B. A person who has problems with thinking, reasoning, and judgment
   C. A person who needs constant care
   D. Someone who is lonely and wants to live with people

5. When a person lives in an ALR, one requirement of the facility would be
   A. The person has at least two rooms and a bath
   B. Both a bathtub and a shower are provided
   C. A door that locks; the person keeps the key
   D. A double or queen-sized bed

6. Environmental requirements in an ALR include
   A. Common bathrooms have toilet paper, soap, and cloth towels, paper towels, or a dryer
   B. Pets or animals must be kept in kennels
   C. Hot water temperatures are between 110°F and 130°F
   D. Garbage is stored in covered containers lined with plastic bags that are removed at least once a day

7. According to the Assisted Living Residents' Rights, the resident
   A. Is required to participate in activities to avoid isolation
   B. Knows that all correspondence, communication, visits, and financial and personal matters will be observed by the staff
   C. Has a doctor or pharmacist assigned by the facility
   D. Make choices about how to receive care

8. A staff member in an ALR would need additional training to
   A. Provide nutrition and menu planning
   B. Know early signs of illness and the need for health care
   C. Know how to prevent and report abuse and neglect
   D. Allow him or her to help with administration of medications

9. Which of these is often a requirement of a resident in an ALR?
   A. The person must be able to leave the building in an emergency
   B. The person requires skilled nursing services
   C. The person has complex nursing problems
   D. The person needs 24-hour nursing care

10. A service plan for a person in an ALR
    A. Is reviewed every 90 days
    B. Lists the services needed by the person and who provides them
    C. States the medications that the person takes each day
    D. Remains the same as long as the person lives in the ALR

11. Which of these is a required service in an ALR?
    A. Clean bed linens every day
    B. A garage for cars owned by residents
    C. A 24-hour emergency communication system
    D. A bank in the facility

12. Meals in an ALR
    A. Are always served in the person's room
    B. Include the noon meal only
    C. Are posted in a menu for residents to see
    D. Cannot meet special dietary needs

13. When you assist with housekeeping, you will be expected to
    A. Clean the tub or shower after each use
    B. Put out clean towels and washcloths every week
    C. Use a disinfectant or water and detergent to clean bathroom surfaces once a week
    D. Dust furniture every day

14. A measure you should follow when handling, preparing, or storing foods is
    A. Use leftover food within 4 or 5 days
    B. Wash all pots and pans in a dishwasher
    C. Date and refrigerate containers of leftovers and refrigerate as soon as possible
    D. Clean kitchen appliances, counters, tables, and other surfaces once a day

15. When practicing food safety, which of these is *incorrect*?
    A. Use a garbage disposal for food and liquid garbage
    B. Place leftover food in the refrigerator as soon as possible
    C. Use leftover food within 4–5 days
    D. Place washed eating and cooking items in a drainer to dry

16. When assisting with laundry, a guideline to follow is
    A. Sort items according to the amount of soil on the items
    B. Wear gloves when handling soiled laundry
    C. Use hot water to wash all items
    D. Use the highest setting on the dryer to sanitize the items

17. When you assist a person with medication, it may involve
    A. Opening containers for a person who cannot do so
    B. Measuring medications for the person
    C. Explaining to a person the action of a medication
    D. Preparing a pill organizer for the person each week

18. If a medication error occurs, you should
    A. Tell the person not to do it again
    B. Make sure the person takes the correct medication at the next scheduled time
    C. Report the error to the nurse
    D. Take all medications away from the person immediately

19. An attendant is needed in an ALR 24 hours a day to
    A. Give care to those who need it
    B. Make sure medications are dispensed when ordered
    C. Assist those who need assistance if an emergency occurs
    D. Provide activities for the residents

20. Which of these is *not* a right of a resident in the ALR?
    A. The right to have financial and other records kept in confidence
    B. The right to have overnight guests whenever the resident wishes
    C. The right to perform work or refuse to perform work for the facility
    D. The right to request to relocate or refuse to relocate within the ALR

FILL IN THE BLANKS

21. Write out the meaning of each abbreviation.
    a. AD _____
    b. ADL _____
    c. ALR _____

22. When working in an assisted living setting, you should follow _____ when contact with blood, body fluids, secretions, excretions, or potentially contaminated items is likely.

23. Persons in assisted living settings usually need help with one or more ADL, such as
    A. _____
    B. _____
    C. _____
    D. _____
    E. _____
    F. _____

24. A bathroom in an ALR must provide privacy and
    A. _____
    B. _____
    C. _____
    D. _____
    E. _____

25. The ALR cannot employ a person with a _____
    _____.

26. The service plan lists
    A. _____
    B. _____
    C. _____

27. The service plan also relates to
    A. _____
    B. _____
    C. _____
    D. _____
    E. _____
    F. _____

28. How many meals are usually provided in an ALR?
    _____
    A. Usually there are no more than _____ hours allowed between the evening meal and breakfast.
    B. The time between the evening meal and breakfast can be longer if there is a _____
    _____.

213

29. When providing housekeeping, bathroom surfaces are cleaned every _____ with a _____ or _____ _____ and _____ _____.

30. When you wash eating and cooking items by hand, what is the order in which they are washed?

   A. _____

   B. _____

   C. _____

   D. _____

   E. _____

31. If you are assisting the person with taking medications, you should know the six rights of medication administration. They are

   A. _____

   B. _____

   C. _____

   D. _____

   E. _____

   F. _____

32. If a person is taking his or her medications and states that a pill looks different, what should you do? _____
   _____

33. If a person needs a medication reminder, it means reminding _____, observing _____, and charting _____ _____.

34. If you are assisting in medication administration, you should report any medication error to the RN. Errors would include:

   A. _____

   B. _____

   C. _____

   D. _____

   E. _____

   F. _____

   G. _____

   H. _____

   I. _____

OPTIONAL LEARNING EXERCISES

You are working in an assisted living facility. What would you do in the following situations?

35. You are providing housekeeping assistance to Mrs. Miller, who lives alone. The stove is on and a pan has burning food in it. Mrs. Miller tells you she did not put the pan on the stove. What should you do? _____
   _____
   _____

   What is a likely reason for her behavior? _____
   _____

36. A resident in the facility has lived there for 2 years and has needed little assistance. He recently had a stroke and now needs care for all of his ADL. Why is he being moved to a nursing facility? _____
   _____

37. Mrs. Jenkins tells you she is expecting an important phone call and wants to eat lunch in her room. What should you do? _____
   _____

38. Mr. Shante asks you to get his medications ready for him to take. What assistance are you allowed to give when the nurse has trained you?

   A. _____

   B. _____

   C. _____

   D. _____

   E. _____

   F. _____

   G. _____

   H. _____

39. When you are assisting Mrs. Clyde with her medications, you notice that two of the labels have an expired date. What should you do? _____
   _____

40. Mrs. Johnson asks you when the next meeting of the quilting group will be held. She also asks on what days the community crafts fair is planned. Where would you direct her to find this information? _____
   _____

INDEPENDENT LEARNING ACTIVITIES

- Find out if your community has any assisted living facilities. They may be part of another facility or may be an independent facility. Visit the facility to answer the following questions.
  - What services are offered in the facility? Who provides the services? Nursing assistants? Other assistants? What training is required?
  - What types of living quarters are provided? What belongings can the person bring from home?
  - What activities are scheduled? How are residents given information about these activities?
  - How do the residents act? Happy? Withdrawn? Sad? How do the staff members act?

- Find out what laws in your state apply to assisted living facilities. Answer the following questions about the laws.
  - What type of license is required for an assisted living facility? Do the laws apply to independent facilities as well as to those attached to other facilities?
  - What laws apply to staff training for these facilities? Does the state require workers to be nursing assistants with special training?
  - What does the state law say about assisting with medications? What non-licensed persons can assist with medications? What training is required?

44 Basic Emergency Care

FILL IN THE BLANKS: KEY TERMS

Anaphylaxis
Cardiac arrest
Convulsion
Fainting

First aid
Hemorrhage
Respiratory arrest
Seizure

Shock
Sudden cardiac arrest

1. In _____, breathing stops but the heart still pumps for several minutes.

2. The sudden loss of consciousness from an inadequate blood supply to the brain is _____.

3. When the heart and breathing stop suddenly and without warning, it is _____.

4. _____ is a condition that results when there is not enough blood supply to organs and tissues.

5. Emergency care given to an ill or injured person before medical help arrives is _____.

6. A convulsion may also be called a _____ _____.

7. _____ is the excessive loss of blood in a short period of time.

8. Violent and sudden contractions or tremors of muscles are a seizure or a _____.

9. A life-threatening sensitivity to an antigen is _____.

10. Another name for sudden cardiac arrest is _____.

CIRCLE THE BEST ANSWER

11. When an emergency occurs in nursing centers, the nurse determines when to
    A. Call the doctor for orders
    B. Activate the EMS system
    C. Call the supervisor
    D. Assist the person to bed

12. If you find a person lying on the floor, you should
    A. Keep the person lying down
    B. Help the person back to bed
    C. Elevate the head
    D. Help the person to a chair

13. If the nurse instructs you to activate the EMS system, you should
    A. Tell the operator your name and title
    B. Explain to the operator what seems to have happened
    C. Give the victim's name and age
    D. Hang up as soon as you have finished giving the information

14. It is important to restore breathing and circulation quickly because
    A. The lungs will be damaged
    B. The person will lose consciousness
    C. Heart, brain, and other organ damage occurs within minutes
    D. Hemorrhage will occur

15. Which of these is *not* a major sign of sudden cardiac arrest (SCA)?
    A. Complaints of chest pain
    B. No pulse
    C. No breathing
    D. No response

16. The purpose of the head tilt–chin lift maneuver is to
    A. Make the person more comfortable
    B. Open the airway
    C. Practice Standard Precautions
    D. Stimulate the heart to beat

17. When you use mouth-to-mouth breathing, you should
    A. Allow the person's chin to relax against the neck
    B. Place your mouth loosely over the person's mouth
    C. Blow into the person's mouth. You should see the chest rise
    D. Apply pressure on the chin to close the mouth

18. Before starting chest compressions
    A. Make sure the person is breathing
    B. Check for a pulse
    C. Wait 30 seconds to see if the person regains consciousness
    D. Turn the person to the side

19. When chest compressions are started, you give compressions at a rate of
    A. 5 compressions, then check for a pulse
    B. 60–100 compressions per minute
    C. 100–120 compressions per minute
    D. 15 compressions per minute

20. The purpose of chest compressions is to
    A. Deflate the lungs
    B. Increase oxygen in the blood
    C. Force blood through the circulatory system
    D. Help the heart work more effectively
21. In order for chest compressions to be effective, the person must be
    A. In prone position
    B. On a soft surface
    C. Supine on a hard, flat surface
    D. In a semi-Fowler position
22. When preparing to give chest compressions, locate the heel of the hands
    A. On the sternum between the nipples
    B. On the lower half of the sternum
    C. Side by side over the sternum
    D. Slightly below the end of the sternum
23. When giving chest compressions to an adult, depress the sternum
    A. About 1 to 1½ inches
    B. About ½ to 1 inch
    C. About 1½ inches
    D. At least 2 inches
24. CPR is done only when the person
    A. Does not respond when you shout, "Are you okay?"
    B. Is not breathing
    C. Is unconscious
    D. Does not respond, is not breathing, and has no pulse
25. Hands-only CPR is useful for persons who
    A. Have taken a BLS course
    B. Are not sure the victim is in cardiac arrest
    C. Have not been trained in BLS
    D. Do not like to do mouth-to-mouth resuscitation
26. If the person is not breathing or not breathing adequately, give two breaths that
    A. Last about 1 second each
    B. Last about 5 seconds each
    C. Last 5–10 seconds each
    D. Last 15 seconds each
27. When performing one rescuer CPR, the cycle of chest compressions and breaths is at a rate of
    A. 15 compressions followed by 2 breaths
    B. 30 compressions followed by 2 breaths
    C. 60 compressions per minute followed by 5 breaths
    D. 12 compressions per minute followed by 1 breath
28. When performing one rescuer CPR, the rate of compressions is
    A. 15 compressions in 5 minutes
    B. 100–120 compressions per minute
    C. 30 compressions per minute
    D. 4 cycles of 15 compressions and 2 breaths
29. Side-lying position is the recovery position when the person is breathing and has a pulse but is not responding because
    A. The position helps keep the airway open and prevents aspiration
    B. It makes the person respond more quickly
    C. You can observe the person more easily
    D. The person will be more comfortable

30. When an automated external defibrillator (AED) is used, it
    A. Stops the heart
    B. Slows the heartbeat down
    C. Stops ventricular fibrillation (VF) and restores a regular heartbeat
    D. Starts the heartbeat
31. Which of these is a sign of internal hemorrhage?
    A. Steady flow of blood from a wound
    B. Pain, shock, vomiting blood, or coughing up blood
    C. Bleeding that occurs in spurts
    D. Dried blood at the site of an injury
32. To control external bleeding, you should
    A. Remove any objects that have pierced or stabbed the person
    B. Keep the injured part flat or below the level of the body
    C. Apply pressure with your hand directly over the bleeding site
    D. Give the person warm or cool fluids to drink
33. If a person tells you she feels faint
    A. Have the person lie down in a supine position
    B. Let the person walk around to increase circulation
    C. Have the person sit or lie down before fainting occurs
    D. Raise the head with pillows if the person is already lying down
34. If a person is in shock, it is helpful if you
    A. Have the person sit in a chair
    B. Keep the person cool by removing some of his or her clothing
    C. Keep the person lying down, maintain an open airway, and control bleeding
    D. Give the person something to drink or eat
35. Anaphylactic shock occurs because of
    A. Hemorrhage
    B. An allergy to foods, insects, chemicals, or medications
    C. Sudden cardiac arrest
    D. Seizures
36. When a stroke occurs, position the person in the recovery position
    A. On the affected side
    B. On the unaffected side
    C. In the supine position
    D. In a semi-Fowler position
37. If a person has a seizure, you should
    A. Place an object between the teeth
    B. Distract the person to stop the seizure
    C. Position the person in bed
    D. Move furniture, equipment, and sharp objects away from the person
38. If you are assisting a person with burns
    A. Remove burned clothing
    B. Cover the burn wounds with a sterile or clean, cool, moist covering
    C. Give the person plenty of fluids
    D. Apply oils or ointments to the burns

217

39. Write the meaning of each abbreviation

    A. ACS _____

    B. AED _____

    C. AHA _____

    D. BLS _____

    E. CPR _____

    F. DNR _____

    G. EMS _____

    H. FAST _____

    I. FBAO _____

    J. SCA _____

    K. VF or V-fib _____

40. If you activate the EMS system, what information should you give to the operator?

    A. _____

    B. _____

    C. _____

    D. _____

    E. _____

    F. _____

41. Chain of Survival actions for adults are

    A. _____

    B. _____

    C. _____

    D. _____

    E. _____

42. Cardiopulmonary resuscitation has four parts. They are

    a. C _____

    b. A _____

    c. B _____

    d. D _____

43. When opening the airway with the head tilt–chin lift maneuver, explain the steps needed

    A. Place _____

    B. Tilt _____

    C. Place _____

    D. Lift _____

    E. Do not _____

44. When you perform mouth-to-mouth breathing, it is likely you will have contact with _____ _____.

45. You determine a person is choking. List the steps of performing abdominal thrusts.

    A. _____

    B. _____

    C. _____

    D. _____

    E. _____

    F. _____

    G. _____

46. If a person is obese or pregnant, give _____ _____.

47. To find the carotid pulse, place _____. Slide your fingers down _____.

48. When giving one- or two-rescuer CPR, give _____ compressions followed by _____ rescue breaths. The rate of compressions should be _____ compressions per minute.

49. When giving 2-person CPR, change positions every _____ minutes or after _____ cycles of _____ compressions and _____ breaths.

50. If direct pressure does not stop hemorrhage, apply pressure over the artery _____.

51. Stop the Bleed cabinets or kits contain

    A. _____

    B. _____

    C. _____

52. Common causes of fainting are

    A. _____

    B. _____

    C. _____

    D. _____

53. List the signs and symptoms of shock.

    A. _____

    B. _____

    C. _____

    D. _____

    E. _____

    F. _____

    G. _____

54. Anaphylaxis is an emergency because it occurs within _____.

55. What signs or symptoms will be present on the affected side with a stroke?

    A. _____

    B. _____

56. Describe the two phases of a generalized tonic-clonic seizure.

    A. Tonic phase _____

    _____

    B. Clonic phase _____

    _____

57. The following relate to the emergency care of a person having a seizure.

    A. How do you protect the person's head? _____

    _____

    _____

    B. How is the person positioned? _____

    _____

    _____

    C. Why is furniture moved? _____

    _____

    D. What times are noted? _____

    _____

58. Partial-thickness burns involve the _____
    _____.

59. Full-thickness burns involve _____
    _____.

60. A _____ burn is very painful because _____.

OPTIONAL LEARNING EXERCISES

You are visiting a neighbor and she is washing dishes. As she washes a glass, it breaks and she sustains a deep cut on her wrist. Answer Questions 61 to 66 about how you would respond.

61. How would you determine whether the bleeding was from an artery or vein? _____
    _____.

62. Your neighbor is crying and walking around the room. What is the best thing you can do to help her?
    A. Stay _____
    _____.

B. Position the arm in an _____
    _____.

C. Instead of walking around, she should be kept _____ until help arrives.

63. Clean rubber gloves are on the counter. How can they be useful to you? _____
    _____

64. What materials in the home could be used to place over the wound? _____
    _____

65. Your neighbor is restless and has a rapid and weak pulse. You notice her skin is cold, moist, and pale. These signs indicate she may be in _____.

66. Her wound is still bleeding and she loses consciousness. What should you do before you continue to give first aid? _____
    _____

INDEPENDENT LEARNING ACTIVITIES

- You have learned some basic emergency care in this chapter. Find out where in your community a more advanced first aid course is available. Answer the following questions about the course.
  - What agency or agencies offer a course in first aid?
  - How long does the course last? How much does it cost?
  - Who may take the course? The public? Medical personnel? Others, such as police, firefighters, etc.?
  - What subjects are covered in the course?
  - Would taking this course help you in your job? In your family? In your community?
- Most health care facilities require that employees take a course in basic CPR. You may be required to take CPR as part of this course. Answer these questions about CPR training in your community.
  - What agency or agencies offer CPR courses?
  - How long does the course take? How much does it cost?
  - Who can take the courses? The public? Medical personnel? Are different classes offered to medical personnel? If so, what is the difference?
  - How often does the person need to be re-certified? How does the re-certification course differ from the beginning class?
- Take a tour of the halls of your school or other public building. Note where emergency equipment is located.
  - Did you find an AED? Stop the Bleed cabinet? First aid kit?
  - Make a point of looking for these when you are in a public building such as an airport, library or hospital.

45 End-of-Life Care

FILL IN THE BLANKS: KEY TERMS

Advance directive
Autopsy
End-of-life care

Hospice care
Palliative care
Postmortem care

Reincarnation
Rigor mortis
Terminal illness

1. The support and care given during the time surrounding death is _____.

2. _____ involves relieving or reducing the intensity of uncomfortable symptoms without producing a cure.

3. The stiffness or rigidity of skeletal muscles that occurs after death is _____.

4. An _____ is a document stating a person's wishes about health care when that person cannot make his or her own decisions.

5. Care of the body after death is _____ _____.

6. An illness or injury for which there is no reasonable expectation of recovery is a _____.

7. _____ is the belief that the spirit or soul is reborn in another human body or in another form of life.

8. The examination of the body after death is an _____.

9. _____ is care that focuses on comfort and quality of life of a person with a serious illness who is approaching the end of life.

CIRCLE THE BEST ANSWER

10. When a person has a terminal illness
    A. The doctor is able to accurately predict when the person will die
    B. Modern medicine can cure the disease
    C. The person may live longer than expected or die sooner than expected
    D. He or she will die when expected

11. When a person is receiving palliative care, he or she will
    A. Not receive any pain medications
    B. Probably recover from the illness
    C. Receive care to relieve uncomfortable symptoms
    D. Not be allowed to live at home

12. A person generally receives hospice care when
    A. He or she has less than 6 months to live
    B. Life-saving measures can cure the disease
    C. The family can no longer care for the person
    D. The doctor refuses to treat the person and the illness any longer

13. Cultural and spiritual beliefs about death
    A. Are all very similar
    B. Do not usually affect the person's reaction to death
    C. Are important to the person and family as death approaches
    D. Should be ignored when giving care

14. Children between ages 2 and 6 years see death as
    A. Final
    B. Punishment for being bad
    C. Suffering and pain
    D. A reunion with those who have died

15. Older persons see death as
    A. A temporary state
    B. Freedom from pain, suffering, and disability
    C. Something that happens to other people
    D. Something that affects plans, hopes, dreams, and ambitions

16. In which stage of dying does the person make promises and "just one more" requests?
    A. Acceptance
    B. Anger
    C. Depression
    D. Bargaining

17. If a dying person begins to talk about worries and concerns, you should
    A. Call a spiritual leader
    B. Tell the nurse
    C. Be there and listen quietly
    D. Change the subject to more pleasant topics

18. When a person is dying, care should be given
    A. Only if the person requests it
    B. To meet basic needs
    C. Often, to keep the person active
    D. Only while the person is conscious

19. Because vision fails as death approaches, you should
   A. Explain what you are doing to the person when you are in the room
   B. Have the room lit very brightly
   C. Turn out all lights
   D. Keep the eyes covered at all times
20. Hearing is one of the last functions lost, so it is important to
   A. Speak in whispers
   B. Give care without talking to avoid disturbing the person
   C. Ask family and friends to speak loudly in the person's room
   D. Provide reassurance and explanations about care
21. As death nears, oral hygiene is
   A. Given during regular care
   B. Given frequently because taking oral fluids is difficult
   C. Given very infrequently to avoid disturbing the person
   D. Never given because the person cannot swallow
22. Which of these does *not* occur as death nears?
   A. Body temperature rises
   B. The skin is cool, pale, and mottled
   C. Perspiration decreases
   D. Circulation fails
23. Because of breathing difficulties, the dying person is generally more comfortable in
   A. The supine position
   B. A side-lying position
   C. A prone position
   D. A semi-Fowler position
24. When a person is dying, you can help the family by
   A. Allowing the family to stay for as long as they wish
   B. Staying away from the room and delaying care
   C. Telling the family that they need to leave so you can give care
   D. Telling the family that the person dying is not in pain
25. If a person has a living will, it instructs doctors to
   A. Start measures that will save the person's life
   B. Start CPR whenever necessary
   C. Not start measures that prolong dying
   D. Activate the EMS system for a person
26. If the doctor writes a "Do Not Resuscitate" (DNR) order it means that
   A. The person will not be resuscitated
   B. The person will be resuscitated if it is an emergency
   C. The doctor will decide whether or not to resuscitate
   D. The RN may decide that in a particular situation resuscitation is needed
27. A sign that death is near would be
   A. Deep, rapid respirations
   B. The blood pressure starts to fall
   C. Muscles tense and contract in spasms
   D. Peristalsis increases

28. After death, an ID tag is attached to the right big toe or
   A. Wrist
   B. Ankle
   C. Upper arm
   D. Upper leg
29. The dying patient's bill of last rights includes
   A. The right to freedom from restraint
   B. The right to be free from abuse, mistreatment, and neglect.
   C. The right to have a private room
   D. All of the above

FILL IN THE BLANKS

30. Write out the meaning of these abbreviations.

   A. AD _____

   B. CPR _____

   C. DNR _____

   D. EMS _____

   E. ID _____

   F. POLST _____

31. It is important to examine your own feelings about death because they will affect _____ _____.

32. When you understand the dying process, you can approach the dying person with _____ _____.

33. The intent of palliative care is to _____ _____.

34. List the services that hospice provides to these persons or groups.

   A. Dying person _____ _____

   B. Survivors _____ _____

   C. Health team _____ _____

35. Religious beliefs strengthen when dying and often provide _____.

36. Adults fear death because they fear

   A. _____

   B. _____

   C. _____

   D. _____

   E. _____

   F. _____

   G. _____

37. Name the five stages of dying.

A. _____

B. _____

C. _____

D. _____

E. _____

38. When caring for a dying person, comfort goals are

A. _____

B. _____

39. By listening to the dying person, it lets the person _____ in his or her own way.

40. Touch shows _____
_____.

41. Signs and symptoms of pain should be reported at once because _____ is easier than relieving pain.

42. Where can you find measures used to prevent and control pain for the person? _____

43. Ways to help a person with breathing problems include the following.

A. Position the person in _____
_____
_____

B. The doctor may order _____
_____
_____

C. Open a _____

D. Circulate air with a _____
_____
_____

44. Because hearing is one of the last functions lost, do not _____ the person.

45. When caring for a dying person, do not ask questions that need long answers because _____
_____.

46. Because crusting and irritation of the nostrils can occur, you should _____.

47. If the person refuses to eat, you should _____
_____.

48. What kinds of elimination problems are common in the dying person? _____

49. The Patient Self-Determination Act and OBRA give two rights that affect the rights of a dying person. They are:

A. _____

B. _____

50. A living will instructs doctors

A. _____

B. _____

51. When a person cannot make health care decisions, the authority to do so is given to the person with ___
_____
_____.

52. What are the signs that death is near?

A. _____

B. _____

C. _____

D. _____

E. _____

F. _____

53. The signs of death include no _____,
no _____, and no _____
_____
_____. The pupils are _____ and
_____.

54. Postmortem care is not done when an _____
_____ is to be done.

55. When assisting with postmortem care, you need this information from the nurse:

A. _____

B. _____

C. _____

D. _____

E. _____

56. The right to confidentiality before and after death provides that _____
_____.

OPTIONAL LEARNING EXERCISES

You are assigned to care for Mrs. Adams, who is dying. Answer Questions 57 to 64 regarding this situation.

57. You find Mrs. Adams crying in her room. When you ask her what is wrong, she tells you no one gave her fresh water this morning and she has not had her bath yet. She tells you to just go away. What stage of dying is she displaying? _____

58. Later in the day, Mrs. Adams tells you she can't wait until she is better so she can go home and plant her garden. She states that she knows the tests done last week were wrong and she will recover quickly from her illness. Now what stage is she displaying? _____ Why is she displaying two different stages so rapidly? _____ _____ _____

59. A minister comes to visit Mrs. Adams while you are giving care. What should you do? _____ _____ _____.

60. You are working overnight and find Mrs. Adams awake during the night. She asks you to sit with her. She begins to talk about her fears, worries, and anxieties. What are two things you can do to convey caring to her? _____ _____

61. As Mrs. Adams becomes weaker, a family member is always at her bedside. When they ask to assist with her care, you know that this is acceptable because _____.

62. Mrs. Adams has very noisy breathing. This occurs as death nears and is called the _____. It is due to _____.

63. Mrs. Adams dies while you are working and the nurse asks you to assist with postmortem care. As you clean soiled areas, you assist the nurse to turn the body and air is expelled. This occurs because _____ _____.

64. You wear gloves during postmortem care because they will _____ _____.

INDEPENDENT LEARNING ACTIVITIES

- It is important to explore your own beliefs about death and dying before you care for persons who are dying. Answer the following questions to understand your own feelings.
  - Have you attended a funeral or visited a funeral home? How did you feel?
  - Has anyone close to you died? How did you assist with any of the funeral arrangements? What kinds of preparation did the family do?
  - What cultural or religious practices in your family affect death and funeral arrangements? How do you think these practices will affect you when you care for those who are dying?
  - Have you ever been present when someone died? In your personal life? As a student? At your job? How did you respond? What were you asked to do in this situation?
  - What is your personal belief about a living will? How will you respond if a person or family refuses a feeding tube or a ventilator? How will you respond if they ask to have these measures discontinued and the person dies?
  - What is your personal belief about a "Do Not Resuscitate" order? How would you feel if a person you are caring for has this order? How will you respond when the person dies and no effort is made to help the person?
- Consider talking with a hospice nurse or volunteer about their work. Why do they find this type of work rewarding? Would you consider enrolling in a volunteer hospice training program?

46 Getting a Job

FILL IN THE BLANKS: KEY TERMS

Application   Preceptor
Cover letter   Résumé

1. A summary of personal information is a _____.

2. An _____ is a form used by an employer to collect information from a potential employee.

3. A staff member who guides another staff member is a mentor or a _____.

4. A _____ is a letter written with the purpose of obtaining an interview.

CIRCLE THE BEST ANSWER

5. Displaying good work ethics at your clinical experience site may help you find a job because
   A. You will pass the course
   B. It will show you care
   C. You will get better grades
   D. The staff may look at students as future employees

6. You should be well-groomed when looking for a job because it
   A. Shows you are cooperative
   B. Makes a good first impression
   C. Shows you are respectful
   D. Shows you have values and attitudes that fit with the center

7. How does an employer know you can perform required job skills?
   A. They will request proof of training and will check your record in the state nursing assistant registry.
   B. They will ask you to give a demonstration of your skills.
   C. You will be asked many questions about performing certain skills.
   D. You will be required to take a written test.

8. You usually get a job application from
   A. The personnel office or the human resources office
   B. A friend who works at the center
   C. The director of nursing
   D. The receptionist in the lobby of the center

9. A résumé includes
   A. A letter of reference from your friend
   B. A summary of your hobbies and interests
   C. Information about your personal life
   D. Contact information such as address, phone number, and email

10. Practicing getting to the job interview site before the day of your interview is a good idea so you can
    A. Show you follow directions well
    B. Show you listen well
    C. Make sure you will be on time for the interview
    D. Look over the center to see if you want to work there

11. When you are interviewing, it is correct to
    A. Touch or read things on the person's desk
    B. Use good eye contact when speaking to the interviewer
    C. Wear a sweatsuit and athletic shoes
    D. Shake hands very gently

12. What is a good way to share your list of skills with the interviewer?
    A. Tell the person verbally what you can do
    B. Ask for a list of skills and check off the ones you know
    C. Bring a list of your skills and give it to the interviewer
    D. Tell the interviewer you will send a list of your skills as soon as possible

13. It is important to ask questions at the end of the interview because it
    A. Will show the interviewer you are interested in the job
    B. Will help you decide if the job is right for you
    C. Shows you have good communication skills
    D. Shows you are dependable

14. If you are assigned a preceptor, the person may be
    A. An RN or LPN/LVN
    B. Another nursing assistant
    C. A doctor
    D. Any member of the health care team

15. A common reason for losing a job is
    A. Being unable to perform a new skill
    B. Taking the bus to work instead of having a car
    C. Being late one time because of an accident on the road
    D. Having several absences or being tardy frequently

16. If you resign from a job, it is good practice to give
    A. One-week's notice
    B. Two-weeks' notice
    C. Four-weeks' notice
    D. No notice

17. Write the meaning of each abbreviation

    A. CNA _____

    B. DON _____

    C. NATCEP _____

    D. RN _____

18. List places you can find out about job openings.

    A. _____

    B. _____

    C. _____

    D. _____

    E. _____

    F. _____

    G. _____

    H. _____

19. When you apply for a job, the employer will require you to provide documents that prove you are qualified. They are

    A. _____

    B. _____

    C. _____

20. If a job application asks you to print in black ink, why is it a poor idea to use blue ink? _____

21. How can writing illegibly on a job application affect getting a job? _____

22. Why is it important to give information about employment gaps or leaving a job? _____

23. If you lie on a job application, it is _____ _____. If you do this, what can happen? _____

OPTIONAL LEARNING EXERCISES

24. When you apply for a job, you will need references for the potential employer. What should you do before giving the references? _____

25. When you send a cover letter and your résumé, what type of envelope should be used? _____

26. When you are considering applying to an organization, what information can you find when you look at the organization's website? _____

27. What should be sent within 24 hours after the interview? _____
    Why? _____

28. When you resign from a job, you should do one of the following:

    A. _____

    B. _____

    C. _____

29. What information should you give with your notice to resign?

    A. _____

    B. _____

    C. _____

INDEPENDENT LEARNING ACTIVITIES

- Have you ever applied for a job? How did you feel when you were being interviewed? After reading this chapter, how would you handle a future interview?
- Role-play a job interview with a classmate. Take turns playing the interviewer and the job applicant. Use the lists in this chapter to ask questions. Practice answers that you can use in a real interview.
- Think of three people you could use as references when applying for a job. Ask their permission to use them as references. If they agree, make a list of the people and their titles, addresses, and telephone numbers to use when you apply for a job. Why would each of these people be a good reference?

Procedure Checklists

Using a Fire Extinguisher

Name: —————————————— Date: ——————————————

Procedure	S	U	Comments
1. Pulled the fire alarm.	——	——	——————
2. Got the nearest fire extinguisher.	——	——	——————
3. Carried it upright.	——	——	——————
4. Took it to the fire.	——	——	——————
5. Followed the word *PASS*:			
a. P—*Pulled* the safety pin to unlock the handle.	——	——	——————
b. A—*Aimed* low. Directed the hose or nozzle at the base of the fire. Did not try to spray the tops of flames.	——	——	——————
c. S—*Squeezed* the lever. Squeezed or pushed down on the lever, handle, or button to start the stream. Released the level, handle, or button to stop the stream.	——	——	——————
d. S—*Swept* back and forth. Swept the stream back and forth (side to side) at the base of the fire.	——	——	——————

Applying a Transfer/Gait Belt

Name: _____ Date: _____

Quality of Life	S	U	Comments
Remembered to:			
• Knock before entering the person's room.	____	____	_____
• Address the person by name.	____	____	_____
• Introduce yourself by name and title.	____	____	_____
• Explain the procedure to the person before beginning and during the procedure.	____	____	_____
• Protect the person's rights during the procedure.			
• Handle the person gently during the procedure.			

Procedure

	S	U	Comments
1. Saw *Promoting Safety and Comfort: Transfer/Gait Belts.*	____	____	_____
2. Practiced hand hygiene.	____	____	_____
3. Identified the person. Checked the identification (ID) bracelet against the assignment sheet. Also called the person by name.	____	____	_____
4. Provided for privacy.	____	____	_____
5. Assisted the person to a sitting position.	____	____	_____
6. Applied the belt around the person's waist over clothing. Did not apply it over bare skin.	____	____	_____
7. Secured the buckle. The buckle was in front.	____	____	_____
8. Tightened the belt so it was snug. It did not cause discomfort or impaired breathing. Slid open, flat hand under the belt.	____	____	_____
9. Made sure that a woman's breasts were not caught under the belt.	____	____	_____
10. Turned the belt so the quick-release buckle was at the person's back. The buckle was not over the spine.	____	____	_____
11. Tucked any excess strap under the belt.	____	____	_____

Helping the Falling Person

Name: _____ Date: _____

Procedure	S	U	Comments
1. Stood behind the person with your feet apart. Kept your back straight.	___	___	_____
2. Brought the person close to your body as fast as possible. Used the transfer/gait belt. Or wrapped your arms around the person's waist. If necessary (but not preferred), held the person under the arms.	___	___	_____
3. Moved your leg so the person's buttocks rested on it. Moved the leg near the person.	___	___	_____
4. Lowered the person to the floor. The person slid down your leg to the floor. Bent at your hips and knees while lowering the person.	___	___	_____
5. Called a nurse to check the person. Stayed with the person.	___	___	_____
6. Helped the nurse return the person to bed. Asked other staff to help if needed.	___	___	_____

Postprocedure

	S	U	Comments
7. Provided for comfort.	___	___	_____
8. Placed the call light within reach.	___	___	_____
9. Raised or lowered the bed rails. Followed the care plan.	___	___	_____
10. Completed a safety check of the room.	___	___	_____
11. Reported and recorded the following:			
a. How the fall occurred.	___	___	_____
b. How far the person walked.	___	___	_____
c. How activity was tolerated before the fall.	___	___	_____
d. Complaints before the fall.	___	___	_____
e. How much help the person needed while walking.	___	___	_____
12. Completed an incident report.	___	___	_____

Applying Restraints

Name: _____ Date: _____

	S	U	Comments
Quality of Life			
Remembered to:			
• Knock before entering the person's room.	___	___	_____
• Address the person by name.	___	___	_____
• Introduce yourself by name and title.	___	___	_____
• Explain the procedure to the person before beginning and during the procedure.	___	___	_____
• Protect the person's rights during the procedure.	___	___	_____
• Handle the person gently during the procedure.	___	___	_____

Preprocedure

1. Followed *Delegation Guidelines: Applying Restraints. Saw Promoting Safety and Comfort: Applying Restraints.* ___ ___ _____
2. Collected the following as instructed by the nurse:
   a. Correct type and size of restraints ___ ___ _____
   b. Padding for skin and bony areas ___ ___ _____
   c. Bed rail pads or gap protectors (if needed) ___ ___ _____
3. Practiced hand hygiene. ___ ___ _____
4. Identified the person. Checked the identification (ID) bracelet against the assignment sheet. Also called the person by name. ___ ___ _____
5. Provided for privacy. ___ ___ _____

Procedure

6. Made sure the person was comfortable and in good alignment. ___ ___ _____
7. Put the bed rail pads or gap protectors (if needed) on the bed if the person was in bed. Followed the manufacturer's instructions. ___ ___ _____
8. Padded bony areas. Followed the nurse's instructions and the care plan. ___ ___ _____
9. Read the manufacturer's instructions. Noted the front and back of the restraint. ___ ___ _____
10. *For wrist restraints*:
    a. Applied the restraint following the manufacturer's instructions. Placed the soft or foam part toward the skin. ___ ___ _____
    b. Secured the restraint so it was snug but not tight. Made sure you could slide one finger under the restraint. Followed the manufacturer's instructions. Adjusted the straps if the restraint was too loose or too tight. Checked for snugness again. ___ ___ _____
    c. Buckled or tied the straps to the movable part of the bed frame out of the person's reach. Used a quick-release tie. ___ ___ _____
    d. Repeated steps 10 a–c for the other wrist.
       i. Applied the restraint following the manufacturer's instructions. Placed the soft or foam part toward the skin. ___ ___ _____
       ii. Secured the restraint so it was snug but not tight. Made sure you could slide one finger under the restraint. Followed the manufacturer's instructions. Adjusted the straps if the restraint was too loose or too tight. Checked for snugness again. ___ ___ _____
       iii. Buckled or tied the straps to the movable part of the bed frame out of the person's reach. Used a quick-release tie. ___ ___ _____
11. *For mitt restraints:*
    a. Made sure the person's hands were clean and dry. ___ ___ _____
    b. Applied the mitt restraint. Followed the manufacturer's instructions. ___ ___ _____
    c. Secured the restraint to the bed if directed to do so by the nurse. Buckled or tied the straps to the movable part of the bed frame. Used a quick-release tie. ___ ___ _____

   d. Made sure the restraint was snug. Slid one finger between the restraint and the wrist. Followed the manufacturer's instructions. Adjusted the straps if the restraint was too loose or too tight. Checked for snugness again.   ___   ___   _____

   e. Repeated steps 11 b–d for the other hand.   ___   ___   _____

     1. Applied the mitt restraint. Followed the manufacturer's instructions.   ___   ___   _____

     2. Secured the restraint to the bed if directed to do so by the nurse. Buckled or tied the straps to the movable part of the bed frame. Used a quick-release tie.   ___   ___   _____

     3. Made sure the restraint was snug. Slid one finger between the restraint and the wrist. Followed the manufacturer's instructions. Adjusted the straps if the restraint was too loose or too tight. Checked for snugness again.   ___   ___   _____

12. *For a belt restraint:*

   a. Assisted the person to a sitting position.   ___   ___   _____

   b. Applied the restraint with your free hand. Followed the manufacturer's instructions.   ___   ___   _____

   c. Removed wrinkles or creases from the front and back of the restraint.   ___   ___   _____

   d. Brought the ties through the slots in the belt.   ___   ___   _____

   e. Positioned the straps at a 45-degree angle between the wheelchair seats and sides.   ___   ___   _____

   f. Helped the person lie down if he or she was in bed.   ___   ___   _____

   g. Made sure the person was comfortable and in good alignment.   ___   ___   _____

   h. Buckled or tied the straps to the movable part of the bed frame out of the person's reach. For a wheelchair, crisscrossed and secured the straps as seen in Fig. 13.10 in the book. Used a quick-release tie.   ___   ___   _____

   i. Made sure the belt was snug. Slid an open hand between the restraint and the person. Adjusted the restraint if it was too loose or too tight. Checked for snugness again.   ___   ___   _____

13. *For a vest restraint:*

   a. Assisted the person to a sitting position.   ___   ___   _____

   b. Applied the restraint with your free hand. Followed the manufacturer's instructions. The "V" part of the vest crossed in front.   ___   ___   _____

   c. Brought the straps through the slots.   ___   ___   _____

   d. Positioned the straps at a 45-degree angle between the wheelchair seats and sides (omitted this step if the person was in bed).   ___   ___   _____

   e. Made sure the vest was free of wrinkles in the front and back.   ___   ___   _____

   f. Helped the person lie down if he or she was in bed.   ___   ___   _____

   g. Made sure the person was comfortable and in good alignment.   ___   ___   _____

   h. Buckled or tied the straps to the movable part of the bed frame. Used a quick-release tie. Made sure the buckle or tie was out of the person's reach. For a wheelchair, crisscrossed and secured the straps as shown in Fig. 13.10 in the book.   ___   ___   _____

   i. Ensured the vest was snug. Slid an open hand between the restraint and the person. Adjusted the restraint if it was too loose or too tight. Checked for snugness again.   ___   ___   _____

14. *For a jacket restraint:*

   a. Assisted the person to a sitting position.   ___   ___   _____

Procedure—cont'd	S	U	Comments

b. Applied the restraint with your free hand. Followed the manufacturer's instructions. The jacket opening was in the back. ___ ___ _____

c. Closed the back with the zipper, ties, or hook and loop closures. ___ ___ _____

d. Made sure the side seams were under the arms. Removed any wrinkles in the front and back. ___ ___ _____

e. Positioned the straps at a 45-degree angle between the wheelchair seat and sides. ___ ___ _____

f. Helped the person lie down if in bed. ___ ___ _____

g. Made sure the person was comfortable and in good alignment. ___ ___ _____

h. Buckled or tied the straps to the movable part of the bed frame. Used a quick-release tie. Made sure the buckle or tie was out of the person's reach. For a wheelchair, crisscrossed and secured straps as shown in Fig. 13.10 in the book. ___ ___ _____

i. Made sure the jacket was snug. Slid an open hand between the restraint and the person. Adjusted the restraint if it was too loose or too tight. Checked for snugness again. ___ ___ _____

Postprocedure

15. Positioned the person as the nurse directed. ___ ___ _____
16. Provided for comfort. ___ ___ _____
17. Placed the call light within the person's reach. ___ ___ _____
18. Raised or lowered bed rails. Followed the care plan and the manufacturer's instructions for the restraint. ___ ___ _____
19. Unscreened the person. ___ ___ _____
20. Completed a safety check of the room. ___ ___ _____
21. Decontaminated your hands. ___ ___ _____
22. Checked the person and the restraint at least every 15 minutes. Reported and recorded your observations:

a. For wrist or mitt restraints: Checked the pulse, color, and temperature of the restrained parts. ___ ___ _____

b. For vest, jacket, or belt restraint: Checked the person's breathing. *Called for the nurse at once if the person was not breathing or was having problems breathing.* Made sure the restraint was properly positioned in the front and back. ___ ___ _____

23. Did the following at least every 2 hours for at least 10 minutes:

a. Removed or released the restraint. ___ ___ _____

b. Measured vital signs. ___ ___ _____

c. Repositioned the person. ___ ___ _____

d. Met food, fluid, hygiene, and elimination needs. ___ ___ _____

e. Gave skin care. ___ ___ _____

f. Performed range of motion exercises or helped the person walk. Followed the care plan. ___ ___ _____

g. Provided for physical and emotional comfort. ___ ___ _____

h. Reapplied the restraints. ___ ___ _____

24. Completed a safety check of the room. ___ ___ _____
25. Reported and recorded your observations and the care given. ___ ___ _____

Hand Washing (NATCEP)

Name: _____ Date: _____

Procedure	S	U	Comments
1. Saw *Promoting Safety and Comfort: Hand Hygiene*.	___	___	_____
2. Made sure you had soap, paper towels, an orangewood stick or nail file, and a wastebasket. Collected missing items.	___	___	_____
3. Pushed your watch up your arm 4–5 inches. If your uniform sleeves were long, pushed them up.	___	___	_____
4. Stood away from the sink so your clothes did not touch the sink. Stood so the soap and faucet were easy to reach. Did not touch the inside of the sink at any time.	___	___	_____
5. Turned on and adjusted the water until it felt warm.	___	___	_____
6. Wet your wrists and hands. Kept your hands lower than your elbows. Was sure to wet the area 3–4 inches above your wrists.	___	___	_____
7. Applied about one teaspoon of soap to your hands.	___	___	_____
8. Rubbed your palms together and interlaced your fingers to work up a good lather. This step lasted at least 20 seconds or the amount of time required by your state competency test. Knew this number.	___	___	_____
9. Washed each hand and wrist thoroughly. Cleaned well between the fingers.	___	___	_____
10. Cleaned under the fingernails. Rubbed your fingertips against your palms.	___	___	_____
11. Cleaned under fingernails with a nail file or orangewood stick. This step was done for the first hand washing of the day and when hands were very soiled.	___	___	_____
12. Rinsed your wrists and hands well. Water flowed from the arms to the hands.	___	___	_____
13. Repeated, if needed:			
a. Applied about one teaspoon of soap to your hands.	___	___	_____
b. Rubbed your palms together and interlaced your fingers to work up a good lather. This step lasted at least 20 seconds or the amount of time required by your state competency test. Knew this number.	___	___	_____
c. Washed each hand and wrist thoroughly. Cleaned well between the fingers.	___	___	_____
d. Cleaned under the fingernails. Rubbed your fingertips against your palms.	___	___	_____
e. Cleaned under the fingernails with a nail file or orangewood stick. This step was done for the first hand washing of the day and when your hands were very soiled.	___	___	_____
f. Rinsed your wrists and hands well. Water flowed from the arms to the hands.	___	___	_____
14. Dried your wrists and hands well with a clean, dry paper towel. Patted dry, starting at fingertips.	___	___	_____
15. Discarded the paper towel into the wastebasket.	___	___	_____
16. Turned off faucets with clean, dry paper towels. This prevented you from contaminating your hands. Used a clean paper towel for each faucet.	___	___	_____
17. Discarded the paper towels in the wastebasket.	___	___	_____

Hand Hygiene Using an Alcohol-Based Hand Rub (NATCEP)

Name: —————————————— Date: ——————————————

Procedure	S	U	Comments
1. Saw *Promoting Safety and Comfort: Hand Hygiene*.	——	——	————
2. Applied the product to the palm of one hand. Followed the manufacturer's instructions for the amount to use.	——	——	————
3. Rubbed palms together in a circular manner.	——	——	————
4. Interlaced fingers to spread hand rub on all surfaces of fingers.	——	——	————
5. Rubbed tips of fingers up and down on palm of opposite hand.	——	——	————
6. Coated surface of each thumb with hand rub.	——	——	————
7. Rubbed fingertips in palm of opposite hand using circular motions.	——	——	————
8. Continued rubbing in product until hands were dry (at least 15 seconds or according to manufacturer's recommendation). Did not use water or paper towels when using alcohol-based hand rubs.	——	——	————
9. Applied hand lotion or cream after hand hygiene. Helped prevent the skin from chapping and drying.	——	——	————

233

Procedure Checklists

Removing Gloves (NATCEP)

Name: _____   Date: _____

Procedure	S	U	Comments
1. *Saw Promoting Safety and Comfort: Gloves.*	____	____	_____
2. Made sure that glove touched only glove.	____	____	_____
3. Grasped a glove just below the cuff. Grasped it on the outside.	____	____	_____
4. Pulled the glove down over your hand so it was inside out.	____	____	_____
5. Held the removed glove with your other gloved hand.	____	____	_____
6. Reached inside the other glove. Used the first two fingers of the ungloved hand.	____	____	_____
7. Pulled the glove down (inside out) over your hand and the other glove.	____	____	_____
8. Discarded the gloves. Followed center policy.	____	____	_____
9. Decontaminated your hands.	____	____	_____

Donning and Removing a Gown (NATCEP)

Name:—————————————— Date: ——————————————

Procedure	S	U	Comments
1. Removed your watch and all jewelry.	——	——	———————
2. Rolled up uniform sleeves.	——	——	———————
3. Practiced hand hygiene.	——	——	———————
4. Held a clean gown out in front of you. Allowed it to unfold. Did not shake the gown.	——	——	———————
5. Put your hands and arms through the sleeves.	——	——	———————
6. Made sure the gown covered you from your neck to your knees. Made sure it covered your arms to the ends of your wrists.	——	——	———————
7. Tied the strings at the back of the neck.	——	——	———————
8. Overlapped the back of the gown. Made sure it covered your uniform. The gown was snug, not loose. (If gown did not cover your back, second gown was put on with the opening in the front.)	——	——	———————
9. Tied the waist strings. Tied them at the back or the side. Did not tie them in front.	——	——	———————
10. Put on other personal protective equipment (PPE).			
a. Mask or respirator, if needed.	——	——	———————
b. Goggles or face shield, if needed.	——	——	———————
c. Gloves. Made sure gloves covered the gown cuffs.	——	——	———————
11. Provided care.	——	——	———————
12. Removed and discarded the gloves.	——	——	———————
13. Removed and discarded the goggles or face shield if worn.	——	——	———————
14. Removed the gown. Did not touch the outside of the gown.			
a. Untied the neck and waist strings.	——	——	———————
b. Pulled the gown down from each shoulder toward the same hand.	——	——	———————
c. Turned the gown inside out as it was removed. Held it at the inside shoulder seams and brought your hands together.	——	——	———————
15. Held and rolled up the gown away from you. Kept it inside out.	——	——	———————
16. Discarded the gown.	——	——	———————
17. Removed and discarded the mask if worn.	——	——	———————
18. Decontaminated your hands.	——	——	———————

Donning and Removing a Mask

Name:——————————   Date: ———————————

Procedure	S	U	Comments
1. Practiced hand hygiene.	———	———	—————
2. Put on a gown if required.	———	———	—————
3. Picked up a mask by its upper ties or ear loops. Did not touch the part that covers your face.	———	———	—————
4. Placed the mask over your nose and mouth.	———	———	—————
5. Placed the upper strings above your ears. Tied them at the back in the middle of your head.	———	———	—————
6. Tied the lower strings at the back of your neck. The lower part of the mask was under your chin (some types of masks have elastic that slips over the ears instead of ties. Secure those over both ears.)	———	———	—————
7. Pinched the metal band around your nose. The top of the mask was snug over your nose. If eyeglasses were worn, the mask was snug under the bottom of the eyeglasses.	———	———	—————
8. Made sure the mask was snug over your face and under your chin.	———	———	—————
9. Put on goggles or a face shield if needed and not part of the mask.	———	———	—————
10. Put on gloves.	———	———	—————
11. Provided care. Avoided coughing, sneezing, and unnecessary talking.	———	———	—————
12. Changed the mask if it became wet or contaminated.	———	———	—————
13. Removed the mask.			
a. Removed the gloves.	———	———	—————
b. Removed the goggles or face shield and gown if worn.	———	———	—————
c. Untied the lower strings of the mask.	———	———	—————
d. Untied the top strings.	———	———	—————
e. Held the top strings. Removed the mask.			
f. If mask has ear elastic loops, grasp one loop, remove mask, and discard into waste container.	———	———	—————
14. Discarded the mask.	———	———	—————
15. Decontaminated your hands.	———	———	—————

Sterile Gloving

Name: —————————————— Date: ——————————————

Procedure	S	U	Comments
1. *Followed Delegation Guidelines: Assisting with Sterile Procedures.* *Saw Promoting Safety and Comfort:*			
a. *Assisting with Sterile Procedures*	———	———	———————
b. *Sterile Gloving*	———	———	———————
2. Practiced hand hygiene.	———	———	———————
3. Inspected the package of sterile gloves for sterility:			
a. Checked the expiration date.	———	———	———————
b. Saw if the package was dry.	———	———	———————
c. Checked for tears, holes, punctures, and water marks.	———	———	———————
4. Arranged a work surface:			
a. Made sure you had enough room.	———	———	———————
b. Arranged the work surface at waist level and within your vision.	———	———	———————
c. Cleaned and dried the work surface.	———	———	———————
d. Did not reach over or turn your back on the work surface.	———	———	———————
5. Opened the package. Grasped the flaps. Gently peeled them back.	———	———	———————
6. Removed the inner package. Placed it on the work surface.	———	———	———————
7. Read the manufacturer's instructions on the inner package. It may be labeled with *left, right, up*, and *down*.			
8. Arranged the inner package for left, right, up, and down. The left glove was on your left. The right glove was on your right. The cuffs were near you with the fingers pointing away from you.	———	———	———————
9. Grasped the folded edges of the inner package. Used the thumb and index finger of each hand.	———	———	———————
10. Folded back the inner package to expose the gloves. Did not touch or otherwise contaminate the inside of the package or the gloves. The inside of the inner package is a sterile field.	———	———	———————
11. Noted that each glove had a cuff about 2–3 inches wide. The cuffs and insides of the gloves are *not considered sterile*.	———	———	———————
12. Put on the right glove if you are right-handed. Put on the left glove if you are left-handed.			
a. Picked up the glove with your other hand. Used your thumb, index, and middle fingers.	———	———	———————
b. Touched only the cuff and inside of the glove.	———	———	———————
c. Turned the hand to be gloved palm side up.	———	———	———————
d. Lifted the cuff up. Slid your fingers and hand into the glove.	———	———	———————
e. Pulled the glove up over your hand. If some fingers got stuck, left them that way until the other glove was on. *Did not use your ungloved hand to straighten the glove. Did not let the outside of the glove touch any nonsterile surface.*	———	———	———————
f. Left the cuff turned down.	———	———	———————
13. Put on the other glove. Used your gloved hand.			
a. Reached under the cuff of the second glove. Used the four fingers of your gloved hand. Kept your gloved thumb close to your gloved palm.	———	———	———————
b. Pulled on the second glove. Your gloved hand did not touch the cuff or any surface. Held the thumb of your first gloved hand away from the gloved palm.	———	———	———————

Procedure—cont'd

	S	U	Comments
14. Adjusted each glove with the other hand. The gloves were smooth and comfortable.	―――	―――	―――――――
15. Slid your fingers under the cuffs to pull them up.	―――	―――	―――――――
16. Touched only sterile items.	―――	―――	―――――――
17. Removed the gloves.	―――	―――	―――――――
18. Decontaminated your hands.	―――	―――	―――――――

Raising the Person's Head and Shoulders

Name: ———————————————— Date: ————————————————

	S	U	Comments
Quality of Life			
Remembered to:			
• Knock before entering the person's room.	——	——	————
• Address the person by name.	——	——	————
• Introduce yourself by name and title.	——	——	————
• Explain the procedure to the person before beginning and during the procedure.	——	——	————
• Protect the person's rights during the procedure.	——	——	————
• Handle the person gently during the procedure.	——	——	————

Preprocedure

	S	U	Comments
1. Followed *Delegation Guidelines*:			
a. *Preventing Work-Related Injuries*	——	——	————
b. *Moving Persons in Bed*	——	——	————
2. Saw *Promoting Safety and Comfort:*			
a. *Safe Resident Handling, Moving, and Transfers*	——	——	————
b. *Preventing Work-Related Injuries*	——	——	————
3. Asked a coworker to assist if needed help.	——	——	————
4. Practiced hand hygiene.	——	——	————
5. Identified the person. Checked the identification (ID) bracelet against the assignment sheet. Also called the person by name.	——	——	————
6. Provided for privacy.	——	——	————
7. Locked the bed wheels.	——	——	————
8. Raised the bed for body mechanics. Bed rails were up if used.	——	——	————

Procedure

	S	U	Comments
9. Asked a coworker to stand on the other side of the bed. Lowered the bed rails if up.	——	——	————
10. Asked the person to put his or her near arm under your near arm and behind your shoulder. His or her hand rested on top of your shoulder. If you stood on the right side, the person's right hand rested on your shoulder. The person did the same with the coworker. The person's left hand rested on the coworker's left shoulder.	——	——	————
11. Put your arm nearest to the person under his or her arm. Your hand was on the person's shoulder. The coworker did the same.	——	——	————
12. Put your free arm under the person's neck and shoulders. The coworker did the same. Supported the neck.	——	——	————
13. Helped the person rise to a sitting or semi-sitting position on the "count of 3."	——	——	————
14. Used the arm and hand that supported the person's neck and shoulders to give care. The coworker supported the person.	——	——	————
15. Helped the person lie down. Provided support with your locked arm. Supported the person's neck and shoulders with your other arm. The coworker did the same.	——	——	————

Postprocedure

	S	U	Comments
16. Provided for comfort.	——	——	————
17. Placed the call light within reach.	——	——	————
18. Lowered the bed to its lowest position.	——	——	————
19. Raised or lowered bed rails. Followed the care plan.	——	——	————
20. Unscreened the person.	——	——	————
21. Completed a safety check of the room.	——	——	————
22. Decontaminated your hands.	——	——	————
23. Reported and recorded your observations.	——	——	————

Moving the Person Up in Bed

Name: ————————————   Date: ————————————

Quality of Life	S	U	Comments
Remembered to:			
• Knock before entering the person's room.	———	———	—————
• Address the person by name.	———	———	—————
• Introduce yourself by name and title.	———	———	—————
• Explain the procedure to the person before beginning and during the procedure.	———	———	—————
• Protect the person's rights during the procedure.	———	———	—————
• Handle the person gently during the procedure.	———	———	—————

Preprocedure

	S	U	Comments
1. Followed *Delegation Guidelines*:			
a. *Preventing Work-Related Injuries*	———	———	—————
b. *Moving Persons in Bed*	———	———	—————
2. Saw *Promoting Safety and Comfort*:			
a. *Safe Resident Handling, Moving, and Transfers*	———	———	—————
b. *Preventing Work-Related Injuries*	———	———	—————
c. *Moving the Person Up in Bed*	———	———	—————
3. Asked a coworker to help you.	———	———	—————
4. Practiced hand hygiene.	———	———	—————
5. Identified the person. Checked the identification (ID) bracelet against the assignment sheet. Also called the person by name.	———	———	—————
6. Provided for privacy.	———	———	—————
7. Locked the bed wheels.	———	———	—————
8. Raised the bed for body mechanics. Bed rails were up if used.	———	———	—————

Procedure

	S	U	Comments
9. Lowered the head of the bed to a level appropriate for the person. It was as flat as possible.	———	———	—————
10. Stood on one side of the bed. The coworker stood on the other side.	———	———	—————
11. Lowered the bed rails if up.	———	———	—————
12. Removed pillows as directed by the nurse. Placed a pillow upright against the headboard if the person could be without it.	———	———	—————
13. Stood with a wide base of support. Pointed the foot near the head of the bed toward the head of the bed. Faced the head of the bed.	———	———	—————
14. Bent your hips and knees. Kept your back straight.	———	———	—————
15. Placed one arm under the person's shoulders and one arm under the thighs. The coworker did the same. Grasped each other's forearms.	———	———	—————
16. Asked the person to grasp the trapeze.	———	———	—————
17. Had the person flex both knees.	———	———	—————
18. Explained the following:			
a. You will count "1, 2, 3."	———	———	—————
b. The move will be on "3."	———	———	—————
c. On "3," the person pushes against the bed with the feet if able. And the person pulls up with the trapeze.			
19. Moved the person to the head of the bed on the count of "3." Shifted your weight from your rear leg to your front leg. Your coworker did the same.	———	———	—————
20. Repeated steps 13–19 if necessary.			
a. Stood with a wide base of support. Pointed the foot near the head of the bed toward the head of the bed. Faced the head of the bed.	———	———	—————

Procedure—cont'd   S   U   Comments

    b. Bent your hips and knees. Kept your back straight.

    c. Placed one arm under the person's shoulder and one arm under the thighs. The coworker did the same. Grasped each other's forearms.

    d. Asked the person to grasp the trapeze.

    e. Had the person flex both knees.

    f. Explained the following:

       i. You will count "1, 2, 3."

      ii. The move will be on "3."

     iii. On "3," the person pushes against the bed with the feet if able. And the person pulls up with the trapeze.

    g. Moved the person to the head of the bed on the count of "3." Shifted your weight from your rear leg to your front leg. The coworker did the same.

Postprocedure

21. Put the pillow under the person's head and shoulders. Straightened linens.

22. Positioned the person in good alignment. Raised the head of the bed to a level appropriate for the person.

23. Provided for comfort.

24. Placed the call light within reach.

25. Lowered the bed to its lowest position.

26. Raised or lowered bed rails. Followed the care plan.

27. Unscreened the person.

28. Completed a safety check of the room.

29. Decontaminated your hands.

30. Reported and recorded your observations.

Moving the Person Up in Bed with an Assist Device

Name: _____ Date: _____

	S	U	Comments
Quality of Life			
Remembered to:			
• Knock before entering the person's room.	____	____	_____
• Address the person by name.	____	____	_____
• Introduce yourself by name and title.	____	____	_____
• Explain the procedure to the person before beginning and during the procedure.	____	____	_____
• Protect the person's rights during the procedure.	____	____	_____
• Handle the person gently during the procedure.	____	____	_____

Preprocedure

	S	U	Comments
1. Followed *Delegation Guidelines:*			
a. *Preventing Work-Related Injuries*	____	____	_____
b. *Moving Persons in Bed*	____	____	_____
2. Saw *Promoting Safety and Comfort:*			
a. *Safe Resident Handling, Moving, and Transfers*	____	____	_____
b. *Preventing Work-Related Injuries*	____	____	_____
c. *Moving the Person Up in Bed*	____	____	_____
d. *Moving the Person Up in Bed with an Assist Device*	____	____	_____
3. Asked a coworker to help you.	____	____	_____
4. Practiced hand hygiene.	____	____	_____
5. Identified the person. Checked the identification (ID) bracelet against the assignment sheet. Also called the person by name.	____	____	_____
6. Provided for privacy.	____	____	_____
7. Locked the bed wheels.	____	____	_____
8. Raised the bed for body mechanics. Bed rails were up if used.	____	____	_____

Procedure

	S	U	Comments
9. Lowered the head of the bed to a level appropriate for the person. It was as flat as possible.	____	____	_____
10. Stood on one side of the bed. The coworker stood on the other side.	____	____	_____
11. Lowered the bed rails if up.	____	____	_____
12. Removed pillows as directed by the nurse. Placed a pillow upright against the headboard if the person could be without it.	____	____	_____
13. Stood with a broad base of support. Pointed the foot near the head of the bed toward the head of the bed. Faced that direction.	____	____	_____
14. Rolled the sides of the assist device up close to the person. (Note: Omitted this step if the device had handles.)	____	____	_____
15. Grasped the rolled-up assist device firmly near the person's shoulders and hips. Or grasped it by the handles. Supported the head.	____	____	_____
16. Bent your hips and knees.	____	____	_____
17. Moved the person up in bed on the count of "3." Shifted your weight from your rear leg to your front leg.	____	____	_____
18. Repeated steps 13–17 if necessary.			
a. Stood with a broad base of support. Pointed the foot near the head of the bed toward the head of the bed. Faced that direction.	____	____	_____
b. Rolled the sides of the assist device up close to the person. (Note: Omitted this step if the device had handles.)	____	____	_____
c. Grasped the rolled-up assist device firmly near the person's shoulders and hips. Or grasped it by the handles. Supported the head.	____	____	_____

Procedure—cont'd	S	U	Comments
d. Bent your hips and knees.	___	___	_____
e. Moved the person up in bed on the count of "3." Shifted your weight from your rear leg to your front leg.	___	___	_____
19. Unrolled the assist device. (Note: Omitted this step if the device had handles.)	___	___	_____

Postprocedure

	S	U	Comments
20. Put the pillow under the person's head and shoulders.	___	___	_____
21. Positioned the person in good alignment. Raised the head of the bed to a level appropriate for the person.	___	___	_____
22. Provided for comfort.	___	___	_____
23. Placed the call light within reach.	___	___	_____
24. Lowered the bed to its lowest position.	___	___	_____
25. Raised or lowered bed rails. Followed the care plan.	___	___	_____
26. Unscreened the person.	___	___	_____
27. Completed a safety check of the room.	___	___	_____
28. Decontaminated your hands.	___	___	_____
29. Reported and recorded your observations.	___	___	_____

Moving the Person to the Side of the Bed

Name: _____ Date: _____

Quality of Life	**S**	**U**	**Comments**
Remembered to:			
• Knock before entering the person's room.	_____	_____	_____
• Address the person by name.	_____	_____	_____
• Introduce yourself by name and title.	_____	_____	_____
• Explain the procedure to the person before beginning and during the procedure.	_____	_____	_____
• Protect the person's rights during the procedure.	_____	_____	_____
• Handle the person gently during the procedure.	_____	_____	_____

Preprocedure

	S	**U**	**Comments**
1. Followed *Delegation Guidelines:*			
a. *Preventing Work-Related Injuries*	_____	_____	_____
b. *Moving Persons in Bed*	_____	_____	_____
2. Saw *Promoting Safety and Comfort:*			
a. *Safe Resident Handling, Moving, and Transfers*	_____	_____	_____
b. *Preventing Work-Related Injuries*	_____	_____	_____
c. *Moving the Person to the Side of the Bed*	_____	_____	_____
3. Asked a coworker to help if using an assist device.	_____	_____	_____
4. Practiced hand hygiene.	_____	_____	_____
5. Identified the person. Checked the identification (ID) bracelet against the assignment sheet. Also called the person by name.	_____	_____	_____
6. Provided for privacy.	_____	_____	_____
7. Locked the bed wheels.	_____	_____	_____
8. Raised the bed for body mechanics. Bed rails were up if used.	_____	_____	_____

Procedure

	S	**U**	**Comments**
9. Lowered the head of the bed to a level appropriate for the person. It was as flat as possible.	_____	_____	_____
10. Stood on the side of the bed to which the person was moved.	_____	_____	_____
11. Lowered the bed rail near you if bed rails were used. (Both bed rails were lowered for step 16).	_____	_____	_____
12. Removed pillows as directed by the nurse.	_____	_____	_____
13. Stood with your feet about 12 inches apart. One foot was in front of the other. Flexed your knees.	_____	_____	_____
14. Crossed the person's arms over his or her chest.	_____	_____	_____
15. *Method 1—Moving the person in segments*: (If person had back or spinal injury, this method was not used.)			
a. Placed your arm under the person's neck and shoulders. Grasped the far shoulder.	_____	_____	_____
b. Placed your other arm under the midback.	_____	_____	_____
c. Moved the upper part of the person's body toward you. Rocked backward and shifted your weight to your rear leg.	_____	_____	_____
d. Placed one arm under the person's waist and one under the thighs.	_____	_____	_____
e. Rocked backward to move the lower part of the person toward you.	_____	_____	_____
f. Repeated the procedure for the legs and feet. Your arms were under the person's thighs and calves.	_____	_____	_____
16. *Method 2—Moving the person with a drawsheet:*			
a. Rolled up the drawsheet close to the person.	_____	_____	_____
b. Grasped the rolled-up drawsheet near the person's shoulders and hips. The coworker did the same. Supported the person's head.	_____	_____	_____

Procedure—cont'd	S	U	Comments
c. Rocked backward on the count of "3" and moved the person toward you. The coworker rocked backward slightly and then forward toward you with arms kept straight.	____	____	_____
d. Unrolled the drawsheet. Removed any wrinkles.	____	____	_____

Postprocedure

	S	U	Comments
17. Positioned the person in good alignment.	____	____	_____
18. Provided for comfort.	____	____	_____
19. Placed the call light within reach.	____	____	_____
20. Lowered the bed to its lowest position.	____	____	_____
21. Raised or lowered bed rails. Followed the care plan.	____	____	_____
22. Unscreened the person.	____	____	_____
23. Completed a safety check of the room.	____	____	_____
24. Decontaminated your hands.	____	____	_____
25. Reported and recorded your observations.	____	____	_____

Turning and Repositioning the Person (NATCEP)

Name: _____   Date: _____

Quality of Life	**S**	**U**	**Comments**

Remembered to:
- Knock before entering the person's room. _____ _____ _____
- Address the person by name. _____ _____ _____
- Introduce yourself by name and title. _____ _____ _____
- Explain the procedure to the person before beginning and during the procedure. _____ _____ _____
- Protect the person's rights during the procedure. _____ _____ _____
- Handle the person gently during the procedure. _____ _____ _____

Preprocedure

1. Followed *Delegation Guidelines:*
   a. *Preventing Work-Related Injuries* _____ _____ _____
   b. *Moving Persons in Bed* _____ _____ _____
   c. *Turning Persons* _____ _____ _____
2. Saw *Promoting Safety and Comfort:*
   a. *Safe Resident Handling, Moving, and Transfers* _____ _____ _____
   b. *Preventing Work-Related Injuries* _____ _____ _____
   c. *Moving the Person to the Side of the Bed* _____ _____ _____
   d. *Turning Persons* _____ _____ _____
3. Practiced hand hygiene. _____ _____ _____
4. Identified the person. Checked the identification (ID) bracelet against the assignment sheet. Also called the person by name. _____ _____ _____
5. Provided for privacy. _____ _____ _____
6. Locked the bed wheels. _____ _____ _____
7. Raised the bed for body mechanics. Bed rails were up. _____ _____ _____

Procedure

8. Lowered the head of the bed to a level appropriate for the person. It was as flat as possible. _____ _____ _____
9. Stood on the side of the bed opposite to where you turned the person. _____ _____ _____
10. Lowered the bed rail near you. _____ _____ _____
11. Moved the person to the side near you. _____ _____ _____
12. Crossed the person's arms over his or her chest. Crossed the leg near you over the far leg. _____ _____ _____
13. *Turned the person away from you*:
    a. Stood with a wide base of support. Flexed the knees. _____ _____ _____
    b. Placed one hand on the person's shoulder. Placed the other on the hip near you. _____ _____ _____
    c. Rolled the person gently away from you toward the raised bed rail. Shifted your weight from your rear leg to your front leg. _____ _____ _____
14. *Turned the person toward you:*
    a. Raised the bed rail. _____ _____ _____
    b. Went to the other side of the bed. Lowered the bed rail. _____ _____ _____
    c. Stood with a wide base of support. Flexed your knees. _____ _____ _____
    d. Placed one hand on the person's far shoulder. Placed the other on the far hip. _____ _____ _____
    e. Rolled the person toward you gently. _____ _____ _____
15. Positioned the person. Followed the nurse's directions, the care plan, and these common measures:
    a. Placed a pillow under the head and neck. _____ _____ _____
    b. Adjusted the shoulder. The person did not lie on an arm. _____ _____ _____
    c. Placed a small pillow under the upper hand and arm. _____ _____ _____
    d. Positioned a pillow against the back. _____ _____ _____

Procedure—cont'd	**S**	**U**	**Comments**
e. Flexed the upper knee. Positioned the upper leg in front of the lower leg.	——	——	————
f. Supported the upper leg and thigh on pillows. Made sure the ankle was supported.	——	——	————

Postprocedure

	S	**U**	**Comments**
16. Provided for comfort.	——	——	————
17. Placed the call light within reach.	——	——	————
18. Lowered the bed to its lowest position.	——	——	————
19. Raised or lowered bed rails. Followed the care plan.	——	——	————
20. Unscreened the person.	——	——	————
21. Completed a safety check of the room.	——	——	————
22. Decontaminated your hands.	——	——	————
23. Reported and recorded your observations.	——	——	————

Logrolling the Person

Name: _____ Date: _____

	S	U	Comments
Quality of Life			
Remembered to:			
• Knock before entering the person's room.	____	____	_____
• Address the person by name.	____	____	_____
• Introduce yourself by name and title.	____	____	_____
• Explain the procedure to the person before beginning and during the procedure.	____	____	_____
• Protect the person's rights during the procedure.	____	____	_____
• Handle the person gently during the procedure.	____	____	_____
Preprocedure			
1. Followed *Delegation Guidelines:*			
a. *Preventing Work-Related Injuries*	____	____	_____
b. *Moving Persons in Bed*	____	____	_____
c. *Turning Persons*	____	____	_____
2. Saw *Promoting Safety and Comfort:*			
a. *Safe Resident Handling, Moving, and Transfers*	____	____	_____
b. *Preventing Work-Related Injuries*	____	____	_____
c. *Turning Persons*	____	____	_____
d. *Logrolling*	____	____	_____
3. Asked a coworker to help you.	____	____	_____
4. Practiced hand hygiene.	____	____	_____
5. Identified the person. Checked the identification (ID) bracelet against the assignment sheet. Also called the person by name.	____	____	_____
6. Provided for privacy.	____	____	_____
7. Locked the bed wheels.	____	____	_____
8. Raised the bed for body mechanics. Bed rails were up if used.	____	____	_____
Procedure			
9. Made sure the bed was flat.	____	____	_____
10. Stood on the side opposite to which you turned the person. The coworker stood on the other side.	____	____	_____
11. Lowered the bed rails if used.	____	____	_____
12. Moved the person as a unit to the side of the bed near you. Used the assist device. (If the person had a spinal cord injury, assisted the nurse as directed.)	____	____	_____
13. Placed the person's arms across the chest. Placed a pillow between the knees.	____	____	_____
14. Raised the bed rail if used.	____	____	_____
15. Went to the other side.	____	____	_____
16. Stood near the shoulders and chest. The coworker stood near the hips and thighs.	____	____	_____
17. Stood with a broad base of support. One foot was in front of the other.	____	____	_____
18. Asked the person to hold his or her body rigid.	____	____	_____
19. Rolled the person toward you. Or used the assist device. Turned the person as a unit.	____	____	_____
20. Positioned the person in good alignment. Used pillows as directed by the nurse and the care plan. Followed these common measures (unless the spinal cord was involved):			
a. One pillow against the back for support.	____	____	_____
b. One pillow under the head and neck if allowed.	____	____	_____
c. One pillow or a folded bath blanket between the legs.	____	____	_____
d. A small pillow under the upper arm and hand.	____	____	_____

Procedure—cont'd	**S**	**U**	**Comments**
22. Lowered the head of the bed after the person returned to bed. Helped him or her move to the center of the bed.	_____	_____	_____
23. Positioned the person in good alignment.	_____	_____	_____

Postprocedure

	S	**U**	**Comments**
24. Provided for comfort.	_____	_____	_____
25. Placed the call light within reach.	_____	_____	_____
26. Lowered the bed to its lowest position.	_____	_____	_____
27. Raised or lowered bed rails. Followed the care plan.	_____	_____	_____
28. Returned furniture to its proper place.	_____	_____	_____
29. Unscreened the person.	_____	_____	_____
30. Completed a safety check of the room.	_____	_____	_____
31. Decontaminated your hands.	_____	_____	_____
32. Reported and recorded your observations.	_____	_____	_____

Transferring the Person to a Chair or Wheelchair (NATCEP)

Name: _____ Date: _____

	S	U	Comments
Quality of Life			
Remembered to:			
• Knock before entering the person's room.	___	___	_____
• Address the person by name.	___	___	_____
• Introduce yourself by name and title.	___	___	_____
• Explain the procedure to the person before beginning and during the procedure.	___	___	_____
• Protect the person's rights during the procedure.	___	___	_____
• Handle the person gently during the procedure.	___	___	_____

Preprocedure

	S	U	Comments
1. Followed *Delegation Guidelines*:			
a. *Preventing Work-Related Injuries*	___	___	_____
b. *Transferring Persons*	___	___	_____
2. Saw Promoting Safety and Comfort:			
a. *Transfer/Gait Belts*	___	___	_____
b. *Safe Resident Handling, Moving, and Transfers*	___	___	_____
c. *Preventing Work-Related Injuries*	___	___	_____
d. *Transferring Persons*	___	___	_____
e. *Bed to Chair or Wheelchair Transfers*	___	___	_____
3. Collected:			
a. Wheelchair or arm chair	___	___	_____
b. Bath blanket	___	___	_____
c. Lap blanket	___	___	_____
d. Robe and nonskid footwear	___	___	_____
e. Paper or sheet	___	___	_____
f. Transfer belt (if needed)	___	___	_____
g. Seat cushion (if needed)	___	___	_____
4. Practiced hand hygiene.	___	___	_____
5. Identified the person. Checked the identification (ID) bracelet against the assignment sheet. Also called the person by name.	___	___	_____
6. Provided for privacy.	___	___	_____
7. Decided what side of the bed to use. Moved furniture for a safe transfer.	___	___	_____

Procedure

	S	U	Comments
8. Positioned the chair:			
a. The chair was near the head of bed on the person's strong side.	___	___	_____
b. The chair faced the foot of the bed.	___	___	_____
c. The arm of the chair almost touched the bed.	___	___	_____
9. Placed a folded bath blanket or cushion on the seat (if needed).	___	___	_____
10. Locked the wheelchair wheels. Raised the footplates. Removed or swung the front rigging out of the way.	___	___	_____
11. Lowered the bed to its lowest position. Locked the bed wheels.	___	___	_____
12. Fan-folded top linens to the foot of the bed.	___	___	_____
13. Placed the paper or sheet under the person's feet. Put footwear on the person.	___	___	_____
14. Helped the person sit on the side of bed. His or her feet touched the floor.	___	___	_____
15. Helped the person put on a robe.	___	___	_____
16. Applied the transfer belt if needed.	___	___	_____
17. *Method 1—Using a transfer belt*:			
a. Stood in front of the person.	___	___	_____
b. Had the person hold on to the mattress.	___	___	_____

Procedure—cont'd	**S**	**U**	**Comments**
c. Made sure the person's feet were flat on the floor.	____	____	_____
d. Had the person lean forward.	____	____	_____
e. Grasped the transfer belt at each side. Grasped the handles or grasped the belt from underneath.	____	____	_____
f. Prevented the person from sliding or falling by doing one of the following:			
i. Braced your knees against the person's knees. Blocked his or her feet with your feet.	____	____	_____
ii. Used the knee and foot of one leg to block the person's weak leg or foot. Placed your other foot slightly behind you for balance.	____	____	_____
iii. Straddled your legs around the person's weak leg.	____	____	_____
g. Explained the following:			
i. You will count "1, 2, 3."	____	____	_____
ii. The move will be on "3."	____	____	_____
iii. On "3," the person pushes down on the mattress and stands.	____	____	_____
h. Asked the person to push down on the mattress and stand on the count of "3." Pulled the person to a standing position as you straightened your knees.	____	____	_____
18. *Method 2—No transfer belt*: (Note: Used this method only if directed by the nurse and the care plan.)			
a. Followed steps 17 a–c			
i. Stood in front of the person.	____	____	_____
ii. Had the person hold on to the mattress.	____	____	_____
iii. Made sure the person's feet were flat on the floor.	____	____	_____
b. Placed your hands under the person's arms. Your hands were around the person's shoulder blades.	____	____	_____
c. Had the person lean forward.	____	____	_____
d. Prevented the person from sliding or falling by doing one of the following:			
i. Braced your knees against the person's knees. Blocked his or her feet with your feet.	____	____	_____
ii. Used the knee and foot of one leg to block the person's weak leg or foot. Placed your other foot slightly behind you for balance.	____	____	_____
iii. Straddled your legs around the person's weak leg.	____	____	_____
e. Explained the "count of 3."			
i. You will count "1, 2, 3."	____	____	_____
ii. The move will be on "3."	____	____	_____
iii. On "3," the person pushes down on the mattress and stands.	____	____	_____
f. Asked the person to push down on the mattress and stand on the count of "3." Pulled the person to a standing position as you straightened your knees.	____	____	_____
19. Supported the person in the standing position. Held the transfer belt, or kept your hands around the person's shoulder blades. Continued to prevent the person from sliding or falling.	____	____	_____
20. Turned the person so he or she could grasp the far arm of the chair. The legs touched the edge of the chair.	____	____	_____
21. Continued to turn the person until the other armrest was grasped.	____	____	_____
22. Lowered the person into the chair as you bent your hips and knees. The person assisted by leaning forward and bending his or her elbows and knees.	____	____	_____
23. Made sure the person's hips were to the back of the seat. Positioned the person in good alignment.	____	____	_____
24. Attached the wheelchair front rigging. Positioned the person's feet on the wheelchair footplates.	____	____	_____

Procedure Checklists

Procedure—cont'd	S	U	Comments
25. Covered the person's lap and legs with a lap blanket. Kept the blanket off the floor and the wheels.	——	——	————
26. Removed the transfer belt if used.	——	——	————
27. Positioned the chair as the person preferred. Locked the wheelchair wheels according to the care plan.	——	——	————

Postprocedure

	S	U	Comments
28. Provided for comfort.	——	——	————
29. Placed the call light and other needed items within reach.	——	——	————
30. Unscreened the person.	——	——	————
31. Completed a safety check of the room.	——	——	————
32. Decontaminated your hands.	——	——	————
33. Reported and recorded your observations.	——	——	————

Transferring the Person from a Chair or Wheelchair to Bed

Name: _____   Date: _____

	S	U	Comments
Quality of Life			
Remembered to:			
• Knock before entering the person's room.	___	___	_____
• Address the person by name.	___	___	_____
• Introduce yourself by name and title.	___	___	_____
• Explain the procedure to the person before beginning and during the procedure.	___	___	_____
• Protect the person's rights during the procedure.	___	___	_____
• Handle the person gently during the procedure.	___	___	_____

Preprocedure

	S	U	Comments
1. Followed *Delegation Guidelines:*			
a. *Preventing Work-Related Injuries*	___	___	_____
b. *Transferring Persons*	___	___	_____
2. Saw *Promoting Safety and Comfort:*			
a. *Transfer/Gait Belts*	___	___	_____
b. *Safe Resident Handling, Moving, and Transfers*	___	___	_____
c. *Preventing Work-Related Injuries*	___	___	_____
d. *Transferring Persons*	___	___	_____
e. *Bed to Chair or Wheelchair Transfers*	___	___	_____
3. Collected a transfer belt if needed.	___	___	_____
4. Practiced hand hygiene.	___	___	_____
5. Identified the person. Checked the identification (ID) bracelet against the assignment sheet. Also called the person by name.	___	___	_____
6. Provided for privacy.	___	___	_____

Procedure

	S	U	Comments
7. Moved furniture for moving space.	___	___	_____
8. Raised the head of the bed to a sitting position. The bed was in the lowest position.	___	___	_____
9. Moved the call light so it was on the strong side when the person was in bed.	___	___	_____
10. Positioned the chair or wheelchair so the person's strong side was next to the bed. Had a coworker help you if necessary.	___	___	_____
11. Locked the wheelchair and bed wheels.	___	___	_____
12. Removed and folded the lap blanket.	___	___	_____
13. Removed the person's feet from the footplates. Raised the footplates. Removed or swung the front rigging out of the way. (The person had on nonskid footwear.)	___	___	_____
14. Applied the transfer belt (if needed).	___	___	_____
15. Made sure the person's feet were flat on the floor.	___	___	_____
16. Stood in front of the person.	___	___	_____
17. Asked the person to hold on to the armrests. (If directed to do so by the nurse, placed your arms under the person's arms. Your hands were around the shoulder blades.)	___	___	_____
18. Had the person lean forward.	___	___	_____
19. Grasped the transfer belt on each side, if used. Grasped underneath the belt.	___	___	_____
20. Prevented the person from sliding or falling by doing one of the following:			
a. Braced your knees against the person's knees. Blocked his or her feet with your feet.	___	___	_____
b. Used the knee and foot of one leg to block the person's weak leg or foot. Placed your other foot slightly behind you for balance.	___	___	_____
c. Straddled your legs around the person's weak leg.	___	___	_____

Procedure—cont'd	S	U	Comments

21. Explained "the count of 3":
    a. You will count "1, 2, 3."
    b. The move will be on "3."
    c. On "3," the person pushes down on the mattress and stands.
22. Asked the person to push down on the armrests on the count of "3." Pulled the person into a standing position as you straightened your knees.
23. Supported the person in the standing position. Held the transfer belt or kept your hands around the person's shoulder blades. Continued to prevent the person from sliding or falling.
24. Turned the person so he or she could reach the edge of the mattress. The person's legs touched the mattress.
25. Continued to turn the person until he or she could reach the mattress with both hands.
26. Lowered him or her onto the bed as you bent your hips and knees. The person assisted by leaning forward and bending his or her elbows and knees.
27. Removed the transfer belt.
28. Removed the robe and footwear.
29. Helped the person lie down.

Postprocedure

30. Provided for comfort.
31. Placed the call light and other needed items within reach.
32. Raised or lowered bed rails. Followed the care plan.
33. Arranged furniture to meet the person's needs.
34. Unscreened the person.
35. Completed a safety check of the room.
36. Decontaminated your hands.
37. Reported and recorded your observations.

Transferring the Person using a Mechanical Lift

Name: _____   Date: _____

	S	U	Comments
Quality of Life			

Remembered to:
- Knock before entering the person's room.
- Address the person by name.
- Introduce yourself by name and title.
- Explain the procedure to the person before beginning and during the procedure.
- Protect the person's rights during the procedure.
- Handle the person gently during the procedure.

Preprocedure

1. Followed *Delegation Guidelines:*
   a. *Preventing Work-Related Injuries*
   b. *Transferring Persons*
   c. *Using Mechanical Lifts*
2. Saw *Promoting Safety and Comfort:*
   a. *Safe Resident Handling, Moving, and Transfers*
   b. *Preventing Work-Related Injuries*
   c. *Transferring Persons*
   d. *Using Mechanical Lifts*
3. Asked a coworker to help you.
4. Collected:
   a. Mechanical lift and sling
   b. Arm chair or wheelchair
   c. Footwear
   d. Bath blanket or cushion
   e. Lap blanket
5. Practiced hand hygiene.
6. Identified the person. Checked the identification (ID) bracelet against the assignment sheet. Also called the person by name.
7. Provided for privacy.

Procedure

8. Raised the bed for body mechanics. Bed rails were up if used.
9. Lowered the head of the bed to a level appropriate for the person. It was as flat as possible.
10. Stood on one side of the bed. The coworker stood on the other side.
11. Lowered the bed rails if up.
12. Centered the sling under the person. To position the sling, turned the person from side to side as if making an occupied bed. Positioned the sling according to the manufacturer's instructions.
13. Positioned the person in semi-Fowler position.
14. Placed the chair at the head of the bed. It was even with the headboard and about 1 foot away from the bed. Placed a folded bath blanket or cushion in the chair.
15. Locked the bed wheels. Lowered the bed to its lowest position.
16. Raised the lift so you could position it over the person.
17. Positioned the lift over the person.
18. Locked the lift wheels in position.
19. Attached the sling to the sling hooks.
20. Raised the head of the bed to a sitting position.
21. Crossed the person's arms over the chest.

Procedure—cont'd	S	U	Comments
22. Raised the lift high enough until the person and the sling were free of the bed.	——	——	————
23. Had the coworker support the person's legs as you moved the lift and the person away from the bed.	——	——	————
24. Positioned the lift so the person's back was toward the chair.	——	——	————
25. Positioned the chair so you could lower the person into it.	——	——	————
26. Lowered the person into the chair. Guided the person into the chair.	——	——	————
27. Lowered the spreader bar to unhook the sling. Removed the sling from under the person unless otherwise indicated.	——	——	————
28. Put footwear on the person. Positioned the person's feet on the wheelchair footplates.	——	——	————
29. Covered the person's lap and legs with a lap blanket. Kept it off the floor and wheels.	——	——	————
30. Positioned the chair as the person preferred. Locked the wheelchair wheels according to the care plan.	——	——	————

Postprocedure

	S	U	Comments
31. Provided for comfort.	——	——	————
32. Placed the call light and other needed items within the person's reach.	——	——	————
33. Unscreened the person.	——	——	————
34. Completed a safety check of the room.	——	——	————
35. Decontaminated your hands.	——	——	————
36. Reported and recorded your observations.	——	——	————
37. Reversed the procedure to return the person to bed.	——	——	————

Transferring the Person to and from the Toilet

Name: _____   Date: _____

Quality of Life	**S**	**U**	**Comments**
Remembered to:			
• Knock before entering the person's room.	____	____	_____
• Address the person by name.	____	____	_____
• Introduce yourself by name and title.	____	____	_____
• Explain the procedure to the person before beginning and during the procedure.	____	____	_____
• Protect the person's rights during the procedure.	____	____	_____
• Handle the person gently during the procedure.	____	____	_____

Preprocedure

	S	U	Comments
1. Followed *Delegation Guidelines:*			
a. *Preventing Work-Related Injuries*	____	____	_____
b. *Transferring Persons*	____	____	_____
2. Saw *Promoting Safety and Comfort:*			
a. *Transfer/Gait Belts*	____	____	_____
b. *Safe Resident Handling, Moving, and Transfers*	____	____	_____
c. *Preventing Work-Related Injuries*	____	____	_____
d. *Transferring Persons*	____	____	_____
e. *Bed to Chair or Wheelchair Transfers*	____	____	_____
f. *Transferring the Person to and from the Toilet*	____	____	_____
3. Practiced hand hygiene.	____	____	_____

Procedure

	S	U	Comments
4. Had the person wear nonskid footwear.	____	____	_____
5. Positioned the wheelchair next to the toilet if there was enough room. If not, positioned the chair at a right angle (90 degrees) to the toilet. If possible, the person's strong side was near the toilet.	____	____	_____
6. Locked the wheelchair wheels.	____	____	_____
7. Raised the footplates. Removed or swung the front rigging out of the way.	____	____	_____
8. Applied the transfer belt.	____	____	_____
9. Helped the person unfasten clothing.	____	____	_____
10. Used the transfer belt to help the person stand and turn to the toilet. The person used the grab bars to turn to the toilet.	____	____	_____
11. Supported the person with the transfer belt while he or she lowered clothing. Or had the person hold on to the grab bars for support. Lowered the person's pants and undergarments.	____	____	_____
12. Used the transfer belt to lower the person onto the toilet seat. Made sure he or she was properly positioned on the toilet.	____	____	_____
13. Told the person you would stay nearby. Reminded the person to use the call light or call for you when help was needed. Stayed with the person if required by the care plan.	____	____	_____
14. Closed the bathroom door to provide privacy.	____	____	_____
15. Stayed near the bathroom. Completed other tasks in the person's room. Checked on the person every 5 minutes.	____	____	_____
16. Knocked on the bathroom door when the person called for you.	____	____	_____
17. Helped with wiping, perineal care, flushing, and hand washing as needed. Wore gloves and practiced hand hygiene after removing the gloves.	____	____	_____
18. Used the transfer belt to help the person stand.	____	____	_____
19. Helped the person raise and secure clothing.	____	____	_____
20. Used the transfer belt to transfer the person to the wheelchair.	____	____	_____
21. Made sure the person's buttocks were to the back of the seat. Positioned the person in good alignment.	____	____	_____

Procedure—cont'd

		S	U	Comments
22.	Positioned the person's feet on the footplates.	⸺	⸺	⸺
23.	Removed the transfer belt.	⸺	⸺	⸺
24.	Covered the person's lap and legs with a lap blanket. Kept the blanket off the floor and wheels.	⸺	⸺	⸺
25.	Positioned the chair as the person preferred. Locked the wheelchair wheels according to the care plan.	⸺	⸺	⸺

Postprocedure

		S	U	Comments
26.	Provided for comfort.	⸺	⸺	⸺
27.	Placed the call light and other needed items within the person's reach.	⸺	⸺	⸺
28.	Unscreened the person.	⸺	⸺	⸺
29.	Completed a safety check of the room.	⸺	⸺	⸺
30.	Practiced hand hygiene.	⸺	⸺	⸺
31.	Reported and recorded your observations.	⸺	⸺	⸺

Moving the Person to a Stretcher

Name: _____ Date: _____

	S	U	Comments
Quality of Life			

Remembered to:
- Knock before entering the person's room.
- Address the person by name.
- Introduce yourself by name and title.
- Explain the procedure to the person before beginning and during the procedure.
- Protect the person's rights during the procedure.
- Handle the person gently during the procedure.

Preprocedure

1. Followed *Delegation Guidelines:*
   a. *Preventing Work-Related Injuries*
   b. *Transferring Persons*
2. Saw *Promoting Safety and Comfort:*
   a. *Safe Resident Handling, Moving, and Transfers*
   b. *Preventing Work-Related Injuries*
   c. *Transferring Persons*
   d. *Moving the Person to a Stretcher*
3. Asked 1 or 2 staff members to help.
4. Collected:
   a. Stretcher covered with a sheet or bath blanket
   b. Bath blanket
   c. Pillow(s) if needed
   d. Slide sheet, slide board, drawsheet, or other assist devices
5. Practiced hand hygiene.
6. Identified the person. Checked the identification (ID) bracelet against the assignment sheet. Also called the person by name.
7. Provided for privacy.
8. Raised the bed and stretcher for body mechanics.

Procedure

9. Positioned yourself and coworkers.
   a. One or two workers stood on the side of the bed where the stretcher was.
   b. One worker stood on the other side of the bed.
10. Lowered the head of the bed. It was as flat as possible.
11. Lowered the bed rails if used.
12. Covered the person with a bath blanket. Fan-folded top linens to the foot of the bed.
13. Positioned the assist device. Or loosened the drawsheet on each side.
14. Used the assist device to move the person to the side of the bed where the stretcher was.
15. Protected the person from falling. Held the far arm and leg.
16. Had the coworkers position the stretcher next to the bed. They stood behind the stretcher.
17. Locked the bed and stretcher wheels.
18. Grasped the assist device.
19. Transferred the person to the stretcher on the count of "3." Centered the person on the stretcher.
20. Placed a pillow or pillows under the person's head and shoulders if allowed. Raised the head of the stretcher if allowed.
21. Covered the person. Provided privacy.
22. Fastened the safety straps. Raised the side rails.
23. Unlocked the stretcher wheels. Transported the person.

261

Postprocedure	S	U	Comments
24. Decontaminated your hands.	———	———	———————
25. Reported and recorded:			
a. The time of the transport	———	———	———————
b. Where the person was transported to	———	———	———————
c. Who went with the person	———	———	———————
d. How the transfer was tolerated	———	———	———————
26. Reversed the procedure to return the person to bed.	———	———	———————

Making a Closed Bed

Name: _____   Date: _____

Quality of Life	S	U	Comments

Remembered to:
- Knock before entering the person's room.
- Address the person by name.
- Introduce yourself by name and title.
- Explain the procedure to the person before beginning and during the procedure.
- Protect the person's rights during the procedure.
- Handle the person gently during the procedure.

Preprocedure

1. Followed *Delegation Guidelines: Making Beds*
   Saw *Promoting Safety and Comfort: Making Beds*
2. Practiced hand hygiene.
3. Collected clean linens:
   a. Mattress pad (if needed)
   b. Bottom sheet (flat or fitted)
   c. Waterproof drawsheet or waterproof pad (if needed)
   d. Cotton drawsheet (if needed)
   e. Top sheet
   f. Blanket
   g. Bedspread
   h. Pillowcase for each pillow
   i. Bath towel(s)
   j. Hand towel
   k. Washcloth
   l. Gown or pajamas
   m. Bath blanket
   n. Gloves
   o. Laundry bag
   p. Paper towels if a barrier for clean linens was needed
4. Placed linens on a clean surface. Used paper towels as a barrier between the clean surface and clean linens if required by center policy.
5. Raised the bed for body mechanics. Bed rails were down.

Procedure

6. Put on the gloves.
7. Removed linens. Rolled each piece away from you. Placed each piece in a laundry bag. (Note: Discarded incontinence products or disposable bed protectors in the trash. Did not put them in the laundry bag.)
8. Cleaned the bed frame and mattress (if this was your job).
9. Removed and discarded gloves. Decontaminated your hands.
10. Moved the mattress to the head of the bed.
11. Put the mattress pad on the mattress. It was even with the top of the mattress.
12. Placed the bottom sheet on the mattress pad. Unfolded it lengthwise. Placed the center crease in the middle of the bed. If using a flat sheet:
    a. Positioned the lower edge even with the bottom of the mattress.
    b. Placed the large hem at the top and the small hem at the bottom.
    c. Faced hemstitching downward, away from the person.
13. Opened the sheet. Fan-folded it to the other side of the bed.

Procedure—cont'd   **S**   **U**   **Comments**

14. Tucked the corners of a fitted sheet over the mattress at the top and then the foot of the bed. If using a flat sheet, tucked the top of the sheet under the mattress. The sheet was tight and smooth. ____ ____ _____

15. Made a mitered corner if using a flat sheet. ____ ____ _____

16. Placed the waterproof drawsheet on the bed. It was in the middle of the mattress. Or put the waterproof pad on the bed. ____ ____ _____

17. Opened the waterproof drawsheet. Fan-folded it to the other side of the bed. ____ ____ _____

18. Placed a cotton drawsheet over the waterproof drawsheet. It covered the entire waterproof drawsheet. ____ ____ _____

19. Opened the cotton drawsheet. Fan-folded it to the other side of the bed. ____ ____ _____

20. Tucked both drawsheets under the mattress. Or tucked each in separately. ____ ____ _____

21. Went to the other side of the bed. ____ ____ _____

22. Mitered the top corner of the flat bottom sheet. ____ ____ _____

23. Pulled the bottom sheet tight so there were no wrinkles. Tucked in the sheet. ____ ____ _____

24. Pulled the drawsheets tight so there were no wrinkles. Tucked both in together or separately. ____ ____ _____

25. Went to the other side of the bed. ____ ____ _____

26. Put the top sheet on the bed. Unfolded it lengthwise. Placed the center crease in the middle. If using a flat sheet:
    a. Placed the large hem even with the top of the mattress. ____ ____ _____
    b. Opened the sheet. Fan-folded it to the other side. ____ ____ _____
    c. Faced hemstitching outward, away from the person. ____ ____ _____
    d. Did not tuck the bottom in yet. ____ ____ _____
    e. Never tucked top linens in on the sides. ____ ____ _____

27. Placed the blanket on the bed:
    a. Unfolded it so the center crease was in the middle. ____ ____ _____
    b. Put the upper hem about 6–8 inches from the top of the mattress. ____ ____ _____
    c. Opened the blanket. Fan-folded it to the other side. ____ ____ _____
    d. If no bedspread, turned the top sheet down over the blanket. Hemstitching was down, away from the person. ____ ____ _____

28. Placed the bedspread on the bed:
    a. Unfolded it so the center crease was in the middle. ____ ____ _____
    b. Placed the upper hem even with the top of the mattress. ____ ____ _____
    c. Opened and fan-folded the bedspread to the other side. ____ ____ _____
    d. Made sure the bedspread facing the door was even. It covered all top linens. ____ ____ _____

29. Tucked in top linens together at the foot of the bed. They were smooth and tight. Made a mitered corner. ____ ____ _____

30. Went to the other side. ____ ____ _____

31. Straightened all top linens. Worked from the head of the bed to the foot. ____ ____ _____

32. Tucked in top linens together at the foot of the bed. Made a mitered corner. ____ ____ _____

33. Turned the top hem of the bedspread under the blanket to make a cuff. ____ ____ _____

34. Turned the top sheet down over the bedspread. Hemstitching was down. (Note: Steps 33 and 34 are not done in some centers. The bedspread covered the pillow. If so, tucked the bedspread under the pillow.) ____ ____ _____

35. Put the pillowcase on the pillow. Folded extra material under the pillow at the seam end of the pillowcase. ____ ____ _____

Procedure—cont'd	S	U	Comments
36. Placed the pillow on the bed. The open end of the pillowcase was away from the door. The seam was toward the head of the bed.	——	——	————

Postprocedure

	S	U	Comments
37. Provided for comfort. Note: Omitted this step if the bed was prepared for a new person.	——	——	————
38. Attached the call light to the bed. Or placed it within the person's reach.	——	——	————
39. Lowered bed to its lowest position. Locked the bed wheels.	——	——	————
40. Put the towels, washcloth, gown or pajamas, and bath blanket in the bedside stand.	——	——	————
41. Completed a safety check of the room.	——	——	————
42. Followed center policy for dirty linens.	——	——	————
43. Decontaminated your hands.	——	——	————

Making an Open Bed

Name: _____   Date: _____

Quality of Life	S	U	Comments
Remembered to:			
• Knock before entering the person's room.	____	____	_____
• Address the person by name.	____	____	_____
• Introduce yourself by name and title.	____	____	_____
• Explain the procedure to the person before beginning and during the procedure.	____	____	_____
• Protect the person's rights during the procedure.	____	____	_____
• Handle the person gently during the procedure.	____	____	_____

Procedure

	S	U	Comments
1. Followed *Delegation Guidelines: Making Beds*	____	____	_____
Saw *Promoting Safety and Comfort: Making Beds*	____	____	_____
2. Practiced hand hygiene.	____	____	_____
3. Collected linens for a closed bed:			
a. Mattress pad (if needed)	____	____	_____
b. Bottom sheet (flat or fitted)	____	____	_____
c. Waterproof drawsheet or waterproof pad (if needed)	____	____	_____
d. Cotton drawsheet (if needed)	____	____	_____
e. Top sheet	____	____	_____
f. Blanket	____	____	_____
g. Bedspread	____	____	_____
h. Pillowcase for each pillow	____	____	_____
i. Bath towel(s)	____	____	_____
j. Hand towel	____	____	_____
k. Washcloth	____	____	_____
l. Gown or pajamas	____	____	_____
m. Bath blanket	____	____	_____
n. Gloves	____	____	_____
o. Laundry bag	____	____	_____
p. Paper towels (if a barrier for clean linens is needed)	____	____	_____
4. Made a closed bed:			
a. Placed linens on a clean surface. Used the paper towels as a barrier between the clean surface and clean linens if required by center policy.	____	____	_____
b. Raised the bed for body mechanics. Bed rails were down.	____	____	_____
c. Put on the gloves.	____	____	_____
d. Removed linens. Rolled each piece away from you. Placed each piece in a laundry bag. (Note: Discarded incontinence products or disposable bed protectors in the trash. Did not put them in the laundry bag.)	____	____	_____
e. Cleaned the bed frame and mattress if this was your job.	____	____	_____
f. Removed and discarded gloves. Decontaminated your hands.	____	____	_____
g. Moved the mattress to the head of the bed.	____	____	_____
h. Put the mattress pad on the mattress. It was even with the top of the mattress.	____	____	_____
i. Placed the bottom sheet on the mattress pad. Unfolded it lengthwise. Placed the center crease in the middle of the bed. If using a flat sheet:			
i. Positioned the lower edge even with the bottom of the mattress.	____	____	_____
ii. Placed the large hem at the top and the small hem at the bottom.	____	____	_____
iii. Faced hemstitching downward, away from the person.	____	____	_____

	S	U	Comments

Procedure—cont'd

j. Opened the sheet. Fan-folded it to the other side of the bed.

k. Tucked the corners of a fitted sheet over the mattress at the top and then the foot of the bed. If using a flat sheet, tucked the top of the sheet under the mattress. The sheet was tight and smooth.

l. Made a mitered corner if using a flat sheet.

m. Placed the waterproof drawsheet on the bed. It was in the middle of the mattress. Or put the waterproof pad on the bed.

n. Opened the waterproof drawsheet. Fan-folded it to the other side of the bed.

o. Placed a cotton drawsheet over the waterproof drawsheet. It covered the entire waterproof drawsheet.

p. Opened the cotton drawsheet. Fan-folded it to the other side of the bed.

q. Tucked both drawsheets under the mattress. Or tucked each in separately.

r. Went to the other side of the bed.

s. Mitered the top corner of the flat bottom sheet.

t. Pulled the bottom sheet tight so there were no wrinkles. Tucked in the sheet.

u. Pulled the drawsheets tight so there were no wrinkles. Tucked both in together or separately.

v. Went to the other side of the bed.

w. Put the top sheet on the bed. Unfolded it lengthwise. Placed the center crease in the middle. Did the following if using a flat sheet:
 i. Placed the large hem even with the top of the mattress.
 ii. Opened the sheet. Fan-folded it to the other side.
 iii. Faced hemstitching outward, away from the person.
 iv. Did not tuck the bottom in yet.
 v. Never tucked top linens in on the sides.

x. Placed the blanket on the bed:
 i. Unfolded it so the center crease was in the middle.
 ii. Put the upper hem about 6–8 inches from the top of the mattress.
 iii. Opened the blanket. Fan-folded it to the other side.
 iv. If no bedspread, turned the top sheet down over the blanket. Hemstitching was down, away from the person. (Note: Followed center procedure.)

y. Placed the bedspread on the bed:
 i. Unfolded it so the center crease was in the middle.
 ii. Placed the upper hem even with the top of the mattress.
 iii. Opened and fan-folded the spread to the other side.
 iv. Made sure the bedspread facing the door was even. It covered all top linens.

z. Tucked in top linens together at the foot of the bed. They were smooth and tight. Made a mitered corner.
 i. Went to the other side.
 ii. Straightened all top linens. Worked from the head of the bed to the foot.
 iii. Tucked in top linens together at the foot of the bed. Made a mitered corner.
 iv. Turned the top hem of the bedspread under the blanket to make a cuff. (Note: Followed center procedure.)
 v. Turned the top sheet down over the bedspread.
 vi. Hemstitching was down. (Note: Not done in some centers.) The bedspread covered the pillow and it was tucked under the pillow.

Procedure—cont'd	S	U	Comments

Procedure—cont'd

vii. Put the pillowcase on the pillow. Folded extra material under the pillow at the seam end of the pillowcase.

viii. Placed the pillow on the bed. The open end of the pillowcase was away from the door. The seam was toward the head of the bed.

5. Fan-folded top linens to the foot of the bed.
6. Attached the call light to the bed.
7. Lowered the bed to its lowest position.
8. Put towels, washcloth, gown or pajamas, and bath blanket in the bedside stand.

Postprocedure

9. Provided for comfort.
10. Placed the call light within the person's reach.
11. Completed a safety check of the room.
12. Followed center policy for dirty linen.
13. Decontaminated your hands.

Making an Occupied Bed

Name: _____   Date: _____

	S	U	Comments

Quality of Life
Remembered to:
- Knock before entering the person's room.
- Address the person by name.
- Introduce yourself by name and title.
- Explain the procedure to the person before beginning and during the procedure.
- Protect the person's rights during the procedure.
- Handle the person gently during the procedure.

Preprocedure

1. Followed *Delegation Guidelines: Making Beds*
   Saw *Promoting Safety and Comfort:*
   a. *Making Beds*
   b. *The Occupied Bed*
2. Practiced hand hygiene.
3. Collected the following:
   a. Gloves
   b. Laundry bag
   c. Clean linens
   d. Paper towels, if a barrier was needed for clean linens
4. Placed linens on a clean surface. Placed paper towels between the clean surface and clean linens if required by center policy.
5. Identified the person. Checked the identification (ID) bracelet against the assignment sheet. Also called the person by name.
6. Provided for privacy.
7. Removed the call light.
8. Raised the bed for body mechanics. Bed rails were up if used. Bed wheels were locked.
9. Lowered the head of the bed. It was as flat as possible.

Procedure

10. Decontaminated your hands. Put on gloves.
11. Loosened top linens at the foot of the bed.
12. Lowered the bed rail near you if up.
13. Removed the bedspread. Then removed the blanket in the same way. Placed each over the chair.
14. Covered the person with a bath blanket. Used the blanket in the bedside stand.
    a. Unfolded the bath blanket over the top sheet.
    b. Asked the person to hold on to the bath blanket. If he or she could not, tucked the top part under the person's shoulders.
    c. Grasped the top sheet under the bath blanket at the shoulders. Brought the sheet down to the foot of the bed. Removed the sheet from under the blanket.
15. Positioned the person on the side of the bed away from you. Adjusted the pillow for comfort.
16. Loosened bottom linens from the head to the foot of the bed.
17. Fan-folded bottom linens one at a time toward the person. Started with the cotton drawsheet. If reusing the mattress pad, did not fan-fold it.
18. Placed a clean mattress pad on the bed. Unfolded it lengthwise. The center crease was in the middle. Fan-folded the top part toward the person. If reusing the mattress pad, straightened and smoothed any wrinkles.

269

Procedure Checklists

Procedure—cont'd	S	U	Comments

19. Placed the bottom sheet on the mattress pad. Hemstitching was away from the person. Unfolded the sheet so the crease was in the middle. If using a flat sheet, the small hem was even with the bottom of the mattress. Fan-folded the top part toward the person.   ___ ___ _____
20. Tucked the corners of a fitted sheet over the mattress. If using a flat sheet, made a mitered corner at the head of the bed. Tucked the sheet under the mattress from the head to the foot.   ___ ___ _____
21. Pulled the waterproof drawsheet toward you over the bottom sheet. Tucked excess material under the mattress. Did the following for a clean waterproof drawsheet:
    a. Placed the waterproof drawsheet on the bed. It was in the middle of the mattress.   ___ ___ _____
    b. Fan-folded the top part toward the person.   ___ ___ _____
    c. Tucked in excess fabric.   ___ ___ _____
22. Placed the cotton drawsheet over the waterproof drawsheet. It covered the entire waterproof drawsheet. Fan-folded the top part toward the person. Tucked in excess fabric.   ___ ___ _____
23. Explained to the person that he or she will roll over a "bump." Assured the person that he or she would not fall.   ___ ___ _____
24. Helped the person turn to the other side. Adjusted the pillow for comfort.   ___ ___ _____
25. Raised the bed rail. Went to the other side and lowered the bed rail.   ___ ___ _____
26. Loosened bottom linens. Removed one piece at a time. Placed each piece in the laundry bag. (Note: Discarded disposable bed protectors and incontinence products in the trash. Did not put them in the laundry bag.)   ___ ___ _____
27. Removed and discarded the gloves. Decontaminated your hands.   ___ ___ _____
28. Straightened and smoothed the mattress pad.   ___ ___ _____
29. Pulled the clean bottom sheet toward you. Tucked the corners of a fitted sheet over the mattress. If using a flat sheet, made a mitered corner at the top. Tucked the sheet under the mattress from the head to the foot of the bed.   ___ ___ _____
30. Pulled the drawsheets tightly toward you. Tucked both under together or separately.   ___ ___ _____
31. Positioned the person supine in the center of the bed. Adjusted the pillow for comfort.   ___ ___ _____
32. Put the top sheet on the bed. Unfolded it lengthwise. The crease was in the middle. The large hem was even with the top of the mattress. Hemstitching was on the outside.   ___ ___ _____
33. Asked the person to hold the top sheet so you could remove the bath blanket. Or tucked the top sheet under the person's shoulders. Removed and discarded the bath blanket.   ___ ___ _____
34. Placed the blanket on the bed. Unfolded it so the center crease was in the middle and it covered the person. The upper hem was 6–8 inches from the top of the mattress.   ___ ___ _____
35. Placed the bedspread on the bed. Unfolded it so the center crease was in the middle and it covered the person. The top hem was even with the mattress top.   ___ ___ _____
36. Turned the top hem of the bedspread under the blanket to make a cuff.   ___ ___ _____
37. Brought the top sheet down over the bedspread to form a cuff.   ___ ___ _____
38. Went to the foot of the bed.   ___ ___ _____
39. Made a toe pleat. Made a 2-inch pleat across the foot of the bed. The pleat was about 6–8 inches from the foot of the bed.   ___ ___ _____

Procedure—cont'd	S	U	Comments
40. Lifted the mattress corner with one arm. Tucked all top linens under the mattress. Made a mitered corner.	——	——	——————
41. Raised the bed rail. Went to the other side and lowered the bed rail.	——	——	——————
42. Straightened and smoothed top linens.	——	——	——————
43. Tucked all top linens under the mattress. Made a mitered corner.	——	——	——————
44. Changed the pillowcase(s).	——	——	——————

Postprocedure

	S	U	Comments
45. Provided for comfort.	——	——	——————
46. Placed the call light within reach.	——	——	——————
47. Lowered the bed to its lowest position. Bed wheels were locked.	——	——	——————
48. Raised or lowered bed rails. Followed the care plan.	——	——	——————
49. Put the clean towels, washcloth, gown or pajamas, and bath blanket in the bedside stand.	——	——	——————
50. Unscreened the person.	——	——	——————
51. Completed a safety check of the room.	——	——	——————
52. Followed center policy for dirty linens.	——	——	——————
53. Decontaminated your hands.	——	——	——————

Name: ———————————— Date: ————————————

Procedure	S	U	Comments
1. Followed *Delegation Guidelines: Making Beds*			
Saw *Promoting Safety and Comfort:*			
a. *Making Beds*	——	——	————
b. *The Surgical Bed*	——	——	————
2. Practiced hand hygiene.	——	——	————
3. Collected the following:			
a. Clean linens	——	——	————
b. Gloves	——	——	————
c. Laundry bag	——	——	————
d. Equipment requested by the nurse	——	——	————
e. Paper towel, if a barrier for clean linens is needed	——	——	————
4. Placed linens on a clean surface. Placed paper towels between the clean surface and clean linens if a barrier is required by center policy.	——	——	————
5. Removed the call light.	——	——	————
6. Raised the bed for body mechanics.	——	——	————
7. Removed all linens from the bed. Wore gloves. Decontaminated your hands after removing gloves.	——	——	————
8. Made a closed bed. Did not tuck top linens under the mattress.			
a. Moved the mattress to the head of the bed.			
b. Put the mattress pad on the mattress. It was even with the top of the mattress.	——	——	————
c. Placed the bottom sheet on the mattress pad. Unfolded it lengthwise. Placed the center crease in the middle of the bed. If using a flat sheet:			
i. Positioned the lower edge even with the bottom of the mattress.	——	——	————
ii. Placed the large hem at the top and the small hem at the bottom.	——	——	————
iii. Faced hemstitching downward, away from the person.	——	——	————
d. Opened the sheet. Fan-folded it to the other side of the bed.	——	——	————
e. Tucked the corners of a fitted sheet at the top and then the foot of the bed. If using a flat sheet, tucked the top of the sheet under the mattress. The sheet was tight and smooth.	——	——	————
f. Made a mitered corner if using a flat sheet.	——	——	————
g. Placed the waterproof drawsheet on the bed. It was in the middle of the mattress. Or put the waterproof pad on the bed.	——	——	————
h. Opened the waterproof drawsheet. Fan-folded it to the other side of the bed.	——	——	————
i. Placed a cotton drawsheet over the waterproof drawsheet. It covered the entire waterproof drawsheet.	——	——	————
j. Opened the cotton drawsheet. Fan-folded it to the other side of the bed.	——	——	————
k. Tucked both drawsheets under the mattress. Or tucked each in separately.	——	——	————
l. Went to the other side of the bed.	——	——	————
m. Mitered the top corner of the flat bottom sheet.	——	——	————
n. Pulled the bottom sheet tight so there were no wrinkles. Tucked in the sheet.	——	——	————
o. Pulled the drawsheet tight so there were no wrinkles. Tucked both in together or separately.	——	——	————

Procedure—cont'd   **S**   **U**   **Comments**

    p. Went to the other side of the bed.

    q. Put the top sheet on the bed. Unfolded it lengthwise. Placed the center crease in the middle. If using a flat sheet:

       i. Placed the large hem even with the top of the mattress.

      ii. Opened the sheet. Fan-folded it to the other side.

     iii. Faced hemstitching outward, away from the person.

9. Folded all top linens at the foot of the bed back onto the bed. The fold was even with the edge of the mattress.

10. Fan-folded linens lengthwise to the side of the bed farthest from the door.

11. Put the pillowcase(s) on the pillow(s).

12. Placed the pillow(s) on a clean surface.

13. Left the bed in its highest position.

14. Left both bed rails down.

15. Put the clean towels, washcloth, gown or pajamas, and bath blanket in the bedside stand.

16. Moved furniture away from the bed. Allowed room for the stretcher and staff.

17. Did not attach the call light to the bed.

18. Completed a safety check of the room.

19. Followed center policy for soiled linen.

20. Decontaminated your hands.

Assisting the Person to Brush and Floss the Teeth

Name:—————————————— Date:——————————————

	S	U	Comments
Quality of Life			

Remembered to:
- Knock before entering the person's room. ⎯⎯ ⎯⎯ ⎯⎯⎯⎯
- Address the person by name. ⎯⎯ ⎯⎯ ⎯⎯⎯⎯
- Introduce yourself by name and title. ⎯⎯ ⎯⎯ ⎯⎯⎯⎯
- Explain the procedure to the person before beginning and during the procedure. ⎯⎯ ⎯⎯ ⎯⎯⎯⎯
- Protect the person's rights during the procedure. ⎯⎯ ⎯⎯ ⎯⎯⎯⎯
- Handle the person gently during the procedure. ⎯⎯ ⎯⎯ ⎯⎯⎯⎯

Preprocedure

1. Followed *Delegation Guidelines: Oral Hygiene* ⎯⎯ ⎯⎯ ⎯⎯⎯⎯
   Saw *Promoting Safety and Comfort: Oral Hygiene* ⎯⎯ ⎯⎯ ⎯⎯⎯⎯
2. Practiced hand hygiene. ⎯⎯ ⎯⎯ ⎯⎯⎯⎯
3. Collected the following:
   a. Toothbrush ⎯⎯ ⎯⎯ ⎯⎯⎯⎯
   b. Toothpaste ⎯⎯ ⎯⎯ ⎯⎯⎯⎯
   c. Mouthwash (or solution noted in care plan) ⎯⎯ ⎯⎯ ⎯⎯⎯⎯
   d. Dental floss (if used) ⎯⎯ ⎯⎯ ⎯⎯⎯⎯
   e. Water glass with cool water ⎯⎯ ⎯⎯ ⎯⎯⎯⎯
   f. Straw ⎯⎯ ⎯⎯ ⎯⎯⎯⎯
   g. Kidney basin ⎯⎯ ⎯⎯ ⎯⎯⎯⎯
   h. Hand towel ⎯⎯ ⎯⎯ ⎯⎯⎯⎯
   i. Paper towels ⎯⎯ ⎯⎯ ⎯⎯⎯⎯
   j. Gloves ⎯⎯ ⎯⎯ ⎯⎯⎯⎯
4. Placed the paper towels on the overbed table. Arranged items on top of them. ⎯⎯ ⎯⎯ ⎯⎯⎯⎯
5. Identified the person. Checked the identification (ID) bracelet against the assignment sheet. Also called the person by name. ⎯⎯ ⎯⎯ ⎯⎯⎯⎯
6. Provided for privacy. ⎯⎯ ⎯⎯ ⎯⎯⎯⎯
7. Lowered the bed rail near you if up. ⎯⎯ ⎯⎯ ⎯⎯⎯⎯

Procedure

8. Positioned the person so he or she could brush with ease. ⎯⎯ ⎯⎯ ⎯⎯⎯⎯
9. Placed the towel over the person's chest. This protected garments and linens from spills. ⎯⎯ ⎯⎯ ⎯⎯⎯⎯
10. Adjusted the overbed table in front of the person. ⎯⎯ ⎯⎯ ⎯⎯⎯⎯
11. Let the person perform oral hygiene. This included brushing the teeth and tongue, rinsing the mouth, flossing, and using mouthwash or other solution. ⎯⎯ ⎯⎯ ⎯⎯⎯⎯
12. Removed the towel when the person was done. ⎯⎯ ⎯⎯ ⎯⎯⎯⎯
13. Moved the overbed table to the side of the bed. ⎯⎯ ⎯⎯ ⎯⎯⎯⎯

Postprocedure

14. Provided for comfort. ⎯⎯ ⎯⎯ ⎯⎯⎯⎯
15. Placed the call light within reach. ⎯⎯ ⎯⎯ ⎯⎯⎯⎯
16. Raised or lowered bed rails. Followed the care plan. ⎯⎯ ⎯⎯ ⎯⎯⎯⎯
17. Cleaned and returned items to their proper place. Wore gloves. ⎯⎯ ⎯⎯ ⎯⎯⎯⎯
18. Wiped off the overbed table with the paper towels. Discarded the paper towels. ⎯⎯ ⎯⎯ ⎯⎯⎯⎯
19. Removed the gloves. Decontaminated your hands. ⎯⎯ ⎯⎯ ⎯⎯⎯⎯
20. Unscreened the person. ⎯⎯ ⎯⎯ ⎯⎯⎯⎯
21. Completed a safety check of the room. ⎯⎯ ⎯⎯ ⎯⎯⎯⎯
22. Followed center policy for dirty linens. ⎯⎯ ⎯⎯ ⎯⎯⎯⎯
23. Decontaminated your hands. ⎯⎯ ⎯⎯ ⎯⎯⎯⎯
24. Reported and recorded your observations. ⎯⎯ ⎯⎯ ⎯⎯⎯⎯

Brushing and Flossing the Person's Teeth

Name:_____   Date:_____

	S	U	Comments
Quality of Life			

Remembered to:
- Knock before entering the person's room.
- Address the person by name.
- Introduce yourself by name and title.
- Explain the procedure to the person before beginning and during the procedure.
- Protect the person's rights during the procedure.
- Handle the person gently during the procedure.

Preprocedure

1. Followed *Delegation Guidelines: Oral Hygiene*
   Saw *Promoting Safety and Comfort: Oral Hygiene*
2. Practiced hand hygiene.
3. Collected the following:
   a. Toothbrush with soft bristles
   b. Toothpaste
   c. Mouthwash (or solution noted in care plan)
   d. Dental floss (if used)
   e. Water glass with cool water
   f. Straw
   g. Kidney basin
   h. Hand towel
   i. Paper towels
   j. Gloves
4. Placed the paper towels on the overbed table. Arranged items on top of them.
5. Identified the person. Checked the identification (ID) bracelet against the assignment sheet. Also called the person by name.
6. Provided for privacy.
7. Raised the bed for body mechanics. Bed rails were up if used.

Procedure

8. Lowered the bed rail near you if up.
9. Assisted the person to a sitting position or to a side-lying position near you.
10. Placed the towel across the person's chest.
11. Adjusted the overbed table so you could reach it with ease.
12. Decontaminated your hands. Put on gloves.
13. Held the toothbrush over the kidney basin. Poured some water over the brush.
14. Applied toothpaste to the toothbrush.
15. Brushed the teeth gently.
16. Brushed the tongue gently.
17. Let the person rinse the mouth with water. Held the kidney basin under the person's chin. Repeated this step as needed.
18. Flossed the person's teeth (optional):
    a. Broke off an 18-inch piece of floss from the dispenser.
    b. Held the floss between the middle fingers of each hand.
    c. Stretched the floss with your thumbs.
    d. Started at the upper back tooth on the right side. Worked around to the left side.
    e. Moved the floss gently up and down between the teeth. Moved the floss up and down against the side of the tooth. Worked from the top of the crown to the gum line.
    f. Moved to a new section of floss after every second tooth.

275

Procedure—cont'd	S	U	Comments

g. Flossed the lower teeth. Used up-and-down motions for the upper teeth. Started on the right side. Worked around to the left side.

19. Let the person use mouthwash or other solution. Held the kidney basin under the chin.
20. Wiped the person's mouth. Removed the towel.
21. Removed and discarded the gloves. Decontaminated your hands.

Postprocedure

22. Provided for comfort.
23. Placed the call light within reach.
24. Lowered the bed to its lowest position.
25. Raised or lowered bed rails. Followed the care plan.
26. Cleaned and returned equipment to its proper place. Wore gloves.
27. Wiped off the overbed table with the paper towels. Discarded the paper towels.
28. Unscreened the person.
29. Completed a safety check of the room.
30. Followed center policy for dirty linens.
31. Removed the gloves. Decontaminated your hands.
32. Reported and recorded your observations.

Providing Mouth Care for the Unconscious Person

Name: ———————————— Date:————————————

Quality of Life	S	U	Comments
Remembered to:			
• Knock before entering the person's room.	———	———	———————
• Address the person by name.	———	———	———————
• Introduce yourself by name and title.	———	———	———————
• Explain the procedure to the person before beginning and during the procedure.	———	———	———————
• Protect the person's rights during the procedure.	———	———	———————
• Handle the person gently during the procedure.	———	———	———————

Preprocedure

	S	U	Comments
1. Followed *Delegation Guidelines: Oral Hygiene*			
Saw *Promoting Safety and Comfort:*	———	———	———————
a. *Oral Hygiene*	———	———	———————
b. *Mouth Care for the Unconscious Person*	———	———	———————
2. Practiced hand hygiene.	———	———	———————
3. Collected the following:			
a. Cleaning agent (checked the care plan)	———	———	———————
b. Sponge swabs	———	———	———————
c. Padded tongue blade	———	———	———————
d. Water glass or cup with cool water	———	———	———————
e. Hand towel	———	———	———————
f. Kidney basin	———	———	———————
g. Lip lubricant	———	———	———————
h. Paper towels	———	———	———————
i. Gloves	———	———	———————
4. Placed the paper towels on the overbed table. Arranged items on top of them.	———	———	———————
5. Identified the person. Checked the identification (ID) bracelet against the assignment sheet. Also called the person by name.	———	———	———————
6. Provided for privacy.	———	———	———————
7. Raised the bed for body mechanics. Bed rails were up if used.	———	———	———————

Procedure

	S	U	Comments
8. Lowered the bed rail near you if up.	———	———	———————
9. Decontaminated your hands. Put on gloves.	———	———	———————
10. Positioned the person in a side-lying position near you. Turned his or her head well to the side.	———	———	———————
11. Placed the towel under the person's face.	———	———	———————
12. Placed the kidney basin under the chin.	———	———	———————
13. Separated the upper and lower teeth. Used the padded tongue blade. Was gentle. Never used force. If you had problems, asked the nurse for help.	———	———	———————
14. Cleaned the mouth using sponge swabs moistened with the cleaning agent.			
a. Cleaned the chewing and inner surfaces of the teeth.	———	———	———————
b. Cleaned the gums and outer surfaces of the teeth.	———	———	———————
c. Swabbed the roof of the mouth, inside of the cheeks, and lips.	———	———	———————
d. Swabbed the tongue.	———	———	———————
e. Moistened a clean swab with water. Swabbed the mouth to rinse.	———	———	———————
f. Placed used swabs in the kidney basin.	———	———	———————
15. Removed the kidney basin and supplies.	———	———	———————
16. Wiped the person's mouth. Removed the towel.	———	———	———————
17. Applied lubricant to the lips.	———	———	———————

Procedure—cont'd	S	U	Comments
18. Removed and discarded the gloves. Decontaminated your hands.	——	——	

Postprocedure

	S	U	Comments
19. Provided for comfort.	——	——	————
20. Placed the call light within reach.	——	——	————
21. Lowered the bed to its lowest position.	——	——	————
22. Raised or lowered bed rails. Followed the care plan.	——	——	————
23. Cleaned and returned equipment to its proper place. Discarded disposable items. (Wore gloves.)	——	——	————
24. Wiped off the overbed table with the paper towels. Discarded the paper towels.	——	——	————
25. Unscreened the person.	——	——	————
26. Completed a safety check of the room.	——	——	————
27. Told the person when you were leaving the room. Told him or her when you would return.	——	——	————
28. Followed center policy for dirty linens.	——	——	————
29. Removed the gloves. Decontaminated your hands.	——	——	————
30. Reported and recorded your observations.	——	——	————

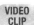

Name: —————————————— Date: ——————————————

	S	U	Comments

Quality of Life

Remembered to:
- Knock before entering the person's room.
- Address the person by name.
- Introduce yourself by name and title.
- Explain the procedure to the person before beginning and during the procedure.
- Protect the person's rights during the procedure.
- Handle the person gently during the procedure.

Preprocedure

1. Followed *Delegation Guidelines: Oral Hygiene*
   Saw *Promoting Safety and Comfort:*
   a. *Oral Hygiene*
   b. *Denture Care*
2. Practiced hand hygiene.
3. Collected the following:
   a. Denture brush or toothbrush (for cleaning dentures)
   b. Denture cup labeled with the person's name and room and bed number
   c. Denture cleaning agent
   d. Soft-bristled toothbrush or sponge swabs (for oral hygiene)
   e. Toothpaste
   f. Water glass with cool water
   g. Straw
   h. Mouthwash (or other noted solution)
   i. Kidney basin
   j. Two hand towels
   k. Gauze squares
   l. Paper towels
   m. Gloves
4. Placed the paper towels on the overbed table. Arranged items on top of them.
5. Identified the person. Checked the identification (ID) bracelet against the assignment sheet. Also called the person by name.
6. Provided for privacy.
7. Raised the bed for body mechanics.

Procedure

8. Lowered the bed rail near you if used.
9. Decontaminated your hands. Put on gloves.
10. Placed a towel over the person's chest.
11. Asked the person to remove the dentures. Carefully placed them in the kidney basin.
12. Removed the dentures if the person could not do so. Used gauze squares to get a good grip on the slippery dentures.
    a. Grasped the denture with your thumb and index finger. Moved it up and down slightly to break the seal. Gently removed the denture. Placed it in the kidney basin.
    b. Grasped and removed the lower denture with thumb and index finger. Turned it slightly and lifted it out of the person's mouth. Placed it in the kidney basin.
13. Followed the care plan for raising side rails.
14. Took the kidney basin, denture cup, denture brush, and denture cleaning agent to the sink.
15. Lined the sink with a towel. Filled the sink halfway with water.

279

Procedure—cont'd	S	U	Comments

16. Rinsed each denture under cool or warm running water. Followed center policy for water temperature. ___ ___ _____
17. Returned dentures to the kidney basin or denture cup. ___ ___ _____
18. Applied the denture cleaning agent to the brush. ___ ___ _____
19. Brushed the dentures. Brushed the inner, outer, and chewing surfaces. ___ ___ _____
20. Rinsed the dentures under running water. Used warm or cool water as directed by the cleaning agent manufacturer. (Some state competency tests require cool water.) ___ ___ _____
21. Rinsed the denture cup and lid. Placed dentures in the denture cup. Covered the dentures with cool or warm water. Followed center policy for water temperature. ___ ___ _____
22. Cleaned the kidney basin. ___ ___ _____
23. Took the denture cup and kidney basin to the overbed table. ___ ___ _____
24. Lowered the bed rail if up. ___ ___ _____
25. Positioned the person for oral hygiene. ___ ___ _____
26. Cleaned the person's gums and tongue. Used toothpaste and the toothbrush (or sponge swabs). ___ ___ _____
27. Had the person use mouthwash (or noted solution). Held the kidney basin under the chin. ___ ___ _____
28. Asked the person to insert the dentures. Inserted them if the person could not:
    a. Held the upper denture firmly with your thumb and index finger. Raised the upper lip with the other hand. Inserted the denture. Gently pressed the denture with your index fingers to make sure it was in place. ___ ___ _____
    b. Held the lower denture with your thumb and index finger. Pulled the lower lip down slightly. Inserted the denture. Gently pressed down on it to make sure it was in place. ___ ___ _____
29. Placed the denture cup in the top drawer of the bedside stand if the dentures were not worn. If not worn, the dentures were in water or a denture soaking solution. ___ ___ _____
30. Wiped the person's mouth. Removed the towel. ___ ___ _____
31. Removed the gloves. Decontaminated your hands. ___ ___ _____

Postprocedure

32. Assisted with hand washing. ___ ___ _____
33. Provided for comfort. ___ ___ _____
34. Placed the call light within reach. ___ ___ _____
35. Lowered the bed to its lowest position. ___ ___ _____
36. Raised or lowered bed rails. Followed the care plan. ___ ___ _____
37. Removed the towel from the sink. Drained the sink. ___ ___ _____
38. Cleaned and returned equipment to its proper place. Discarded disposable items. (Wore gloves for this step.) ___ ___ _____
39. Wiped off the overbed table with the paper towels. Discarded the paper towels. ___ ___ _____
40. Unscreened the person. ___ ___ _____
41. Completed a safety check of the room. ___ ___ _____
42. Followed center policy for dirty linens. ___ ___ _____
43. Removed the gloves. Decontaminated your hands. ___ ___ _____
44. Reported and recorded your observations. ___ ___ _____

Giving a Complete Bed Bath (NATCEP)

Name: ————————————— Date: —————————————

	S	U	Comments
Quality of Life			

Remembered to:
- Knock before entering the person's room.
- Address the person by name.
- Introduce yourself by name and title.
- Explain the procedure to the person before beginning and during the procedure.
- Protect the person's rights during the procedure.
- Handle the person gently during the procedure.

Preprocedure

1. Followed *Delegation Guidelines: Bathing*
   Saw *Promoting Safety and Comfort: Bathing*
2. Practiced hand hygiene.
3. Identified the person. Checked the identification (ID) bracelet against the assignment sheet. Also called the person by name.
4. Collected clean linens for a closed bed (saw *Making a Closed Bed*) and placed linens on a clean surface:
   a. Mattress pad (if needed)
   b. Bottom sheet (flat or fitted)
   c. Waterproof drawsheet or waterproof pad (if used)
   d. Cotton drawsheet (if needed)
   e. Top sheet
   f. Blanket
   g. Bedspread
   h. Pillowcase for each pillow
   i. Bath towel
   j. Hand towel
   k. Gloves
   l. Laundry bag
5. Collected the following:
   a. Wash basin
   b. Soap
   c. Bath thermometer
   d. Orangewood stick or nail file
   e. Washcloth
   f. Two bath towels and two hand towels
   g. Bath blanket
   h. Clothing or sleepwear
   i. Lotion
   j. Powder
   k. Deodorant or antiperspirant
   l. Brush and comb
   m. Other grooming items as requested
   n. Paper towels
   o. Gloves
6. Covered the overbed table with paper towels. Arranged items on the overbed table. Adjusted the height as needed.
7. Provided for privacy.
8. Raised the bed for body mechanics. Bed rails were up if used.

Procedure

9. Removed the call light.
10. Decontaminated your hands. Put on gloves.

281

Procedure—cont'd   S   U   Comments

11. Covered the person with a bath blanket. Removed top linens. (Saw procedure: *Making an Occupied Bed* in Chapter 17.)

12. Lowered the head of the bed. It was as flat as possible. The person had at least one pillow.

13. Filled the wash basin ⅔ (two-thirds) full with water. Followed the care plan for water temperature, usually 110°F–115°F (43.3°C–46.1°C) for adults. Measured water temperature. Used the bath thermometer. Or tested the water by dipping your elbow or inner wrist into the basin.

14. Lowered the bed rail near you if up.

15. Asked the person to check the water temperature. Adjusted the water temperature if it was too hot or too cold. Raised the bed rail before leaving the bedside. Lowered it when you returned.

16. Placed the basin on the overbed table.

17. Removed the sleepwear. Did not expose the person.

18. Placed a hand towel over the person's chest.

19. Made a mitt with the washcloth. Used a mitt for the entire bath.

20. Washed around the person's eyes with water. Did not use soap.
    a. Cleaned the far eye. Gently wiped from the inner to the outer aspect of the eye with a corner of the mitt.
    b. Cleaned the eye near you. Used a clean part of the washcloth for each stroke.

21. Asked the person if you should use soap to wash the face.

22. Washed the face, ears, and neck. Rinsed and patted dry with the towel on the chest.

23. Helped the person move to the side of the bed near you.

24. Exposed the far arm. Placed a bath towel lengthwise under the arm. Applied soap to the washcloth.

25. Supported the arm with your palm under the person's elbow. His or her forearm rested on your forearm.

26. Washed the arm, shoulder, and underarm. Used long, firm strokes. Rinsed and patted dry.

27. Placed the basin on the towel. Put the person's hand into the water. Washed it well. Cleaned under the fingernails with an orangewood stick or nail file.

28. Had the person exercise the hand and fingers.

29. Removed the basin. Dried the hand well. Covered the arm with the bath blanket.

30. Repeated steps 24–29 for the near arm:
    a. Exposed the near arm. Placed a bath towel lengthwise under the arm. Applied soap to the washcloth.
    b. Supported the arm with your palm under the person's elbow. His or her forearm rested on your forearm.
    c. Washed the arm, shoulder, and underarm. Used long, firm strokes. Rinsed and patted dry.
    d. Placed the basin on the towel. Put the person's hand into the water. Washed it well. Cleaned under the fingernails with an orangewood stick or nail file.
    e. Had the person exercise the hand and fingers.
    f. Removed the basin. Dried the hand well. Covered the arm with the bath blanket.

31. Placed a bath towel over the chest crosswise. Held the towel in place. Pulled the bath blanket from under the towel to the waist. Applied soap to the washcloth.

32. Lifted the towel slightly and washed the chest. Did not expose the person. Rinsed and patted dry, especially under the breasts. ——— ——— —————

33. Moved the towel lengthwise over the chest and abdomen. Did not expose the person. Pulled the bath blanket down to the pubic area. Applied soap to the washcloth. ——— ——— —————

34. Lifted the towel slightly and washed the abdomen. Rinsed and patted dry. ——— ——— —————

35. Pulled the bath blanket up to the shoulders. Covered both arms. Removed the towel. ——— ——— —————

36. Changed soapy or cool water. Measured water temperature. Followed the care plan for water temperature, usually 110°F–115°F (43.3°C–46.1°C) for adults. Measured water temperature. Used the bath thermometer. Or tested the water by dipping your elbow or inner wrist into the basin. If bed rails used, raised the bed rail near you before you left the bedside. Lowered it when you returned. ——— ——— —————

37. Uncovered the far leg. Did not expose the genital area. Placed a towel lengthwise under the foot and leg. Applied soap to the washcloth. ——— ——— —————

38. Bent the knee and supported the leg with your arm. Washed it with long, firm strokes. Rinsed and patted dry. ——— ——— —————

39. Placed the basin on the towel near the foot. ——— ——— —————

40. Lifted the leg slightly. Slid the basin under the foot. ——— ——— —————

41. Placed the foot in the basin. Used an orangewood stick or nail file to clean under toenails if necessary. If the person could not bend the knees:
    a. Washed the foot. Carefully separated the toes. Rinsed and patted dry. ——— ——— —————
    b. Cleaned under the toenails with an orangewood stick or nail file if necessary. ——— ——— —————

42. Removed the basin. Dried the leg and foot. Applied lotion to the foot if directed by the nurse and care plan. Covered the leg with the bath blanket. Removed the towel. ——— ——— —————

43. Repeated for the near leg:
    a. Uncovered the near leg. Did not expose the genital area. Placed a towel lengthwise under the foot and leg. ——— ——— —————
    b. Bent the knee and supported the leg with your arm. Washed it with long, firm strokes. Rinsed and patted dry. ——— ——— —————
    c. Placed the basin on the towel near the foot. ——— ——— —————
    d. Lifted the leg slightly. Slid the basin under the foot. ——— ——— —————
    e. Placed the foot in the basin. Used an orangewood stick or nail file to clean under toenails if necessary. If the person could not bend the knees:
       i. Washed the foot. Carefully separated the toes. Rinsed and patted dry. ——— ——— —————
       ii. Cleaned under the toenails with an orangewood stick or nail file if necessary. ——— ——— —————
    f. Removed the basin. Dried the leg and foot. Applied lotion to the foot if directed by the nurse and care plan. Covered the leg with the bath blanket. Removed the towel. ——— ——— —————

44. Changed the water. Measured water temperature. Followed the care plan for water temperature, usually 110°F–115°F (43.3°C–46.1°C) for adults. Measured water temperature. Used the bath thermometer. Or tested the water by dipping your elbow or inner wrist into the basin. If bed rails used, raised the bed rail near you before you left the bedside. Lowered it when you returned. ——— ——— —————

Procedure—cont'd	S	U	Comments

Procedure—cont'd

45. Turned the person onto the side away from you. The person was covered with the bath blanket.

46. Uncovered the back and buttocks. Did not expose the person. Placed a towel lengthwise on the bed along the back. Applied soap to the washcloth.

47. Washed the back. Worked from the back of the neck to the lower end of the buttocks. Used long, firm, continuous strokes. Rinsed and dried well.

48. Gave a back massage. (The person may want the back massage after the bath.)

49. Turned the person onto his or her back.

50. Changed the water for perineal care. Water temperature is usually 105°F–109°F (40.5°C–42.7°C). Followed the care plan for water temperature. Measured water temperature according to center policy. (Some state competency tests require changing gloves and hand hygiene at this time.) If bed rails used, raised the bed rail near you before you left the bedside. Lowered it when you returned.

51. Let the person wash the genital area. Adjusted the overbed table so he or she could reach the wash basin, soap, and towels with ease. Placed the call light within reach. Asked the person to signal when finished. Made sure the person understood what to do.

52. Removed the gloves. Decontaminated your hands.

53. Answered the call light promptly. Knocked before entering the room. Provided perineal care if the person could not do so. (Decontaminated your hands and wore gloves for perineal care.)

54. Gave a back massage if you had not already done so.

55. Applied deodorant or antiperspirant. Applied lotion and powder as requested. Saw *Promoting Safety and Comfort: Bathing*

56. Put clean garments on the person.

57. Combed and brushed the hair.

58. Made the bed.

Postprocedure

59. Provided for comfort.

60. Placed the call light within reach.

61. Lowered the bed to its lowest position.

62. Raised or lowered bed rails. Followed the care plan.

63. Put on clean gloves.

64. Emptied, cleaned, and dried the wash basin. Returned it and other supplies to their proper place.

65. Wiped off the overbed table with the paper towels. Discarded the paper towels.

66. Unscreened the person.

67. Completed a safety check of the room.

68. Followed center policy for dirty linens.

69. Removed the gloves. Decontaminated your hands.

70. Reported and recorded your observations.

Assisting with the Partial Bath

Name: _____   Date: _____

Quality of Life	**S**	**U**	**Comments**

Remembered to:
- Knock before entering the person's room.
- Address the person by name.
- Introduce yourself by name and title.
- Explain the procedure to the person before beginning and during the procedure.
- Protect the person's rights during the procedure.
- Handle the person gently during the procedure.

Preprocedure

1. Followed *Delegation Guidelines: Bathing*
   Saw *Promoting Safety and Comfort: Bathing*
2. Did the following:
   a. Practiced hand hygiene.
   b. Identified the person. Checked the identification (ID) bracelet against the assignment sheet. Also called the person by name.
   c. Collected clean linens for a closed bed. Saw procedure: *Making a Closed Bed*. Placed linens on a clean surface:
      i. Mattress pad (if needed)
      ii. Bottom sheet (flat fit or fitted sheet)
      iii. Waterproof drawsheet or waterproof pad (if needed)
      iv. Cotton drawsheet (if needed)
      v. Top sheet
      vi. Blanket
      vii. Bedspread
      viii. A pillowcase for each pillow
      ix. Gloves
      x. Laundry bag
   d. Collected the following:
      i. Wash basin
      ii. Soap
      iii. Bath thermometer
      iv. Orangewood stick or nail file
      v. Washcloth
      vi. Two bath towels and two hand towels
      vii. Bath blanket
      viii. Clothing or sleepwear
      ix. Lotion
      x. Powder
      xi. Deodorant or antiperspirant
      xii. Brush and comb
      xiii. Other grooming items as requested
      xiv. Paper towels
      xv. Gloves
   e. Covered the overbed table with paper towels. Arranged items on the overbed table. Adjusted the height as needed.
   f. Provided for privacy.
   g. Raised the bed for body mechanics. Bed rails were up if used.

Procedure

3. Made sure the bed was in the lowest position.
4. Decontaminated your hands. Put on gloves.
5. Covered the person with a bath blanket. Removed top linens.

285

Procedure—cont'd	S	U	Comments

Procedure—cont'd

6. Filled the wash basin ⅔ (two-thirds) full with water. Water temperature was 110°F–115°F (43.3°C–46.1°C) or as directed by the nurse. Measured water temperature with the bath thermometer. Or tested the water by dipping your elbow or inner wrist into the basin.
7. Asked the person to check the water temperature. Adjusted the water temperature if it was too hot or too cold.
8. Placed the basin on the overbed table.
9. Positioned the person in Fowler position. Or assisted him or her to sit at the bedside.
10. Adjusted the overbed table so the person could reach the basin and supplies.
11. Helped the person undress. Provided for privacy and warmth with the bath blanket.
12. Asked the person to wash easy-to-reach body parts. Explained that you would wash the back and areas the person could not reach.
13. Placed the call light within reach. Asked the person to signal when help was needed or bathing was complete.
14. Decontaminated your hands. Left the room.
15. Returned when the call light was on. Knocked before entering. Decontaminated your hands.
16. Changed the bath water. Measured bath water temperature: 110°F–115°F (43.3°C–46.1°C) or as directed by the nurse. Used the bath thermometer. Or tested the water by dipping your elbow or inner wrist into the basin.
17. Raised the bed for body mechanics. The far bed rail was up if used.
18. Asked what was washed. Put on gloves. Washed and dried areas the person could not reach. The face, hands, underarms, back, buttocks, and perineal area were washed for the partial bath.
19. Removed the gloves. Decontaminated your hands.
20. Gave a back massage.
21. Applied lotion, powder, and deodorant or antiperspirant as requested.
22. Helped the person put on clean garments.
23. Assisted with hair care and other grooming needs.
24. Assisted the person to a chair. (Lowered the bed if the person transferred to a chair.) Or turned the person onto the side away from you.
25. Made the bed. (Raised the bed for body mechanics.)

Postprocedure

26. Provided for comfort.
27. Placed the call light within reach.
28. Lowered the bed to its lowest position.
29. Raised or lowered bed rails. Followed the care plan.
30. Put on clean gloves.
31. Emptied, cleaned, and dried the bath basin. Returned the basin and supplies to their proper place.
32. Wiped off the overbed table with the paper towels. Discarded the paper towels.
33. Unscreened the person.
34. Completed a safety check of the room.
35. Followed center policy for dirty linens.
36. Removed your gloves. Decontaminated your hands.
37. Reported and recorded your observations.

Assisting with a Tub Bath or Shower

Name: _____ Date: _____

	S	**U**	**Comments**

Quality of Life

Remembered to:
- Knock before entering the person's room.
- Address the person by name.
- Introduce yourself by name and title.
- Explain the procedure to the person before beginning and during the procedure.
- Protect the person's rights during the procedure.
- Handle the person gently during the procedure.

Preprocedure

1. Followed *Delegation Guidelines:*
   a. *Bathing*
   b. *Tub Baths and Showers*
2. Saw *Promoting Safety and Comfort:*
   a. *Bathing*
   b. *Tub Baths and Showers*
3. Reserved the bathtub or shower.
4. Practiced hand hygiene.
5. Identified the person. Checked the identification (ID) bracelet against the assignment sheet. Also called the person by name.
6. Collected the following:
   a. Two washcloths and two bath towels
   b. Soap
   c. Bath thermometer (for tub bath)
   d. Clothing or sleepwear
   e. Grooming items as requested
   f. Robe and nonskid footwear
   g. Rubber bath mat if needed
   h. Disposable bath mat
   i. Gloves
   j. Wheelchair, shower chair, transfer bench, and so on as needed.

Procedure

7. Placed items in the tub or shower room. Used the space provided or a chair.
8. Cleaned and disinfected the tub or shower.
9. Placed a rubber bath mat in the tub or on the shower floor. Did not block the drain.
10. Placed the disposable bath mat on the floor in front of the tub or shower.
11. Placed the occupied sign on the door.
12. Returned to the person's room. Provided for privacy. Decontaminated your hands.
13. Helped the person sit on the side of the bed.
14. Helped the person put on a robe and nonskid footwear. Or the person left on clothing.
15. Assisted or transported the person to the tub room or shower.
16. Had the person sit on a chair if he or she walked to the tub or shower room.
17. Provided for privacy.
18. *For a tub bath*:
    a. Filled the tub halfway with warm water (usually 105°F [40.5°C]). Followed the care plan for water temperature.
    b. Measured water temperature. Used the bath thermometer or checked the digital display.

Procedure—cont'd	S	U	Comments

Procedure—cont'd

c. Asked the person to check the water temperature. Adjusted the water temperature if it was too hot or too cold. _____ _____ _____

19. *For a shower:*

   a. Turned on the shower. _____ _____ _____

   b. Adjusted water temperature and pressure. Checked the digital display. _____ _____ _____

   c. Asked the person to check the water temperature. Adjusted the water if it was too hot or too cold. _____ _____ _____

20. Helped the person undress and remove footwear. _____ _____ _____

21. Helped the person into the tub or shower. Positioned the shower chair and locked the wheels. _____ _____ _____

22. Asked the person about shampooing his or her hair. If yes, performed this before washing the body. After shampooing, covered the head with a towel to prevent chilling. _____ _____ _____

23. Assisted with washing as necessary. Wore gloves. _____ _____ _____

24. Asked the person to use the call light when done or when help was needed. Reminded the person that a tub bath lasts no longer than 20 minutes. _____ _____ _____

25. Placed a towel across the chair. _____ _____ _____

26. Left the room if the person could bathe alone. If not, stayed in the room or nearby. Removed the gloves and decontaminated your hands if you left the room. _____ _____ _____

27. Checked the person at least every 5 minutes. _____ _____ _____

28. Returned when the person signaled for you. Knocked before entering. Decontaminated your hands. _____ _____ _____

29. Turned off the shower or drained the tub. Covered the person while the tub drained. _____ _____ _____

30. Helped the person out of the shower or tub and onto the chair. _____ _____ _____

31. Helped the person dry off. Patted gently. Dried under the breasts, between skin folds, in the perineal area, and between the toes. _____ _____ _____

32. Assisted with lotion and other grooming items as needed. _____ _____ _____

33. Helped the person dress and put on footwear. _____ _____ _____

34. Helped the person return to the room. Provided for privacy. _____ _____ _____

35. Assisted the person to a chair or into bed. _____ _____ _____

36. Provided a back massage if the person returned to bed. _____ _____ _____

37. Assisted with hair care and other grooming needs. _____ _____ _____

Postprocedure

38. Provided for comfort. _____ _____ _____

39. Placed the call light within reach. _____ _____ _____

40. Raised or lowered bed rails. Followed the care plan. _____ _____ _____

41. Unscreened the person. _____ _____ _____

42. Completed a safety check of the room. _____ _____ _____

43. Cleaned and disinfected the tub or shower. Removed soiled linens. Wore gloves. _____ _____ _____

44. Discarded disposable items. Put the unoccupied sign on the door. Returned supplies to their proper place. _____ _____ _____

45. Followed center policy for dirty linens. _____ _____ _____

46. Removed the gloves. Decontaminated your hands. _____ _____ _____

47. Reported and recorded your observations. _____ _____ _____

Giving a Back Massage

Name: _____   Date: _____

	S	U	Comments

Quality of Life

Remembered to:
- Knock before entering the person's room.
- Address the person by name.
- Introduce yourself by name and title.
- Explain the procedure to the person before beginning and during the procedure.
- Protect the person's rights during the procedure.
- Handle the person gently during the procedure.

Preprocedure

1. Followed *Delegation Guidelines: The Back Massage*
   Saw *Promoting Safety and Comfort: The Back Massage*
2. Practiced hand hygiene.
3. Identified the person. Checked the identification (ID) bracelet against the assignment sheet. Also called the person by name.
4. Collected the following:
   a. Bath blanket
   b. Bath towel
   c. Lotion
5. Provided for privacy.
6. Raised the bed for body mechanics. Bed rails were up if used.

Procedure

7. Lowered the bed rail near you if up.
8. Positioned the person in the prone or side-lying position. The back was toward you.
9. Exposed the back, shoulders, upper arms, and buttocks. Covered the rest of the body with the bath blanket. Exposed the buttocks if person gave consent.
10. Laid the towel on the bed along the back (if the person was in the side-lying position).
11. Warmed the lotion.
12. Explained that the lotion may feel cool and wet.
13. Applied lotion to the lower back area.
14. Stroked up from the buttocks to the shoulders. Then stroked down over the upper arms. Stroked up the upper arms, across the shoulders, and down the back to the buttocks. Used firm strokes. Kept your hands in contact with the person's skin. If the person did not want the buttocks exposed, stroked down the back to the waist and up the back to the shoulders.
15. Repeated stroking up from the buttocks to the shoulders. Then stroked down over the upper arms. Stroked up the upper arms, across the shoulders, and down the back to the buttocks. Used firm strokes. Kept your hands in contact with the person's skin. Did not stroke down to the buttocks without permission. Continued this for at least 3 minutes.
16. Kneaded the back:
    a. Grasped the skin between your thumb and fingers.
    b. Kneaded half of the back. Started at the buttocks and moved up to the shoulder. Then kneaded down from the shoulder to the buttocks.
    c. Repeated on the other half of the back.
17. Applied lotion to bony areas. Used circular motions with the tips of your index and middle fingers. (Did not massage reddened bony areas.)

289

Procedure—cont'd	S	U	Comments
18. Used fast movements to stimulate. Used slow movements to relax the person.	——	——	————————
19. Stroked with long, firm movements to end the massage. Told the person you were finishing.	——	——	————————
20. Straightened and secured clothing or sleepwear.	——	——	————————
21. Covered the person. Removed the towel and bath blanket.	——	——	————————

Postprocedure

	S	U	Comments
22. Provided for comfort.	——	——	————————
23. Placed the call light within reach.	——	——	————————
24. Lowered the bed to its lowest position.	——	——	————————
25. Raised or lowered bed rails. Followed the care plan.	——	——	————————
26. Returned lotion to its proper place.	——	——	————————
27. Unscreened the person.	——	——	————————
28. Completed a safety check of the room.	——	——	————————
29. Followed center policy for dirty linens.	——	——	————————
30. Decontaminated your hands.	——	——	————————
31. Reported and recorded your observations.	——	——	————————

Giving Female Perineal Care (NATCEP)

Name: _____ Date: _____

	S	U	Comments

Quality of Life
Remembered to:
- Knock before entering the person's room.
- Address the person by name.
- Introduce yourself by name and title.
- Explain the procedure to the person before beginning and during the procedure.
- Protect the person's rights during the procedure.
- Handle the person gently during the procedure.

Preprocedure

1. Followed *Delegation Guidelines: Perineal Care*
   Saw *Promoting Safety and Comfort: Perineal Care*
2. Practiced hand hygiene.
3. Collected the following:
   a. Soap or other cleaning agents as directed
   b. At least four washcloths
   c. Bath towel
   d. Bath blanket
   e. Bath thermometer
   f. Wash basin
   g. Waterproof pad
   h. Gloves
   i. Paper towels
4. Covered the overbed table with paper towels. Arranged items on top of them.
5. Identified the person. Checked the identification (ID) bracelet against the assignment sheet. Also called her by name.
6. Provided for privacy.
7. Raised the bed for body mechanics. Bed rails were up if used.

Procedure

8. Lowered the bed rail near you if up.
9. Decontaminated your hands. Put on gloves.
10. Covered the person with a bath blanket. Moved top linens to the foot of the bed.
11. Positioned the person on her back.
12. Draped the person.
13. Raised the bed rail if used.
14. Filled the wash basin. Water temperature was 105°F–109°F (40.5°C–42.7°C) or followed the care plan for water temperature. Measured water temperature according to center policy.
15. Asked the person to check the water temperature. Adjusted the water temperature if it was too hot or too cold. Raised the bed rail before leaving the bedside. Lowered it when you returned.
16. Placed the basin on the overbed table.
17. Lowered the bed rail if up.
18. Helped the person flex her knees and spread her legs. Or helped her spread her legs as much as possible with the knees straight.
19. Placed a waterproof pad under her buttocks. Protected the person and dry linens from the wet or soiled incontinence product.
20. Folded the corner of the bath blanket between her legs onto her abdomen.

Procedure—cont'd	S	U	Comments
21. Wet the washcloths.	——	——	————
22. Squeezed out excess water from a washcloth. Made a mitted washcloth. Applied soap.	——	——	————
23. Separated the labia. Cleaned downward from front to back with one stroke.	——	——	————
24. Repeated steps a and b until the area was clean. Used a clean part of the washcloth for each stroke. Used more than one washcloth if needed.			
a. Squeezed out excess water from a washcloth. Made a mitted washcloth. Applied soap.	——	——	————
b. Separated the labia. Cleaned downward from front to back with one stroke.	——	——	————
25. Rinsed the perineum with a clean washcloth. Separated the labia. Stroked downward from front to back. Repeated as necessary. Used a clean part of the washcloth for each stroke. Used more than one washcloth if needed.	——	——	————
26. Patted the area dry with the towel. Dried from front to back.	——	——	————
27. Folded the blanket back between her legs.	——	——	————
28. Helped her lower her legs and turn onto her side away from you.	——	——	————
29. Applied soap to a mitted washcloth.	——	——	————
30. Cleaned the rectal area. Cleaned from the vagina to the anus with one stroke.	——	——	————
31. Repeated steps a and b until the area was clean. Used a clean part of the washcloth for each stroke. Used more than one washcloth if needed.			
a. Applied soap to a mitted washcloth.	——	——	————
b. Cleaned the rectal area. Cleaned from the vagina to the anus with one stroke.	——	——	————
32. Rinsed the rectal area with a washcloth. Stroked from the vagina to the anus. Repeated as necessary. Used a clean part of the washcloth for each stroke. Used more than one washcloth if needed.	——	——	————
33. Patted the area dry with the towel. Dried from front to back.	——	——	————
34. Removed any wet or soiled incontinence product. Removed the waterproof pad.	——	——	————
35. Removed and discarded the gloves. Decontaminated your hands. Put on clean gloves.	——	——	————
36. Provided clean and dry linens and incontinence products as needed.	——	——	————

Postprocedure

	S	U	Comments
37. Covered the person. Removed the bath blanket.	——	——	————
38. Provided for comfort.	——	——	————
39. Placed the call light within reach.	——	——	————
40. Lowered the bed to its lowest position.	——	——	————
41. Raised or lowered bed rails. Followed the care plan.	——	——	————
42. Emptied, cleaned, and dried the wash basin.	——	——	————
43. Returned the basin and supplies to their proper place.	——	——	————
44. Wiped off the overbed table with the paper towels. Discarded the paper towels.	——	——	————
45. Unscreened the person.	——	——	————
46. Completed a safety check of the room.	——	——	————
47. Followed center policy for dirty linens.	——	——	————
48. Removed the gloves. Decontaminated your hands.	——	——	————
49. Reported and recorded your observations.	——	——	————

Giving Male Perineal Care

Name: _____ Date: _____

	S	U	Comments
Quality of Life			

Remembered to:
- Knock before entering the person's room.
- Address the person by name.
- Introduce yourself by name and title.
- Explain the procedure to the person before beginning and during the procedure.
- Protect the person's rights during the procedure.
- Handle the person gently during the procedure.

Procedure

1. Followed steps 1–17 in *Giving Female Perineal Care*.
   a. Followed *Delegation Guidelines: Perineal Care*
      Saw *Promoting Safety and Comfort: Perineal Care*
   b. Practiced hand hygiene.
   c. Collected the following:
      i.   Soap or other cleaning agents as directed
      ii. At least four washcloths
      iii. Bath towel
      iv. Bath blanket
      v.   Bath thermometer
      vi. Wash basin
      vii. Waterproof pad
      viii. Gloves
      ix. Paper towels
   d. Covered the overbed table with paper towels. Arranged items on top of them.
   e. Identified the person. Checked the identification (ID) bracelet against the assignment sheet. Also called him by name.
   f. Provided for privacy.
   g. Raised the bed for body mechanics. Bed rails were up if used.
   h. Lowered the bed rail near you if up.
   i. Decontaminated your hands. Put on gloves.
   j. Covered the person with a bath blanket. Moved top linens to the foot of the bed.
   k. Positioned the person on his back.
   l. Draped the person.
   m. Raised the bed rail if used.
   n. Filled the wash basin. Water temperature was 105°F–109°F (40.5°C–42.7°C). Followed the care plan for water temperature. Measured water temperature according to center policy.
   o. Asked the person to check the water temperature. Adjusted the water temperature if it was too hot or too cold. Raised the bed rail before leaving bedside. Lowered it when you returned.
   p. Placed the basin on the overbed table.
   q. Lowered the bed rail if up.
2. Placed a waterproof pad under his buttocks. Protected the person and dry linens from the wet or soiled incontinence product.
3. Retracted the foreskin if the person was uncircumcised.
4. Grasped the penis.

Procedure—cont'd

	S	U	Comments

5. Cleaned the tip. Used a circular motion. Started at the meatus of the urethra and worked outward. Repeated as needed. Used a clean part of the washcloth each time. _____ _____ _____

6. Rinsed the area with another washcloth. _____ _____ _____

7. Returned the foreskin immediately after rinsing to its natural position. _____ _____ _____

8. Cleaned the shaft of the penis. Used firm downward strokes. Rinsed the area. _____ _____ _____

9. Helped the person flex his knees and spread his legs. Or helped him spread his legs as much as possible with his knees straight.

10. Cleaned the scrotum. Rinsed well. Observed for redness and irritation of the skin folds. _____ _____ _____

11. Patted dry the penis and the scrotum. Used the towel. _____ _____ _____

12. Folded the bath blanket back between his legs. _____ _____ _____

13. Helped the person lower his legs and turn onto his side away from you. _____ _____ _____

14. Cleaned the rectal area:

   a. Applied soap to a mitted washcloth. _____ _____ _____

   b. Cleaned from behind the scrotum to the anus with one stroke. _____ _____ _____

   c. Repeated until the area was clean. Used a clean part of the washcloth for each stroke. Used more than one washcloth if needed. _____ _____ _____

   d. Rinsed the rectal area with a washcloth. Stroked from the scrotum to the anus. Repeated as necessary. Used a clean part of the washcloth for each stroke. Used more than one washcloth if needed. _____ _____ _____

   e. Rinsed and dried well. Patted the area dry with the towel. Dried from front to back. _____ _____ _____

15. Removed any wet or soiled incontinence product. Removed the waterproof pad. _____ _____ _____

16. Removed and discarded the gloves. Decontaminated your hands. Put on clean gloves. _____ _____ _____

17. Provided clean and dry linens and incontinence products. _____ _____ _____

Postprocedure

18. Covered the person. Removed the bath blanket. _____ _____ _____

19. Provided for comfort. _____ _____ _____

20. Placed call light within reach. _____ _____ _____

21. Lowered the bed to its lowest position. _____ _____ _____

22. Raised or lowered bed rails. Followed the care plan. _____ _____ _____

23. Emptied, cleaned, and dried the wash basin. _____ _____ _____

24. Returned the basin and supplies to their proper place. _____ _____ _____

25. Wiped off the overbed table with the paper towels. Discarded the paper towels. _____ _____ _____

26. Unscreened the person. _____ _____ _____

27. Completed a safety check of the room. _____ _____ _____

28. Followed center policy for dirty linens. _____ _____ _____

29. Removed the gloves. Decontaminated your hands. _____ _____ _____

30. Reported and recorded your observations. _____ _____ _____

Brushing and Combing the Person's Hair

Name: _____ Date: _____

	S	U	Comments
Quality of Life			

Remembered to:
- Knock before entering the person's room.
- Address the person by name.
- Introduce yourself by name and title.
- Explain the procedure to the person before beginning and during the procedure.
- Protect the person's rights during the procedure.
- Handle the person gently during the procedure.

Preprocedure

1. Followed *Delegation Guidelines: Brushing and Combing Hair*
   Saw *Promoting Safety and Comfort: Brushing and Combing Hair*
2. Practiced hand hygiene.
3. Identified the person. Checked the identification (ID) bracelet against the assignment sheet. Also called the person by name.
4. Asked the person how to style hair.
5. Collected the following:
   a. Comb and brush
   b. Bath towel
   c. Other hair items as requested
6. Arranged items on the bedside stand.
7. Provided for privacy.

Procedure

8. Lowered the bed rail if up.
9. Helped the person to the chair. The person put on a robe and nonskid footwear while up. (If the person was in bed, raised the bed for body mechanics. Bed rails were up if used. Lowered the bed rail near you. Assisted the person to a semi-Fowler position if allowed.)
10. Placed a towel across the person's back and shoulders or across the pillow.
11. Asked the person to remove eyeglasses. Put them in the eyeglass case. Put the case inside the bedside stand.
12. *Brushed and combed hair that was not matted or tangled*:
    a. Used the comb to part the hair.
       i. Parted hair down the middle into two sides.
       ii. Divided one side into two smaller sections.
    b. Brushed one of the small sections of hair. Started at the scalp and brushed toward the hair ends. Did the same for the other small section of hair.
    c. Repeated for the other side:
       i. Divided other side into two smaller sections.
       ii. Brushed one of the small sections of hair. Started at the scalp and brushed toward the hair ends. Did the same for the other small section of hair.
13. *Brushed and combed matted and tangled hair*:
    a. Took a small section of hair near the ends.
    b. Combed or brushed through to the hair ends.
    c. Added small sections of hair as you worked up to the scalp.
    d. Combed or brushed through each longer section to the hair ends.
    e. Brushed or combed from the scalp to the hair ends.
14. Styled the hair as the person preferred.

295

Procedure—cont'd	S	U	Comments
15. Removed the towel.	———	———	———————
16. Let the person put on the eyeglasses.	———	———	———————

Postprocedure

	S	U	Comments
17. Provided for comfort.	———	———	———————
18. Placed the call light within reach.	———	———	———————
19. Lowered the bed to its lowest position.	———	———	———————
20. Raised or lowered bed rails. Followed the care plan.	———	———	———————
21. Cleaned and returned hair care items to their proper place.	———	———	———————
22. Unscreened the person.	———	———	———————
23. Completed a safety check of the room.	———	———	———————
24. Followed center policy for dirty linens.	———	———	———————
25. Decontaminated your hands.	———	———	———————

Shampooing the Person's Hair

Name: _____   Date: _____

Quality of Life	**S**	**U**	**Comments**

Remembered to:
- Knock before entering the person's room.
- Address the person by name.
- Introduce yourself by name and title.
- Explain the procedure to the person before beginning and during the procedure.
- Protect the person's rights during the procedure.
- Handle the person gently during the procedure.

Preprocedure

1. Followed *Delegation Guidelines: Shampooing*
   Saw *Promoting Safety and Comfort: Shampooing*
2. Practiced hand hygiene.
3. Collected the following:
   a. Two bath towels
   b. Washcloth
   c. Shampoo
   d. Hair conditioner (if requested)
   e. Bath thermometer
   f. Pitcher or handheld nozzle (if needed)
   g. Shampoo tray (if needed)
   h. Basin or pan (if needed)
   i. Waterproof pad (if needed)
   j. Gloves (if needed)
   k. Comb and brush
   l. Hair dryer
4. Arranged items nearby.
5. Identified the person. Checked the identification (ID) bracelet against the assignment sheet. Also called the person by name.
6. Provided for privacy.
7. Removed any hearing aids and eyeglasses.
8. Raised the bed for body mechanics for a shampoo in bed. Bed rails were up if used.
9. Decontaminated your hands.

Procedure

10. Lowered the bed rail near you if up.
11. Covered the person's chest with a bath towel.
12. Brushed and combed hair to remove snarls and tangles.
13. Positioned the person for the method you used. To shampoo the person in bed:
    a. Lowered the head of the bed and removed the pillow.
    b. Placed the waterproof pad and shampoo tray under the head and shoulders.
    c. Supported the head and neck with a folded towel if necessary.
14. Raised the bed rail if used.
15. Obtained water. Water temperature usually 105°F (40.5°C). Tested water temperature according to center policy. Also asked the person to check the water. Adjusted water temperature as needed. Raised the bed rail before leaving the bedside.
16. Lowered the bed rail near you if up.
17. Put on gloves (if needed).

297

Procedure—cont'd	S	U	Comments

18. Asked the person to hold a washcloth over the eyes. It did not cover the nose and mouth. (Note: A damp washcloth is easier to hold. It will not slip. However, some state competency tests require a dry washcloth.) _____ _____ _____
19. Used the pitcher or nozzle to wet the hair. _____ _____ _____
20. Applied a small amount of shampoo. _____ _____ _____
21. Worked up a lather with both hands. Started at the hairline. Worked toward the back of the head. _____ _____ _____
22. Massaged the scalp with your fingertips. Did not scratch the scalp. _____ _____ _____
23. Rinsed the hair until the water ran clear. _____ _____ _____
24. Repeated:
   a. Applied a small amount of shampoo. _____ _____ _____
   b. Worked up a lather with both hands. Started at the hairline. Worked toward the back of the head. _____ _____ _____
   c. Massaged the scalp with your fingertips. Did not scratch the scalp. _____ _____ _____
   d. Rinsed the hair until the water ran clear. _____ _____ _____
25. Applied conditioner according to the directions on the container. _____ _____ _____
26. Squeezed water from the person's hair. _____ _____ _____
27. Covered the hair with a bath towel. _____ _____ _____
28. Removed the shampoo tray, basin, and waterproof pad. _____ _____ _____
29. Dried the person's face with the towel. Used the towel on the person's chest. _____ _____ _____
30. Helped the person raise the head if appropriate. For the person in bed, raised the head of the bed. _____ _____ _____
31. If using a disposable shampoo cap:
   a. Combed hair to remove any tangles.
   b. Opened package, applied cap, tucked all hair in cap.
   c. Massaged head through cap, checked that cap was fitted properly.
   d. Massaged for 2–4 minutes or as directed on package.
   e. Removed cap and discarded in trash.
32. Rubbed the hair and scalp with the towel. Used the second towel if the first one was wet. _____ _____ _____
33. Combed the hair to remove snarls and tangles. _____ _____ _____
34. Dried and styled hair as quickly as possible. _____ _____ _____
35. Removed and discarded the gloves if used. Decontaminated your hands. _____ _____ _____

Postprocedure

36. Provided for comfort. _____ _____ _____
37. Assisted person to replace hearing aids and eyeglasses. _____ _____ _____
38. Placed the call light within reach. _____ _____ _____
39. Lowered the bed to its lowest position. _____ _____ _____
40. Raised or lowered bed rails. Followed the care plan. _____ _____ _____
41. Unscreened the person. _____ _____ _____
42. Completed a safety check of the room. _____ _____ _____
43. Cleaned, dried, and returned equipment to its proper place. Remembered to clean the brush and comb. Discarded disposable items. _____ _____ _____
44. Followed center policy for dirty linens. _____ _____ _____
45. Decontaminated your hands. _____ _____ _____
46. Reported and recorded your observations. _____ _____ _____

Shaving the Person's Face with a Safety Razor

Name: _____ Date: _____

	S	**U**	**Comments**

Quality of Life
Remembered to:
- Knock before entering the person's room.
- Address the person by name.
- Introduce yourself by name and title.
- Explain the procedure to the person before beginning and during the procedure.
- Protect the person's rights during the procedure.
- Handle the person gently during the procedure.

Preprocedure

1. Followed *Delegation Guidelines: Shaving*
   Saw *Promoting Safety and Comfort: Shaving*
2. Practiced hand hygiene.
3. Collected the following:
   a. Wash basin
   b. Bath towel
   c. Hand towel
   d. Washcloth
   e. Safety razor
   f. Mirror
   g. Shaving cream, soap, or lotion
   h. Shaving brush
   i. Aftershave or lotion
   j. Tissues
   k. Paper towels
   l. Gloves
4. Arranged paper towels and supplies on the overbed table.
5. Identified the person. Checked the identification (ID) bracelet against the assignment sheet. Also called the person by name.
6. Provided for privacy.
7. Raised the bed for body mechanics. Bed rails were up if used.

Procedure

8. Filled the wash basin with warm water.
9. Placed the basin on the overbed table.
10. Lowered the bed rail near you if up.
11. Decontaminated your hands. Put on gloves.
12. Assisted the person to semi-Fowler position if allowed or to the supine position.
13. Adjusted lighting to clearly see the person's face.
14. Placed the bath towel over the person's chest and shoulders.
15. Adjusted the overbed table for easy reach.
16. Tightened the razor blade to the shaver if necessary.
17. Washed the person's face. Did not dry.
18. Wet the washcloth or towel. Wrung it out.
19. Applied the washcloth or towel to the face for a few minutes.
20. Applied shaving cream with your hands or used a shaving brush to apply lather.
21. Held the skin taut with one hand.
22. Shaved in the direction of hair growth. Used shorter strokes around the chin and lips.
23. Rinsed the razor often. Wiped it with tissues or paper towels.
24. Applied direct pressure to any bleeding areas.
25. Washed off any remaining shaving cream or soap. Patted dry with a towel.

299

Procedure—cont'd	S	U	Comments
26. Applied aftershave or lotion if requested. Did not apply aftershave or lotion if there were nicks or cuts.	⎯⎯	⎯⎯	⎯⎯⎯⎯⎯
27. Removed the towel and gloves. Decontaminated your hands.	⎯⎯	⎯⎯	⎯⎯⎯⎯⎯

Postprocedure

	S	U	Comments
28. Provided for comfort.	⎯⎯	⎯⎯	⎯⎯⎯⎯⎯
29. Placed the call light within reach.	⎯⎯	⎯⎯	⎯⎯⎯⎯⎯
30. Lowered the bed to its lowest position.	⎯⎯	⎯⎯	⎯⎯⎯⎯⎯
31. Raised or lowered bed rails. Followed the care plan.	⎯⎯	⎯⎯	⎯⎯⎯⎯⎯
32. Cleaned and returned equipment and supplies to their proper place. Discarded razor blade or disposable razor into the sharps container. Discarded other disposable items. Wore gloves.	⎯⎯	⎯⎯	⎯⎯⎯⎯⎯
33. Wiped off the overbed table with paper towels. Discarded the paper towels.	⎯⎯	⎯⎯	⎯⎯⎯⎯⎯
34. Unscreened the person.	⎯⎯	⎯⎯	⎯⎯⎯⎯⎯
35. Completed a safety check of the room.	⎯⎯	⎯⎯	⎯⎯⎯⎯⎯
36. Followed center policy for dirty linens.	⎯⎯	⎯⎯	⎯⎯⎯⎯⎯
37. Removed the gloves. Decontaminated your hands.	⎯⎯	⎯⎯	⎯⎯⎯⎯⎯
38. Reported nicks, cuts, irritation, or bleeding to the nurse at once. Also reported and recorded other observations.	⎯⎯	⎯⎯	⎯⎯⎯⎯⎯

Shaving the Person's Face with an Electric Razor

Name: _____   Date: _____

	S	U	Comments
Quality of Life			

Quality of Life

Remembered to:
- Knock before entering the person's room.
- Address the person by name.
- Introduce yourself by name and title.
- Explain the procedure to the person before beginning and during the procedure.
- Protect the person's rights during the procedure.
- Handle the person gently during the procedure.

Preprocedure

1. Followed *Delegation Guidelines: Shaving*
   Saw *Promoting Safety and Comfort: Shaving*
2. Practiced hand hygiene.
3. Collected the following:
   a. Wash basin
   b. Bath towel
   c. Hand towel
   d. Washcloth
   e. Person's own electric razor
   f. Mirror
   g. Soap
   h. Pre-shave or aftershave lotion
   i. Tissues
   j. Paper towels
   k. Gloves
4. Arranged paper towels and supplies on the overbed table.
5. Identified the person. Checked the identification (ID) bracelet against the assignment sheet. Also called the person by name.
6. Provided for privacy.
7. If worn, dentures were in person's mouth.
8. Did not use electric shaver if person was using oxygen. (Note: Could use shaver on battery power if the shaver has that option.)
9. Raised the bed for body mechanics. Bed rails were up if used.

Procedure

10. Filled the wash basin with warm water.
11. Placed the basin on the overbed table.
12. Lowered the bed rail near you if up.
13. Decontaminated your hands. Put on gloves.
14. Assisted the person to semi-Fowler position if allowed or to the supine position.
15. Adjusted lighting to clearly see the person's face.
16. Placed the bath towel over the person's chest and shoulders.
17. Adjusted the overbed table for easy reach.
18. Washed the person's face and rinsed. The beard may have been softened by leaving a moist, warm washcloth or towel in place for a few minutes. Patted dry.
19. Applied pre-shave lotion or talcum powder, if desired.
20. For a rotary-type shaver, held the skin taut with one hand as you shaved in circular motions. For a straight-type electric shaver, gently pressed the shaving edge against the skin and shaved against the direction of the hair growth. (NOTE: Your state and agency may require shaving in the direction of hair growth. Follow the manufacturer's instructions and the rules in your state and agency.)

Procedure—cont'd	S	U	Comments
21. Shaved the cheek area first, then around the mouth.	___	___	_____
22. Shaved the neck area last. Had the person tilt head back if able.	___	___	_____
23. Applied direct pressure to any bleeding areas.	___	___	_____
24. Applied aftershave lotion if requested. (Did not apply aftershave lotion if there were nicks or cuts.)	___	___	_____
25. Removed the towel and gloves. Decontaminated your hands.	___	___	_____

Postprocedure

	S	U	Comments
26. Provided for comfort.	___	___	_____
27. Placed the call light within reach.	___	___	_____
28. Lowered the bed to its lowest position.	___	___	_____
29. Raised or lowered bed rails. Followed the care plan.	___	___	_____
30. Cleaned equipment and put in proper place. Cleaned shaver by removing head and using a soft brush to remove the whiskers. Wiped off head of shaver with alcohol prep. Put shaver back in case.	___	___	_____
31. Wiped off the overbed table with paper towels. Discarded the paper towels.	___	___	_____
32. Unscreened the person.	___	___	_____
33. Completed a safety check of the room.	___	___	_____
34. Followed center policy for dirty linens.	___	___	_____
35. Removed the gloves. Decontaminated your hands.	___	___	_____
36. Reported nicks, cuts, irritation, or bleeding to the nurse at once. Also reported and recorded other observations.	___	___	_____

Giving Nail and Foot Care (NATCEP)

Name: _____   Date: _____

	S	U	Comments
Quality of Life			

Remembered to:
- Knock before entering the person's room.
- Address the person by name.
- Introduce yourself by name and title.
- Explain the procedure to the person before beginning and during the procedure.
- Protect the person's rights during the procedure.
- Handle the person gently during the procedure.

Preprocedure

1. Followed *Delegation Guidelines: Nail and Foot Care*
   Saw *Promoting Safety and Comfort: Nail and Foot Care*
2. Practiced hand hygiene.
3. Collected the following:
   a. Wash basin or whirlpool foot bath
   b. Soap
   c. Bath thermometer
   d. Bath towel
   e. Hand towel
   f. Washcloth
   g. Kidney basin
   h. Nail clippers
   i. Orangewood stick
   j. Emery board or nail file
   k. Lotion for the hands
   l. Lotion or petroleum jelly for the feet
   m. Paper towels
   n. Bath mat
   o. Gloves
4. Arranged paper towels and other items on the overbed table.
5. Identified the person. Checked the identification (ID) bracelet against the assignment sheet. Also called the person by name.
6. Provided for privacy.
7. Assisted the person to the bedside chair. Placed the call light within reach.

Procedure

8. Placed the bath mat under the feet.
9. Filled the wash basin or whirlpool foot bath ⅔ (two-thirds) full with water. The nurse told you what water temperature to use. (Measured water temperature with a bath thermometer. Or tested it by dipping your elbow or inner wrist into the basin. Followed center policy.) Also asked the person to check the water temperature. Adjusted the water temperature as needed.
10. Placed the basin or foot bath on the bath mat.
11. Put on gloves.
12. Helped the person put the feet into the basin or foot bath. Made sure both feet were completely covered by water.
13. Adjusted the overbed table in front of the person.
14. Filled the kidney basin ⅔ (two-thirds) full with water. The nurse told you what water temperature to use. (Measured water temperature with a bath thermometer. Or tested it by dipping your elbow or inner wrist into the basin. Followed center policy.) Also asked the person to check the water temperature. Adjusted the water temperature as needed.
15. Placed the kidney basin on the overbed table.

303

Procedure—cont'd   S   U   Comments

16. Placed the person's fingers into the basin. Positioned the arms for comfort. ____ ____ _____
17. Let the fingers soak for 5–10 minutes. Let the feet soak for 15–20 minutes. Rewarmed water as needed. ____ ____ _____
18. Removed the kidney basin. ____ ____ _____
19. Cleaned under the fingernails with the flat end of the orangewood stick. Used a towel to wipe the orangewood stick after each nail. ____ ____ _____
20. Dried the hands and between the fingers thoroughly. ____ ____ _____
21. Clipped fingernails straight across with the nail clippers. (Followed center policy.) ____ ____ _____
22. Shaped nails with an emery board or nail file. Nails were smooth with no rough edges. Checked each nail for smoothness. Filed as needed. ____ ____ _____
23. Gently pushed cuticles back with the orangewood stick or a washcloth. (Followed center policy.) ____ ____ _____
24. Applied lotion to the hands. Warmed the lotion before applying it. ____ ____ _____
25. Moved the overbed table to the side. ____ ____ _____
26. Lifted a foot out of the water. Supported the foot and ankle with one hand. With the other hand, washed the foot and between the toes with soap and a washcloth. Returned the foot to the water for rinsing. Rinsed between the toes. ____ ____ _____
27. Repeated for the other foot: Lifted the other foot out of the water. Supported the foot and ankle with one hand. With the other hand, washed the foot and between the toes with soap and a washcloth. Returned the foot to the water for rinsing. Rinsed between the toes. ____ ____ _____
28. Removed the feet from the basin or foot bath. Dried thoroughly, especially between the toes. ____ ____ _____
29. Applied lotion or petroleum jelly to the tops and soles of the feet. Did not apply between the toes. Warmed lotion or petroleum jelly before applying it. Removed excess lotion or petroleum jelly with a towel. ____ ____ _____
30. Removed and discarded the gloves. Decontaminated your hands. ____ ____ _____
31. Assisted the person to put on stockings. ____ ____ _____
32. Helped the person put on nonskid footwear. ____ ____ _____

Postprocedure

33. Provided for comfort. ____ ____ _____
34. Placed the call light within reach. ____ ____ _____
35. Raised or lowered bed rails. Followed the care plan. ____ ____ _____
36. Cleaned, dried, and returned equipment and supplies to their proper place. Discarded disposable items. Wore gloves for this step. ____ ____ _____
37. Unscreened the person. ____ ____ _____
38. Completed a safety check of the room. ____ ____ _____
39. Followed center policy for dirty linens. ____ ____ _____
40. Removed the gloves. Decontaminated your hands. ____ ____ _____
41. Reported and recorded your observations. ____ ____ _____

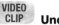

Name: _____   Date: _____

	S	U	Comments

Quality of Life

Remembered to:
- Knock before entering the person's room.
- Address the person by name.
- Introduce yourself by name and title.
- Explain the procedure to the person before beginning and during the procedure.
- Protect the person's rights during the procedure.
- Handle the person gently during the procedure.

Preprocedure

1. Followed *Delegation Guidelines: Dressing and Undressing*
2. Practiced hand hygiene.
3. Collected a bath blanket and clothing requested by the person.
4. Identified the person. Checked the identification (ID) bracelet against the assignment sheet. Also called the person by name.
5. Provided for privacy.
6. Raised the bed for body mechanics. Bed rails were up if used.
7. Lowered the bed rail on the person's weak side.
8. Positioned the person supine.
9. Covered the person with a bath blanket. Fan-folded linens to the foot of the bed.

Procedure

10. Removed garments that opened in the back:
    a. Raised the head and shoulders. Or turned the person onto the side away from you.
    b. Undid buttons, zippers, ties, or snaps.
    c. Brought the sides of the garment to the sides of the person. If he or she was in a side-lying position, tucked the far side under the person. Folded the near side onto the chest.
    d. Positioned the person supine.
    e. Slid the garment off the shoulder on the strong side. Removed it from the arm.
    f. Removed the garment from the weak side.
11. Removed garments that opened in the front:
    a. Undid buttons, zippers, ties, or snaps.
    b. Slid the garment off the shoulder and arm on the strong side.
    c. Assisted the person to sit up or raised the head and shoulders. Brought the garment over to the weak side.
    d. Lowered the head and shoulders. Removed the garment from the weak side.
    e. If you could not raise the head and shoulders:
        i. Turned the person toward you. Tucked the removed part under the person.
        ii. Turned him or her onto the side away from you.
        iii. Pulled the side of the garment out from under the person. Made sure he or she was not lying on it when supine.
        iv. Returned the person to the supine position.
        v. Removed the garment from the weak side.
12. Removed pullover garments:
    a. Undid any buttons, zippers, ties, or snaps.

305

Procedure—cont'd   S   U   **Comments**

    b. Removed the garment from the strong side. ____ ____ _____
    c. Raised the head and shoulders. Or turned the person onto the side
       away from you. Brought the garment up to the person's neck. ____ ____ _____
    d. Removed the garment from the weak side. ____ ____ _____
    e. Brought the garment over the person's head. ____ ____ _____
    f. Positioned him or her in the supine position. ____ ____ _____
13. Removed pants or slacks:
    a. Removed footwear and socks. ____ ____ _____
    b. Positioned the person supine. ____ ____ _____
    c. Undid buttons, zippers, ties, snaps, or buckles. ____ ____ _____
    d. Removed the belt. ____ ____ _____
    e. Asked the person to lift the buttocks off the bed. Slid the pants
       down over the hips and buttocks. Had the person lower the hips and
       buttocks. ____ ____ _____
    f. If the person could not raise the hips off the bed:
      i. Turned the person toward you. ____ ____ _____
      ii. Slid the pants off the hip and buttock on the strong side. ____ ____ _____
      iii. Turned the person away from you. ____ ____ _____
      iv. Slid the pants off the hip and buttock on the weak side. ____ ____ _____
    g. Slid the pants down the legs and over the feet. ____ ____ _____
14. Dressed the person. ____ ____ _____

Postprocedure

15. Provided for comfort. ____ ____ _____
16. Placed the call light within reach. ____ ____ _____
17. Lowered the bed to its lowest position. ____ ____ _____
18. Raised or lowered bed rails. Followed the care plan. ____ ____ _____
19. Unscreened the person. ____ ____ _____
20. Completed a safety check of the room. ____ ____ _____
21. Followed center policy for soiled clothing. ____ ____ _____
22. Decontaminated your hands. ____ ____ _____
23. Reported and recorded your observations. ____ ____ _____

Dressing the Person (NATCEP)

Name: _____   Date: _____

	S	U	Comments
Quality of Life			
Remembered to:			
• Knock before entering the person's room.	___	___	_____
• Address the person by name.	___	___	_____
• Introduce yourself by name and title.	___	___	_____
• Explain the procedure to the person before beginning and during the procedure.	___	___	_____
• Protect the person's rights during the procedure.	___	___	_____
• Handle the person gently during the procedure.	___	___	_____
Preprocedure			
1. Followed *Delegation Guidelines: Dressing and Undressing*	___	___	_____
2. Practiced hand hygiene.	___	___	_____
3. Asked the person what he or she would like to wear.	___	___	_____
4. Got a bath blanket and clothing requested by the person.	___	___	_____
5. Identified the person. Checked the identification (ID) bracelet against the assignment sheet. Also called the person by name.	___	___	_____
6. Provided for privacy.	___	___	_____
7. Raised the bed for body mechanics. Bed rails were up if used.	___	___	_____
8. Lowered the bed rail (if up) on the person's strong side.	___	___	_____
9. Positioned the person supine.	___	___	_____
10. Covered the person with a bath blanket. Fan-folded linens to the foot of the bed.	___	___	_____
11. Undressed the person.	___	___	_____
Procedure			
12. Put on garments that opened in the back:			
a. Slid the garment onto the arm and shoulder of the weak side.	___	___	_____
b. Slid the garment onto the arm and shoulder of the strong side.	___	___	_____
c. Raised the person's head and shoulders.	___	___	_____
d. Brought the sides to the back.	___	___	_____
e. If you could not raise the person's head and shoulders:			
i. Turned the person toward you.	___	___	_____
ii. Brought one side of the garment to the person's back.	___	___	_____
iii. Turned the person away from you.	___	___	_____
iv. Brought the other side to the person's back.	___	___	_____
f. Fastened buttons, snaps, zippers, or other closures.	___	___	_____
g. Positioned the person supine.	___	___	_____
13. Put on garments that opened in the front:			
a. Slid the garment onto the arm and shoulder on the weak side.	___	___	_____
b. Raised the head and shoulders. Brought the side of the garment around to the back. Lowered the person down. Slid the garment onto the arm and shoulder of the strong arm.	___	___	_____
c. If the person could not raise the head and shoulders:			
i. Turned the person away from you.	___	___	_____
ii. Tucked the garment under the person.	___	___	_____
iii. Turned the person toward you.	___	___	_____
iv. Pulled the garment out from under the person.	___	___	_____
v. Turned the person back to the supine position.	___	___	_____
vi. Slid the garment over the arm and shoulder of the strong arm.	___	___	_____
d. Fastened buttons, ties, snaps, zippers, or other closures.	___	___	_____

Procedure—cont'd   S   U   **Comments**

14. Put on pullover garments:
    a. Positioned the person supine.   _____   _____   _____
    b. Brought the neck of the garment over the head.   _____   _____   _____
    c. Slid the arm and shoulder of the garment onto the weak side.   _____   _____   _____
    d. Raised the person's head and shoulders.   _____   _____   _____
    e. Brought the garment down.   _____   _____   _____
    f. Slid the arm and shoulder of the garment onto the strong side.   _____   _____   _____
    g. If the person could not assume a semi-sitting position:
        i. Turned the person away from you.   _____   _____   _____
        ii. Tucked the garment under the person.   _____   _____   _____
        iii. Turned the person toward you.   _____   _____   _____
        iv. Pulled the garment out from under the person.   _____   _____   _____
        v. Positioned the person supine.   _____   _____   _____
        vi. Slid the arm and shoulder of the garment onto the strong side.   _____   _____   _____
    h. Fastened buttons, ties, snaps, zippers, or other closures.   _____   _____   _____

15. Put on pants or slacks:
    a. Slid the pants over the feet and up the legs.   _____   _____   _____
    b. Asked the person to raise the hips and buttocks off the bed.   _____   _____   _____
    c. Brought the pants up over the buttocks and hips.   _____   _____   _____
    d. Asked the person to lower the hips and buttocks.   _____   _____   _____
    e. If the person could not raise the hips and buttocks:
        i. Turned the person onto the strong side.   _____   _____   _____
        ii. Pulled the pants over the buttock and hip on the weak side.   _____   _____   _____
        iii. Turned the person onto the weak side.   _____   _____   _____
        iv. Pulled the pants over the buttock and hip on the strong side.   _____   _____   _____
        v. Positioned the person supine.   _____   _____   _____
    f. Fastened buttons, ties, snaps, zippers, belt buckle, or other closures.   _____   _____   _____

16. Put socks and nonskid footwear on the person. Made sure socks were up all the way and smooth.   _____   _____   _____

17. Helped the person get out of bed. If the person stayed in bed, covered the person. Removed the bath blanket.   _____   _____   _____

Postprocedure

18. Provided for comfort.   _____   _____   _____
19. Placed the call light within reach.   _____   _____   _____
20. Lowered the bed to its lowest position.   _____   _____   _____
21. Raised or lowered bed rails. Followed the care plan. _____   _____   _____
22. Unscreened the person.   _____   _____   _____
23. Completed a safety check of the room.   _____   _____   _____
24. Followed center policy for soiled clothing.   _____   _____   _____
25. Decontaminated your hands.   _____   _____   _____
26. Reported and recorded your observations.   _____   _____   _____

Changing the Gown of the Person with an IV

Name: _____   Date: _____

	S	U	Comments
Quality of Life			

Remembered to:
- Knock before entering the person's room.
- Address the person by name.
- Introduce yourself by name and title.
- Explain the procedure to the person before beginning and during the procedure.
- Protect the person's rights during the procedure.
- Handle the person gently during the procedure.

Preprocedure

1. Followed *Delegation Guidelines: Changing Hospital Gowns*
   Saw *Promoting Safety and Comfort: Changing Hospital Gowns*
2. Practiced hand hygiene.
3. Got a clean gown and a bath blanket.
4. Identified the person. Checked the identification (ID) bracelet against the assignment sheet. Also called the person by name.
5. Provided for privacy.
6. Raised the bed for body mechanics. Bed rails were up if used.

Procedure

7. Lowered the bed rail near you (if up).
8. Covered the person with a bath blanket. Fan-folded linens to the foot of the bed.
9. Untied the gown. Freed parts the person was lying on.
10. Removed the gown from the arm with *no IV*.
11. Gathered up the sleeve of the arm *with the IV*. Slid it over the IV site and tubing. Removed the arm and hand from the sleeve.
12. Kept the sleeve gathered. Slid your arm along the tubing to the bag.
13. Removed the bag from the pole. Slid the bag and tubing through the sleeve. Did not pull on the tubing. Kept the bag above the person.
14. Hung the IV bag on the pole.
15. Gathered the sleeve of the clean gown that went on the arm with the IV infusion.
16. Removed the bag from the pole. Slipped the sleeve over the bag at the shoulder part of the gown. Hung the bag.
17. Slid the gathered sleeve over the tubing, hand, arm, and IV site. Then slid it onto the shoulder.
18. Put the other side of the gown on the person. Fastened the gown.
19. Covered the person. Removed the bath blanket.

Postprocedure

20. Provided for comfort.
21. Placed the call light within reach.
22. Lowered the bed to its lowest position.
23. Raised or lowered bed rails. Followed the care plan.
24. Unscreened the person.
25. Completed a safety check of the room.
26. Followed center policy for dirty linen.
27. Decontaminated your hands.
28. Asked the nurse to check the flow rate.
29. Reported and recorded your observations.

Measuring Intake and Output (NATCEP)

Name: _____   Date: _____

Quality of Life	S	U	Comments
Remembered to:			
• Knock before entering the person's room.	___	___	_____
• Address the person by name.	___	___	_____
• Introduce yourself by name and title.	___	___	_____
• Explain the procedure to the person before beginning and during the procedure.	___	___	_____
• Protect the person's rights during the procedure.	___	___	_____
• Handle the person gently during the procedure.	___	___	_____

Preprocedure

	S	U	Comments
1. Followed *Delegation Guidelines: Intake and Output*	___	___	_____
Saw *Promoting Safety and Comfort: Intake and Output*	___	___	_____
2. Practiced hand hygiene.	___	___	_____
3. Collected the following:			
a. Intake and output (I&O) record	___	___	_____
b. Graduates	___	___	_____
c. Gloves	___	___	_____

Procedure

	S	U	Comments
4. Put on gloves.	___	___	_____
5. Measured intake as follows:			
a. Poured liquid remaining in the container into the graduate.	___	___	_____
b. Measured the amount at eye level or on a flat surface. Kept the container level.	___	___	_____
c. Checked the serving amount on the I&O record.	___	___	_____
d. Subtracted the remaining amount from the full serving amount. Noted the amount.	___	___	_____
e. Poured fluid in the graduate back into the container.	___	___	_____
f. Repeated steps for each liquid:			
i. Poured liquid remaining in the container into the graduate.	___	___	_____
ii. Measured the amount at eye level or on a flat surface. Kept the container level.	___	___	_____
iii. Checked the serving amount on the I&O record.	___	___	_____
iv. Subtracted the remaining amount from the full serving amount. Noted the amount.	___	___	_____
v. Poured fluid in the graduate back into the container.	___	___	_____
g. Added the amounts from each liquid together.	___	___	_____
h. Recorded the time and amount on the I&O record.	___	___	_____
6. Measured output as follows:			
a. Poured fluid into the graduate used to measure output.	___	___	_____
b. Measured the amount at eye level or on a flat surface. Kept the container level.	___	___	_____
c. Disposed of fluid in the toilet. Avoided splashes.	___	___	_____
7. Cleaned and rinsed the graduates. Disposed of rinse into the toilet. Returned the graduates to their proper place.	___	___	_____
8. Cleaned and rinsed the voiding receptacle or drainage container. Disposed of rinse in the toilet. Returned item to its proper place.	___	___	_____
9. Removed the gloves. Practiced hand hygiene.	___	___	_____
10. Recorded the output on the I&O record.	___	___	_____

Postprocedure

	S	U	Comments
11. Provided for comfort.	___	___	_____
12. Made sure the call light was within reach.	___	___	_____
13. Completed a safety check of the room.	___	___	_____
14. Reported and recorded your observations.	___	___	_____

Preparing the Person for a Meal

Name: _____ Date: _____

	S	U	Comments
Quality of Life			
Remembered to:			
• Knock before entering the person's room.	___	___	_____
• Address the person by name.	___	___	_____
• Introduce yourself by name and title.	___	___	_____
• Explain the procedure to the person before beginning and during the procedure.	___	___	_____
• Protect the person's rights during the procedure.	___	___	_____
• Handle the person gently during the procedure.	___	___	_____
Preprocedure			
1. Followed *Delegation Guidelines: Preparing for Meals*	___	___	_____
Saw *Promoting Safety and Comfort: Preparing for Meals*	___	___	_____
2. Practiced hand hygiene.	___	___	_____
3. Collected the following:			
a. Equipment for oral hygiene	___	___	_____
b. Bedpan and cover, urinal, commode, or specimen pan	___	___	_____
c. Toilet tissue	___	___	_____
d. Wash basin	___	___	_____
e. Soap	___	___	_____
f. Washcloth	___	___	_____
g. Towel	___	___	_____
h. Gloves	___	___	_____
4. Provided for privacy.	___	___	_____
Procedure			
5. Made sure eyeglasses and hearing aids were in place.	___	___	_____
6. Assisted with oral hygiene. Made sure dentures were in place. Wore gloves and decontaminated your hands after removing them.	___	___	_____
7. Assisted with elimination. Made sure the incontinent person was clean and dry. Wore gloves and practiced hand hygiene after removing them.	___	___	_____
8. Assisted with hand washing. Wore gloves and practiced hand hygiene after removing them.	___	___	_____
9. Did the following if the person ate in bed:			
a. Raised the head of the bed to a comfortable position. (Fowler position preferred.)	___	___	_____
b. Removed items from the overbed table. Cleaned the overbed table.	___	___	_____
c. Adjusted the overbed table in front of the person.	___	___	_____
10. Did the following if the person was sitting in a chair:			
a. Positioned the person in a chair or wheelchair.	___	___	_____
b. Removed items from the overbed table. Cleaned the overbed table.	___	___	_____
c. Adjusted the overbed table in front of the person.	___	___	_____
11. Assisted the person to the dining area, if person ate in dining area.	___	___	_____
Postprocedure			
12. Provided for comfort.	___	___	_____
13. Placed the call light within reach.	___	___	_____
14. Emptied, cleaned, and disinfected equipment. Returned equipment to its proper place. Wore gloves and practiced hand hygiene after removing them.	___	___	_____
15. Straightened the room. Eliminated unpleasant noises, odors, or equipment.	___	___	_____
16. Unscreened the person.	___	___	_____
17. Completed a safety check of the room.	___	___	_____
18. Decontaminated your hands.	___	___	_____

VIDEO CLIP **Serving Meal Trays**

Name: _____   Date: _____

	S	**U**	**Comments**

Quality of Life

Remembered to:
- Knock before entering the person's room.
- Address the person by name.
- Introduce yourself by name and title.
- Explain the procedure to the person before beginning and during the procedure.
- Protect the person's rights during the procedure.
- Handle the person gently during the procedure.

Preprocedure

1. Followed *Delegation Guidelines: Serving Meal Trays*
   Saw *Promoting Safety and Comfort: Serving Meal Trays*
2. Practiced hand hygiene.

Procedure

3. Made sure the tray was complete. Checked items on the tray with the dietary card. Was aware of any allergies. Made sure assist devices were included.
4. Identified the person. Checked the identification (ID) bracelet against the dietary card. Also called person by name.
5. Placed the tray within the person's reach. Adjusted the overbed table as needed.
6. Removed food covers. Opened cartons, cut food into bite-sized pieces, buttered bread, and so on as needed. Seasoned food as person preferred and as allowed on the care plan.
7. Placed the napkin, clothes protector, assist devices, and eating utensils within reach.
8. Placed the call light within reach.
9. Did the following when the person was done eating:
   a. Measured and recorded intake if ordered.
   b. Noted the amount and type of foods eaten.
   c. Checked for and removed any food in the person's mouth (pocketing). Wore gloves. Decontaminated your hands after removing gloves.
   d. Removed the tray.
   e. Cleaned spills. Changed soiled linens and clothing.
   f. Helped the person return to bed if needed.
   g. Assisted with oral hygiene and hand washing. Wore gloves. Decontaminated your hands after removing the gloves.

Postprocedure

10. Provided for comfort.
11. Placed the call light within reach.
12. Raised or lowered bed rails. Followed the care plan.
13. Completed a safety check of the room.
14. Followed center policy for soiled linen.
15. Decontaminated your hands.
16. Reported and recorded your observations.

Feeding the Person

Name: _____ Date: _____

Quality of Life	**S**	**U**	**Comments**

Remembered to:
- Knock before entering the person's room.
- Address the person by name.
- Introduce yourself by name and title.
- Explain the procedure to the person before beginning and during the procedure.
- Protect the person's rights during the procedure.
- Handle the person gently during the procedure.

Preprocedure

1. Followed *Delegation Guidelines: Feeding the Person*
   Saw *Promoting Safety and Comfort: Feeding the Person*
2. Practiced hand hygiene.
3. Positioned the person in a comfortable position for eating (usually sitting or Fowler).
4. Got the tray. Placed it on the overbed table or dining table.

Procedure

5. Identified the person. Checked the identification (ID) bracelet against the dietary card. Also called the person by name.
6. Draped a napkin or clothes protector across the person's chest and underneath the chin. Always referred to this as a napkin or clothes protector, not a "bib," to protect the person's dignity.
7. Told the person what foods and fluids were on the tray.
8. Prepared food for eating. Cut food into bite-sized pieces. Seasoned foods as the person preferred and was allowed on the care plan.
9. Placed a chair where you could sit comfortably. Sat facing the person.
10. Served foods in the order the person preferred. Identified foods as you served them. If the person had a dry mouth, began by offering a drink of water. Then alternated between solid and liquid foods. Used a spoon for safety. Allowed enough time for chewing and swallowing. Did not rush the person. Also offered water, coffee, tea, or other beverage on the tray.
11. Checked the person's mouth before offering more food or fluids. Made sure the person's mouth was empty between bites and swallows.
12. Used straws for liquids if person could not drink out of a glass or cup. Had one straw for each liquid. Provided short straws for weak persons.
13. Wiped the person's hands, face, and mouth as needed during the meal. Used the napkin.
14. Followed the care plan if the person had dysphagia (checked if person could use a straw). Gave thickened liquids with a spoon.
15. Conversed with the person in a pleasant manner.
16. Encouraged the person to eat as much as possible.
17. Wiped the person's mouth with a napkin. Discarded the napkin.
18. Noted how much and which foods were eaten.
19. Measured and recorded intake if ordered.
20. Removed the tray.
21. Took the person back to his or her room, if in dining area.

Procedure—cont'd	S	U	Comments
22. Assisted with oral hygiene and hand washing. Wore gloves. Provided for privacy. Decontaminated your hands after removing the gloves.	___	___	

Postprocedure

	S	U	Comments
23. Provided for comfort.	___	___	_____
24. Placed the call light within reach.	___	___	_____
25. Raised or lowered bed rails. Followed the care plan.	___	___	_____
26. Completed a safety check of the room.	___	___	_____
27. Returned the food tray to the food cart.	___	___	_____
28. Decontaminated your hands.	___	___	_____
29. Reported and recorded your observations.	___	___	_____

Providing Drinking Water

Name: _____   Date: _____

	S	U	Comments
Quality of Life			

Remembered to:
- Knock before entering the person's room.
- Address the person by name.
- Introduce yourself by name and title.
- Explain the procedure to the person before beginning and during the procedure.
- Protect the person's rights during the procedure.
- Handle the person gently during the procedure.

Preprocedure

1. Followed *Delegation Guidelines: Providing Drinking Water* Saw *Promoting Safety and Comfort: Providing Drinking Water*
2. Obtained a list of persons who have special fluid orders from the nurse. Or used your assignment sheet.
3. Practiced hand hygiene.
4. Collected the following:
   a. Cart
   b. Ice chest filled with ice
   c. Cover for ice chest
   d. Scoop
   e. Water cups
   f. Straws
   g. Paper towels
   h. Water pitchers for resident use
   i. Large water pitcher filled with cold water (optional, depending on center procedure)
   j. Towel for the scoop
5. Covered the cart with paper towels. Arranged equipment on top of the paper towels.

Procedure

6. Took the cart to the person's room door. Did not take the cart into the room.
7. Checked the person's fluid orders. Used the list from the nurse.
8. Identified the person. Checked the identification (ID) bracelet against the fluid orders sheet or your assignment sheet. Also called the person by name.
9. Took the pitcher from the person's overbed table. Emptied it into the bathroom sink.
10. Determined if a new water pitcher was needed.
11. Used the scoop to fill the pitcher with ice. Did not let the scoop touch the rim or inside of the pitcher. Did not place the person's pitcher on the cart.
12. Placed the ice scoop on the towel.
13. Filled the water pitcher with water. Got water from the bathroom or used the larger water pitcher on the cart.
14. Placed the pitcher, cup, and straw (if used) on the overbed table. Filled the cup with water. Did not let the water pitcher touch the rim or inside of the cup.
15. Made sure the pitcher, cup, and straw (if used) were within the person's reach.

Postprocedure

16. Provided for comfort.
17. Placed the call light within reach.
18. Completed a safety check of the room.
19. Decontaminated your hands.

Postprocedure—cont'd　　　　　　　　　　　　　　　　　　　　　　S　　U　　**Comments**

20. Repeated for each resident:

   a. Took the cart to the person's room door. Did not take the cart into the room.   ———— ———— ————————

   b. Checked the person's fluid orders. Used the list from the nurse.   ———— ———— ————————

   c. Identified the person. Checked the ID bracelet against the fluid orders sheet or your assignment sheet. Also called the person by name.   ———— ———— ————————

   d. Took the pitcher from the person's overbed table. Emptied it into the bathroom sink.   ———— ———— ————————

   e. Determined if a new water pitcher was needed.   ———— ———— ————————

   f. Used the scoop to fill the pitcher with ice. Did not let the scoop touch the rim or inside of the pitcher. Did not place the person's pitcher on the cart.   ———— ———— ————————

   g. Placed the ice scoop on the towel.   ———— ———— ————————

   h. Filled the water pitcher with water. Got water from the bathroom or used the larger water pitcher on the cart.   ———— ———— ————————

   i. Placed the pitcher, cup, and straw (if used) on the overbed table.   ———— ———— ————————

   j. Filled the cup with water. Did not let the water pitcher touch the rim or inside of the cup.   ———— ———— ————————

   k. Made sure the pitcher, cup, and straw (if used) were within the person's reach.   ———— ———— ————————

   l. Provided for comfort.   ———— ———— ————————

   m. Placed the call light within reach.   ———— ———— ————————

   n. Completed a safety check of the room.   ———— ———— ————————

   o. Decontaminated your hands.   ———— ———— ————————

Name: _____   Date: _____

Quality of Life	**S**	**U**	**Comments**

Remembered to:
- Knock before entering the person's room.
- Address the person by name.
- Introduce yourself by name and title.
- Explain the procedure to the person before beginning and during the procedure.
- Protect the person's rights during the procedure.
- Handle the person gently during the procedure.

Preprocedure

1. Followed *Delegation Guidelines: Bedpans*
   Saw *Promoting Safety and Comfort: Bedpans*
2. Provided for privacy.
3. Practiced hand hygiene.
4. Put on gloves.
5. Collected the following:
   a. Bedpan
   b. Bedpan cover
   c. Toilet tissue
   d. Waterproof pad (if required by center)
6. Arranged equipment on the chair or bed.

Procedure

7. Lowered the bed rail near you if up.
8. Positioned the person supine. Raised the head of the bed slightly.
9. Folded the top linens and gown out of the way. Kept the lower body covered.
10. Asked the person to flex the knees and raise the buttocks by pushing against the mattress with his or her feet.
11. Slid a hand under the lower back. Helped raise the buttocks. If using waterproof pad, placed it under the person's buttocks.
12. Slid the bedpan under the person.
13. If the person could not assist in getting on the bedpan:
    a. Placed the waterproof pad under the person's buttocks if using one.
    b. Turned the person onto the side away from you.
    c. Placed the bedpan firmly against the buttocks.
    d. Pushed the bedpan down and toward the person.
    e. Held the bedpan securely. Turned the person onto his or her back.
    f. Made sure the bedpan was centered under the person.
14. Covered the person.
15. Raised the head of the bed so the person was in a sitting position (Fowler position) if using standard bedpan. (Note: Removed gloves and washed your hands before raising head of bed if required by the state competency test.)
16. Made sure the person was correctly positioned on the bedpan.
17. Raised the bed rail if used.
18. Placed the toilet tissue and call light within reach.
19. Asked the person to signal when done or when help was needed.
20. Removed the gloves. Practiced hand hygiene.
21. Left the room and closed the door.
22. Returned when the person signaled. Or checked on the person every 5 minutes. Knocked before entering.
23. Practiced hand hygiene. Put on gloves.

317

Procedure—cont'd

	S	U	Comments
24. Raised the bed for body mechanics. Lowered the bed rail (if used) and lowered the head of the bed.	___	___	_____
25. Asked the person to raise the buttocks. Removed the bedpan. Or held the bedpan and turned the person onto the side away from you.	___	___	_____
26. Cleaned the genital area if the person could not do so. Cleaned from front (urethra) to back (anus) with toilet tissue. Used fresh tissue for each wipe. Provided perineal care if needed. Removed and discarded the waterproof pad if using.	___	___	_____
27. Covered the bedpan. Took it to the bathroom. Raised the bed rail (if used) before leaving the bedside.	___	___	_____
28. Noted the color, amount, and character of the urine or feces.	___	___	_____
29. Emptied the bedpan contents into the toilet and flushed.	___	___	_____
30. Rinsed the bedpan. Poured the rinse into the toilet and flushed.	___	___	_____
31. Cleaned the bedpan with a disinfectant.	___	___	_____
32. Removed soiled gloves. Practiced hand hygiene and put on clean gloves.	___	___	_____
33. Returned the bedpan and clean cover to the bedside stand.	___	___	_____
34. Helped the person with hand washing. Wore gloves.	___	___	_____
35. Removed the gloves. Practiced hand hygiene.	___	___	_____

Postprocedure

	S	U	Comments
36. Provided for comfort.	___	___	_____
37. Placed the call light within reach.	___	___	_____
38. Lowered the bed to its lowest position.	___	___	_____
39. Raised or lowered bed rails. Followed the care plan.	___	___	_____
40. Unscreened the person.	___	___	_____
41. Completed a safety check of the room.	___	___	_____
42. Followed center policy for soiled linens.	___	___	_____
43. Practiced hand hygiene.	___	___	_____
44. Reported and recorded your observations.	___	___	_____

VIDEO CLIP **Giving the Urinal**

Name: _____   Date: _____

	S	U	Comments
Quality of Life			

Remembered to:
- Knock before entering the person's room.
- Address the person by name.
- Introduce yourself by name and title.
- Explain the procedure to the person before beginning and during the procedure.
- Protect the person's rights during the procedure.
- Handle the person gently during the procedure.

Preprocedure

1. Followed *Delegation Guidelines: Urinals*
   Saw *Promoting Safety and Comfort: Urinals*
2. Provided for privacy.
3. Determined if the person will stand, sit, or lie in bed.
4. Practiced hand hygiene.
5. Put on gloves.
6. Collected the following:
   a. Urinal
   b. Nonskid footwear if the person will stand to void

Procedure

7. Gave the person the urinal if he or she was in bed. Reminded the person to tilt the bottom down to prevent spills.
8. If the person stood:
   a. Helped him or her sit on the side of the bed.
   b. Put nonskid footwear on the person.
   c. Helped the person stand. Provided support if he or she was unsteady.
   d. Gave the person the urinal.
9. Positioned the urinal if necessary. For a male, positioned his penis in the urinal if he could not do so. For a female, positioned the urinal closely against her genitalia.
10. Placed the call light within reach. Asked the person to signal when done or when he or she needed help.
11. Provided for privacy.
12. Removed the gloves. Practiced hand hygiene.
13. Left the room and closed the door.
14. Returned when the person signaled for you. Or checked on him or her every 5 minutes. Knocked before entering.
15. Practiced hand hygiene. Put on gloves.
16. Provided perineal care if needed.
17. Closed the cap on the urinal. Took it to the bathroom.
18. Noted the color and clarity of urine. Noted the amount of urine in milliliters.
19. Emptied the urine into the toilet and flushed.
20. Rinsed the urinal with cold water. Poured rinse into the toilet and flushed.
21. Cleaned the urinal with a disinfectant.
22. Returned the urinal to its proper place.
23. Removed soiled gloves. Practiced hand hygiene and put on clean gloves.
24. Assisted with hand washing.
25. Removed the gloves. Practiced hand hygiene.

Postprocedure

26. Provided for comfort.
27. Placed the call light within reach.
28. Raised or lowered bed rails. Followed the care plan.

319

Postprocedure—cont'd   S   U   **Comments**

29. Unscreened the person.   ____   ____   _____
30. Completed a safety check of the room.   ____   ____   _____
31. Followed center policy for soiled linens.   ____   ____   _____
32. Practiced hand hygiene.   ____   ____   _____
33. Reported and recorded your observations. Recorded on the intake and output
    (I&O) record if necessary.   ____   ____   _____

Helping the Person to the Commode

Name: _____   Date: _____

	S	**U**	**Comments**

Quality of Life

Remembered to:
- Knock before entering the person's room.   ____ ____ _____
- Address the person by name.   ____ ____ _____
- Introduce yourself by name and title.   ____ ____ _____
- Explain the procedure to the person before beginning and during the procedure.   ____ ____ _____
- Protect the person's rights during the procedure.   ____ ____ _____
- Handle the person gently during the procedure.   ____ ____ _____

Preprocedure

1. Followed *Delegation Guidelines: Commodes*
   Saw *Promoting Safety and Comfort: Commodes*   ____ ____ _____
2. Provided for privacy.   ____ ____ _____
3. Practiced hand hygiene.   ____ ____ _____
4. Put on gloves.   ____ ____ _____
5. Collected the following:
   a. Commode   ____ ____ _____
   b. Toilet tissue   ____ ____ _____
   c. Bath blanket   ____ ____ _____
   d. Transfer belt   ____ ____ _____
   e. Robe and nonskid footwear   ____ ____ _____

Procedure

6. Brought the commode next to the bed. Removed the chair seat and container lid.   ____ ____ _____
7. Helped the person sit on the side of the bed. Lowered the bed rail if used.   ____ ____ _____
8. Helped the person put on a robe and nonskid footwear.   ____ ____ _____
9. Assisted the person to the commode. Used the transfer belt.   ____ ____ _____
10. Removed the transfer belt. Covered the person with a bath blanket for warmth.   ____ ____ _____
11. Placed the toilet tissue and call light within reach.   ____ ____ _____
12. Asked the person to signal when done or when help was needed. (Stayed with the person if necessary. Was respectful. Provided as much privacy as possible.)   ____ ____ _____
13. Removed the gloves. Practiced hand hygiene.   ____ ____ _____
14. Left the room. Closed the door.   ____ ____ _____
15. Returned when the person signaled. Or checked on the person every 5 minutes. Knocked before entering.   ____ ____ _____
16. Decontaminated your hands. Put on gloves.   ____ ____ _____
17. Helped the person clean the genital area as needed. Removed the gloves and practiced hand hygiene.   ____ ____ _____
18. Applied the transfer belt. Helped the person back to bed using the transfer belt. Removed the transfer belt, robe, and footwear. Raised the bed rail if used.   ____ ____ _____
19. Put on clean gloves. Removed and covered the commode container. Cleaned the commode.   ____ ____ _____
20. Took the container to the bathroom.   ____ ____ _____
21. Observed urine and feces for color, amount, and character.   ____ ____ _____
22. Poured into graduate container if the person's output is to be measured.   ____ ____ _____
23. Emptied the container contents into the toilet and flushed.   ____ ____ _____
24. Rinsed the container. Poured rinse into the toilet and flushed.   ____ ____ _____
25. Cleaned and disinfected the container.   ____ ____ _____
26. Returned the container to the commode. Returned other supplies to their proper place.   ____ ____ _____

    Procedure Checklists

Procedure—cont'd	S	U	Comments
27. Removed soiled gloves. Practiced hand hygiene and put on clean gloves.	——	——	———————
28. Assisted with hand washing.	——	——	———————
29. Removed the gloves. Practiced hand hygiene.	——	——	———————

Postprocedure

	S	U	Comments
30. Provided for comfort.	——	——	———————
31. Placed the call light within reach.	——	——	———————
32. Raised or lowered bed rails. Followed the care plan.	——	——	———————
33. Unscreened the person.	——	——	———————
34. Completed a safety check of the room.	——	——	———————
35. Followed center policy for soiled linens.	——	——	———————
36. Practiced hand hygiene.	——	——	———————
37. Reported and recorded your observations. Recorded on I&O sheet if necessary.	——	——	———————

Applying an Incontinence Brief

Name: _____   Date: _____

Quality of Life	S	U	Comments
Remembered to:			
• Knock before entering the person's room.	___	___	_____
• Address the person by name.	___	___	_____
• Introduce yourself by name and title.	___	___	_____
• Explain the procedure to the person before beginning and during the procedure.	___	___	_____
• Protect the person's rights during the procedure.	___	___	_____
• Handle the person gently during the procedure.	___	___	_____

Preprocedure

	S	U	Comments
1. Followed *Delegation Guidelines: Perineal Care*	___	___	_____
Saw *Promoting Safety and Comfort: Perineal Care*	___	___	_____
2. Provided for privacy.	___	___	_____
3. Practiced hand hygiene.	___	___	_____
4. Put on gloves.	___	___	_____
5. Collected the following:			
a. Correct type and size of brief for resident	___	___	_____
b. Gloves	___	___	_____
c. Supplies for perineal care (basin of warm water, soap, washcloth, towel) or disposable periwipes	___	___	_____
d. Waterproof pad	___	___	_____
e. Bath blanket	___	___	_____
f. Plastic trash bag	___	___	_____

Procedure

	S	U	Comments
6. Lowered the head of the bed. The bed was as flat as possible.	___	___	_____
7. Lowered the bed rail near you if up.	___	___	_____
8. Covered the person with a bath blanket. Lowered top linens to the foot of the bed.	___	___	_____
9. To apply an incontinence brief with the person in bed:			
a. Placed a waterproof pad under the buttocks. Asked the person to raise the buttocks off the bed. Or turned the person from side to side.	___	___	_____
b. Loosened the tabs on each side of the soiled brief.	___	___	_____
c. Turned the person onto the side away from you.	___	___	_____
d. Removed the soiled brief from front to back. Observed the urine or feces as you rolled the brief up.	___	___	_____
e. Placed the soiled brief in the trash bag. Set the bag aside.	___	___	_____
f. Removed gloves. Practiced hand hygiene.	___	___	_____
g. Put on gloves.	___	___	_____
h. Performed perineal care. Was sure to use facility-approved perineal cleanser and barrier cream if ordered.	___	___	_____
i. Removed gloves. Practiced hand hygiene.	___	___	_____
j. Put on gloves.	___	___	_____
k. Opened the new brief. Folded it in half lengthwise along the center.	___	___	_____
l. Inserted the brief between the legs from front to back.	___	___	_____
m. Unfolded and spread the back panel.	___	___	_____
n. Centered the brief in the perineal area.	___	___	_____
o. Turned the person onto his or her back.	___	___	_____
p. Unfolded and spread the front panel. Provided a "cup" shape in the perineal area. For a male, positioned the penis downward.	___	___	_____
q. Made sure the brief was positioned high in the groin folds. This allowed it to fit the shape of the body.	___	___	_____

Procedure—cont'd	S	U	Comments

r. Secured the brief by fastening the tape tabs. Pulled the lower tab forward on the side near you. Attached it at a slightly upward angle. Did the same for the other side. Repeated for the upper tabs, attaching in a horizontal manner. _____ _____ _____

s. Smoothed out all wrinkles and folds. _____ _____ _____

t. Removed and discarded gloves. _____ _____ _____

u. Practiced hand hygiene. _____ _____ _____

10. To apply a pad and undergarment with the person in bed:

a. Placed a waterproof pad under the buttocks. Asked the person to raise the buttocks off the bed. Or turned the person from side to side. _____ _____ _____

b. Turned the person onto the side away from you. _____ _____ _____

c. Pulled the undergarment down. The waistband was over the knee. _____ _____ _____

d. Removed the pad from front to back. Observed the urine or feces as you rolled the pad up. _____ _____ _____

e. Placed the soiled pad in the trash bag. Removed gloves. Set the bag aside. _____ _____ _____

f. Performed hand hygiene. _____ _____ _____

g. Put on gloves. _____ _____ _____

h. Performed perineal care. Was sure to use facility-approved perineal cleanser and barrier cream if ordered. _____ _____ _____

i. Removed gloves. Practiced hand hygiene. _____ _____ _____

j. Put on gloves. _____ _____ _____

k. Folded the new pad in half lengthwise along the center. _____ _____ _____

l. Inserted the pad between the legs from front to back. _____ _____ _____

m. Unfolded and spread the back panel. _____ _____ _____

n. Centered the pad in the perineal area. _____ _____ _____

o. Pulled the undergarment up at the back. _____ _____ _____

p. Checked and adjusted the pad and undergarment for a good fit. _____ _____ _____

11. To apply pull-on underwear (briefs) with the person standing:

a. Helped the person put on nonskid footwear. _____ _____ _____

b. Helped the person stand. _____ _____ _____

c. Tore the side seams to remove the soiled pull-on brief. _____ _____ _____

d. Removed the brief from front to back. Observed the urine or feces as you rolled the brief up. _____ _____ _____

e. Placed the brief in the trash bag. Removed your gloves. Set the bag aside. _____ _____ _____

f. Practiced hand hygiene. _____ _____ _____

g. Performed perineal care. Was sure to use facility-approved perineal cleanser and barrier cream if ordered. _____ _____ _____

h. Removed gloves. Practiced hand hygiene. _____ _____ _____

i. Put on gloves. Placed a waterproof pad on the bed. _____ _____ _____

j. Had the person sit on the side of the bed on a waterproof pad. _____ _____ _____

k. Slid the pull-on brief over the feet to past the knees. _____ _____ _____

l. Helped the person stand. _____ _____ _____

m. Pulled the brief up. _____ _____ _____

n. Checked for a good fit. _____ _____ _____

o. Discarded waterproof pad. Removed and discarded gloves. _____ _____ _____

p. Practiced hand hygiene. _____ _____ _____

Postprocedure

12. Provided for comfort. _____ _____ _____

13. Placed the call light within reach. _____ _____ _____

14. Lowered the bed to its lowest position. _____ _____ _____

Postprocedure—cont'd

	S	U	Comments
15. Raised or lowered bed rails. Followed the care plan.			
16. Cleaned, dried, and returned equipment to its proper place. Discarded disposable items. (Wore gloves for this step.) Did not leave a trash bag with a soiled brief in the person's room. Tied up the plastic bag and took it to the proper place for disposal.			
17. Unscreened the person.			
18. Completed a safety check of the room.			
19. Followed center policy for soiled linens.			
20. Removed the gloves. Practiced hand hygiene.			
21. Reported and recorded your observations.			

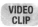 **Giving Catheter Care (NATCEP)**

Name: _____ Date: _____

	S	U	Comments
Quality of Life			

Remembered to:
- Knock before entering the person's room. ___ ___ _____
- Address the person by name. ___ ___ _____
- Introduce yourself by name and title. ___ ___ _____
- Explain the procedure to the person before beginning and during the procedure. ___ ___ _____
- Protect the person's rights during the procedure. ___ ___ _____
- Handle the person gently during the procedure. ___ ___ _____

Preprocedure

1. Followed *Delegation Guidelines:*
   a. *Perineal Care* ___ ___ _____
   b. *Catheters* ___ ___ _____
   Saw *Promoting Safety and Comfort:*
   a. *Perineal Care* ___ ___ _____
   b. *Catheters* ___ ___ _____
2. Practiced hand hygiene. ___ ___ _____
3. Collected the following:
   a. Items for perineal care:
      i. Soap or other cleaning agents as directed ___ ___ _____
      ii. At least four washcloths ___ ___ _____
      iii. Bath towel ___ ___ _____
      iv. Bath thermometer ___ ___ _____
      v. Wash basin ___ ___ _____
      vi. Waterproof pad ___ ___ _____
      vii. Paper towels ___ ___ _____
   b. Gloves ___ ___ _____
   c. Bath blanket ___ ___ _____
4. Covered the overbed table with paper towels. Arranged items on top of paper towels. ___ ___ _____
5. Identified the person. Checked the identification (ID) bracelet against the assignment sheet. Also called the person by name. ___ ___ _____
6. Provided for privacy. ___ ___ _____
7. Filled the wash basin. Water temperature was about 105°F (40.5°C). Measured water temperature according to center policy. Asked the person to check the water temperature. Adjusted water temperature as needed. ___ ___ _____
8. Raised the bed for body mechanics. Bed rails were up if used. ___ ___ _____

Procedure

9. Lowered the bed rail near you if up. ___ ___ _____
10. Decontaminated your hands. Put on gloves. ___ ___ _____
11. Covered the person with a bath blanket. Fan-folded top linens to the foot of the bed. ___ ___ _____
12. Draped the person for perineal care. ___ ___ _____
13. Folded back the bath blanket to expose the genital area. ___ ___ _____
14. Placed the waterproof pad under the buttocks. Asked the person to flex the knees and raise the buttocks off the bed. ___ ___ _____
15. Separated the labia (female). In an uncircumcised male, retracted the foreskin. Checked for crusts, abnormal drainage, or secretions. ___ ___ _____
16. Gave perineal care. ___ ___ _____
17. Applied soap to clean, wet washcloth. ___ ___ _____
18. Held the catheter near the meatus. ___ ___ _____

Procedure—cont'd	S	U	Comments

19. Cleaned the catheter from the meatus down the catheter about 4 inches. Cleaned downward, away from the meatus with 1 stroke. Did not tug or pull on the catheter. Repeated as needed with a clean area of the washcloth. Used a clean washcloth if needed. _____ _____ _____

20. Rinsed the catheter with a clean washcloth. Rinsed from the meatus down the catheter about 4 inches. Rinsed downward, away from the meatus, with 1 stroke. Did not tug or pull on the catheter. Repeated as needed with a clean area of the washcloth. Used a clean washcloth if needed. _____ _____ _____

21. Dried the catheter with a towel. Dried from the meatus down the catheter about 4 inches. Did not tug or pull on the catheter. _____ _____ _____

22. Patted the perineal area dry. Dried from front to back. _____ _____ _____

23. Returned the foreskin to its natural position. _____ _____ _____

24. Secured the catheter. Coiled and secured tubing. _____ _____ _____

25. Removed the waterproof pad. _____ _____ _____

26. Covered the person. Removed the bath blanket. _____ _____ _____

27. Removed the gloves. Practiced hand hygiene. _____ _____ _____

Postprocedure

28. Provided for comfort. _____ _____ _____

29. Placed the call light within reach. _____ _____ _____

30. Lowered the bed to its lowest position. _____ _____ _____

31. Raised or lowered bed rails. Followed the care plan. _____ _____ _____

32. Cleaned, dried, and returned equipment to its proper place. Discarded disposable items. (Wore gloves for this step.) _____ _____ _____

33. Unscreened the person. _____ _____ _____

34. Completed a safety check of the room. _____ _____ _____

35. Followed center policy for soiled linens. _____ _____ _____

36. Removed the gloves. Practiced hand hygiene. _____ _____ _____

37. Reported and recorded your observations. _____ _____ _____

Name: _____   Date: _____

	S	U	Comments

Quality of Life
Remembered to:
- Knock before entering the person's room.
- Address the person by name.
- Introduce yourself by name and title.
- Explain the procedure to the person before beginning and during the procedure.
- Protect the person's rights during the procedure.
- Handle the person gently during the procedure.

Preprocedure

1. Followed *Delegation Guidelines: Drainage Systems*
   Saw *Promoting Safety and Comfort: Drainage Systems*
2. Practiced hand hygiene.
3. Collected the following:
   a. Gloves
   b. Drainage bag and tubing
   c. Antiseptic wipes
   d. Waterproof pad
   e. Sterile cap and plug
   f. Catheter clamp
   g. Paper towels
   h. Bedpan
   i. Bath blanket
4. Arranged paper towels and equipment on the overbed table.
5. Identified the person. Checked the identification (ID) bracelet against the assignment sheet. Also called the person by name.
6. Provided for privacy.

Procedure

7. Had the person sit on the side of the bed.
8. Practiced hand hygiene. Put on gloves.
9. Exposed the catheter and leg bag.
10. Clamped the catheter. This prevented urine from draining from the catheter into the drainage tubing.
11. Let urine drain from below the clamp into the drainage tubing. This emptied the lower end of the catheter.
12. Helped the person lie down.
13. Raised the bed rails if used. Raised the bed for body mechanics.
14. Lowered the bed rail near you if up.
15. Covered the person with a bath blanket. Fan-folded top linens to the foot of the bed. Exposed the catheter and leg bag.
16. Placed the waterproof pad under the person's leg.
17. Opened the antiseptic wipes. Set them on paper towels.
18. Opened the package with the sterile cap and plug. Placed the package on the paper towels. Did not let anything touch the sterile cap or plug.
19. Opened the package with the drainage bag and tubing.
20. Attached the drainage bag to the bed frame.
21. Disconnected the catheter from the drainage tubing. Did not allow anything to touch the ends.

Procedure—cont'd	S	U	Comments

22. Inserted the sterile plug into the catheter end. Touched only the end of the plug. Did not touch the part that went inside the catheter. (If you contaminated the end of the catheter, wiped the end with an antiseptic wipe. Did so before you inserted the sterile plug.) ___ ___ _____
23. Placed the sterile cap on the end of the leg bag drainage tube. (If you contaminated the end of the tubing, wiped the end with an antiseptic wipe. Did so before you put on the sterile cap.) ___ ___ _____
24. Removed the cap from the new drainage tubing. ___ ___ _____
25. Removed the sterile plug from the catheter. ___ ___ _____
26. Inserted the end of the drainage tubing into the catheter. ___ ___ _____
27. Removed the clamp from the catheter. ___ ___ _____
28. Looped the drainage tubing on the bed. Secured the tubing to the bottom linens. ___ ___ _____
29. Removed the leg bag. Placed it in the bedpan. ___ ___ _____
30. Removed and discarded the waterproof pad. ___ ___ _____
31. Covered the person. Removed the bath blanket. ___ ___ _____
32. Took the bedpan to the bathroom. ___ ___ _____
33. Removed the gloves. Practiced hand hygiene. ___ ___ _____

Postprocedure

34. Provided for comfort. ___ ___ _____
35. Placed the call light within reach. ___ ___ _____
36. Lowered the bed to its lowest position. ___ ___ _____
37. Raised or lowered bed rails. Followed the care plan. ___ ___ _____
38. Unscreened the person. ___ ___ _____
39. Put on clean gloves. Discarded disposable items. ___ ___ _____
40. Emptied the drainage bag. ___ ___ _____
41. Discarded the drainage tubing and bag following center policy. Or cleaned the bag following center policy. ___ ___ _____
42. Cleaned and disinfected the bedpan. Placed it in a clean cover. ___ ___ _____
43. Returned the bedpan and other supplies to their proper place. ___ ___ _____
44. Removed the gloves. Practiced hand hygiene. ___ ___ _____
45. Completed a safety check of the room. ___ ___ _____
46. Followed center policy for soiled linens. ___ ___ _____
47. Practiced hand hygiene. ___ ___ _____
48. Reported and recorded your observations. ___ ___ _____

Emptying a Urinary Drainage Bag

Name: _____   Date: _____

	S	U	Comments
Quality of Life			
Remembered to:			
• Knock before entering the person's room.	___	___	_____
• Address the person by name.	___	___	_____
• Introduce yourself by name and title.	___	___	_____
• Explain the procedure to the person before beginning and during the procedure.	___	___	_____
• Protect the person's rights during the procedure.	___	___	_____
• Handle the person gently during the procedure.	___	___	_____

Preprocedure

1. Followed *Delegation Guidelines: Drainage Systems*   ___ ___ _____
   Saw *Promoting Safety and Comfort: Drainage Systems*   ___ ___ _____
2. Collected the following:
   a. Graduate (measuring container)   ___ ___ _____
   b. Waterproof pad or plastic bag to place on the floor under the graduate   ___ ___ _____
   c. Gloves   ___ ___ _____
   d. Paper towels   ___ ___ _____
   e. Antiseptic wipes (if used by your nursing center)   ___ ___ _____
3. Practiced hand hygiene.   ___ ___ _____
4. Identified the person. Checked the identification (ID) bracelet against the assignment sheet. Also called the person by name.   ___ ___ _____
5. Provided for privacy.   ___ ___ _____

Procedure

6. Put on the gloves.   ___ ___ _____
7. Placed paper towel on the floor. Placed graduate on top of it.   ___ ___ _____
8. Positioned the graduate under the collection bag and on a waterproof pad.   ___ ___ _____
9. Opened the clamp on the drain.   ___ ___ _____
10. Let all urine to drain into the graduate. Did not let the drain touch the graduate.   ___ ___ _____
11. Closed and positioned the clamp.   ___ ___ _____
12. Wiped the drain with an antiseptic wipe. (Not all facilities include this step.)   ___ ___ _____
13. Measured the urine.   ___ ___ _____
14. Removed and discarded the paper towel.   ___ ___ _____
15. Emptied the contents of the graduate into the toilet and flushed.   ___ ___ _____
16. Rinsed the graduate. Emptied the rinse into the toilet and flushed.   ___ ___ _____
17. Cleaned and disinfected the graduate.   ___ ___ _____
18. Returned the graduate to its proper place.   ___ ___ _____
19. Removed the gloves. Practiced hand hygiene.   ___ ___ _____
20. Recorded the time and amount on the intake and output (I&O) record.   ___ ___ _____

Postprocedure

21. Provided for comfort.   ___ ___ _____
22. Placed the call light within reach.   ___ ___ _____
23. Unscreened the person.   ___ ___ _____
24. Completed a safety check of the room.   ___ ___ _____
25. Reported and recorded the amount and other observations.   ___ ___ _____

Applying a Condom Catheter

Name: _____   Date: _____

	S	**U**	**Comments**

Quality of Life

Remembered to:
- Knock before entering the person's room.
- Address the person by name.
- Introduce yourself by name and title.
- Explain the procedure to the person before beginning and during the procedure.
- Protect the person's rights during the procedure.
- Handle the person gently during the procedure.

Preprocedure

1. Followed *Delegation Guidelines:*
   a. *Perineal Care*
   b. *Condom Catheters*
   Saw *Promoting Safety and Comfort:*
   a. *Perineal Care*
   b. *Condom Catheters*
2. Practiced hand hygiene.
3. Collected the following:
   a. Condom catheter
   b. Elastic tape
   c. Drainage bag or leg bag
   d. Cap for the drainage bag
   e. Basin of warm water
   f. Soap
   g. Towel and washcloths
   h. Bath blanket
   i. Gloves
   j. Waterproof pad
   k. Paper towels
4. Covered the overbed table with paper towels. Arranged items on top of paper towels.
5. Identified the person. Checked the identification (ID) bracelet against the assignment sheet. Also called the person by name.
6. Provided for privacy.
7. Filled the wash basin. Water temperature was about 105°F (40.5°C). Measured water temperature according to center policy. Asked the person to check the water temperature. Adjusted water temperature as needed.
8. Raised the bed for body mechanics. Bed rails were up if used.

Procedure

9. Lowered the bed rail near you if up.
10. Practiced hand hygiene. Put on gloves.
11. Covered the person with a bath blanket. Lowered top linens to the knees.
12. Asked the person to raise his buttocks off the bed. Or turned him onto his side away from you.
13. Slid the waterproof pad under his buttocks.
14. Had the person lower his buttocks. Or turned him onto his back.
15. Secured the drainage bag to the bed frame. Or had a leg bag ready. Closed the drain.
16. Exposed the genital area.

Procedure—cont'd	S	U	Comments
17. Removed the condom catheter:			
a. Removed the tape. Rolled the sheath off the penis.	____	____	_____
b. Disconnected the drainage tubing from the condom. Capped the drainage tube.	____	____	_____
c. Discarded the tape and condom.	____	____	_____
18. Provided perineal care. Observed the penis for reddened areas, skin breakdown, and irritation.	____	____	_____
19. Removed gloves and practiced hand hygiene. Put on clean gloves.	____	____	_____
20. Removed the protective backing from the condom. This exposed the adhesive strip.	____	____	_____
21. Held the penis firmly. Rolled the condom onto the penis. Left a 1-inch space between the penis and the end of the catheter.	____	____	_____
22. Secured the condom:			
a. For a self-adhering condom, pressed the condom to the penis.	____	____	_____
b. For a condom secured with elastic tape, applied elastic tape in a spiral fashion. Did not apply tape completely around the penis.	____	____	_____
23. Made sure the penis tip did not touch the condom. Made sure the condom was not twisted.	____	____	_____
24. Connected the condom to the drainage tubing. Coiled and secured excess tubing on the bed. Or attached a leg bag.	____	____	_____
25. Removed the waterproof pad and gloves. Discarded them. Practiced hand hygiene.	____	____	_____
26. Covered the person. Removed the bath blanket.	____	____	_____

Postprocedure

	S	U	Comments
27. Provided for comfort.	____	____	_____
28. Placed the call light within reach.	____	____	_____
29. Lowered the bed to its lowest position.	____	____	_____
30. Raised or lowered bed rails. Followed the care plan.	____	____	_____
31. Unscreened the person.	____	____	_____
32. Practiced hand hygiene. Put on clean gloves.	____	____	_____
33. Measured and recorded the amount of urine in the bag. Cleaned or discarded the collection bag.	____	____	_____
34. Cleaned, dried, and returned the wash basin and other equipment. Returned items to their proper place.	____	____	_____
35. Removed the gloves. Practiced hand hygiene.	____	____	_____
36. Completed a safety check of the room.	____	____	_____
37. Reported and recorded your observations.	____	____	_____

Giving a Cleansing Enema

Name: _____   Date: _____

	S	U	Comments
Quality of Life			
Remembered to:			
• Knock before entering the person's room.	___	___	_____
• Address the person by name.	___	___	_____
• Introduce yourself by name and title.	___	___	_____
• Explain the procedure to the person before beginning and during the procedure.	___	___	_____
• Protect the person's rights during the procedure.	___	___	_____
• Handle the person gently during the procedure.	___	___	_____

Preprocedure

	S	U	Comments
1. Followed *Delegation Guidelines: Enemas*	___	___	_____
Saw *Promoting Safety and Comfort: Enemas*	___	___	_____
2. Practiced hand hygiene.	___	___	_____
3. Collected the following before going to the person's room:			
a. Disposable enema kit as directed by the nurse (enema bag, tube, clamp, and waterproof pad)	___	___	_____
b. Bath thermometer	___	___	_____
c. Waterproof pad (if not part of the enema kit)	___	___	_____
d. Water-soluble lubricant	___	___	_____
e. 3–5 mL (1 teaspoon) castile soap or 1–2 teaspoons of salt	___	___	_____
f. Intravenous (IV) pole	___	___	_____
g. Gloves	___	___	_____
4. Arranged items in the person's room and bathroom.	___	___	_____
5. Decontaminated your hands.	___	___	_____
6. Identified the person. Checked the identification (ID) bracelet against the assignment sheet. Also called the person by name.	___	___	_____
7. Put on gloves.	___	___	_____
8. Collected the following:			
a. Commode or bedpan and cover	___	___	_____
b. Toilet tissue	___	___	_____
c. Bath blanket	___	___	_____
d. Robe and nonskid footwear	___	___	_____
e. Paper towels	___	___	_____
9. Provided for privacy.	___	___	_____
10. Raised the bed for body mechanics. Bed rails were up if used.	___	___	_____

Procedure

	S	U	Comments
11. Removed the gloves and decontaminated your hands. Put on clean gloves.	___	___	_____
12. Lowered the bed rail near you if up.	___	___	_____
13. Covered the person with a bath blanket. Fan-folded top linens to the foot of the bed.	___	___	_____
14. Positioned the IV pole so the enema bag was 12 inches above the anus. Or it was at the height directed by the nurse.	___	___	_____
15. Raised the bed rail if used.	___	___	_____
16. Prepared the enema:			
a. Closed the clamp on the tube.	___	___	_____
b. Adjusted water flow until it was lukewarm.	___	___	_____
c. Filled the enema bag for the amount ordered.	___	___	_____
d. Measured water temperature with the bath thermometer. Followed the nurse's directions for water temperature.	___	___	_____

Procedure—cont'd	S	U	Comments
e. Prepared the solution as directed by the nurse:			
i. Tap water enema (TWE): added nothing	____	____	_____
ii. Saline enema: added salt as directed	____	____	_____
iii. Soapsuds enema (SSE): added castile soap as directed.	____	____	_____
f. Stirred the solution with the bath thermometer. Scooped off any suds (SSE).	____	____	_____
g. Sealed the bag.	____	____	_____
h. Hung the bag on the IV pole.	____	____	_____
17. Lowered the bed rail near you if up.	____	____	_____
18. Positioned the person in a left side-lying position.	____	____	_____
19. Placed a waterproof pad under the buttocks.	____	____	_____
20. Exposed the anal area.	____	____	_____
21. Placed the bedpan behind the person.	____	____	_____
22. Positioned the enema tube in the bedpan. Removed the cap from the tubing.	____	____	_____
23. Opened the clamp. Let solution flow through the tube to remove air. Clamped the tube.	____	____	_____
24. Lubricated the tube 2–4 inches from the tip.	____	____	_____
25. Separated the buttocks to see the anus.	____	____	_____
26. Asked the person to take a deep breath through the mouth.	____	____	_____
27. Inserted the tube gently 2–4 inches into the adult's rectum. Did this when the person was exhaling. Stopped if the person complained of pain, you felt resistance, or bleeding occurred.	____	____	_____
28. Checked the amount of solution in the bag.	____	____	_____
29. Unclamped the tube. Gave the solution slowly.	____	____	_____
30. Asked the person to take slow, deep breaths. This helped the person relax.	____	____	_____
31. Clamped the tube if the person needed to have a bowel movement (BM), had cramping, or started to expel solution. Also clamped the tube if the person was sweating or complained of nausea or weakness. Unclamped when symptoms subsided.	____	____	_____
32. Gave the amount of solution ordered. Stopped if the person could not tolerate the procedure.	____	____	_____
33. Clamped the tube before it emptied. This prevented air from entering the bowel.	____	____	_____
34. Held toilet tissue around the tube and against the anus. Removed the tube.	____	____	_____
35. Discarded toilet tissue in the bedpan.	____	____	_____
36. Wrapped the tubing tip with paper towels. Placed it inside the enema bag.	____	____	_____
37. Assisted the person to the bathroom or commode. The person wore a robe and nonskid footwear while up. The bed was in the lowest position. Or helped the person onto the bedpan. Raised the head of the bed. Raised or lowered bed rail according to the care plan.	____	____	_____
38. Placed the call light and toilet tissue within reach. Reminded the person not to flush the toilet.	____	____	_____
39. Discarded disposable items.	____	____	_____
40. Removed the gloves. Practiced hand hygiene.	____	____	_____
41. Left the room if the person could be left alone.	____	____	_____
42. Returned when the person signaled. Or checked on the person every 5 minutes. Knocked before entering the room or bathroom.	____	____	_____
43. Decontaminated your hands and put on gloves. Lowered the bed rail if up.	____	____	_____

Procedure—cont'd   S   U   **Comments**

44. Observed enema results for amount, color, consistency, shape, and odor. Called the nurse to observe results. _____ _____ _____
45. Provided perineal care as needed. _____ _____ _____
46. Removed the waterproof pad. _____ _____ _____
47. Emptied, cleaned, and disinfected equipment. Flushed the toilet after the nurse observed the results. _____ _____ _____
48. Returned equipment to its proper place. _____ _____ _____
49. Removed the gloves and practiced hand hygiene. _____ _____ _____
50. Assisted with hand washing. Wore gloves for this step. _____ _____ _____
51. Covered the person. Removed the bath blanket. _____ _____ _____

Postprocedure

52. Provided for comfort. _____ _____ _____
53. Placed the call light within reach. _____ _____ _____
54. Lowered the bed to its lowest position. _____ _____ _____
55. Raised or lowered bed rails. Followed the care plan. _____ _____ _____
56. Unscreened the person. _____ _____ _____
57. Completed a safety check of the room. _____ _____ _____
58. Followed center policy for dirty linens and used supplies. _____ _____ _____
59. Practiced hand hygiene. _____ _____ _____
60. Reported and recorded your observations. _____ _____ _____

Name: _____ Date: _____

	S	U	Comments
Quality of Life			

Remembered to:
- Knock before entering the person's room.
- Address the person by name.
- Introduce yourself by name and title.
- Explain the procedure to the person before beginning and during the procedure.
- Protect the person's rights during the procedure.
- Handle the person gently during the procedure.

Preprocedure

1. Followed *Delegation Guidelines: Enemas*
   Saw *Promoting Safety and Comfort: Enemas*
2. Practiced hand hygiene.
3. Collected the following before going to the person's room:
   a. Small-volume enema
   b. Waterproof pad
   c. Gloves
4. Arranged items in the person's room.
5. Practiced hand hygiene.
6. Identified the person. Checked the identification (ID) bracelet against the assignment sheet. Also called the person by name.
7. Put on gloves.
8. Collected the following:
   a. Commode or bedpan
   b. Waterproof pad
   c. Toilet tissue
   d. Robe and nonskid footwear
   e. Bath blanket
9. Provided for privacy.
10. Raised the bed for body mechanics. Bed rails were up if used.

Procedure

11. Removed the gloves and practiced hand hygiene. Put on clean gloves.
12. Lowered the bed rail near you if up.
13. Covered the person with a bath blanket. Fan-folded top linens to the foot of the bed.
14. Positioned the person in left side-lying position.
15. Placed a waterproof pad under the buttocks.
16. Exposed the anal area.
17. Positioned the bedpan near the person.
18. Removed the cap from the enema tip.
19. Separated the buttocks to see the anus.
20. Asked the person to take a deep breath through the mouth.
21. Inserted the enema tip 2 inches into the adult's rectum. Did this when the person was exhaling. Inserted the tip gently. Stopped if the person complained of pain, you felt resistance, or bleeding occurred.
22. Squeezed and rolled the bottle gently. Released pressure on the bottle after you removed the tip from the rectum.
23. Placed the bottle into the box, tip first.

Procedure—cont'd   S   U   Comments

24. Assisted the person to the bathroom or commode when he or she had the urge to have a bowel movement (BM). The person wore a robe and nonskid footwear while up. The bed was in the lowest position. Or helped the person onto the bedpan and raised the head of the bed. Raised or lowered bed rails according to the care plan.   _____   _____   _____

25. Placed the call light and toilet tissue within reach. Reminded the person not to flush the toilet.   _____   _____   _____

26. Discarded disposable items.   _____   _____   _____

27. Removed the gloves. Practiced hand hygiene.   _____   _____   _____

28. Left the room if the person could be left alone.   _____   _____   _____

29. Returned when the person signaled. Or checked on the person every 5 minutes. Knocked before entering the room or bathroom.   _____   _____   _____

30. Practiced hand hygiene. Put on gloves.   _____   _____   _____

31. Lowered the bed rail if up.   _____   _____   _____

32. Observed enema results for amount, color, consistency, shape, and odor. Called the nurse to observe results.   _____   _____   _____

33. Provided perineal care as needed.   _____   _____   _____

34. Removed the waterproof pad.   _____   _____   _____

35. Emptied, cleaned, and disinfected equipment. Flushed the toilet after the nurse observed the results.   _____   _____   _____

36. Returned equipment to its proper place.   _____   _____   _____

37. Removed the gloves and practiced hand hygiene.   _____   _____   _____

38. Assisted with hand washing. Wore gloves for this step.   _____   _____   _____

39. Covered the person. Removed the bath blanket.   _____   _____   _____

Postprocedure

40. Provided for comfort.   _____   _____   _____

41. Placed the call light within reach.   _____   _____   _____

42. Lowered the bed to its lowest position.   _____   _____   _____

43. Raised or lowered bed rails. Followed the care plan.   _____   _____   _____

44. Unscreened the person.   _____   _____   _____

45. Completed a safety check of the room.   _____   _____   _____

46. Followed center policy for dirty linens and used supplies.   _____   _____   _____

47. Practiced hand hygiene.   _____   _____   _____

48. Reported and recorded your observations.   _____   _____   _____

Giving an Oil-Retention Enema

Name: _____ Date: _____

	S	U	Comments
Quality of Life			
Remembered to:			
• Knock before entering the person's room.	___	___	_____
• Address the person by name.	___	___	_____
• Introduce yourself by name and title.	___	___	_____
• Explain the procedure to the person before beginning and during the procedure.	___	___	_____
• Protect the person's rights during the procedure.	___	___	_____
• Handle the person gently during the procedure.	___	___	_____

Preprocedure

1. Followed *Delegation Guidelines: Enemas*	___	___	_____
Saw *Promoting Safety and Comfort:*			
a. *Enemas*	___	___	_____
b. *The Oil-Retention Enema.*	___	___	_____
2. Practiced hand hygiene.	___	___	_____
3. Collected the following before going to the person's room:			
a. Oil-retention enema	___	___	_____
b. Waterproof pads	___	___	_____
4. Arranged items in the person's room.	___	___	_____
5. Practiced hand hygiene.	___	___	_____
6. Identified the person. Checked the identification (ID) bracelet against the assignment sheet. Also called the person by name.	___	___	_____
7. Put on gloves.	___	___	_____
8. Collected the following:			
a. Gloves	___	___	_____
b. Bath blanket	___	___	_____
9. Provided for privacy.	___	___	_____
10. Raised the bed for body mechanics. Bed rails were up if used.	___	___	_____

Procedure

11. Removed gloves and practiced hand hygiene. Put on clean gloves.	___	___	_____
12. Followed these steps:			
a. Lowered the bed rail near you if up.	___	___	_____
b. Removed the gloves and practiced hand hygiene. Put on clean gloves.	___	___	_____
c. Covered the person with a bath blanket. Fan-folded top linens to the foot of the bed.	___	___	_____
d. Positioned the person in left side-lying position.	___	___	_____
e. Placed a waterproof pad under the buttocks.	___	___	_____
f. Exposed the anal area.	___	___	_____
g. Positioned the bedpan near the person.	___	___	_____
h. Removed the cap from the enema tip.	___	___	_____
i. Separated the buttocks to see the anus.	___	___	_____
j. Asked the person to take a deep breath through the mouth.	___	___	_____
k. Inserted the enema tip 2 inches into the adult's rectum. Did this when the person was exhaling. Inserted the tip gently. Stopped if the person complained of pain, you felt resistance, or bleeding occurred.	___	___	_____
l. Squeezed and rolled the bottle gently. Released pressure on the bottle after you removed the tip from the rectum.	___	___	_____
m. Placed the bottle into the box, tip first.	___	___	_____

Procedure—cont'd   S   U   **Comments**

13. Covered the person. Left the person in left side-lying position. ___   ___   _____
14. Encouraged the person to retain the enema for the time ordered. ___   ___   _____
15. Placed more waterproof pads on the bed if needed.   ___   ___   _____
16. Removed the gloves. Practiced hand hygiene.   ___   ___   _____

Postprocedure

17. Provided for comfort.   ___   ___   _____
18. Placed the call light within reach.   ___   ___   _____
19. Lowered the bed to its lowest position.   ___   ___   _____
20. Raised or lowered bed rails. Followed the care plan.   ___   ___   _____
21. Unscreened the person.   ___   ___   _____
22. Completed a safety check of the room.   ___   ___   _____
23. Followed center policy for dirty linens and used supplies.   ___   ___   _____
24. Practiced hand hygiene.   ___   ___   _____
25. Reported and recorded your observations.   ___   ___   _____
26. Checked the person often.   ___   ___   _____

Changing an Ostomy Pouch

Name: _____ Date: _____

	S	U	Comments
Quality of Life			
Remembered to:			
• Knock before entering the person's room.	___	___	___
• Address the person by name.	___	___	___
• Introduce yourself by name and title.	___	___	___
• Explain the procedure to the person before beginning and during the procedure.	___	___	___
• Protect the person's rights during the procedure.	___	___	___
• Handle the person gently during the procedure.	___	___	___

Preprocedure

	S	U	Comments
1. Followed *Delegation Guidelines: Ostomy Pouches*	___	___	___
Saw *Promoting Safety and Comfort: Ostomy Pouches*	___	___	___
2. Practiced hand hygiene.	___	___	___
3. Collected the following before going to the person's room:			
a. Clean pouch with skin barrier	___	___	___
b. Pouch clamp, clip, or wire closure	___	___	___
c. Clean ostomy belt (if used)	___	___	___
d. Gauze pads or washcloths	___	___	___
e. Adhesive remover wipes	___	___	___
f. Skin paste (optional)	___	___	___
g. Pouch deodorant	___	___	___
h. Disposable bag	___	___	___
4. Arranged your work area.	___	___	___
5. Practiced hand hygiene.	___	___	___
6. Identified the person. Checked the ID bracelet against the assignment sheet. Also called the person by name.	___	___	___
7. Put on gloves.	___	___	___
8. Collected the following:			
a. Bedpan with cover	___	___	___
b. Waterproof pad	___	___	___
c. Bath blanket	___	___	___
d. Wash basin with warm water	___	___	___
e. Paper towels	___	___	___
f. Gloves	___	___	___
9. Provided for privacy.	___	___	___
10. Raised the bed for body mechanics. Bed rails were up if used.	___	___	___

Procedure

	S	U	Comments
11. Removed the gloves and practiced hand hygiene. Put on clean gloves.	___	___	___
12. Lowered the bed rail near you if up.	___	___	___
13. Covered the person with a bath blanket. Fan-folded linens to the foot of the bed.	___	___	___
14. Placed the waterproof pad under the buttocks.	___	___	___
15. Disconnected the pouch from the belt if one is worn. Removed the belt.	___	___	___
16. Removed and placed the pouch and skin barrier in the bedpan. Gently pushed the skin down and lifted up on the barrier. Used the adhesive remover wipes if necessary.	___	___	___
17. Wiped the stoma and around it with a gauze pad. This removed excess stool and mucous. Discarded the gauze pad into the disposable bag.	___	___	___
18. Wet the gauze pads or the washcloth.	___	___	___
19. Washed the stoma and the skin around it with a gauze pad or washcloth. Washed gently. Did not scrub or rub the skin.	___	___	___
20. Patted dry with a gauze pad or the towel.	___	___	___

340

Procedure—cont'd | S | U | Comments

21. Observed the stoma and the skin around the stoma. Reported bleeding, skin irritation, or skin breakdown to the nurse. ____ ____ _____
22. Remove the backing from the new pouch. ____ ____ _____
23. Applied a thin layer of paste around the pouch opening. Let it dry following the manufacturer's instructions. ____ ____ _____
24. Pulled the skin around the stoma taut. The skin was wrinkle-free. ____ ____ _____
25. Centered the pouch over the stoma. The drain pointed downward. ____ ____ _____
26. Pressed around the pouch and skin barrier so it sealed to the skin. Applied gentle pressure with your fingers. Started at the bottom and worked up around the sides to the top. ____ ____ _____
27. Maintained the pressure for 1–2 minutes. Followed the manufacturer's instructions. ____ ____ _____
28. Tugged downward on the pouch gently. Made sure the pouch was secure. ____ ____ _____
29. Added deodorant to the pouch. ____ ____ _____
30. Closed the pouch at the bottom. Used a clamp, clip, or wire closure. ____ ____ _____
31. Attached the ostomy belt if used. The belt was not too tight. You were able to slide two fingers under the belt. ____ ____ _____
32. Removed the waterproof pad. ____ ____ _____
33. Discarded disposable supplies into the disposable bag. ____ ____ _____
34. Remove the gloves. Practiced hand hygiene. ____ ____ _____
35. Covered the person. Removed the bath blanket. ____ ____ _____

Postprocedure

36. Provided for comfort. ____ ____ _____
37. Placed the call light within reach. ____ ____ _____
38. Lowered the bed to its lowest position. ____ ____ _____
39. Raised or lowered bed rails. Followed the care plan. ____ ____ _____
40. Unscreened the person. ____ ____ _____
41. Practiced hand hygiene. Put on gloves. ____ ____ _____
42. Took the bedpan and disposable bag into the bathroom. ____ ____ _____
43. Emptied the pouch and bedpan into the toilet. Observed the color, amount, consistency, and odor of stools. Flushed the toilet. ____ ____ _____
44. Discarded the pouch into the disposable bag. Discarded the disposable bag. ____ ____ _____
45. Emptied, cleaned, and disinfected equipment. Returned equipment to its proper place. ____ ____ _____
46. Removed the gloves. Practiced hand hygiene. ____ ____ _____
47. Completed a safety check of the room. ____ ____ _____
48. Followed center policy for dirty linens. ____ ____ _____
49. Practiced hand hygiene. ____ ____ _____
50. Reported and recorded your observations. ____ ____ _____

Performing Range of Motion Exercises (NATCEP)

Name: _____   Date: _____

	S	U	Comments

Quality of Life

Remembered to:
- Knock before entering the person's room.
- Address the person by name.
- Introduce yourself by name and title.
- Explain the procedure to the person before beginning and during the procedure.
- Protect the person's rights during the procedure.
- Handle the person gently during the procedure.

Preprocedure

1. Followed *Delegation Guidelines: Range of Motion Exercises*
   Saw *Promoting Safety and Comfort: Range of Motion Exercises*
2. Practiced hand hygiene.
3. Identified the person. Checked the identification (ID) bracelet against the assignment sheet. Also called the person by name.
4. Obtained a bath blanket.
5. Provided for privacy.
6. Raised the bed for body mechanics. Bed rails were up if used.

Procedure

7. Lowered the bed rail near you if up.
8. Positioned the person supine.
9. Covered the person with a bath blanket. Fan-folded top linens to the foot of the bed.
10. Exercised the neck *if allowed by the center and if instructed to do so by the nurse*:
    a. Placed your hands over the person's ears to support the head. Supported the jaws with your fingers.
    b. Flexion—brought the head forward. The chin touched the chest.
    c. Extension—straightened the head.
    d. Hyperextension—brought the head backward until the chin pointed up.
    e. Rotation—turned the head from side to side.
    f. Lateral flexion—moved the head to the right and to the left.
    g. Repeated flexion, extension, hyperextension, rotation, and lateral flexion five times—or the number of times stated on the care plan.
11. Exercised the shoulder:
    a. Grasped the wrist with one hand. Grasped the elbow with the other hand.
    b. Flexion—raised the arm straight in front and over the head.
    c. Extension—brought the arm down to the side.
    d. Hyperextension—moved the arm behind the body. (Did this if the person was sitting in a straight-backed chair or was standing.)
    e. Abduction—moved the straight arm away from the side of the body.
    f. Adduction—moved the straight arm to the side of the body.
    g. Internal rotation—bent the elbow. Placed it at the same level as the shoulder. Moved the forearm down toward the body.

Procedure—cont'd	S	U	Comments

   h. External rotation—moved the forearm toward the head.

   i. Repeated flexion, extension, hyperextension, abduction, adduction, and internal and external rotation five times—or the number of times stated on the care plan.

12. Exercised the elbow:

   a. Grasped the person's wrist with one hand. Grasped the elbow with your other hand.

   b. Flexion—bent the arm so the same-side shoulder was touched.

   c. Extension—straightened the arm.

   d. Repeated flexion and extension five times—or the number of times stated on the care plan.

13. Exercised the forearm:

   a. Continue to support the wrist and elbow.

   b. Pronation—turned the hand so the palm was down.

   c. Supination—turned the hand so the palm was up.

   d. Repeated pronation and supination five times—or the number of times stated on the care plan.

14. Exercised the wrist:

   a. Held the wrist with both of your hands.

   b. Flexion—bent the hand down.

   c. Extension—straightened the hand.

   d. Hyperextension—bent the hand back.

   e. Radial flexion—turned the hand toward the thumb.

   f. Ulnar flexion—turned the hand toward the little finger.

   g. Repeated flexion, extension, hyperextension, radial flexion, and ulnar flexion five times—or the number of times stated on the care plan.

15. Exercised the thumb:

   a. Held the person's hand with one hand. Held the thumb with your other hand.

   b. Abduction—moved the thumb out from the inner part of the index finger.

   c. Adduction—moved the thumb back next to the index finger.

   d. Opposition—touched each fingertip with the thumb.

   e. Flexion—bent the thumb into the hand.

   f. Extension—moved the thumb out to the side of the fingers.

   g. Repeated abduction, adduction, opposition, flexion, and extension five times—or the number of times stated on the care plan.

16. Exercised the fingers:

   a. Abduction—spread the fingers and the thumb apart.

   b. Adduction—bought the fingers and thumb together.

   c. Flexion—made a fist.

   d. Extension—straightened the fingers so the fingers, hand, and arm were straight.

   e. Repeated abduction, adduction, flexion, and extension five times—or the number of times stated on the care plan.

17. Exercised the hip:

   a. Supported the leg. Placed one hand under the knee. Placed your other hand under the ankle.

   b. Flexion—raised the leg.

   c. Extension—straightened the leg.

   d. Abduction—moved the leg away from the body.

   e. Adduction—moved the leg toward the other leg.

   f. Internal rotation—turned the leg inward.

   g. External rotation—turned the leg outward.

Procedure—cont'd	S	U	Comments

Procedure—cont'd

h. Repeated flexion, extension, abduction, adduction, and internal and external rotation five times—or the number of times stated on the care plan. ＿＿＿ ＿＿＿ ＿＿＿＿＿

18. Exercised the knee:
   a. Supported the knee. Placed one hand under the knee. Placed your other hand under the ankle. ＿＿＿ ＿＿＿ ＿＿＿＿＿
   b. Flexion—bent the knee. ＿＿＿ ＿＿＿ ＿＿＿＿＿
   c. Extension—straightened the knee. ＿＿＿ ＿＿＿ ＿＿＿＿＿
   d. Repeated flexion and extension of the knee five times— or the number of times stated on the care plan. ＿＿＿ ＿＿＿ ＿＿＿＿＿

19. Exercised the ankle:
   a. Supported the foot and ankle. Placed one hand under the foot. Placed your other hand under the ankle. ＿＿＿ ＿＿＿ ＿＿＿＿＿
   b. Dorsiflexion—pulled the foot upward. Pushed down on the heel at the same time. ＿＿＿ ＿＿＿ ＿＿＿＿＿
   c. Plantar flexion—turned the foot down. Or pointed the toes. ＿＿＿ ＿＿＿ ＿＿＿＿＿
   d. Repeated dorsiflexion and plantar flexion five times— or the number of times stated on the care plan. ＿＿＿ ＿＿＿ ＿＿＿＿＿

20. Exercised the foot:
   a. Continued to support the foot and ankle. ＿＿＿ ＿＿＿ ＿＿＿＿＿
   b. Pronation—turned the outside of the foot up and the inside down. ＿＿＿ ＿＿＿ ＿＿＿＿＿
   c. Supination—turned the inside of the foot up and the outside down. ＿＿＿ ＿＿＿ ＿＿＿＿＿
   d. Repeated pronation and supination five times—or the number of times stated on the care plan. ＿＿＿ ＿＿＿ ＿＿＿＿＿

21. Exercised the toes:
   a. Flexion—curled the toes. ＿＿＿ ＿＿＿ ＿＿＿＿＿
   b. Extension—straightened the toes. ＿＿＿ ＿＿＿ ＿＿＿＿＿
   c. Abduction—spread the toes apart. ＿＿＿ ＿＿＿ ＿＿＿＿＿
   d. Adduction—pulled the toes together. ＿＿＿ ＿＿＿ ＿＿＿＿＿
   e. Repeated flexion, extension, abduction, and adduction five times—or the number of times stated on the care plan. ＿＿＿ ＿＿＿ ＿＿＿＿＿

22. Covered the leg. Raised the bed rail if used. ＿＿＿ ＿＿＿ ＿＿＿＿＿

23. Went to the other side. Lowered the bed rail near you if up. ＿＿＿ ＿＿＿ ＿＿＿＿＿

24. Repeated exercises:
   a. Exercised the shoulder:
      i. Grasped the wrist with one hand. Grasped the elbow with the other hand. ＿＿＿ ＿＿＿ ＿＿＿＿＿
      ii. Flexion—raised the arm straight in front and over the head. ＿＿＿ ＿＿＿ ＿＿＿＿＿
      iii. Extension—brought the arm down to the side. ＿＿＿ ＿＿＿ ＿＿＿＿＿
      iv. Hyperextension—moved the arm behind the body. (Did this if the person was sitting in a straight-backed chair or was standing.) ＿＿＿ ＿＿＿ ＿＿＿＿＿
      v. Abduction—moved the straight arm away from the side of the body. ＿＿＿ ＿＿＿ ＿＿＿＿＿
      vi. Adduction—moved the straight arm to the side of the body. ＿＿＿ ＿＿＿ ＿＿＿＿＿
      vii. Internal rotation—bent the elbow. Placed it at the same level as the shoulder. Moved the forearm down toward the body. ＿＿＿ ＿＿＿ ＿＿＿＿＿
      viii. External rotation—moved the forearm toward the head. ＿＿＿ ＿＿＿ ＿＿＿＿＿
      ix. Repeated flexion, extension, hyperextension, abduction, adduction, and internal and external rotation five times— or the number of times stated on the care plan. ＿＿＿ ＿＿＿ ＿＿＿＿＿

Procedure—cont'd   S   U   Comments

   b. Exercised the elbow:
      i.   Grasped the person's wrist with one hand. Grasped the elbow with
           your other hand.   _____   _____   _____
      ii. Flexion—bent the arm so the same-side shoulder was touched.   _____   _____   _____
      iii. Extension—straightened the arm.   _____   _____   _____
      iv. Repeated flexion and extension five times—or the number of
           times stated on the care plan.   _____   _____   _____
   c. Exercised the forearm:
      i.   Continued to support the wrist and elbow.   _____   _____   _____
      ii. Pronation—turned the hand so the palm was down.   _____   _____   _____
      iii. Supination—turned the hand so the palm was up.   _____   _____   _____
      iv. Repeated pronation and supination five times—or the number of
           times stated on the care plan.   _____   _____   _____
   d. Exercised the wrist:
      i.   Held the wrist with both of your hands.   _____   _____   _____
      ii. Flexion—bent the hand down.   _____   _____   _____
      iii. Extension—straightened the hand.   _____   _____   _____
      iv. Hyperextension—bent the hand back.   _____   _____   _____
      v.   Radial flexion—turned the hand toward the thumb.   _____   _____   _____
      vi. Ulnar flexion—turned the hand toward the little finger.   _____   _____   _____
      vii. Repeated flexion, extension, hyperextension, radial flexion, and
           ulnar flexion five times—or the number of times stated on the care
           plan.   _____   _____   _____
   e. Exercised the thumb:
      i.   Held the person's hand with one hand. Held the thumb with your
           other hand.   _____   _____   _____
      ii. Abduction—moved the thumb out from the inner part of the index
           finger.   _____   _____   _____
      iii. Adduction—moved the thumb back next to the index finger.   _____   _____   _____
      iv. Opposition—touched each fingertip with the thumb.   _____   _____   _____
      v.   Flexion—bent the thumb into the hand.   _____   _____   _____
      vi. Extension—moved the thumb out to the side of the fingers.   _____   _____   _____
      vii. Repeated abduction, adduction, opposition, flexion, and extension
           five times—or the number of times stated on the care plan.   _____   _____   _____
   f. Exercised the fingers:
      i.   Abduction—spread the fingers and the thumb apart.   _____   _____   _____
      ii. Adduction—bought the fingers and thumb together.   _____   _____   _____
      iii. Flexion—made a fist.   _____   _____   _____
      iv. Extension—straightened the fingers so the fingers, hand, and arm
           were straight.   _____   _____   _____
      v.   Repeated abduction, adduction, flexion, and extension five
           times—or the number of times stated on the care plan.   _____   _____   _____
   g. Exercised the hip:
      i.   Supported the leg. Placed one hand under the knee. Placed your
           other hand under the ankle.   _____   _____   _____
      ii. Flexion—raised the leg.   _____   _____   _____
      iii. Extension—straightened the leg.   _____   _____   _____
      iv. Abduction—moved the leg away from the body.   _____   _____   _____
      v.   Adduction—moved the leg toward the other leg.   _____   _____   _____
      vi. Internal rotation—turned the leg inward.   _____   _____   _____
      vii. External rotation—turned the leg outward.   _____   _____   _____
      viii. Repeated flexion, extension, abduction, adduction, and internal
           and external rotation five times—or the number of times stated on
           the care plan.   _____   _____   _____

Procedure—cont'd	S	U	Comments

h. Exercised the knee:
   i. Supported the knee. Placed one hand under the knee. Placed your other hand under the ankle. _____ _____ _____
   ii. Flexion—bent the knee. _____ _____ _____
   iii. Extension—straightened the knee. _____ _____ _____
   iv. Repeated flexion and extension of the knee five times— or the number of times stated on the care plan. _____ _____ _____

i. Exercised the ankle:
   i. Supported the foot and ankle. Placed one hand under the foot. Placed your other hand under the ankle. _____ _____ _____
   ii. Dorsiflexion—pulled the foot upward. Pushed down on the heel at the same time. _____ _____ _____
   iii. Plantar flexion—turned the foot down. Or pointed the toes. _____ _____ _____
   iv. Repeated dorsiflexion and plantar flexion five times— or the number of times stated on the care plan. _____ _____ _____

j. Exercised the foot:
   i. Continued to support the foot and ankle. _____ _____ _____
   ii. Pronation—turned the outside of the foot up and the inside down. _____ _____ _____
   iii. Supination—turned the inside of the foot up and the outside down. _____ _____ _____
   iv. Repeated pronation and supination five times—or the number of times stated on the care plan. _____ _____ _____

k. Exercised the toes:
   i. Flexion—curled the toes. _____ _____ _____
   ii. Extension—straightened the toes. _____ _____ _____
   iii. Abduction—spread the toes apart. _____ _____ _____
   iv. Adduction—pulled the toes together. _____ _____ _____
   v. Repeated flexion, extension, abduction, and adduction five times—or the number of times stated on the care plan. _____ _____ _____

Postprocedure

25. Provided for comfort. _____ _____ _____
26. Removed the bath blanket. _____ _____ _____
27. Placed the call light within reach. _____ _____ _____
28. Lowered the bed to its lowest position. _____ _____ _____
29. Raised or lowered bed rails. Followed the care plan. _____ _____ _____
30. Folded and returned the bath blanket its proper place. _____ _____ _____
31. Unscreened the person. _____ _____ _____
32. Completed a safety check of the room. _____ _____ _____
33. Decontaminated your hands. _____ _____ _____
34. Reported and recorded your observations. _____ _____ _____

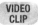 **Helping the Person Walk**

Name: _____   Date: _____

	S	**U**	**Comments**

Quality of Life

Remembered to:
- Knock before entering the person's room.
- Address the person by name.
- Introduce yourself by name and title.
- Explain the procedure to the person before beginning and during the procedure.
- Protect the person's rights during the procedure.
- Handle the person gently during the procedure.

Preprocedure

1. Followed *Delegation Guidelines: Ambulation*
   Saw *Promoting Safety and Comfort: Ambulation*
2. Practiced hand hygiene.
3. Collected the following:
   a. Robe, socks, and nonskid shoes
   b. Paper or sheet to protect bottom linens
   c. Gait (transfer) belt
4. Identified the person. Checked the identification (ID) bracelet against the assignment sheet. Also called the person by name.
5. Provided for privacy.

Procedure

6. Lowered the bed to its lowest position. Locked the bed wheels. Lowered the bed rail if up.
7. Fan-folded top linens to the foot of the bed.
8. Placed the paper or sheet under the person's feet. Put the socks and shoes on the person. Fastened the shoes.
9. Helped the person sit on the side of the bed.
10. Helped the person put on the robe.
11. Made sure the person's feet were flat on the floor.
12. Applied the gait belt.
13. Helped the person stand. Grasped the gait belt at each side. If no gait belt, placed your arms under the person's arms around to the shoulder blades.
14. Stood at the person's weak side while he or she gained balance. Held the belt at the side and back. If not using a gait belt, had one arm around the back and the other at the elbow to support the person.
15. Encouraged the person to stand erect with the head up and back straight.
16. Helped the person walk. Walked to the side and slightly behind the person on the person's weak side. Provided support with the gait belt. If not using a gait belt, had one arm around the back and the other at the elbow to support the person. Encouraged the person to use the handrail on his or her strong side.
17. Encouraged the person to walk normally. The heel struck the floor first. Discouraged shuffling, sliding, or walking on tiptoes.
18. Walked the required distance if the person tolerated the activity. Did not rush the person.
19. Helped the person return to bed. Removed the gait belt.
20. Lowered the head of the bed. Helped the person to the center of the bed.
21. Removed the shoes. Removed the paper or sheet over the bottom sheet.

347

Postprocedure

	S	U	Comments
22. Provided for comfort.	___	___	_____
23. Placed the call light within reach.	___	___	_____
24. Raised or lowered bed rails. Followed the care plan.	___	___	_____
25. Returned the robe and shoes to their proper place.	___	___	_____
26. Unscreened the person.	___	___	_____
27. Completed a safety check of the room.	___	___	_____
28. Decontaminated your hands.	___	___	_____
29. Reported and recorded your observations.	___	___	_____

Using a Pulse Oximeter

Name: _____ Date: _____

Quality of Life	**S**	**U**	**Comments**

Remembered to:
- Knock before entering the person's room.
- Address the person by name.
- Introduce yourself by name and title.
- Explain the procedure to the person before beginning and during the procedure.
- Protect the person's rights during the procedure.
- Handle the person gently during the procedure.

Preprocedure

1. Followed *Delegation Guidelines: Pulse Oximetry*
   Saw *Promoting Safety and Comfort: Pulse Oximetry*
2. Practiced hand hygiene.
3. Collected the following:
   a. Oximeter and sensor
   b. Tape
   c. Towel
4. Arranged your work area.
5. Decontaminated your hands.
6. Identified the person. Checked the identification (ID) bracelet against the assignment sheet. Also called the person by name.
7. Provided for privacy.

Procedure

8. Provided for comfort.
9. Dried the site with a towel.
10. Clipped or taped the sensor to the site.
11. Turned on the oximeter.
12. Set the high and low alarm limits for saturation of peripheral oxygen (SpO_2) and pulse rate. Turned on audio and visual alarms. (This step was done for continuous monitoring.)
13. Checked the person's pulse (apical or radial) with the pulse on the display. The pulses should have been about the same. Noted both pulses on the assignment sheet.
14. Read the SpO_2 on the display. Noted the value on the flow sheet and the assignment sheet. Also recorded if the person received supplemental oxygen and the flow rate.
15. Left the sensor in place for continuous monitoring. Otherwise, turned off the device and removed the sensor. If continuous monitoring, the site sensor was changed at least every 2 hours.

Postprocedure

16. Provided for comfort.
17. Placed the call light within reach.
18. Unscreened the person.
19. Completed a safety check of the room.
20. Returned the device to its proper place (unless monitoring was continuous).
21. Decontaminated your hands.
22. Reported and recorded the SpO_2, the pulse rates, and your other observations.

Assisting with Deep-Breathing and Coughing Exercises

Name: _____   Date: _____

Quality of Life	S	U	Comments
Remembered to:			
• Knock before entering the person's room.	___	___	_____
• Address the person by name.	___	___	_____
• Introduce yourself by name and title.	___	___	_____
• Explain the procedure to the person before beginning and during the procedure.	___	___	_____
• Protect the person's rights during the procedure.	___	___	_____
• Handle the person gently during the procedure.	___	___	_____

Preprocedure			
1. Followed *Delegation Guidelines: Deep Breathing and Coughing*	___	___	_____
Saw *Promoting Safety and Comfort: Deep Breathing and Coughing*	___	___	_____
2. Practiced hand hygiene.	___	___	_____
3. Collected the following before going to the person's room:			
a. Box of tissues	___	___	_____
b. Gloves	___	___	_____
c. Mask (needed for persons with respiratory infections)	___	___	_____
4. Identified the person. Checked the identification (ID) bracelet against the assignment sheet. Also called the person by name.	___	___	_____
5. Provided for privacy.	___	___	_____

Procedure			
6. Lowered the bed rail if up.	___	___	_____
7. Helped the person to a comfortable sitting position: sitting on the side of the bed, semi-Fowler, or Fowler.	___	___	_____
8. Put on gloves and mask if required.	___	___	_____
9. Had the person deep breathe:			
a. Had the person place the hands over the rib cage.	___	___	_____
b. Had the person take a deep breath. It was as deep as possible. Reminded the person to inhale through the nose.	___	___	_____
c. Asked the person to hold the breath for 2–3 seconds.	___	___	_____
d. Asked the person to exhale slowly through pursed lips. Asked the person to exhale until the ribs moved as far down as possible.	___	___	_____
e. Repeated four more times:			
i. Deep breathed in through the nose.	___	___	_____
ii. Held 2–3 seconds.	___	___	_____
iii. Exhaled slowly with pursed lips until the ribs moved as far down as possible.	___	___	_____
10. Asked the person to cough:			
a. Had the person place both hands over the incision. One hand was on top of the other. The person could have held a pillow or folded towel over the incision.	___	___	_____
b. Had the person take a deep breath through the nose.	___	___	_____
c. Asked the person to cough strongly twice with the mouth open.	___	___	_____
d. Had box of tissues within person's reach for productive cough.	___	___	_____

Postprocedure			
11. Provided for comfort.	___	___	_____
12. Placed the call light within reach.	___	___	_____
13. Raised or lowered the bed rails. Followed the care plan.	___	___	_____

Postprocedure—cont'd   S   U   Comments

14. Unscreened the person.   ___   ___   _____
15. Completed a safety check of the room.   ___   ___   _____
16. Removed gloves and decontaminated your hands.   ___   ___   _____
17. Reported and recorded your observations.   ___   ___   _____

Assisting with Incentive Spirometry

Name: _____ Date: _____

	S	U	Comments

Quality of Life

Remembered to:
- Knock before entering the person's room.
- Address the person by name.
- Introduce yourself by name and title.
- Explain the procedure to the person before beginning and during the procedure.
- Protect the person's rights during the procedure.
- Handle the person gently during the procedure.

Preprocedure

1. Followed *Delegation Guidelines: Incentive Spirometry*
2. Practiced hand hygiene.
3. Collected the following before going into the person's room:
   a. Box of tissues
   b. Gloves
   c. Spirometer
4. Identified the person. Checked the identification (ID) bracelet against the assignment sheet. Also called the person by name.
5. Provided for privacy.

Procedure

6. Lowered the bed rail if up.
7. Helped the person to a comfortable sitting position: sitting on the side of the bed, semi-Fowler, or Fowler.
8. Had the person hold the spirometer upright.
9. Asked the person to exhale normally.
10. Had the person seal his or her lips around the mouthpiece of the spirometer.
11. Asked the person to take a slow, deep breath until the balls rose to the desired height.
12. Asked the person to hold the breath for 3–6 seconds to keep the balls floating.
13. Had the person remove the mouthpiece and exhale slowly. The person coughed at this time, if necessary.
14. Asked the person to take some normal breaths, then use device again.
15. The nurse or care plan will direct how many times the person should repeat the breaths with the spirometer (often 10 times).

Postprocedure

16. Provided for comfort.
17. Placed the call light within reach.
18. Raised or lowered the bed rails. Followed the care plan.
19. Unscreened the person.
20. Completed a safety check of the room.
21. Decontaminated your hands.
22. Reported and recorded your observations.

Setting up for Oxygen Administration

Name: _____   Date: _____

	S	U	Comments
Quality of Life			

Remembered to:
- Knock before entering the person's room.
- Address the person by name.
- Introduce yourself by name and title.
- Explain the procedure to the person before beginning and during the procedure.
- Protect the person's rights during the procedure.
- Handle the person gently during the procedure.

Preprocedure

1. Followed *Delegation Guidelines: Oxygen Administration Set-Up*
   Saw *Promoting Safety and Comfort: Oxygen Administration Set-Up*
2. Practiced hand hygiene.
3. Collected the following before going to the person's room:
   a. Oxygen device with connection tubing
   b. Flowmeter
   c. Humidifier (if ordered)
   d. Distilled water (if using humidifier)
4. Arranged your work area.
5. Decontaminated your hands.
6. Identified the person. Checked the identification (ID) bracelet against the assignment sheet. Also called the person by name.

Procedure

7. Made sure the flowmeter was in the OFF position.
8. Attached the flowmeter to the wall outlet or to the tank.
9. Filled the humidifier with distilled water.
10. Attached the humidifier to the bottom of the flowmeter.
11. Attached the oxygen device and connected tubing to the humidifier. *Did not set the flowmeter. Did not apply the oxygen device on the person.*
12. Placed the cap securely on the distilled water. Stored the water according to center policy.
13. Discarded the packaging from the oxygen device and connecting tubing.

Postprocedure

14. Provided for comfort.
15. Placed the call light within reach.
16. Decontaminated your hands.
17. Completed a safety check of the room.
18. Told the nurse when you were done. *The nurse then*:
    a. *Turned on the oxygen and set the flow rate.*
    b. *Applied the oxygen device on the person.*

Taking a Temperature With an Electronic Thermometer (NATCEP)

Name: _____   Date: _____

Quality of Life	S	U	Comments

Remembered to:
- Knock before entering the person's room.
- Address the person by name.
- Introduce yourself by name and title.
- Explain the procedure to the person before beginning and during the procedure.
- Protect the person's rights during the procedure.
- Handle the person gently during the procedure.

Preprocedure

1. Followed *Delegation Guidelines: Taking Temperatures*
   Saw *Promoting Safety and Comfort: Taking Temperatures*
2. For an oral temperature, asked the person not to eat, drink, smoke, or chew gum for at least 15–20 minutes before measurement or as required by center policy.
3. Practiced hand hygiene.
4. Collected the following:
   a. Thermometer—electronic, tympanic membrane, or temporal
   b. Probe (blue for an oral or axillary temperature; red for a rectal temperature)
   c. Probe covers
   d. Toilet tissue (rectal temperature)
   e. Water-soluble lubricant (rectal temperature)
   f. Gloves
   g. Towel (axillary temperature)
5. Plugged the probe into the thermometer, if using an electronic thermometer.
6. Decontaminated your hands.
7. Identified the person. Checked the identification (ID) bracelet against the assignment sheet. Also called the person by name.

Procedure

8. Provided for privacy. Positioned the person for an oral, rectal, axillary, or tympanic membrane temperature.
9. Put on the gloves if contact with blood, body fluid, secretions, or excretions was likely.
10. Inserted the probe into a probe cover.
11. For an *oral temperature*:
    a. Asked the person to open the mouth and raise the tongue.
    b. Placed the covered probe at the base of the tongue and to one side.
    c. Asked the person to lower the tongue and close the mouth.
12. For a rectal *temperature*:
    a. Placed some lubricant on toilet tissue.
    b. Lubricated the end of the covered probe.
    c. Exposed the anal area.
    d. Raised the upper buttock.
    e. Inserted the probe ½ inch into the rectum.
    f. Held the probe in place.
13. For an *axillary temperature*:
    a. Helped the person remove an arm from the gown. Did not expose the person.
    b. Dried the axilla with a towel.
    c. Placed the covered probe in the center of the axilla.

Procedure—cont'd	S	U	Comments
d. Placed the person's arm over the chest.	———	———	—————
e. Held the probe in place.	———	———	—————
14. For a *tympanic membrane temperature*:			
a. Asked the person to turn his or her head so the ear was in front of you.	———	———	—————
b. Pulled up and back on the adult's ear to straighten the ear canal.	———	———	—————
c. Inserted the covered probe gently.	———	———	—————
15. Started the thermometer.	———	———	—————
16. Held the probe in place until you heard a tone or saw a flashing or steady light.	———	———	—————
17. Read the temperature on the display.	———	———	—————
18. Removed the probe. Pressed the eject button to discard the cover.	———	———	—————
19. For a *temporal artery temperature*:			
a. Asked the person to turn his or her face toward you.	———	———	—————
b. Placed the device near the center of the forehead. Pressed the button.	———	———	—————
c. While keeping the button depressed, slid the device across the forehead and over the temporal artery, ending in front of the ear. (If the person had perspiration on the forehead, continued sliding the device to the back of the ear.) Followed manufacturer's instructions.	———	———	—————
20. Noted the person's name and temperature on your notepad or assignment sheet. Noted the temperature site.	———	———	—————
21. Returned the probe to the holder.	———	———	—————
22. Helped the person put the gown back on (axillary temperature). For a rectal temperature:	———	———	—————
a. Wiped the anal area with toilet tissue to remove lubricant.	———	———	—————
b. Covered the person.	———	———	—————
c. Disposed of used toilet tissue.	———	———	—————
d. Removed the gloves. Practiced hand hygiene.	———	———	—————
23. For a *noncontact infrared thermometer*:			
a. Asked the person to pull back any hair from forehead.	———	———	—————
b. Held thermometer the recommended distance from the person's forehead.	———	———	—————
c. Pressed the button on thermometer.	———	———	—————
d. Noted the reading.	———	———	—————

Postprocedure

	S	U	Comments
24. Provided for comfort.	———	———	—————
25. Placed the call light within reach.	———	———	—————
26. Unscreened the person.	———	———	—————
27. Completed a safety check of the room.	———	———	—————
28. Returned the thermometer to the charging unit.	———	———	—————
29. Decontaminated your hands.	———	———	—————
30. Reported and recorded the temperature. Noted the temperature site when reporting and recording. A rectal temperature was noted with an "R" after the value. An axillary temperature was recorded with an "Ax" after the value. Reported an abnormal temperature at once.	———	———	—————

Taking a Radial Pulse (NATCEP)

Name: _____ Date: _____

Quality of Life	S	U	Comments
Remembered to:			
• Knock before entering the person's room.	____	____	_____
• Address the person by name.	____	____	_____
• Introduce yourself by name and title.	____	____	_____
• Explain the procedure to the person before beginning and during the procedure.	____	____	_____
• Protect the person's rights during the procedure.	____	____	_____
• Handle the person gently during the procedure.	____	____	_____

Preprocedure

	S	U	Comments
1. Followed *Delegation Guidelines: Taking Pulses*	____	____	_____
Saw *Promoting Safety and Comfort: Taking Pulses*	____	____	_____
2. Practiced hand hygiene.	____	____	_____
3. Identified the person. Checked the identification (ID) bracelet against the assignment sheet. Also called the person by name.	____	____	_____
4. Provided for privacy.	____	____	_____

Procedure

	S	U	Comments
5. Had the person sit or lie down.	____	____	_____
6. Located the radial pulse on the thumb side of the person's wrist. Used your first 2 or 3 middle fingertips.	____	____	_____
7. Noted if the pulse was strong or weak, regular or irregular.	____	____	_____
8. Counted the pulse for 30 seconds. Multiplied the number of beats by 2. Or counted the pulse for 1 minute if:	____	____	_____
a. Directed by the nurse and care plan.	____	____	_____
b. Required by center policy.	____	____	_____
c. The pulse was irregular.	____	____	_____
d. Required for your state competency test.	____	____	_____
9. Noted the person's name and pulse on your notepad or assignment sheet. Noted the strength of the pulse. Noted if it was regular or irregular.	____	____	_____

Postprocedure

	S	U	Comments
10. Provided for comfort.	____	____	_____
11. Placed the call light within reach.	____	____	_____
12. Unscreened the person.	____	____	_____
13. Completed a safety check of the room.	____	____	_____
14. Decontaminated your hands.	____	____	_____
15. Reported and recorded the pulse rate and your observations. Reported an abnormal pulse at once.	____	____	_____

Taking an Apical Pulse

Name: _____   Date: _____

	S	U	Comments
Quality of Life			
Remembered to:			
• Knock before entering the person's room.	___	___	_____
• Address the person by name.	___	___	_____
• Introduce yourself by name and title.	___	___	_____
• Explain the procedure to the person before beginning and during the procedure.	___	___	_____
• Protect the person's rights during the procedure.	___	___	_____
• Handle the person gently during the procedure.	___	___	_____

Preprocedure

	S	U	Comments
1. Followed *Delegation Guidelines: Taking Pulses*	___	___	_____
Saw *Promoting Safety and Comfort: Using a Stethoscope*	___	___	_____
2. Practiced hand hygiene.	___	___	_____
3. Collected a stethoscope and antiseptic wipes.	___	___	_____
4. Decontaminated your hands.	___	___	_____
5. Identified the person. Checked the identification (ID) bracelet against the assignment sheet. Also called the person by name.	___	___	_____
6. Provided for privacy.	___	___	_____

Procedure

	S	U	Comments
7. Cleaned the earpieces and diaphragm with the wipes.	___	___	_____
8. Had the person sit or lie down.	___	___	_____
9. Exposed the nipple area of the left chest. Exposed a woman's breasts to the extent necessary.	___	___	_____
10. Warmed the diaphragm in your palm.	___	___	_____
11. Placed the earpieces in your ears.	___	___	_____
12. Found the apical pulse. Placed the diaphragm 2–3 inches to the left of the breastbone and below the left nipple.	___	___	_____
13. Counted the pulse for 1 minute. Noted if the pulse was regular or irregular.	___	___	_____
14. Covered the person. Removed the earpieces.	___	___	_____
15. Noted the person's name and pulse on your notepad or assignment sheet. Noted if the pulse was regular or irregular.	___	___	_____

Postprocedure

	S	U	Comments
16. Provided for comfort.	___	___	_____
17. Placed the call light within reach.	___	___	_____
18. Unscreened the person.	___	___	_____
19. Completed a safety check of the room.	___	___	_____
20. Cleaned the earpieces and diaphragm with the wipes.	___	___	_____
21. Returned the stethoscope to its proper place.	___	___	_____
22. Decontaminated your hands.	___	___	_____
23. Reported and recorded your observations. Recorded the pulse rate with *Ap* for apical. Reported an abnormal pulse rate at once.	___	___	_____

Taking an Apical-Radial Pulse

Name: _____ Date: _____

	S	U	Comments
Quality of Life			
Remembered to:			
• Knock before entering the person's room.	___	___	_____
• Address the person by name.	___	___	_____
• Introduce yourself by name and title.	___	___	_____
• Explain the procedure to the person before beginning and during the procedure.	___	___	_____
• Protect the person's rights during the procedure.	___	___	_____
• Handle the person gently during the procedure.	___	___	_____

Preprocedure

	S	U	Comments
1. Followed *Delegation Guidelines: Taking Pulses*	___	___	_____
Saw *Promoting Safety and Comfort:*			
a. *Using a Stethoscope*	___	___	_____
b. *Taking Pulses*	___	___	_____
2. Asked a coworker to help you.	___	___	_____
3. Practiced hand hygiene.	___	___	_____
4. Collected a stethoscope and antiseptic wipes.	___	___	_____
5. Decontaminated your hands.	___	___	_____
6. Identified the person. Checked the identification (ID) bracelet against the assignment sheet. Also called the person by name.	___	___	_____
7. Provided for privacy.	___	___	_____

Procedure

	S	U	Comments
8. Cleaned the earpieces and diaphragm with the wipes.	___	___	_____
9. Had the person sit or lie down.	___	___	_____
10. Exposed the nipple area of the left chest. Exposed a woman's breasts only to the extent necessary.	___	___	_____
11. Warmed the diaphragm in your palm.	___	___	_____
12. Placed the earpieces in your ears.	___	___	_____
13. Found the apical pulse. The coworker found the radial pulse.	___	___	_____
14. Gave the signal to begin counting.	___	___	_____
15. Counted the pulse for 1 minute.	___	___	_____
16. Gave the signal to stop counting.	___	___	_____
17. Covered the person. Removed the stethoscope earpieces.	___	___	_____
18. Noted the person's name and apical and radial pulses on your notepad or assignment sheet. Subtracted the radial pulse from the apical pulse for the pulse deficit. Noted if the pulses were regular or irregular.	___	___	_____

Postprocedure

	S	U	Comments
19. Provided for comfort.	___	___	_____
20. Placed the call light within reach.	___	___	_____
21. Unscreened the person.	___	___	_____
22. Completed a safety check of the room.	___	___	_____
23. Cleaned the earpieces and diaphragm with the wipes.	___	___	_____
24. Returned the stethoscope to its proper place.	___	___	_____
25. Decontaminated your hands.	___	___	_____
26. Reported and recorded your observations. (Reported an abnormal pulse at once.) Included:			
a. The apical and radial pulse rates	___	___	_____
b. The pulse deficit	___	___	_____

Counting Respirations (NATCEP)

Name: _____ Date: _____

	S	U	Comments

Preprocedure

1. Followed *Delegation Guidelines: Respirations*
2. Kept your fingers or stethoscope over the pulse site.
3. Did not tell the person you were counting respirations.
4. Began counting when the chest rose. Counted each rise and fall of the chest as 1 respiration.
5. Noted the following:
   a. If respirations were regular
   b. If both sides of the chest rose equally
   c. The depth of the respirations
   d. If the person had any pain or difficulty breathing
   e. An abnormal respiratory pattern
6. Counted respirations for 30 seconds. Multiplied the number by 2. Counted respirations for 1 minute if:
   a. Directed by the nurse and care plan.
   b. Required by center policy.
   c. Respirations were abnormal or irregular.
   d. Required for the state competency test.
7. Noted the person's name, respiratory rate, and other observations on your notepad or assignment sheet.

Postprocedure

8. Provided for comfort.
9. Placed the call light within reach.
10. Unscreened the person.
11. Completed a safety check of the room.
12. Decontaminated your hands.
13. Reported and recorded the respiratory rate and your observations. Reported abnormal respirations at once.

Name: _____   Date: _____

Quality of Life	S	U	Comments
Remembered to:			
• Knock before entering the person's room.	___	___	_____
• Address the person by name.	___	___	_____
• Introduce yourself by name and title.	___	___	_____
• Explain the procedure to the person before beginning and during the procedure.	___	___	_____
• Protect the person's rights during the procedure.	___	___	_____
• Handle the person gently during the procedure.	___	___	_____

Preprocedure

	S	U	Comments
1. Followed *Delegation Guidelines: Measuring Blood Pressure*	___	___	_____
Saw *Promoting Safety and Comfort: Using a Stethoscope*	___	___	_____
2. Practiced hand hygiene.	___	___	_____
3. Collected the following:			
a. Sphygmomanometer	___	___	_____
b. Stethoscope	___	___	_____
c. Antiseptic wipes	___	___	_____
4. Decontaminated your hands.	___	___	_____
5. Identified the person. Checked the identification (ID) bracelet against the assignment sheet. Also called the person by name.	___	___	_____
6. Provided for privacy.	___	___	_____

Procedure

	S	U	Comments
7. Wiped the stethoscope earpieces and diaphragm with the wipes. Warmed the diaphragm in your palm.	___	___	_____
8. Had the person sit or lie down. If sitting in a chair, asked the person to put both feet on the floor.	___	___	_____
9. Positioned the person's arm level with the heart. The palm was up.	___	___	_____
10. Stood no more than 3 feet away from the manometer. The aneroid type was directly in front of you or mounted on the wall.	___	___	_____
11. Exposed the upper arm.	___	___	_____
12. Squeezed the cuff to expel any remaining air. Closed the valve on the bulb.	___	___	_____
13. Found the brachial artery at the inner aspect of the elbow (on the little finger side of the arm). Used your fingertips.	___	___	_____
14. Located the arrow on the cuff. Placed the arrow on the cuff over the brachial artery. Wrapped the cuff around the upper arm at least 1 inch above the elbow. It was even and snug.	___	___	_____
15. Placed the stethoscope earpieces in your ears.	___	___	_____
16. Placed the diaphragm of the stethoscope over the brachial artery. Did not place it under the cuff.	___	___	_____
17. Inflated the cuff between 160 and 180 mm Hg.	___	___	_____
18. Deflated the cuff at an even rate of 2–4 mm per second. Turned the valve counterclockwise to deflate the cuff.	___	___	_____
19. If a beat was heard immediately upon deflation, completely deflated the cuff. Waited for 30–60 seconds. Reinflated the cuff to no more than 200 mm Hg.	___	___	_____
20. Noted the point where you heard the first sound. This was the systolic reading.	___	___	_____
21. Continued to deflate the cuff. Noted the point where the sound disappeared. This was the diastolic reading.	___	___	_____
22. Deflated the cuff completely. Removed it from the person's arm. Removed the stethoscope earpieces from your ears.	___	___	_____

Procedure—cont'd	S	U	Comments
23. Noted the person's name and blood pressure on your notepad or assignment sheet.	____	____	_____
24. Returned the cuff to the case or wall holder.	____	____	_____

Postprocedure

	S	U	Comments
25. Provided for comfort.	____	____	_____
26. Placed the call light within reach.	____	____	_____
27. Unscreened the person.	____	____	_____
28. Completed a safety check of the room.	____	____	_____
29. Cleaned the earpieces and diaphragm with the wipes.	____	____	_____
30. Returned the equipment to its proper place.	____	____	_____
31. Decontaminated your hands.	____	____	_____
32. Reported and recorded the blood pressure. Noted which arm was used. Reported an abnormal blood pressure at once.	____	____	_____

Name: _____   Date: _____

Quality of Life	S	U	Comments
Remembered to:			
• Knock before entering the person's room.	___	___	_____
• Address the person by name.	___	___	_____
• Introduce yourself by name and title.	___	___	_____
• Explain the procedure to the person before beginning and during the procedure.	___	___	_____
• Protect the person's rights during the procedure.	___	___	_____
• Handle the person gently during the procedure.	___	___	_____

Preprocedure

	S	U	Comments
1. Followed *Delegation Guidelines: Weight and Height*	___	___	_____
Saw *Promoting Safety and Comfort: Weight and Height*	___	___	_____
2. Asked the person to void.	___	___	_____
3. Practiced hand hygiene.	___	___	_____
4. Brought the scale and paper towels (for standing scale) to the person's room, or transported the person by wheelchair to the wheelchair platform scale.	___	___	_____
5. Decontaminated your hands.	___	___	_____
6. Identified the person. Checked the identification (ID) bracelet against the assignment sheet. Also called the person by name.	___	___	_____
7. Provided for privacy.	___	___	_____

Procedure

	S	U	Comments
8. Placed the paper towels on the scale platform.	___	___	_____
9. Raised the height rod.	___	___	_____
10. Moved the weights to zero (0). The pointer was in the middle.	___	___	_____
11. Had the person remove the robe and footwear. Assisted as needed.	___	___	_____
12. Helped the person stand on the scale. The person stood in the center of the scale. Arms were at the sides.	___	___	_____
13. Moved the weights until the balance pointer was in the middle.	___	___	_____
14. If using a wheelchair scale, pushed the person sitting in the wheelchair onto the scale. Noted the weight. Safely moved the person in the wheelchair off the platform. Subtracted the weight of the wheelchair from the total weight. That was the value recorded.	___	___	_____
15. Noted the weight on your notepad or assignment sheet. Recorded in pounds or kilograms according to your center's policy.	___	___	_____
16. Asked the person to stand very straight.	___	___	_____
17. Lowered the height rod until it rested on the person's head.	___	___	_____
18. Noted the height on your notepad or assignment sheet. Recorded in inches or centimeters according to your center's policy.	___	___	_____
19. Raised the height rod. Helped the person step off of the scale.	___	___	_____
20. Helped the person put on a robe and nonskid footwear if he or she was to be up. Or helped the person back to bed.	___	___	_____
21. Lowered the height rod. Adjusted the weights to zero (0) if this was center policy.	___	___	_____

Postprocedure   S   U   Comments

22. Provided for comfort.   ____   ____   _____
23. Placed the call light within reach.   ____   ____   _____
24. Raised or lowered bed rails. Followed the care plan. ____   ____   _____
25. Unscreened the person.   ____   ____   _____
26. Completed a safety check of the room.   ____   ____   _____
27. Discarded the paper towels.   ____   ____   _____
28. Returned the scale to its proper place.   ____   ____   _____
29. Decontaminated your hands.   ____   ____   _____
30. Reported and recorded the measurements.   ____   ____   _____

Measuring Height—The Person is in Bed

Name: _____   Date: _____

	S	**U**	**Comments**
Quality of Life			
Remembered to:			
• Knock before entering the person's room.	____	____	_____
• Address the person by name.	____	____	_____
• Introduce yourself by name and title.	____	____	_____
• Explain the procedure to the person before beginning and during the procedure.	____	____	_____
• Protect the person's rights during the procedure.	____	____	_____
• Handle the person gently during the procedure.	____	____	_____

Preprocedure

	S	U	Comments
1. Followed *Delegation Guidelines: Weight and Height*	____	____	_____
Saw *Promoting Safety and Comfort: Weight and Height*	____	____	_____
2. Practiced hand hygiene.	____	____	_____
3. Asked a coworker to help you.	____	____	_____
4. Collected a measuring tape and ruler.	____	____	_____
5. Decontaminated your hands.	____	____	_____
6. Identified the person. Checked the identification (ID) bracelet against the assignment sheet. Also called the person by name.	____	____	_____
7. Provided for privacy.	____	____	_____
8. Raised the bed for body mechanics. Bed rails were up if used.	____	____	_____

Procedure

	S	U	Comments
9. Lowered the bed rails (if up).	____	____	_____
10. Positioned the person supine if the position was allowed.	____	____	_____
11. Had your coworker hold the end of the measuring tape so it extended to the person's heel.	____	____	_____
12. Pulled the measuring tape along the person's body. Pulled until it extended past the head.	____	____	_____
13. Placed the ruler flat across the top of the person's head. It extended from the person's head to the measuring tape. Made sure the ruler was level.	____	____	_____
14. Noted the height on your notepad or assignment sheet. Recorded in either inches or centimeters according to your center's policy.	____	____	_____

Postprocedure

	S	U	Comments
15. Provided for comfort.	____	____	_____
16. Placed the call light within reach.	____	____	_____
17. Lowered the bed to its lowest position.	____	____	_____
18. Raised or lowered bed rails. Followed the care plan.	____	____	_____
19. Completed a safety check of the room.	____	____	_____
20. Returned equipment to its proper place.	____	____	_____
21. Decontaminated your hands.	____	____	_____
22. Reported and recorded the height.	____	____	_____

Preparing the Person for an Examination

Name: _____   Date: _____

	S	U	Comments
Quality of Life			
Remembered to:			
• Knock before entering the person's room.	___	___	_____
• Address the person by name.	___	___	_____
• Introduce yourself by name and title.	___	___	_____
• Explain the procedure to the person before beginning and during the procedure.	___	___	_____
• Protect the person's rights during the procedure.	___	___	_____
• Handle the person gently during the procedure.	___	___	_____
Preprocedure			
1. Followed *Delegation Guidelines: Preparing the Person*	___	___	_____
Saw *Promoting Safety and Comfort: Preparing the Person*	___	___	_____
2. Practiced hand hygiene.	___	___	_____
3. Collected the following:			
a. Flashlight	___	___	_____
b. Sphygmomanometer	___	___	_____
c. Stethoscope	___	___	_____
d. Thermometer	___	___	_____
e. Tongue depressors (blades)	___	___	_____
f. Laryngeal mirror	___	___	_____
g. Ophthalmoscope	___	___	_____
h. Otoscope	___	___	_____
i. Nasal speculum	___	___	_____
j. Percussion (reflex) hammer	___	___	_____
k. Tuning fork	___	___	_____
l. Tape measure	___	___	_____
m. Gloves	___	___	_____
n. Water-soluble lubricant	___	___	_____
o. Vaginal speculum	___	___	_____
p. Cotton-tipped applicators	___	___	_____
q. Specimen containers and labels	___	___	_____
r. Disposable bag	___	___	_____
s. Kidney basin	___	___	_____
t. Towel	___	___	_____
u. Bath blanket	___	___	_____
v. Tissues	___	___	_____
w. Drape (sheet, bath blanket, drawsheet, or paper drape)	___	___	_____
x. Paper towels	___	___	_____
y. Cotton balls	___	___	_____
z. Waterproof pad	___	___	_____
a. Eye chart (Snellen chart)	___	___	_____
b. Slides	___	___	_____
c. Gown	___	___	_____
d. Alcohol wipes	___	___	_____
e. Wastebasket	___	___	_____
f. Container for soiled instruments	___	___	_____
g. Marking pencils or pens	___	___	_____
4. Decontaminated your hands.	___	___	_____
5. Identified the person. Checked the identification (ID) bracelet against the assignment sheet. Also called the person by name.	___	___	_____
6. Provided for privacy.	___	___	_____
Procedure			
7. Told the person to remove all clothes. Had the person put on the gown. Assisted as needed.	___	___	_____

365

Procedure—cont'd   S   U   **Comments**

8. Asked the person to void. Collected a urine specimen if needed. Provided for privacy. _____ _____ _____

9. Transported the person to the exam room. (This was not done for an exam in the person's room.) _____ _____ _____

10. Measured weight and height. Recorded the measurements on the exam form. _____ _____ _____

11. Helped the person onto the exam table. Provided a step stool if necessary. (Omitted this step for an exam in the person's room.) _____ _____ _____

12. Raised the far bed rail (if used). Raised the bed to its highest level. (This step was not done if an exam table was used.) _____ _____ _____

13. Measured vital signs. Recorded them on the exam form. _____ _____ _____

14. Positioned the person as directed. _____ _____ _____

15. Draped the person. _____ _____ _____

16. Placed a waterproof pad under the buttocks. _____ _____ _____

17. Raised the bed rail near you (if used). _____ _____ _____

18. Provided adequate lighting. _____ _____ _____

19. Put the call light on for the examiner. Did not leave the person alone. _____ _____ _____

Postprocedure

20. Assisted the examiner as needed. _____ _____ _____

21. Processed specimens (if any) according to directions. _____ _____ _____

22. Performed hand hygiene. _____ _____ _____

23. Assisted the person to get dressed, if necessary. _____ _____ _____

24. Assisted the person off the exam table, or, if in bed, helped the person to a comfortable position. _____ _____ _____

25. After the person left the exam room, cleaned the area and put away all equipment and supplies. _____ _____ _____

26. Completed a safety check of the room. _____ _____ _____

Collecting a Random Urine Specimen

Name: _____   Date: _____

Quality of Life	**S**	**U**	**Comments**

Remembered to:
- Knock before entering the person's room.
- Address the person by name.
- Introduce yourself by name and title.
- Explain the procedure to the person before beginning and during the procedure.
- Protect the person's rights during the procedure.
- Handle the person gently during the procedure.

Preprocedure

1. Followed *Delegation Guidelines: Urine Specimens*
   Saw *Promoting Safety and Comfort: Urine Specimens*
2. Practiced hand hygiene.
3. Collected the following before going to the person's room:
   a. Laboratory requisition slip
   b. Specimen container and lid
   c. Specimen label
   d. Plastic bag(s)
   e. *BIOHAZARD* label (if needed)
   f. Gloves
4. Arranged collected items in the person's bathroom.
5. Decontaminated your hands.
6. Identified the person. Checked the identification (ID) bracelet against the requisition slip. Also called the person by name.
7. Labeled the container in the person's presence.
8. Put on gloves.
9. Collected the following:
   a. Voiding receptacle—bedpan and cover, urinal, commode, or specimen pan
   b. Graduate to measure output
10. Provided for privacy.

Procedure

11. Asked the person to void into the receptacle. Reminded the person to put toilet tissue in the wastebasket or toilet. Toilet tissue was not put in the bedpan or specimen pan.
12. Took the receptacle to the bathroom.
13. Poured about 120 mL (milliliters) (4 oz [ounces]) into the specimen container.
14. Placed the lid on the specimen container. Put the container in the plastic bag. Did not let the container touch the outside of the bag. (Double-bagged the specimen if required by facility.) Applied a *BIOHAZARD* label according to center policy.
15. Measured urine intake and output (I&O) if ordered. Included the amount in the specimen container.
16. Emptied, cleaned, and disinfected equipment. Returned equipment to its proper place.
17. Removed the gloves and practiced hand hygiene. Put on clean gloves.
18. Assisted with hand washing.
19. Removed the gloves. Practiced hand hygiene.

Postprocedure

20. Provided for comfort.
21. Placed the call light within reach.
22. Raised or lowered bed rails. Followed the care plan.
23. Unscreened the person.

367

Postprocedure—cont'd

	S	U	Comments
24. Completed a safety check of the room.	⎯⎯	⎯⎯	⎯⎯⎯⎯⎯
25. Decontaminated your hands.	⎯⎯	⎯⎯	⎯⎯⎯⎯⎯
26. Took the specimen and the requisition slip to the storage area. Followed center policy. Wore gloves.	⎯⎯	⎯⎯	⎯⎯⎯⎯⎯
	⎯⎯	⎯⎯	⎯⎯⎯⎯⎯
27. Reported and recorded your observations.	⎯⎯	⎯⎯	⎯⎯⎯⎯⎯

Collecting a Midstream Specimen

Name: _____ Date: _____

	S	U	Comments

Quality of Life

Remembered to:
- Knock before entering the person's room.
- Address the person by name.
- Introduce yourself by name and title.
- Explain the procedure to the person before beginning and during the procedure.
- Protect the person's rights during the procedure.
- Handle the person gently during the procedure.

Preprocedure

1. Followed *Delegation Guidelines: Urine Specimens*
   Saw *Promoting Safety and Comfort: Urine Specimens*
2. Practiced hand hygiene.
3. Collected the following before going to the person's room:
   a. Laboratory requisition slip
   b. Midstream specimen kit—included specimen container, label, and towelettes; may include sterile gloves
   c. Plastic bag(s)
   d. Sterile gloves (if not part of kit)
   e. *BIOHAZARD* label (if needed)
4. Arranged your work area.
5. Decontaminated your hands.
6. Identified the person. Checked the identification (ID) bracelet against the requisition slip. Also called the person by name.
7. Put on disposable gloves.
8. Collected the following:
   a. Voiding receptacle—bedpan and cover, urinal, commode, or specimen pan if needed
   b. Supplies for perineal care
   c. Graduate to measure output
   d. Paper towel
9. Provided for privacy.

Procedure

10. Provided perineal care. (Wore gloves for this step. Decontaminated your hands after removing gloves.)
11. Opened the sterile kit.
12. Put on the sterile gloves.
13. Opened the packet of towelettes inside the kit.
14. Opened the sterile specimen container. Did not touch the inside of the container or the lid. Set the lid down so the inside was up.
15. *For a female*—cleaned the perineal area with the towelettes.
    a. Spread the labia with your thumb and index finger. Used your nondominant hand. (This hand was then contaminated and did not touch anything sterile.)
    b. Cleaned the urethral area from front to back. Used a clean towelette for each stroke.
    c. Kept the labia separated to collect the urine specimen.
16. *For a male*—cleaned the penis with towelettes.
    a. Held the penis with your nondominant hand. (This hand was then contaminated and did not touch anything sterile.)
    b. Cleaned the penis starting at the meatus. Cleaned in a circular motion. Started at the center and worked outward.
    c. Kept holding the penis until the specimen was collected.

369

Procedure—cont'd   S   U   Comments

17. Asked the person to void into the receptacle.

18. Passed the specimen container into the stream of urine. (For a female, kept the labia separated.)

19. Collected about 30–60 mL (1–2 oz) of urine.

20. Removed the specimen container before the person stopped voiding.

21. Released the labia or penis. Allowed the person to finish voiding into the receptacle.

22. Put the lid on the specimen container. Touched only the outside of the container and lid. Wiped the outside of the container. Set the container on a paper towel.

23. Provided toilet tissue after the person was done voiding.

24. Took the receptacle to the bathroom.

25. Measured urine if intake and output (I&O) were ordered. Included the amount in the specimen container.

26. Emptied, cleaned, and disinfected equipment. Returned equipment to its proper place.

27. Removed the gloves and practiced hand hygiene. Put on clean disposable gloves.

28. Labeled the specimen container in the person's presence. Placed the container in the plastic bag. Did not let the container touch the outside of the bag. (Double-bagged the specimen if required by facility.) Applied a *BIOHAZARD* label according to center policy.

29. Assisted with hand washing.

30. Removed the gloves. Practiced hand hygiene.

Postprocedure

31. Provided for comfort.

32. Placed the call light within reach.

33. Raised or lowered bed rails. Followed the care plan.

34. Unscreened the person.

35. Completed a safety check of the room.

36. Decontaminated your hands.

37. Took the specimen and the requisition slip to the storage area. Followed center policy. Wore gloves.

38. Reported and recorded your observations.

Collecting a 24-Hour Urine Specimen

Name: _____   Date: _____

	S	U	Comments
Quality of Life			

Remembered to:
- Knock before entering the person's room. ____ ____ _____
- Address the person by name. ____ ____ _____
- Introduce yourself by name and title. ____ ____ _____
- Explain the procedure to the person before beginning and during the procedure. ____ ____ _____
- Protect the person's rights during the procedure. ____ ____ _____
- Handle the person gently during the procedure. ____ ____ _____

Preprocedure

1. Followed *Delegation Guidelines: Urine Specimens* Saw *Promoting Safety and Comfort:* ____ ____ _____
   a. *Urine Specimens* ____ ____ _____
   b. *The 24-Hour Urine Specimen* ____ ____ _____
2. Practiced hand hygiene. ____ ____ _____
3. Collected the following: ____ ____ _____
   a. Laboratory requisition slip ____ ____ _____
   b. Urine container for a 24-hour collection ____ ____ _____
   c. Specimen label ____ ____ _____
   d. Preservative if needed ____ ____ _____
   e. Bucket with ice if needed ____ ____ _____
   f. Two 24-hour urine labels ____ ____ _____
   g. Funnel ____ ____ _____
   h. BIOHAZARD label ____ ____ _____
4. Arranged collected items in the person's bathroom. ____ ____ _____
5. Placed one 24-hour urine label in the bathroom. Placed the other near the bed. ____ ____ _____
6. Decontaminated your hands. ____ ____ _____
7. Identified the person. Checked the identification (ID) bracelet against the requisition slip. Also called the person by name. ____ ____ _____
8. Labeled the urine container in the person's presence. Applied the BIOHAZARD label. ____ ____ _____
9. Put on gloves. ____ ____ _____
10. Collected the following: ____ ____ _____
    a. Voiding receptacle—bedpan and cover, urinal, commode, or specimen pan ____ ____ _____
    b. Gloves ____ ____ _____
    c. Graduate to measure output ____ ____ _____
11. Provided for privacy. ____ ____ _____

Procedure

12. Asked the person to void. Provided a voiding receptacle. ____ ____ _____
13. Measured and discarded the urine. Noted the time. This started the 24-hour collection period. ____ ____ _____
14. Marked the time on the collection container. ____ ____ _____
15. Emptied, cleaned, and disinfected equipment. Returned equipment to its proper place. ____ ____ _____
16. Removed the gloves and practiced hand hygiene. Put on clean gloves. ____ ____ _____
17. Assisted with hand washing. ____ ____ _____
18. Removed the gloves. Practiced hand hygiene. ____ ____ _____
19. Marked the time the test began and the time it will end on the room and bathroom labels. ____ ____ _____
20. Reminded the person to: ____ ____ _____
    a. Use the voiding receptacle when voiding during the next 24 hours. ____ ____ _____
    b. Not have a bowel movement (BM) when voiding. ____ ____ _____

371

Procedure—cont'd	S	U	Comments
c. Put toilet tissue in the toilet or wastebasket.	——	——	————
d. Put on the call light after voiding.	——	——	————
21. Returned to the room when the person signaled for you. Knocked before entering the room.	——	——	————
22. Did the following after every voiding:			
a. Decontaminated your hands. Put on gloves.	——	——	————
b. Measured urine if intake and output (I&O) were ordered.	——	——	————
c. Poured urine into the container using the funnel. Did not spill any urine. Restarted the test if you spilled or discarded the urine.	——	——	————
d. Emptied, cleaned, and disinfected equipment. Returned equipment to its proper place.	——	——	————
e. Removed the gloves and practiced hand hygiene. Put on clean gloves.	——	——	————
f. Assisted with hand washing.	——	——	————
g. Removed the gloves. Practiced hand hygiene.	——	——	————
h. Provided for comfort.	——	——	————
i. Placed the call light within reach.	——	——	————
j. Raised or lowered bed rails. Followed the care plan.	——	——	————
k. Put on gloves.	——	——	————
l. Cleaned and returned equipment to its proper place. Discarded disposable items.	——	——	————
m. Removed the gloves. Practiced hand hygiene.	——	——	————
n. Unscreened the person.	——	——	————
o. Completed a safety check of the room.	——	——	————
p. Reported and recorded your observations.	——	——	————
23. Asked the person to void at the end of the 24-hour period. Did the following:			
a. Decontaminated your hands. Put on gloves.	——	——	————
b. Measured urine if I&O were ordered.	——	——	————
c. Poured urine into the container using the funnel. Did not spill any urine. Restarted the test if you spilled or discarded the urine.	——	——	————
d. Emptied, cleaned, and disinfected equipment. Returned equipment to its proper place.	——	——	————
e. Removed the gloves and practiced hand hygiene. Put on clean gloves.	——	——	————
f. Assisted with hand washing.	——	——	————
g. Removed the gloves. Practiced hand hygiene.	——	——	————

Postprocedure

	S	U	Comments
24. Provided for comfort.	——	——	————
25. Placed the call light within reach.	——	——	————
26. Raised or lowered bed rails. Followed the care plan.	——	——	————
27. Put on gloves.	——	——	————
28. Removed the labels from the room and bathroom.	——	——	————
29. Cleaned and returned equipment to its proper place. Discarded disposable items.	——	——	————
30. Removed the gloves. Practiced hand hygiene.	——	——	————
31. Unscreened the person.	——	——	————
32. Completed a safety check of the room.	——	——	————
33. Took the specimen and the requisition slip to the storage area. Wore gloves.	——	——	————
34. Reported and recorded your observations.	——	——	————

Testing Urine with Reagent Strips

Name: _____   Date: _____

	S	U	Comments
Quality of Life			
Remembered to:			
• Knock before entering the person's room.	___	___	_____
• Address the person by name.	___	___	_____
• Introduce yourself by name and title.	___	___	_____
• Explain the procedure to the person before beginning and during the procedure.	___	___	_____
• Protect the person's rights during the procedure.	___	___	_____
• Handle the person gently during the procedure.	___	___	_____

Preprocedure

	S	U	Comments
1. Followed *Delegation Guidelines: Testing Urine* Saw *Promoting Safety and Comfort:*	___	___	_____
a. *Testing Urine*	___	___	_____
b. *Using Reagent Strips*	___	___	_____
2. Practiced hand hygiene.	___	___	_____
3. Collected gloves and the reagent strips ordered.	___	___	_____
4. Decontaminated your hands.	___	___	_____
5. Identified the person. Checked the identification (ID) bracelet against the assignment sheet. Also called the person by name.	___	___	_____
6. Put on gloves.	___	___	_____
7. Collected equipment for the urine specimen.	___	___	_____
8. Provided for privacy.	___	___	_____

Procedure

	S	U	Comments
9. Collected the urine specimen.	___	___	_____
10. Removed the strip from the bottle. Put the cap on the bottle at once. It was on tight.	___	___	_____
11. Dipped the strip test areas into the urine.	___	___	_____
12. Removed the strip after the correct amount of time. Saw the manufacturer's instructions.	___	___	_____
13. Tapped the strip gently against the container. This removed excess urine.	___	___	_____
14. Waited the required amount of time. Saw the manufacturer's instructions.	___	___	_____
15. Compared the strip with the color chart on the bottle. Read the results.	___	___	_____
16. Discarded disposable items and the specimen.	___	___	_____
17. Emptied, cleaned, and disinfected equipment. Returned equipment to its proper place.	___	___	_____
18. Removed the gloves. Practiced hand hygiene.	___	___	_____

Postprocedure

	S	U	Comments
19. Provided for comfort.	___	___	_____
20. Placed the call light within reach.	___	___	_____
21. Raised or lowered bed rails. Followed the care plan.	___	___	_____
22. Unscreened the person.	___	___	_____
23. Completed a safety check of the room.	___	___	_____
24. Decontaminated your hands.	___	___	_____
25. Reported and recorded the test results and any other observations.	___	___	_____

Straining Urine

Name: _____   Date: _____

Quality of Life	**S**	**U**	**Comments**

Remembered to:
- Knock before entering the person's room. _____ _____ _____
- Address the person by name. _____ _____ _____
- Introduce yourself by name and title. _____ _____ _____
- Explain the procedure to the person before beginning and during the procedure. _____ _____ _____
- Protect the person's rights during the procedure. _____ _____ _____
- Handle the person gently during the procedure. _____ _____ _____

Preprocedure

1. Followed *Delegation Guidelines: Testing Urine* _____ _____ _____
   Saw *Promoting Safety and Comfort: Testing Urine* _____ _____ _____
2. Practiced hand hygiene. _____ _____ _____
3. Collected the following before going to the person's room:
   a. Laboratory requisition slip _____ _____ _____
   b. Gauze or strainer _____ _____ _____
   c. Specimen container _____ _____ _____
   d. Specimen label _____ _____ _____
   e. Two STRAIN ALL URINE labels _____ _____ _____
   f. Plastic bag _____ _____ _____
   g. BIOHAZARD label if needed _____ _____ _____
   h. Gloves _____ _____ _____
4. Arranged collected items in the person's bathroom. _____ _____ _____
5. Placed one STRAIN ALL URINE label in the bathroom. Placed the other near the bed. _____ _____ _____
6. Decontaminated your hands. _____ _____ _____
7. Identified the person. Checked the identification (ID) bracelet against the assignment sheet. Also called the person by name. _____ _____ _____
8. Labeled the specimen container in the person's presence. _____ _____ _____
9. Put on gloves. _____ _____ _____
10. Collected the following:
    a. Voiding receptacle—bedpan and cover, urinal, commode, or specimen pan _____ _____ _____
    b. Graduate _____ _____ _____
    c. Gloves _____ _____ _____
11. Provided for privacy. _____ _____ _____

Procedure

12. Asked the person to use the voiding receptacle for urinating. Asked the person to put on the call light after voiding. _____ _____ _____
13. Removed the gloves. Practiced hand hygiene. _____ _____ _____
14. Returned to the room when the person signaled for you. Knocked before entering the room. _____ _____ _____
15. Decontaminated your hands. Put on gloves. _____ _____ _____
16. Placed the gauze or strainer into the graduate. _____ _____ _____
17. Poured urine into the graduate. Urine passed through the gauze or strainer. _____ _____ _____
18. Placed the gauze or strainer in the specimen container if any crystals, stones, or particles appeared. _____ _____ _____
19. Placed the specimen container in the plastic bag. Did not let the container touch the outside of the bag. Applied a BIOHAZARD label according to center policy. _____ _____ _____
20. Measured urine if intake and output (I&O) were ordered. _____ _____ _____
21. Emptied, cleaned, and disinfected equipment. Returned equipment to its proper place. _____ _____ _____
22. Removed the gloves and practiced hand hygiene. Put on clean gloves. _____ _____ _____

Procedure—cont'd	S	U	Comments
23. Assisted with hand washing.	——	——	————
24. Removed the gloves. Practiced hand hygiene.	——	——	————

Postprocedure

	S	U	Comments
25. Provided for comfort.	——	——	————
26. Placed the call light within reach.	——	——	————
27. Raised or lowered bed rails. Followed the care plan.	——	——	————
28. Unscreened the person.	——	——	————
29. Completed a safety check of the room.	——	——	————
30. Decontaminated your hands.	——	——	————
31. Took the specimen container and requisition slip to the laboratory or storage area. Wore gloves.	——	——	————
32. Reported and recorded your observations.	——	——	————

Collecting a Stool Specimen

Name: _____   Date: _____

Quality of Life	**S**	**U**	**Comments**

Remembered to:
- Knock before entering the person's room. _____ _____ _____
- Address the person by name. _____ _____ _____
- Introduce yourself by name and title. _____ _____ _____
- Explain the procedure to the person before beginning and during the procedure. _____ _____ _____
- Protect the person's rights during the procedure. _____ _____ _____
- Handle the person gently during the procedure. _____ _____ _____

Preprocedure

1. Followed *Delegation Guidelines: Stool Specimens* _____ _____ _____
   Saw *Promoting Safety and Comfort: Stool Specimens* _____ _____ _____
2. Practiced hand hygiene. _____ _____ _____
3. Collected the following before going to the person's room:
   a. Laboratory requisition slip _____ _____ _____
   b. Specimen pan for the toilet _____ _____ _____
   c. Specimen container and lid _____ _____ _____
   d. Specimen label _____ _____ _____
   e. Tongue blade _____ _____ _____
   f. Disposable bag _____ _____ _____
   g. Plastic bag(s) _____ _____ _____
   h. BIOHAZARD label (if needed) _____ _____ _____
   i. Gloves _____ _____ _____
4. Arranged collected items in the person's bathroom. _____ _____ _____
5. Decontaminated your hands. _____ _____ _____
6. Identified the person. Checked the identification (ID) bracelet against the requisition slip. Also called the person by name. _____ _____ _____
7. Labeled the specimen container in the person's presence. _____ _____ _____
8. Put on gloves. _____ _____ _____
9. Collected the following:
   a. Receptacle for voiding—bedpan and cover, urinal, commode, or specimen pan _____ _____ _____
   b. Toilet tissue _____ _____ _____
10. Provided for privacy. _____ _____ _____

Procedure

11. Asked the person to void. Provided the receptacle for voiding if the person did not use the bathroom. Emptied, cleaned, and disinfected the device. Returned it to its proper place. _____ _____ _____
12. Put the specimen pan on the toilet if the person used the bathroom. Placed it at the back of the toilet. Or provided a bedpan or commode. _____ _____ _____
13. Asked the person not to put toilet tissue into the bedpan, commode, or specimen pan. Provided a bag for toilet tissue. _____ _____ _____
14. Placed the call light and toilet tissue within reach. Raised or lowered bed rails. Followed the care plan. _____ _____ _____
15. Removed the gloves. Decontaminated your hands. Left the room. _____ _____ _____
16. Returned when the person signaled. Or checked on the person every 5 minutes. Knocked before entering. _____ _____ _____
17. Decontaminated your hands. Put on clean gloves. _____ _____ _____
18. Lowered the bed rail near you if up. _____ _____ _____
19. Removed the bedpan (if used). Noted the color, amount, consistency, and odor of stools. _____ _____ _____
20. Provided perineal care if needed. _____ _____ _____

Procedure—cont'd	S	U	Comments
21. Collected the specimen:			
a. Used a tongue blade to take about two tablespoons of stool to the specimen container. Took the sample from the middle of a formed stool.	____	____	_____
b. Included pus, mucus, or blood present in the stool.	____	____	_____
c. Took stool from two different places in the bowel movement (BM) if required by center policy.	____	____	_____
d. Put the lid on the specimen container.	____	____	_____
e. Placed the container in the plastic bag. Did not let the container touch the outside of the bag. (Double-bagged if required by facility.) Applied a *BIOHAZARD* label according to center policy.	____	____	_____
22. Wrapped the tongue blade in toilet tissue. Discarded it in the disposable bag.	____	____	_____
23. Emptied, cleaned, and disinfected equipment. Returned equipment to its proper place.	____	____	_____
24. Removed the gloves and practiced hand hygiene. Put on clean gloves.	____	____	_____
25. Assisted with hand washing.	____	____	_____
26. Removed the gloves. Practiced hand hygiene.	____	____	_____

Postprocedure

	S	U	Comments
27. Provided for comfort.	____	____	_____
28. Placed the call light within reach.	____	____	_____
29. Raised or lowered bed rails. Followed the care plan.	____	____	_____
30. Unscreened the person.	____	____	_____
31. Completed a safety check of the room.	____	____	_____
32. Delivered the specimen and requisition slip to the storage area. Followed center policy. Wore gloves.	____	____	_____
33. Reported and recorded your observations.	____	____	_____

Testing a Stool Specimen for Blood

Name: _____ Date: _____

	S	U	Comments
Quality of Life			

Remembered to:
- Knock before entering the person's room.   ___ ___ _____
- Address the person by name.   ___ ___ _____
- Introduce yourself by name and title.   ___ ___ _____
- Explain the procedure to the person before beginning and during the procedure.   ___ ___ _____
- Protect the person's rights during the procedure.   ___ ___ _____
- Handle the person gently during the procedure.   ___ ___ _____

Preprocedure

1. Followed *Delegation Guidelines: Testing Stools for Blood*
   Saw *Promoting Safety and Comfort:*   ___ ___ _____
   a. *Stool Specimens*   ___ ___ _____
   b. *Testing Stools for Blood*   ___ ___ _____
2. Practiced hand hygiene.   ___ ___ _____
3. Collected the following before going to the person's room:
   a. Occult blood test kit   ___ ___ _____
   b. Tongue blades (if needed)   ___ ___ _____
   c. Gloves   ___ ___ _____
4. Arranged collected items in the person's bathroom.   ___ ___ _____
5. Decontaminated your hands.   ___ ___ _____
6. Identified the person. Checked the identification (ID) bracelet against the assignment sheet. Also called the person by name.   ___ ___ _____
7. Put on gloves.   ___ ___ _____
8. Collected the following:
   a. Equipment for a stool specimen   ___ ___ _____
   b. Paper towels   ___ ___ _____
9. Provided for privacy.   ___ ___ _____

Procedure

10. Collected a stool specimen.   ___ ___ _____
11. Practiced hand hygiene. Put on clean gloves.   ___ ___ _____
12. Opened the test kit.   ___ ___ _____
13. Used a tongue blade to obtain a small amount of stool.   ___ ___ _____
14. Applied a thin smear of stool on box A on the test paper.   ___ ___ _____
15. Used another tongue blade to obtain stool from another part of the specimen.   ___ ___ _____
16. Applied a thin smear of stool on box B on the test paper.   ___ ___ _____
17. Closed the packet.   ___ ___ _____
18. Turned the test packet to the other side. Opened the flap. Applied developer (from the kit) to *boxes A and B*. Followed the manufacturer's instructions.   ___ ___ _____
19. Waited for 10–60 seconds as required by the manufacturer's instructions.   ___ ___ _____
20. Noted the color changes on the assignment sheet.   ___ ___ _____
21. Disposed of test packet.   ___ ___ _____
22. Wrapped the tongue blades in toilet tissue. Then discarded them.   ___ ___ _____
23. Emptied, cleaned, and disinfected equipment. Returned equipment to its proper place.   ___ ___ _____
24. Removed the gloves. Practiced hand hygiene.   ___ ___ _____

Postprocedure	**S**	**U**	**Comments**
25. Provided for comfort.	____	____	_____
26. Placed the call light within reach.	____	____	_____
27. Raised or lowered bed rails. Followed the care plan.	____	____	_____
28. Completed a safety check of the room.	____	____	_____
29. Decontaminated your hands.	____	____	_____
30. Reported and recorded the test results and your observations.	____	____	_____

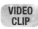**Collecting a Sputum Specimen**

Name: _____   Date: _____

Quality of Life	**S**	**U**	**Comments**

Remembered to:
- Knock before entering the person's room.
- Address the person by name.
- Introduce yourself by name and title.
- Explain the procedure to the person before beginning and during the procedure.
- Protect the person's rights during the procedure.
- Handle the person gently during the procedure.

Preprocedure

1. Followed *Delegation Guidelines: Sputum Specimens*
   Saw *Promoting Safety and Comfort: Sputum Specimens*
2. Practiced hand hygiene.
3. Collected the following before going to the person's room:
   a. Laboratory requisition slip
   b. Sputum specimen container and lid
   c. Specimen label
   d. Plastic bag(s)
   e. BOHAZARD label (if needed)
4. Arranged collected items in the person's bathroom.
5. Decontaminated your hands.
6. Identified the person. Checked the identification (ID) bracelet against the requisition slip. Also called the person by name.
7. Labeled the specimen container in the person's presence.
8. Collected gloves and tissues.
9. Provided for privacy. If able, the person used the bathroom for this procedure.

Procedure

10. Put on gloves.
11. Asked the person to rinse the mouth out with clear water. Did not have them use mouthwash.
12. Had the person hold the container. Only the outside was touched.
13. Asked the person to cover the mouth and nose with tissues when coughing. Followed center policy for used tissues.
14. Asked the person to take 2 or 3 deep breaths and cough up sputum.
15. Had the person expectorate directly into the container. Sputum did not touch the outside of the container.
16. Collected 1–2 teaspoons of sputum unless told to collect more.
17. Put the lid on the container.
18. Placed the container in the plastic bag. Did not let the container touch the outside of the bag. (Double-bagged the container if required by facility.) Applied a BIOHAZARD label according to center policy.
19. Removed gloves and decontaminated your hands. Put on clean gloves.
20. Assisted with hand washing.
21. Removed the gloves. Decontaminated your hands.

Postprocedure

22. Provided for comfort.
23. Placed the call light within reach.
24. Raised or lowered bed rails. Followed the care plan.

Postprocedure—cont'd   S   U   Comments

25. Unscreened the person.   _____   _____   _____
26. Completed a safety check of the room.   _____   _____   _____
27. Decontaminated your hands.   _____   _____   _____
28. Delivered the specimen and requisition slip to the storage
    area. Followed center policy. Wore gloves.   _____   _____   _____
29. Reported and recorded your observations.   _____   _____   _____

Name: _____   Date: _____

	S	U	Comments
Quality of Life			
Remembered to:			
• Knock before entering the person's room.	___	___	_____
• Address the person by name.	___	___	_____
• Introduce yourself by name and title.	___	___	_____
• Explain the procedure to the person before beginning and during the procedure.	___	___	_____
• Protect the person's rights during the procedure.	___	___	_____
• Handle the person gently during the procedure.	___	___	_____

Preprocedure

	S	U	Comments
1. Followed *Delegation Guidelines: Blood Glucose Testing*	___	___	_____
Saw *Promoting Safety and Comfort: Blood Glucose Testing*	___	___	_____
2. Practiced hand hygiene.	___	___	_____
3. Collected the following:			
a. Sterile lancet	___	___	_____
b. Antiseptic wipes	___	___	_____
c. Gloves	___	___	_____
d. Cotton balls	___	___	_____
e. Bandage	___	___	_____
f. Glucose meter	___	___	_____
g. Reagent strips (used correct strips for the meter. Checked expiration date.)	___	___	_____
h. Paper towels	___	___	_____
i. Warm washcloth	___	___	_____
4. Read the manufacturer's instructions for lancet and glucose meter.	___	___	_____
5. Arranged your work area.	___	___	_____
6. Identified the person. Checked the identification (ID) bracelet against the assignment sheet. Also called the person by name.	___	___	_____
7. Provided privacy.	___	___	_____
8. Raised the bed for body mechanics. Far bed rail was up if used.	___	___	_____

Procedure

	S	U	Comments
9. Helped the person to a comfortable position.	___	___	_____
10. Put on gloves.	___	___	_____
11. Prepared the supplies:			
a. Opened the antiseptic wipes.	___	___	_____
b. Removed a reagent strip from the bottle. Placed it on the paper towel. Placed the cap securely on the bottle.	___	___	_____
c. Prepared the lancet.	___	___	_____
d. Turned on the glucose meter.	___	___	_____
e. Followed the prompts. Entered username and person's ID number, if required. Scanned the bar code on the bottle of reagent strips if needed.	___	___	_____
f. Inserted a reagent strip into the glucose meter.	___	___	_____
12. Performed a skin puncture to obtain a drop of blood:			
a. Inspected the person's fingers. Selected a puncture site.	___	___	_____
b. Warmed the finger. Rubbed it gently or applied a warm washcloth.	___	___	_____
c. Lightly massaged twice only the hand and finger toward the puncture site. Lowered the finger below the person's waist. These actions increased blood flow to the site.	___	___	_____
d. Held the finger with your thumb and forefinger. Used your nondominant hand. Held the finger at the point where you applied pressure to the puncture site until bleeding stopped.	___	___	_____

Procedure—cont'd	S	U	Comments

    e. Cleaned the site with antiseptic wipe. *Did not touch the site after cleaning.* ___ ___ _____

    f. Let the site dry. ___ ___ _____

    g. Picked up the sterile lancet. ___ ___ _____

    h. Placed the lancet against the puncture site. ___ ___ _____

    i. Pushed the button on the lancet to puncture the skin. (Followed the manufacturer's instructions.) ___ ___ _____

    j. Wiped away the first blood drop. Used a cotton ball. ___ ___ _____

    k. Applied gentle pressure below the puncture site. ___ ___ _____

    l. Allowed a large drop of blood to form. ___ ___ _____

13. Collected and tested the specimen. Followed the manufacturer's instructions and center procedures for the glucose meter used.

    a. Held the test area of the reagent strip close to the drop of blood. ___ ___ _____

    b. Lightly touched the reagent strip to the drop of blood. Did not smear the blood. The meter tested the sample when enough blood was applied. ___ ___ _____

    c. Applied pressure to the puncture site until the bleeding stopped. Used a cotton ball or gauze. Allowed person, if able, to apply pressure to the site. ___ ___ _____

    d. Read the result on the display. Noted the result on your notepad or assignment sheet. Told person the result. ___ ___ _____

    e. Turned off the glucose meter. ___ ___ _____

    f. Applied a bandage to the area. Told the person the bandage could be removed after 15 minutes. ___ ___ _____

14. Discarded the lancet in the sharps container. ___ ___ _____

15. Discarded the cotton balls and reagent strip following center policy. ___ ___ _____

16. Removed and discarded gloves. Decontaminated your hands. ___ ___ _____

Postprocedure

17. Provided for comfort. ___ ___ _____

18. Placed the call light within reach. ___ ___ _____

19. Lowered the bed to its lowest position. ___ ___ _____

20. Raised or lowered bed rails. Followed the care plan. ___ ___ _____

21. Unscreened the person. ___ ___ _____

22. Discarded used supplies. ___ ___ _____

23. Completed a safety check of the room. ___ ___ _____

24. Followed center policy for soiled linens. ___ ___ _____

25. Decontaminated your hands. ___ ___ _____

26. Reported and recorded the test result and your observations. ___ ___ _____

Preparing the Person's Room

Name: _____   Date: _____

Procedure	S	U	Comments
1. Followed *Delegation Guidelines: Admissions, Transfers, and Discharges*	———	———	———————
2. Practiced hand hygiene.	———	———	———————
3. Collected the following:			
a. Admission kit—wash basin, soap, toothpaste, toothbrush, water pitcher and cup, and so on	———	———	———————
b. Bedpan and urinal (for a man)	———	———	———————
c. Admission form	———	———	———————
d. Thermometer	———	———	———————
e. Sphygmomanometer	———	———	———————
f. Stethoscope	———	———	———————
g. Gown or pajamas (if needed)	———	———	———————
h. Towels and washcloth	———	———	———————
i. IV (intravenous) pole (if needed)	———	———	———————
j. Other items requested by the nurse	———	———	———————
4. Placed the following on the overbed table:			
a. Thermometer	———	———	———————
b. Sphygmomanometer	———	———	———————
c. Stethoscope	———	———	———————
d. Admission form	———	———	———————
5. Placed the water pitcher and cup on the bedside stand or overbed table.	———	———	———————
6. Placed the following in the bedside stand:			
a. Admission kit	———	———	———————
b. Bedpan and urinal	———	———	———————
c. Gown or pajamas	———	———	———————
d. Towels and washcloth	———	———	———————
7. *If the person arrived by stretcher:*			
a. Made a surgical bed.	———	———	———————
b. Raised the bed to its highest level.	———	———	———————
8. *If the person was ambulatory or arrived by wheelchair:*			
a. Left the bed closed.	———	———	———————
b. Lowered the bed to its lowest position.	———	———	———————
9. Attached the call light to the bed linens.	———	———	———————
10. Decontaminated your hands.	———	———	———————

Admitting the Person

Name: _____ Date: _____

	S	U	Comments
Quality of Life			
Remembered to:			
• Knock before entering the person's room.	___	___	_____
• Address the person by name.	___	___	_____
• Introduce yourself by name and title.	___	___	_____
• Explain the procedure to the person before beginning and during the procedure.	___	___	_____
• Protect the person's rights during the procedure.	___	___	_____
• Handle the person gently during the procedure.	___	___	_____
Preprocedure			
1. Followed *Delegation Guidelines: Admissions, Transfers, and Discharges*	___	___	_____
Saw *Promoting Safety and Comfort: Admissions, Transfers, and Discharges*	___	___	_____
2. Practiced hand hygiene.	___	___	_____
3. Prepared the room.	___	___	_____
Procedure			
4. Checked the person's name on the admission form.	___	___	_____
5. Greeted the person by name. Asked if he or she preferred a certain name.	___	___	_____
6. Introduced yourself to the person and others present. Gave your name and title. Explained that you assist the nurses in giving care.	___	___	_____
7. Introduced the roommate.	___	___	_____
8. Provided for privacy. Asked family or friends to leave the room. Told them how much time you needed and directed them to the waiting area. Allowed a family member or friend to stay if the person preferred.	___	___	_____
9. Allowed the person to stay dressed if his or her condition permitted. Or helped the person change into a gown or pajamas.	___	___	_____
10. Provided for comfort. The person was in bed or in a chair as directed by the nurse.	___	___	_____
11. Assisted the nurse with assessment:			
a. Measured vital signs.	___	___	_____
b. Measured weight and height.	___	___	_____
c. Collected information for the admission form as requested by the nurse.	___	___	_____
12. Completed a clothing and personal belongings list.	___	___	_____
13. Helped the person put away clothes and personal items. Put them in the closet, drawers, and bedside stand. (The family may wish to help with this step.)	___	___	_____
14. Explained ordered activity limits.	___	___	_____
15. Oriented the person and family to the area:			
a. Gave names of the nurses and nursing assistants.	___	___	_____
b. Identified items in the bedside stand. Explained the purpose of each.	___	___	_____
c. Explained how to use the overbed table.	___	___	_____
d. Showed how to use the call light.	___	___	_____
e. Showed how to use the bed, TV, and light controls.	___	___	_____
f. Explained how to make phone calls. Placed the phone within reach.	___	___	_____
g. Showed the person the bathroom. Also showed how to use the call light in the bathroom.	___	___	_____
h. Explained visiting hours and policies.	___	___	_____

Procedure Checklists

Procedure—cont'd	S	U	Comments

Procedure—cont'd

    i. Explained where to find the nurses' station, lounge, chapel, dining room, and other areas. ____ ____ _____

    j. Identified staff—housekeeping, dietary, physical therapy, and others. Also identified students in the center. ____ ____ _____

    k. Explained when meals and snacks are served. ____ ____ _____

16. Filled the water pitcher and cup if oral fluids were allowed. ____ ____ _____

17. Placed the call light within reach. ____ ____ _____

18. Placed other controls and needed items within reach. ____ ____ _____

19. Provided a denture container if needed. Labeled it with the person's name and room and bed number. ____ ____ _____

20. Labeled the person's property and personal care items with his or her name (if not completed by the family). ____ ____ _____

Postprocedure

21. Provided for comfort. ____ ____ _____

22. Lowered the bed to its lowest position. ____ ____ _____

23. Raised or lowered bed rails. Followed the care plan. ____ ____ _____

24. Completed a safety check of the room. ____ ____ _____

25. Decontaminated your hands. ____ ____ _____

26. Reported and recorded your observations. ____ ____ _____

Moving the Person to a New Room

Name: _____   Date: _____

	S	U	Comments
Quality of Life			

Remembered to:
- Knock before entering the person's room. ____ ____ _____
- Address the person by name. ____ ____ _____
- Introduce yourself by name and title. ____ ____ _____
- Explain the procedure to the person before beginning and during the procedure. ____ ____ _____
- Protect the person's rights during the procedure. ____ ____ _____
- Handle the person gently during the procedure. ____ ____ _____

Preprocedure

1. Followed *Delegation Guidelines: Admissions, Transfers, and Discharges* Saw *Promoting Safety and Comfort: Admissions, Transfers, and Discharges* ____ ____ _____
2. Asked a coworker to help you. ____ ____ _____
3. Practiced hand hygiene. ____ ____ _____
4. Collected the following:
   a. Wheelchair or stretcher ____ ____ _____
   b. Utility cart ____ ____ _____
   c. Bath blanket ____ ____ _____
5. Decontaminated your hands. ____ ____ _____
6. Identified the person. Checked the identification (ID) bracelet against the assignment sheet. Also called the person by name. ____ ____ _____
7. Provided for privacy. ____ ____ _____

Procedure

8. Collected the person's belongings and care equipment. Placed them on the cart. ____ ____ _____
9. Transferred the person to a wheelchair or a stretcher. Covered the person with a bath blanket. ____ ____ _____
10. Transported the person to the new room. Your coworker brought the cart. ____ ____ _____
11. Helped transfer the person to the bed or chair. Helped position the person. ____ ____ _____
12. Helped arrange the person's belongings and equipment. ____ ____ _____
13. Reported the following to the receiving nurse:
    a. How the person tolerated the transfer ____ ____ _____
    b. Any observations made during the transfer ____ ____ _____
    c. That the nurse will bring the medical record, care plan, Kardex, and medications ____ ____ _____

Postprocedure

14. Returned the wheelchair or stretcher and the cart to the storage area. ____ ____ _____
15. Decontaminated your hands. ____ ____ _____
16. Reported and recorded the following:
    a. The time of the transfer ____ ____ _____
    b. Who helped you with the transfer ____ ____ _____
    c. Where the person was taken ____ ____ _____
    d. How the person was transferred (bed, wheelchair, or stretcher) ____ ____ _____
    e. How the person tolerated the transfer ____ ____ _____
    f. Who received the person ____ ____ _____
    g. Any other observations ____ ____ _____
17. Stripped the bed and cleaned the unit. Decontaminated your hands and put on gloves for this step. (The housekeeping staff may do this step.) ____ ____ _____

Postprocedure—cont'd	S	U	Comments
18. Removed the gloves. Decontaminated your hands.	_____	_____	_____
19. Followed center policy for dirty linen.	_____	_____	_____
20. Made a closed bed.	_____	_____	_____
21. Decontaminated your hands.	_____	_____	_____

Transferring or Discharging the Person

Name: _____   Date: _____

	S	U	Comments
Quality of Life			
Remembered to:			
• Knock before entering the person's room.	___	___	_____
• Address the person by name.	___	___	_____
• Introduce yourself by name and title.	___	___	_____
• Explain the procedure to the person before beginning and during the procedure.	___	___	_____
• Protect the person's rights during the procedure.	___	___	_____
• Handle the person gently during the procedure.	___	___	_____

Preprocedure

	S	U	Comments
1. Followed *Delegation Guidelines: Admissions, Transfers, and Discharges*	___	___	_____
Saw *Promoting Safety and Comfort: Admissions, Transfers, and Discharges*	___	___	_____
2. Asked a coworker to help you.	___	___	_____
3. Practiced hand hygiene.	___	___	_____
4. Identified the person. Checked the identification (ID) bracelet against the assignment sheet. Also called the person by name.	___	___	_____
5. Provided for privacy.	___	___	_____

Procedure

	S	U	Comments
6. Helped the person dress as needed.	___	___	_____
7. Helped the person pack. Checked all drawers and closets. Checked the bathroom. Made sure all items were collected.	___	___	_____
8. Checked off the clothing list and personal belongings list. Made sure the person had eyeglasses, hearing aids, and dentures. Gave the list to the nurse.	___	___	_____
9. Told the nurse that the person was ready for the final visit. The nurse:			
a. Gave prescriptions written by the doctor.	___	___	_____
b. Provided discharge instructions.	___	___	_____
c. Got valuables from the safe.	___	___	_____
d. Had the person sign the clothing and personal belongings list.	___	___	_____
10. *If the person left by wheelchair:*			
a. Got a wheelchair and a utility cart for the person's items. Asked a coworker to help you.	___	___	_____
b. Helped the person into the wheelchair.	___	___	_____
c. Took the person to the exit area.	___	___	_____
d. Locked the wheelchair wheels.	___	___	_____
e. Helped the person out of the wheelchair and into the car.	___	___	_____
f. Helped put the person's items into the car.	___	___	_____
11. *If the person left by ambulance:*			
a. Raised the bed rails.	___	___	_____
b. Raised the bed to its highest level.	___	___	_____
c. Placed the call light within reach.	___	___	_____
d. Waited for the ambulance attendants.	___	___	_____

Postprocedure

	S	U	Comments
12. Returned the wheelchair and cart to the storage area.	___	___	_____
13. Decontaminated your hands.	___	___	_____
14. Reported and recorded the following:			
a. The time of the discharge	___	___	_____
b. Who helped you with the procedure	___	___	_____
c. How the person was transported	___	___	_____
d. Who was with the person	___	___	_____
e. The person's destination	___	___	_____
f. Any other observations	___	___	_____

389

Postprocedure—cont'd   S   U   **Comments**

15. Stripped the bed and cleaned the unit. Decontaminated your hands and
    put on gloves for this step. (The housekeeping staff may do this step.)   _____   _____   _____
16. Removed the gloves. Decontaminated your hands.   _____   _____   _____
17. Followed center policy for dirty linens.   _____   _____   _____
18. Made a closed bed.   _____   _____   _____
19. Decontaminated your hands.   _____   _____   _____

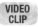 **Applying Compression Stockings (NATCEP)**

Name: _____ Date: _____

	S	U	Comments

Quality of Life

Remembered to:
- Knock before entering the person's room.
- Address the person by name.
- Introduce yourself by name and title.
- Explain the procedure to the person before beginning and during the procedure.
- Protect the person's rights during the procedure.
- Handle the person gently during the procedure.

Preprocedure

1. Followed *Delegation Guidelines: Compression Stockings*
   Saw *Promoting Safety and Comfort: Compression Stockings*
2. Practiced hand hygiene.
3. Obtained compression stockings in the correct size and length. (Checked if nurse measured the leg.)
4. Identified the person. Checked the identification (ID) bracelet against the assignment sheet. Also called the person by name.
5. Provided for privacy.
6. Raised the bed for body mechanics. Bed rails were up if used.

Procedure

7. Lowered the bed rail near you if up.
8. Positioned the person supine.
9. Exposed the legs. Fan-folded top linens toward the thighs.
10. Turned the stocking inside out down to the heel.
11. Slipped the foot of the stocking over the toes, foot, and heel. Made sure the stocking heel was properly positioned on the person's heel.
12. Grasped the stocking top. Pulled the stocking up the leg. It turned right side out as it was pulled up. The stocking was even and snug.
13. Removed twists, creases, or wrinkles.
14. Repeated for the other leg:
    a. Turned the stocking inside out down to the heel.
    b. Slipped the foot of the stocking over the toes, foot, and heel. Made sure the stocking heel was properly positioned on the person's heel.
    c. Grasped the stocking top. Pulled the stocking up the leg. It turned right side out as it was pulled up. The stocking was even and snug.
    d. Removed twists, creases, or wrinkles.

Postprocedure

15. Covered the person.
16. Provided for comfort.
17. Placed the call light within reach.
18. Lowered the bed to its lowest position.
19. Raised or lowered bed rails. Followed the care plan.
20. Unscreened the person.
21. Completed a safety check of the room.
22. Decontaminated your hands.
23. Reported and recorded your observations.

391

Applying Elastic Bandages

Name: _____ Date: _____

	S	U	Comments
Quality of Life			
• Remembered to:			
• Knock before entering the person's room.	___	___	_____
• Address the person by name.	___	___	_____
• Introduce yourself by name and title.	___	___	_____
• Explain the procedure to the person before beginning and during the procedure.	___	___	_____
• Protect the person's rights during the procedure.	___	___	_____
• Handle the person gently during the procedure.	___	___	_____
Preprocedure			
1. Followed *Delegation Guidelines: Elastic Bandages*	___	___	_____
Saw *Promoting Safety and Comfort: Elastic Bandages*	___	___	_____
2. Practiced hand hygiene.	___	___	_____
3. Collected the following:			
a. Elastic bandage as directed by the nurse	___	___	_____
b. Tape or clips (unless the bandage had Velcro)	___	___	_____
4. Identified the person. Checked the identification (ID) bracelet against the assignment sheet. Also called the person by name.	___	___	_____
5. Provided for privacy.	___	___	_____
6. Raised the bed for body mechanics. Bed rails were up if used.	___	___	_____
Procedure			
7. Lowered the bed rail near you if up.	___	___	_____
8. Helped the person to a comfortable position. Exposed the part to be bandaged.	___	___	_____
9. Made sure the area was clean and dry.	___	___	_____
10. Held the bandage so the roll was up. The loose end was on the bottom.	___	___	_____
11. Applied the bandage to the smallest part of the wrist, foot, ankle, or knee.	___	___	_____
12. Made two circular turns around the part.	___	___	_____
13. Made overlapping spiral turns in an upward direction. Each turn overlapped about ½ to ⅔ of the previous turn. Each overlap was equal.	___	___	_____
14. Applied the bandage smoothly with firm, even pressure. It was not tight.	___	___	_____
15. Ended the bandage with two circular turns.	___	___	_____
16. Secured the bandage in place with Velcro, tape, or clips. The clips were not under any body part.	___	___	_____
17. Checked the fingers or toes for coldness or cyanosis (bluish color). Asked about pain, itching, numbness, or tingling. Removed the bandage if any were noted. Reported your observations.	___	___	_____
Postprocedure			
18. Provided for comfort.	___	___	_____
19. Placed the call light within reach.	___	___	_____
20. Lowered the bed to its lowest position.	___	___	_____
21. Raised or lowered bed rails. Followed the care plan.	___	___	_____
22. Unscreened the person.	___	___	_____
23. Completed a safety check of the room.	___	___	_____
24. Decontaminated your hands.	___	___	_____
25. Reported and recorded your observations.	___	___	_____

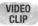 **Applying a Dry, Nonsterile Dressing**

Name: _____   Date: _____

	S	U	Comments

Quality of Life

Remembered to:
- Knock before entering the person's room.
- Address the person by name.
- Introduce yourself by name and title.
- Explain the procedure to the person before beginning and during the procedure.
- Protect the person's rights during the procedure.
- Handle the person gently during the procedure.

Preprocedure

1. Followed *Delegation Guidelines: Applying Dressings*
   Saw *Promoting Safety and Comfort: Applying Dressings*
2. Practiced hand hygiene.
3. Collected the following:
   a. Gloves
   b. Personal protective equipment (PPE) as needed
   c. Tape
   d. Dressings as directed by the nurse
   e. Saline solution as directed by the nurse
   f. Cleansing solution as directed by the nurse
   g. Adhesive remover
   h. Dressing set with scissors and forceps
   i. Plastic bag
   j. Bath blanket
4. Decontaminated your hands.
5. Identified the person. Checked the identification (ID) bracelet against the assignment sheet. Also called the person by name.
6. Provided for privacy.
7. Arranged your work area. You did not have to reach over or turn your back on the work area.
8. Raised the bed for body mechanics. Bed rails were up if used.

Procedure

9. Lowered the bed rail near you if up.
10. Helped the person to a comfortable position.
11. Covered the person with a bath blanket. Fan-folded top linens to the foot of the bed.
12. Exposed the affected body part.
13. Made a cuff on the plastic bag. Placed it within reach.
14. Decontaminated your hands.
15. Put on needed PPE. Put on gloves.
16. Removed tape. Held the skin down. Gently pulled the tape toward the wound.
17. Removed any adhesive from the skin. Wet a 4 × 4 gauze dressing with adhesive remover. Cleaned away from the wound.
18. Removed gauze dressings. Started with the top dressing and removed each layer. Kept the soiled side of each dressing away from the person's sight. Put dressings in the plastic bag. They did not touch the outside of the bag.
19. Removed the dressing over the wound very gently. Moistened the dressing with saline, if it stuck to the wound.
20. Observed the wound, drain site, and wound drainage.
21. Removed the gloves and discarded in the plastic bag. Decontaminated your hands.
22. Opened new dressings.
23. Cut the length of tape needed.

393

Procedure—cont'd   S   U   **Comments**

24. Put on clean gloves. _____ _____ _____
25. Cleaned the wound with saline or as directed by the nurse. _____ _____ _____
26. Applied dressings as directed by the nurse. _____ _____ _____
27. Secured the dressings in place with tape. _____ _____ _____
28. Removed the gloves. Put them in the bag. _____ _____ _____
29. Removed and discarded PPE. _____ _____ _____
30. Decontaminated your hands. _____ _____ _____
31. Covered the person. Removed the bath blanket. _____ _____ _____

Postprocedure

32. Provided for comfort. _____ _____ _____
33. Placed the call light within reach. _____ _____ _____
34. Lowered the bed to its lowest position. _____ _____ _____
35. Raised or lowered bed rails. Followed the care plan. _____ _____ _____
36. Returned equipment and supplies to the proper place. Left extra dressings and tape in the room. _____ _____ _____
37. Discarded used supplies in the bag. Tied the bag closed. Discarded the bag following center policy. (Wore gloves for this step.) _____ _____ _____
38. Cleaned your work area. Followed the Bloodborne Pathogen Standard. _____ _____ _____
39. Unscreened the person. _____ _____ _____
40. Completed a safety check of the room. _____ _____ _____
41. Decontaminated your hands. _____ _____ _____
42. Reported and recorded your observations. _____ _____ _____

Applying Warm and Cold Applications

Name: _____   Date: _____

	S	**U**	**Comments**

Quality of Life

Remembered to:
- Knock before entering the person's room.
- Address the person by name.
- Introduce yourself by name and title.
- Explain the procedure to the person before beginning and during the procedure.
- Protect the person's rights during the procedure.
- Handle the person gently during the procedure.

Preprocedure

1. Followed Delegation Guidelines: Applying Warm and Cold
   Saw *Promoting Safety and Comfort: Applying Warm and Cold*
2. Practiced hand hygiene.
3. Collected needed equipment:
   a. For *a warm compress:*
      i. Basin
      ii. Bath thermometer
      iii. Small towel, washcloth, or gauze squares
      iv. Plastic wrap or Aquathermia pad
      v. Ties, tape, or rolled gauze
      vi. Bath towel
      vii. Waterproof pad
   b. For *a warm soak:*
      i. Water basin or arm or foot bath
      ii. Bath thermometer
      iii. Waterproof pad
      iv. Bath blanket
      v. Towel
   c. For a *sitz bath*:
      i. Disposable sitz bath
      ii. Bath thermometer
      iii. Two bath blankets, bath towels, and a clean gown
   d. For a *warm or cold pack*:
      i. Commercial pack
      ii. Pack cover
      iii. Ties, tape, or rolled gauze (if needed)
      iv. Waterproof pad
   e. For an *Aquathermia pad*:
      i. Aquathermia pad and heating unit
      ii. Distilled water
      iii. Flannel cover or other cover as directed by the nurse
      iv. Ties, tape, or rolled gauze
   f. For an *ice bag, ice collar, ice glove, or dry cold pack*:
      i. Ice bag, collar, glove, or cold pack
      ii. Crushed ice (except for cold pack)
      iii. Flannel cover or other cover as directed by the nurse
      iv. Paper towels
   g. For a *cold compress*:
      i. Large basin with ice
      ii. Small basin with cold water
      iii. Gauze squares, washcloths, or small towels
      iv. Waterproof pad
4. Identified the person. Checked the identification (ID) bracelet against the assignment sheet. Also called the person by name.
5. Provided for privacy.

395

Procedure	S	U	Comments
6. Positioned the person for the procedure.	___	___	___
7. Placed the waterproof pad (if needed) under the body part.	___	___	___
8. For a *warm compress*:			
a. Filled the basin ½ to ⅔ full with warm water as directed by the nurse. Measured water temperature.	___	___	___
b. Placed the compress in the water.	___	___	___
c. Wrung out the compress.	___	___	___
d. Applied the compress over the area. Noted the time.	___	___	___
e. Covered the compress quickly. Used one of the following as directed by the nurse:			
i. Applied plastic wrap and then a bath towel. Secured the towel in place with ties, tape, or rolled gauze. OR	___	___	___
ii. Applied an Aquathermia pad.	___	___	___
9. For a *warm soak*:			
a. Filled a container ½ full with warm water as directed by the nurse. Measured water temperature.	___	___	___
b. Placed the body part into the water. Padded the edge of the container with a towel. Noted the time.	___	___	___
c. Covered the person with a bath blanket for warmth.	___	___	___
10. For a *sitz bath*:			
a. Placed the disposable sitz bath on the toilet seat.	___	___	___
b. Filled the sitz bath ⅔ full with water as directed by the nurse. Measured water temperature.	___	___	___
c. Secured the gown above the waist.	___	___	___
d. Helped the person sit on the sitz bath. Noted the time.	___	___	___
e. Provided for warmth. Placed a bath blanket around the shoulders. Placed another over the legs.	___	___	___
f. Stayed with the person if he or she was weak or unsteady.	___	___	___
11. For a *warm or cold pack:*			
a. Squeezed, kneaded, or struck the pack as directed by the manufacturer.	___	___	___
b. Placed the pack in the cover.	___	___	___
c. Applied the pack. Noted the time.	___	___	___
d. Secured the pack in place with ties, tape, or rolled gauze. Some packs are secured with Velcro straps.	___	___	___
12. For an *Aquathermia pad:*			
a. Filled the heating unit to the fill line with distilled water.	___	___	___
b. Removed the bubbles. Placed the pad and tubing below the heating unit. Tilted the heating unit from side to side.	___	___	___
c. Set the temperature as the nurse directed (usually 105°F [40.5°C]). Removed the key.	___	___	___
d. Placed the pad in the cover.	___	___	___
e. Plugged in the unit. Allowed water to warm to the desired temperature.	___	___	___
f. Set the heating unit on the bedside stand. Kept the pad and connecting hoses level with the unit. Hoses did not have kinks.	___	___	___
g. Applied the pad to the body part. Noted the time.	___	___	___
h. Secured the pad in place with ties, tape, or rolled gauze. Did not use pins.	___	___	___
13. For an *ice bag, collar, or glove:*			
a. Filled the device with water. Put in the stopper. Turned the device upside down and checked for leaks.	___	___	___
b. Emptied the device.	___	___	___
c. Filled the device ½ to ⅔ full with crushed ice or ice chips.	___	___	___
d. Removed excess air. Bent, twisted, or squeezed the device. Or pressed it against a firm surface.	___	___	___
e. Placed the cap or stopper on securely.	___	___	___
f. Dried the device with paper towels.	___	___	___
g. Placed the device in the cover.	___	___	___

Procedure—cont'd	S	U	Comments
h. Applied the device. Noted the time.	——	——	————
i. Secured the device in place with ties, tape, or rolled gauze.	——	——	————
14. For a *cold compress:*			
a. Placed the small basin with cold water into the large basin with ice.	——	——	————
b. Placed the compress into the cold water.	——	——	————
c. Wrung out a compress.	——	——	————
d. Applied the compress to the part. Noted the time.	——	——	————
15. Placed the call light within reach. Unscreened the person.	——	——	————
16. Raised or lowered bed rails. Followed the care plan.	——	——	————
17. Checked the person every 5 minutes. Checked for signs and symptoms of complications. Removed the application if complications occurred. Told the nurse at once.	——	——	————
18. Checked the application every 5 minutes. Changed the application if cooling (warm applications) or warming (cold applications) occurred.	——	——	————
19. Removed the application at the specified time. Warm and cold applications are usually left on for 15–20 minutes. (If bed rails were up, lowered the near one for this step.)	——	——	————

Postprocedure

	S	U	Comments
20. Provided for comfort.	——	——	————
21. Placed the call light within reach.	——	——	————
22. Raised or lowered bed rails. Followed the care plan.	——	——	————
23. Unscreened the person.	——	——	————
24. Cleaned and returned reusable items to the proper place. Followed center policy for soiled linens. Wore gloves for this step.	——	——	————
25. Completed a safety check of the room.	——	——	————
26. Removed and discarded the gloves. Decontaminated your hands.	——	——	————
27. Reported and recorded your observations.	——	——	————

Caring for Hearing Aids

Name: _____   Date: _____

Quality of Life	S	U	Comments
Remembered to:			
• Knock before entering the person's room.	——	——	————
• Address the person by name.	——	——	————
• Introduce yourself by name and title.	——	——	————
• Explain the procedure to the person before beginning and during the procedure.	——	——	————
• Protect the person's rights during the procedure.	——	——	————
• Handle the person gently during the procedure.	——	——	————

Preprocedure

	S	U	Comments
1. Followed *Delegation Guidelines: Hearing Aids*	——	——	————
Saw *Promoting Safety and Comfort: Hearing Aids*	——	——	————
2. Practiced hand hygiene.	——	——	————
3. Collected the following:			
a. Hearing aid case	——	——	————
b. Soft towel to place on work surface	——	——	————
c. Soft, dry cloth	——	——	————

Procedure

	S	U	Comments
4. Placed the towel over the surface where you were working.	——	——	————
5. Asked the resident to remove the hearing aid. If necessary, carefully removed it for the person.	——	——	————
6. With a soft, dry cloth, carefully wiped the surfaces of the hearing aid.			
a. Wiped the hearing aid from top to bottom.	——	——	————
b. Did not use water, alcohol, or any disinfectant unless told to do so.	——	——	————
7. Removed the battery and gently wiped the battery area. Replaced the battery if needed.	——	——	————
8. *If the person wore the hearing aid:*			
a. Made sure the ear was clean and dry.	——	——	————
b. Correctly placed the hearing aid or had the resident place it.	——	——	————
c. Made sure the hearing aid was on and adjusted properly.	——	——	————
d. Asked the resident if he or she was able to hear clearly.	——	——	————
9. *If the person did not wear the hearing aid:*			
a. Opened the hearing aid case.	——	——	————
b. Opened the battery door and removed the battery.	——	——	————
c. Put the hearing aid in the case.	——	——	————
d. Placed the case in the top drawer of the bedside stand.	——	——	————
e. Did not expose the hearing aid to moisture or humidity.	——	——	————

Postprocedure

	S	U	Comments
10. Provided for comfort.	——	——	————
11. Placed the call light within reach.	——	——	————
12. Placed the soiled cloth and towel in the proper place.	——	——	————
13. Completed a safety check of the room.	——	——	————
14. Decontaminated your hands.	——	——	————
15. Reported and recorded your observations.	——	——	————

Caring for Eyeglasses

Name: _____   Date: _____

	S	U	Comments
Quality of Life			

Remembered to:
- Knock before entering the person's room. ___ ___ _____
- Address the person by name. ___ ___ _____
- Introduce yourself by name and title. ___ ___ _____
- Explain the procedure to the person before beginning and during the procedure. ___ ___ _____
- Protect the person's rights during the procedure. ___ ___ _____
- Handle the person gently during the procedure. ___ ___ _____

Preprocedure

1. Followed *Delegation Guidelines: Eyeglasses* ___ ___ _____
   Saw *Promoting Safety and Comfort: Eyeglasses* ___ ___ _____
2. Practiced hand hygiene. ___ ___ _____
3. Collected the following:
   a. Eyeglass case ___ ___ _____
   b. Cleaning solution or warm water ___ ___ _____
   c. Disposable lens cloth or cotton cloth ___ ___ _____

Procedure

4. Removed the eyeglasses:
   a. Held the frames in front of the ears. ___ ___ _____
   b. Lifted the frames from the ears. Brought the eyeglasses down away from the face. ___ ___ _____
5. Cleaned the lenses with cleaning solution or warm water. Cleaned in a circular motion. Dried the lenses with the cloth. ___ ___ _____
6. *If the person did not wear the eyeglasses*:
   a. Opened the eyeglass case. ___ ___ _____
   b. Folded the glasses. Put them in the case. Did not touch the clean lenses. ___ ___ _____
   c. Placed the eyeglass case in the top drawer of the bedside stand. ___ ___ _____
7. *If the person wore the eyeglasses:*
   a. Unfolded the eyeglasses. ___ ___ _____
   b. Held the frames at each side. Placed them over the ears. ___ ___ _____
   c. Adjusted the eyeglasses so the nosepiece rested on the nose. ___ ___ _____
   d. Returned the eyeglass case to the top drawer in the bedside stand. ___ ___ _____

Postprocedure

8. Provided for comfort. ___ ___ _____
9. Placed the call light within reach. ___ ___ _____
10. Returned the cleaning solution to its proper place. ___ ___ _____
11. Discarded the disposable cloth. ___ ___ _____
12. Completed a safety check of the room. ___ ___ _____
13. Decontaminated your hands. ___ ___ _____
14. Reported and recorded your observations. ___ ___ _____

399

Adult CPR—One Rescuer

Name: _____   Date: _____

Procedure	S	U	Comments
1. Made sure the scene was safe.	——	——	——————
2. Took 5–10 seconds to check for a response and breathing:			
a. Checked if the person was responding. Tapped or gently shook the person. Called the person by name, if known. Shouted: "Are you okay?"	——	——	——————
b. Checked for no breathing or no normal breathing (gasping).	——	——	——————
3. Called for help. Activated the Emergency Medical Services (EMS) system or center's emergency response system if the person was not responding and not breathing or not breathing normally (gasping).	——	——	——————
4. Got or asked someone to bring an automated external defibrillator (AED) if available.	——	——	——————
5. Positioned the person supine on a hard, flat surface. Logrolled the person so there was no twisting of the spine. Placed the arms alongside the body.	——	——	——————
6. Checked for a carotid pulse. This took 5–10 seconds. Started chest compressions if you did not feel a pulse.	——	——	——————
7. Exposed the person's chest.	——	——	——————
8. Gave chest compressions at a rate of 100–120 per minute. Pushed hard and fast. Established a regular rhythm. Counted out loud. Pressed down at least 2 inches. Allowed the chest to recoil between compressions. Gave 30 chest compressions.	——	——	——————
9. Opened the airway. Used the head tilt–chin lift method.	——	——	——————
10. Gave two breaths. Each breath took only 1 second. Each breath made the chest rise. (If the first breath did not make the chest rise, tried opening the airway again. Used the head tilt–chin lift method.)	——	——	——————
11. Continued the cycle of 30 compressions followed by 2 breaths. Limited interruptions in compressions to less than 10 seconds. Continued cycles until the AED arrived. Or continued until help arrived or the person began to move. If movement occurred, placed the person in the recovery position.	——	——	——————

Adult CPR—Two Rescuers

Name: _____   Date: _____

Procedure	S	U	Comments
1. Made sure the scene was safe.	___	___	_____
2. *Rescuer 1*: Took 5–10 seconds to check for a response and breathing:			
a. Checked if the person was responding. Tapped or gently shook the person. Called the person by name, if known. Shouted: "Are you okay?"	___	___	_____
b. Checked for no breathing or no normal breathing (gasping).	___	___	_____
3. *Rescuer 2*:			
a. Activated the Emergency Medical Services (EMS) system or center's emergency response system if the person was not responding and not breathing or not breathing normally (gasping).	___	___	_____
b. Got an automated external defibrillator (AED) if one was available.	___	___	_____
4. *Rescuer 1*: Positioned the person supine on a hard, flat surface. Logrolled the person so there was no twisting of the spine. Placed the arms alongside the body. Began one-rescuer CPR until the second rescuer returned.	___	___	_____
5. When the second rescuer returned, performed two person CPR.			
a. *Rescuer 1*: Gave chest compressions at a rate of 100–120 per minute. Pushed hard and fast. Established a regular rhythm. Counted out loud. Pressed down at least 2 inches. Allowed the chest to recoil between compressions. Gave 30 chest compressions. Paused to allow the other rescuer to give two breaths.	___	___	_____
b. *Rescuer 2*:			
1. Opened the airway. Used the head tilt–chin lift method.	___	___	_____
2. Gave 2 breaths after every 30 compressions. Each breath took only 1 second and made the chest rise. (If the first breath did not make the chest rise, tried opening the airway again. Used the head tilt–chin lift method.)	___	___	_____
3. Continued cycles of 30 compressions and 2 breaths.	___	___	_____
c. Changed positions every 2 minutes (after about five cycles of 30 compressions and 2 breaths). The switch took no more than 5 seconds.	___	___	_____
d. Continued until the AED arrived. Or continued until help took over or the person began to move. If movement occurred, placed the person in the recovery position.	___	___	_____

Adult CPR with AED—Two Rescuers

Name: _____ Date: _____

Procedure	S	U	Comments
1. Made sure the scene was safe.	___	___	_____
2. *Rescuer 1*: Took 5–10 seconds to check for a response and breathing. Checked if the person was responding. Tapped or gently shook the person. Called the person by name, if known. Shouted: "Are you okay?"	___	___	_____
3. *Rescuer 2:*			
a. Activated the Emergency Medical Services (EMS) system or the center's emergency response system if the person was not responding and not breathing or not breathing normally (gasping).	___	___	_____
b. Got an automated external defibrillator (AED) if one was available.	___	___	_____
4. *Rescuer 1:*			
a. Positioned the person supine on a hard, flat surface. Logrolled the person so there was no twisting of the spine. Placed the arms alongside the body.	___	___	_____
b. Checked for a carotid pulse. This took 5–10 seconds. Started chest compressions if you did not feel a pulse.	___	___	_____
c. Exposed the person's chest.	___	___	_____
d. Gave chest compressions at a rate of 100–120 per minute. Pushed hard and fast. Established a regular rhythm. Counted out loud. Pressed down at least 2 inches. Allowed the chest to recoil between compressions. Gave 30 chest compressions.	___	___	_____
e. Opened the airway. Used the head tilt–chin lift method.	___	___	_____
f. Gave two breaths. Each breath took only 1 second. Each breath made the chest rise. (If the first breath did not make the chest rise, tried opening the airway again. Used the head tilt–chin lift method.)	___	___	_____
g. Continued the cycle of 30 compressions followed by 2 breaths. Limited interruptions in compressions to less than 10 seconds.	___	___	_____
5. *Rescuer 2:*			
a. Opened the case with the AED.	___	___	_____
b. Turned on the AED.	___	___	_____
c. Applied adult electrode pads to the person's chest. Followed the instructions and diagram provided with the AED.	___	___	_____
d. Attached the connecting cables to the AED.	___	___	_____
e. Cleared away from the person. Made sure no one was touching the person.	___	___	_____
f. Allowed the AED to analyze the person's heart rhythm.	___	___	_____
g. Made sure everyone was clear of the person if the AED advised a "shock." Loudly instructed others not to touch the person. Said: "I am clear, you are clear, everyone is clear!" Looked to make sure no one was touching the person.	___	___	_____
h. Pressed the "SHOCK" button if the AED advised a "shock."	___	___	_____

Procedure—cont'd   S   U   Comments

6. *Rescuers 1 and 2:*
   a. Performed two person CPR:
      1. Began with compressions. One rescuer gave chest compressions
         at a rate of 100–120 per minute. Pushed hard and fast. Established
         a regular rhythm. Counted out loud. Allowed the chest to recoil
         between compressions. Gave 30 chest compressions. Paused to
         allow the other rescuer to give two breaths.   ____   ____   _____
      2. The other rescuer gave 2 breaths after every 30 chest compressions.   ____   ____   _____
7. Repeated the following after 2 minutes of cardiopulmonary respiration
   (CPR) (five cycles of 30 compressions and 2 breaths). Then changed
   positions and continued CPR beginning with compressions.
   a. Cleared away from the person. Made sure no one was touching the
      person.   ____   ____   _____
   b. Allowed the AED to analyze the person's heart rhythm.   ____   ____   _____
   c. Made sure everyone was clear of the person if the AED advised a
      "shock." Loudly instructed others not to touch the person. Said: "I am
      clear, you are clear, everyone is clear!" Looked to make sure no one
      was touching the person.   ____   ____   _____
   d. Pressed the "SHOCK" button if the AED advised a "shock."   ____   ____   _____
8. Continued until help took over or the person began to move. If movement
   occurred, placed the person in the recovery position.   ____   ____   _____

Relieving Choking—Adult or Child (Over 1 Year of Age)

Name: _____ Date: _____

Procedure	S	U	Comments
1. Asked the person if he or she was choking. Helped the person if he or she nodded "yes" and could not talk.	⎯	⎯	⎯⎯⎯⎯
2. Had someone call for help.			
a. *In public area:* Had someone activate the Emergency Medical Services (EMS) system by calling 911. Sent someone to get an automated external defibrillator (AED).	⎯	⎯	⎯⎯⎯⎯
b. *In a center:* Called emergency response system and sent for AED and emergency cart.	⎯	⎯	⎯⎯⎯⎯
3. *If the person was sitting or standing*, gave abdominal thrusts.			⎯⎯⎯⎯
a. Stood or knelt behind the person.	⎯	⎯	
b. Wrapped your arms around the person's waist.	⎯	⎯	⎯⎯⎯⎯
c. Made a fist with one hand.	⎯	⎯	⎯⎯⎯⎯
d. Placed thumb side of fist against the abdomen. The fist was slightly above the navel in the middle of the abdomen and well below the end of the sternum (breastbone).	⎯	⎯	⎯⎯⎯⎯
e. Grasped the fist with your other hand.	⎯	⎯	⎯⎯⎯⎯
f. Pressed your fist into the person's abdomen with a quick, upward thrust.	⎯	⎯	⎯⎯⎯⎯
g. Repeated thrusts until the object was expelled or the person became unresponsive.	⎯	⎯	⎯⎯⎯⎯
4. *If person was obese or pregnant*, gave chest thrusts.			
a. Stood behind the person.	⎯	⎯	⎯⎯⎯⎯
b. Placed your arms under the person's underarms. Wrapped your arms around the person's chest.	⎯	⎯	⎯⎯⎯⎯
c. Made a fist and placed the thumb side of fist on the middle of the sternum (breastbone).	⎯	⎯	⎯⎯⎯⎯
d. Grasped the fist with your other hand.	⎯	⎯	⎯⎯⎯⎯
e. Gave thrusts to the chest until object was expelled or the person became unresponsive.	⎯	⎯	⎯⎯⎯⎯
5. *If object was dislodged*, encouraged the person to go to the hospital.	⎯	⎯	⎯⎯⎯⎯

6. *If person became unresponsive*, lowered person to the floor or ground. Positioned the person supine. Made sure EMS or emergency response system was called (step 2). *If alone*, provided five cycles (2 minutes) of CPR first, then called EMS or emergency response system.   _____   _____   _____

7. Started CPR:
   a. Did not check for a pulse. Began compressions. Gave 30 compressions.   _____   _____   _____
   b. Used the head tilt–chin lift method to open the airway. Opened the person's mouth. Mouth was wide open. Looked for an object. Removed the object if it was seen and could be removed easily. Used fingers.   _____   _____   _____
   c. Gave two breaths.   _____   _____   _____
   d. Continued cycles of 30 compressions and 2 breaths. Looked for an object every time airway was opened for rescue breaths.   _____   _____   _____

8. *If choking was relieved in an unresponsive person*:
   a. Checked for a response, breathing, and pulse.   _____   _____   _____
   1. *If no response, normal breathing, or pulse*, continued CPR. Attached an AED.   _____   _____   _____
   2. *If no response and no normal breathing but there was a pulse*, gave rescue breaths. For adult, gave one breath every 5–6 seconds (10–12 breaths per minute). For child, gave one breath every 3–5 seconds (12–20 breaths per minute). Checked pulse every 2 minutes. If no pulse, began CPR.   _____   _____   _____
   3. *If person had normal breathing and a pulse*, placed the person in recovery position, if there was no response. Continued to check the person until help arrived. Encouraged the person to go to hospital if he or she responded.   _____   _____   _____

Assisting with Postmortem Care

Name: _____   Date: _____

	S	U	Comments
Preprocedure			
1. Followed *Delegation Guidelines: Care of the Body After Death*			
Saw *Promoting Safety and Comfort: Care of the Body After Death*	___	___	_____
2. Practiced hand hygiene.	___	___	_____
3. Collected the following:			
a. Postmortem kit (shroud or body bag, gown, identification [ID] tags, gauze squares, safety pins)	___	___	_____
b. Bed protectors	___	___	_____
c. Wash basin	___	___	_____
d. Bath towel and washcloths	___	___	_____
e. Denture cup	___	___	_____
f. Tape	___	___	_____
g. Dressings	___	___	_____
h. Gloves	___	___	_____
i. Cotton balls	___	___	_____
j. Valuables envelope	___	___	_____
4. Provided for privacy.	___	___	_____
5. Raised the bed for body mechanics.	___	___	_____
6. Made sure the bed was flat.	___	___	_____
Procedure			
7. Put on gloves.	___	___	_____
8. Positioned the body supine. Arms and legs were straight. A pillow was under the head and shoulders. Or raised the head of the bed 15–20 degrees, if center policy.	___	___	_____
9. Closed the eyes. Gently pulled the eyelids over the eyes. Applied moist cotton balls gently over the eyelids if the eyes did not stay closed.	___	___	_____
10. Inserted dentures if it is center policy to do so. If not, placed them in a labeled denture cup.	___	___	_____
11. Closed the mouth. If necessary, placed a rolled towel under the chin to keep the mouth closed.	___	___	_____
12. Followed center policy for jewelry. Removed all jewelry, except for wedding rings if this is center policy. Listed the jewelry that you removed. Placed the jewelry and the list in a valuables envelope.	___	___	_____
13. Placed a cotton ball over the rings. Taped them in place.	___	___	_____
14. Removed drainage containers.	___	___	_____
15. Removed tubes and catheters. Used the gauze squares as needed. (Omitted this step if autopsy will be performed.)	___	___	_____
16. Bathed soiled areas with plain water. Dried thoroughly.	___	___	_____
17. Placed a bed protector under the buttocks.	___	___	_____
18. Removed soiled dressings. Replaced them with clean ones.	___	___	_____
19. Put a clean gown on the body. Positioned the body supine. Arms and legs were straight. A pillow was under the head and shoulders. Or the head of the bed was raised 15–20 degrees if center policy.	___	___	_____
20. Brushed and combed the hair if necessary.	___	___	_____
21. Covered the body to the shoulders with a sheet if the family was to view the body.	___	___	_____
22. Gathered the person's belongings. Put them in a bag labeled with the person's name. Made sure you included eyeglasses, hearing aids, and other valuables.	___	___	_____
23. Removed supplies, equipment, and linens. Straightened the room. Provided soft lighting.	___	___	_____
24. Removed the gloves. Decontaminated your hands.	___	___	_____

Procedure—cont'd   S   U   **Comments**

25. Let the family view the body. Provided for privacy. Returned to the room after they left. — — ———————

26. Decontaminated your hands. Put on gloves. — — ———————

27. Filled out the ID tags. Tied one to the ankle or to the right big toe. — — ———————

28. Placed the body in the body bag or covered it with a sheet. Or applied the shroud.

   a. Positioned the shroud under the body. — — ———————

   b. Brought the top down over the head. — — ———————

   c. Folded the bottom up over the feet. — — ———————

   d. Folded the sides over the body. — — ———————

   e. Pinned or taped the shroud in place. — — ———————

29. Attached the second ID tag to the shroud, sheet, or body bag. — — ———————

30. Left the denture cup with the body. — — ———————

31. Pulled the privacy curtain around the bed. Or closed the door. — — ———————

Postprocedure

32. Removed the gloves. Decontaminated your hands. — — ———————

33. Stripped the unit after the body had been removed. Wore gloves for this step. — — ———————

34. Removed the gloves. Decontaminated your hands. — — ———————

35. Reported the following:

   a. The time the body was taken by the funeral director — — ———————

   b. What was done with jewelry, other valuables, and personal items — — ———————

   c. What was done with dentures — — ———————

Competency Evaluation Review

PREPARING FOR THE COMPETENCY EVALUATION

After completing your state's training program, you need to pass the competency evaluation. The purpose of the competency evaluation is to make sure you can do your job safely. This section will help you prepare for the test.

COMPETENCY EVALUATION

The competency evaluation has a written test and a skills test. The number of questions varies with each state. Each question has four possible answers. Although some questions may appear to have more than one possible answer, there is only one best answer. You will have about 1 minute to read and answer each question. Some questions take less time to read and answer. Other questions take longer. You should have enough time to take the test without feeling rushed.

The content of the written test varies depending on your state. Content may include:

- Activities of Daily Living—hygiene, dressing and grooming, nutrition and hydration, elimination, rest/sleep/comfort
- Basic Nursing Skills—infection control, safety/emergency, therapeutic/technical procedures (e.g., vital signs, bedmaking), data collection and reporting
- Restorative Skills—prevention, self-care/independence
- Emotional and Mental Health Needs
- Spiritual and Cultural Needs
- The Person's Rights
- Legal and Ethical Behavior
- Being a Member of the Health Care Team
- Communication

The written test is given as a paper and pencil test in most states. Some test sites may use computers. You do not need computer experience to take the test on the computer. If you have difficulty reading English, you may request to take an oral test. Talk with your instructor or employer about details for computer testing or oral testing.

The skills test involves performing five nursing skills you learned in your training program. These skills are chosen randomly. You do not select the skills. You are allowed about 30 minutes to do the skills. See pp. 410–411 for more information about the skills test.

TAKING THE COMPETENCY EVALUATION

To register for the test, you need to complete an application. Your instructor or employer tells you when and where the tests are given. There is a fee for the evaluation. If you work in a nursing center, the employer may pay this fee. If you pay the fee, you may need to purchase a money order or certified check. Make sure your name is on the money order or certified check. Cash and personal checks may not be accepted.

Plan to arrive at the test site about 15 to 30 minutes before the evaluation begins. Most centers do not admit you if you are late. Know the exact location of the test site and room. Actually drive or take transportation to the test site a few days or a week before the test. Making a "dry run" lets you know how much time you need to travel, park, and get to the test site. It will also help decrease your anxiety level on the test day.

To be admitted to the test, you need two pieces of identification (ID). The first form of ID is a government-issued document such as a driver's license or passport. It must have a current photo and your signature. The name on the ID must be the same as the name on your application form. If your name has changed and you have not been able to have the name changed on your identification documents, ask your instructor or employer what to do. The second form of ID must include your name and signature. Examples include a library card, hunting license, or credit card.

Take several sharpened Number 2 pencils to the test. For the skills test you will need a watch with a second hand. You may need a person to play the role of the patient or resident. Ask your instructor or employer how this is done in your state.

Taking the written test and skills test may take several hours. You may want to bring snacks or lunch and a beverage to the testing site. Eating and drinking are not allowed during the test. However, you may be told where you can eat while waiting for the test.

You cannot bring textbooks, study notes, or other materials into the testing room. The only exception may be a language translation dictionary that you show to the proctor (a person who monitors the test) before the test begins. Cell phones, calculators, or other electronic devices are not permitted during testing. Children and pets are not allowed in the testing areas.

STUDYING FOR THE COMPETENCY EVALUATION

You began to prepare for the written and skills test during your training program. You learned the basic nursing content and skills needed to provide safe, quality care. The following suggestions can help you study for the competency evaluation:

- Begin to study at least 2 to 3 weeks before the test. Plan to study for 1 to 2 hours each day.
- Decide on a specific time to study. Choose a study time that is best for you. This may be early in the morning before others are awake. It may be in the

evening after others go to sleep. Try to choose a time when you are mentally alert.

- Choose a specific area to study in. This area should be quiet, well-lit, and comfortable. You should have enough room to write and to spread out your books, notes, and other study aids—such as a CD or DVD. The area does not need to be noise-free. The testing site is not completely quiet. You want to concentrate and not be distracted by the noise around you.
- Collect everything you need before settling down to study. This includes your textbook, notes, paper, highlighters, pens or pencils, CDs, and DVDs.
- Take short breaks when you need them. Take a break when your mind begins to wander or if you feel sleepy.
- Develop a study plan. Write your plan down so you can refer to it. Study one content area before going on to the next. For example, study personal hygiene before going on to vital signs. Do not jump from one subject to another.
- Use a variety of ways to study:
  - Use index cards to help you review abbreviations and terminology. Put the abbreviation or term on the front of the card and place the meaning on the back. Take the cards with you and review them whenever you have a break or are waiting.
  - Record key points. You can listen to the recording while cooking or riding in the car.
  - Study groups are another way to prepare for a test. Group members can quiz each other.
- To remember what you are learning, try these ideas:
  - Relax when you study. When relaxed, you learn information quickly and recall it with greater ease.
  - Repeat what you are learning. Say it out loud. This helps you remember the idea.
  - Make the information you are learning meaningful. Think about how the information will help you be a good nursing assistant.
  - Write down what you are learning. Writing helps you remember information. Prepare study sheets.
  - Be positive about what you are learning. You remember what you find interesting.
- Suggestions for studying if you have children:
  - When you first come home from work or school, spend time with your children. Then plan study time.
  - Select educational programs on TV that your children can watch as you study. Or get a DVD from the library.
  - When you take your study breaks, spend time with your children.
  - Ask other adults to take care of the children while you study.
- Take the two 75-question practice tests in this section. Each question has the correct answer and the reason why an answer is correct or incorrect. If you practice taking tests, you are more likely to pass

them. Take the practice tests under conditions similar to the real test. Work within time limits.
- If your state has a practice test and a candidate handbook, study the content. Some states have practice tests online.

MANAGING ANXIETY

Almost everyone dreads taking tests. It is common and normal to experience anxiety before taking a test. If used wisely, anxiety can actually help you do well. When you are anxious, that means you are concerned. You may be concerned about how prepared you are to take the test. Or you may be concerned about how you will feel about yourself if you do not pass the test. Being concerned usually results in some action. To overcome anxiety before the test:

- Study and prepare for the test. That helps increase your confidence as you recall or clarify what you have learned. Anxiety decreases as confidence increases. When you think you know the information, keep studying. This reinforces your learning.
- Develop a positive mental attitude. You can pass this test. You took tests in your training program and passed them. Praise yourself. Talk to yourself in a positive way. If a negative thought enters your mind, stop it at once. Challenge the mental thought and tell yourself you will pass the test.
- Visualize success. Think about how wonderful you will feel when you are notified that you have passed the test.
- Perform breathing exercises. Breathe slowly and deeply.
- Perform regular exercise. Exercise helps you stay physically fit. It also helps keep you calm.
- Good nourishment helps you think clearly. Eat a nourishing meal before the test. Do not skip breakfast. Vitamin C helps fight short-term stress. Protein and calcium help overcome the effects of long-term stress. Complex carbohydrates (pasta, nuts, yogurt) can help settle your nerves. Eat familiar foods the day before and the day of the test. Do not eat foods that could cause stomach or intestinal upset.
- Maintain a normal routine the day before the test.
- Get a good night's sleep before the test. Go to bed early enough so you do not oversleep or are too tired to get up. Set your alarm clock properly. You may want to set two alarm clocks.
- Do not "cram" the evening before or the day of the test. Last-minute cramming increases your anxiety. Do something relaxing with family and friends.
- Avoid drinking large amounts of coffee, colas, water, or other beverages. You do not want to be uncomfortable with a full bladder when you take the test.
- Wear comfortable clothes. Dress in layers so that you are prepared for a cold or warm room. Dress professionally. Have long hair pulled back. Do not wear nail polish. Ask your instructor if a uniform or scrubs should be worn.

409

- If you are a woman, remember that worry and anxiety can affect your menstrual cycle. Wear a panty liner, sanitary napkin, or tampon if you think your period may start. This eliminates worry about soiling your clothing during the test.
- Allow plenty of time for travel, traffic, and parking.
- Arrive early enough to use the restroom before the test begins.
- Do not talk about the test with others. Their panic or anxiety may affect your self-confidence.

TAKING THE TEST

Follow these guidelines for taking the test:
- Listen carefully and follow the instructions given by the proctor (person administering the test).
- When you receive the test, make certain you have all the test pages.
- Read and follow all directions carefully.
- You are not allowed to ask questions about the content of the test questions.
- Do deep-breathing and muscle-relaxation exercises as needed.
- Cheating of any kind is not allowed. If the proctor sees you giving or receiving any type of assistance, your test booklet is taken and you must leave the testing site.
- If using a computer answer sheet, completely fill in the bubble.
- If you make a mistake, erase the wrong answer completely. Do not make any stray marks on the paper. Not erasing completely or leaving stray marks could cause the computer to misread your answer.
- Do not worry or get anxious if people finish the test before you do. Persons who finish a test early do not necessarily score better than those who finish later.
- You cannot take any evaluation materials or notes out of the testing room.

ANSWERING MULTIPLE-CHOICE QUESTIONS

Pace yourself during the test. First, answer all the questions that you know. Then go back and answer skipped questions. Sometimes you will remember the answer later. Or another test question may give you a clue to the one you skipped. Spending too much time on a question can cost you valuable time later. To help you answer the questions or statements:
- Always read the questions or statements carefully. Do not scan or glance at questions. Scanning or glancing can cause you to miss important key words. Read each word of the question.
- Before reading the answers, decide what the answer is in your own words. Then read all four answers to the question. Select the one best answer.
- Do not read into a question. Take the question as it is asked. Do not add your own thoughts and ideas to the question. Do not assume or suppose "what if." Just respond to the information provided.

- Trust your common sense. If unsure of an answer, select your first choice. Do not change your answer unless you are absolutely sure of the correct answer. Your first reaction is usually correct.
- Look for key words in every question. Sometimes key words are in italics, highlighted, or underlined. Common key words are: *always, never, first, except, best, not, correct, incorrect, true,* or *false.*
- Know which words can make a statement correct (e.g., *may, can, usually, most, at least, sometimes*). The word "except" can make a question a false statement.
- Be careful of answers with these key words or phrases: *always, never, every, only, all, none, at all times,* or *at no time.* These words and phrases do not allow for exceptions. In nursing, exceptions are generally present. However, sometimes answers containing these words are correct. For example, which of the following is correct and which are incorrect?
  a. Always use a turning sheet.
  b. Never shake linens.
  c. Soap is used for all baths.
  d. The call light must always be attached to the bed.

The correct answer is b. Incorrect answers are a, c, and d.
- Omit answers that are obviously wrong. Then choose the best of the remaining answers.
- Go back to the questions you skipped. Answer all questions by eliminating or narrowing your choices. Always mark an answer even if you are not sure.
- Review the test a second time for completeness and accuracy before turning it in.
- Make sure you have answered each question. Also check that you have given only one answer for each question.
- Remember, the test is not designed to trick or confuse you. The written competency evaluation tests what you know, not what you do not know. You know more than you are asked.

ONLINE TESTING

The test may be given by computer at the test site. Ask your instructor what computer skills you will need. You usually do not need keyboard or typing skills. You will use a computer mouse to select answers. Also, you will usually receive instruction before the test begins. This will let you practice using the computer before starting the test.

SKILLS EVALUATION REVIEW

Each state has its own policies and procedures for the skills test. The following information is an overview of what to expect:
- To pass the skills evaluation, you will need to perform all five skills correctly.
- A nurse evaluates your performance of certain skills. Having someone watch as you work is not a new experience. Your instructor evaluated your

performance during your training program. While you are working, your supervisor evaluates your skills.

- Mannequins and people are used as "patients" or "residents," depending on the skills you are performing.
- If you make a mistake, tell the evaluator what you did wrong. Then perform the skill correctly. Do not panic.
- Take whatever equipment you normally take or use at work. Wear a watch with a second hand. You may need it to measure vital signs and check how much time you have left. Bring a pen to record vital signs or other observations.

BEFORE AND DURING THE PROCEDURE

- Hand washing is evaluated at the beginning of the skills test. You are expected to know when to wash your hands. Therefore, you may not be told to do so. Follow the rules for hand hygiene during the test.
- Before entering a person's room, knock on the door. Greet the person by name and introduce yourself before beginning a procedure. Check the identification (ID) bracelet or the photo ID to make certain you are giving care to the right person.
- Explain what you are going to do before beginning the procedure and as needed throughout the procedure.
- Always follow the rules of medical asepsis. For example, remove gloves and dispose of them properly. Keep clean linens separated from dirty linens.
- Always protect the person's rights throughout the skills test.
- Communicate with the person as you give care. Focus on the person's needs and interests. Always treat the person with respect. Do not talk about yourself or your personal problems.
- Provide privacy. This involves pulling the privacy curtain around the bed, closing doors, and asking visitors to leave the room.
- Promote safety for the person. For example, lock the wheelchair when you transfer a person to and from it. Use a gait/transfer belt for transfers and ambulation. Place the bed in the lowest horizontal position when the person must get out of bed or when you are done giving care.
- Make sure the call light is within the person's reach. Attaching it to the bed or bed rail does not mean the person can reach it.

- Use good body mechanics. Raise the bed and overbed table to a good working height.
- Provide for comfort:
  ○ Make sure the person and linens are clean and dry. The person may have become incontinent during the procedure.
  ○ Change or straighten bed linens as needed.
  ○ Position the person for comfort and in good alignment.
  ○ Provide pillows as directed by the nurse and the care plan.
  ○ Raise the head of the bed as the person prefers and as is allowed by the nurse and the care plan.
  ○ Provide for warmth. The person may need an extra blanket, a lap blanket, a sweater, socks, and so on.
  ○ Adjust lighting to meet the person's needs.
  ○ Make sure eyeglasses, hearing aids, and other devices are in place as needed.
  ○ Ask the person if he or she is comfortable.
  ○ Ask the person if there is anything else you can do for him or her.
  ○ Make sure the person is covered for warmth and privacy.

SKILLS

You are responsible for following the most current standards, practices, and guidelines of your state. Ask your instructor to tell you which skills are tested in your state. If your state has one, review the candidate's handbook for a listing of the skills. Refer to the Skills Evaluation Review section on Evolve to see a comprehensive list of skills. These skills are offered as a study guide to you. The skills marked with an asterisk (*) are used with permission of the National Council of State Boards of Nursing (NCSBN). Make a note of the skills that are tested in your state.

In the skills, the word "client" refers to the resident or person receiving care. You may also see some steps of the skill shown in boldface type. Steps shown in boldface type are critical element steps. Critical element steps must be done correctly to pass the skill. If you miss a critical element step, you will not pass the skills evaluation. For example, you are to transfer a client from the bed to a wheelchair. You will fail if you do not lock the wheels on the wheelchair before transferring the person. An automatic failure is one that could potentially cause harm to a person. Your state may mark critical element steps in another way—underline or italics.

Textbook Chapters Review

Note: This review covers selected chapters based on Competency Evaluation requirements.

CHAPTER 1 THE NURSING ASSISTANT WORKING IN LONG-TERM CARE

- Provide medical, nursing, dietary, recreational, rehabilitative, social services. Housekeeping and laundry services are also provided.
- Residents are older or disabled.
- Some residents are recovering from illness, injury, or surgery.
- Some residents return home when well enough. Some residents need nursing care until death.
- Long-term care centers include board and care homes (group homes), assisted living residences, skilled nursing facilities (SNFs), hospices, memory care units, and rehabilitation and subacute care units.

THE NURSING TEAM

- Provides quality care to people.
- Care is coordinated by a registered nurse (RN).

Nursing Assistants

- Report to the nurse supervising their work.
- Provide basic nursing care under the supervision of a licensed nurse.
- Need formal training and must pass a competency test.

THE INTERDISCIPLINARY HEALTH CARE TEAM (HEALTH TEAM)

- Involves many health care workers whose skills and knowledge focus on total care.
- Works together to provide coordinated care to meet each person's needs.
- Follows the direction of the RN leading the team.

MEETING STANDARDS

Survey Process

- Surveys are done to see if agencies meet standards for licensure, certification, and accreditation.
  - A license is issued by the state. A center must have a license to operate and provide care.
  - Certification is required to receive Medicare and Medicaid funds.
  - Accreditation is voluntary. It signals quality and excellence.

Your Role

- Provide quality care.
- Protect the person's rights.
- Provide for the person's and your own safety.
- Help keep the center clean and safe.
- Conduct yourself in a professional manner.
- Have good work ethics.
- Follow center policies and procedures.
- Answer questions honestly and completely.

FEDERAL AND STATE LAWS

Nurse Practice Acts

- Each state has a nurse practice act. It regulates nursing practice in that state
- A state's nurse practice act is used to decide what nursing assistants can do. Some nurse practice acts also regulate nursing assistant roles, functions, education, and certification requirements. Some states have separate laws for nursing assistants.
- Nursing assistants must be able to function with skill and safety. They can have their certification, license, or registration denied, revoked, or suspended. The National Council of State Boards of Nursing (NCSBN) lists these reasons for doing so:
- Substance abuse or dependency.
- Abandoning, abusing, or neglecting a resident.
- Fraud or deceit. Examples include:
  - Filing false personal information
  - Providing false information when applying for initial certification or reinstatement.
- Violating professional boundaries.
- Giving unsafe care.
- Performing acts beyond the nursing assistant role.
- Misappropriation (stealing, theft) or misusing property.
- Obtaining money or property from a resident. Fraud, falsely representing oneself, and through force are examples.
- Having been convicted of a crime. Examples include murder, assault, kidnapping, rape or sexual assault, robbery, sexual crimes involving children, criminal mistreatment of children or a vulnerable adult, drug trafficking, embezzlement, theft, and arson.
- Failing to conform to the standards of nursing assistants.
- Putting patients and residents at risk for harm.
- Violating resident's privacy.
- Failing to maintain the confidentiality of resident information.

THE OMNIBUS BUDGET RECONCILIATION ACT OF 1987 (OBRA)

- The purpose of OBRA, a federal law, is to improve the quality of life of nursing center residents.
- OBRA sets minimum training and competency evaluation requirements for nursing assistants. Each state must have a nursing assistant training and competency evaluation program (NATCEP). A nursing assistant must successfully complete a NATCEP to work in a nursing center, hospital, or home care agency receiving Medicare funds.
- OBRA requires at least 75 hours of instruction. Some states have more hours. Sixteen hours of supervised training in a laboratory or clinical setting are required.
- OBRA requires a nursing assistant registry in each state. It is an official record that lists persons who have successfully completed the NATCEP.
- Retraining and a new competency evaluation program are required for nursing assistants who have not worked for 24 months.
- Each state's NATCEP must meet OBRA requirements.

ROLES, RESPONSIBILITIES, AND STANDARDS

- OBRA, state laws, and legal and advisory opinions direct what you can do.
- Rules for you to follow:
  - You are an assistant to the nurse.
  - A nurse assigns and supervises your work.
  - You report observations about the person's physical and mental status to the nurse. Report changes in the person's condition or behavior at once.
  - The nurse decides what should and should not be done for a person. You do not make these decisions.
  - Review directions and the care plan with the nurse before going to the person.
  - Perform only tasks that you are trained to do.
  - Perform only the nursing tasks that your state and job description allow.
  - Ask a nurse to supervise you if you are not comfortable doing a task.
- Role limits for nursing assistants:
  - Never give medications.
  - Never insert tubes or objects into body openings. Do not remove tubes from the body.
  - Never take oral or telephone orders from doctors.
  - Never perform procedures that require sterile technique.
  - Never tell the person or family the person's diagnosis or treatment plans.
  - Never diagnose or prescribe treatments or medications for anyone.
  - Never supervise others, including other nursing assistants.
  - Never ignore an order or request to do something. This includes nursing tasks that you can do, those

you cannot do, and those that are beyond your legal limits.
- Review Box 1.5, Nursing Assistant Standards, in the textbook.
- Always obtain a written job description when you apply for a job. Do not take a job that requires you to:
  - Act beyond the legal limits of your role.
  - Function beyond your training limits.
  - Perform acts that are against your morals or religion.

DELEGATION

- RNs can delegate tasks to you. In some states, licensed practical nurses/licensed vocational nurses (LPNs/LVNs) can delegate tasks to you.
- Nursing assistants cannot delegate. You cannot delegate any task to other nursing assistants or to any other worker.
- Delegation decisions must protect the person's health and safety. The delegating nurse is legally responsible for his or her actions and the actions of others who performed the delegated tasks.
- If you perform a task that places the person at risk, you may face serious legal problems.
- *The Five Rights of Delegation*
  - The right task. Can the task be delegated? Is the nurse allowed to delegate the task? Is the task in your job description?
  - The right circumstances. What are the person's physical, mental, emotional, and spiritual needs at this time?
  - The right person. Do you have the training and experience to safely perform the task for this person?
  - The right directions and communication. Did the nurse give clear directions and instructions? Did you review the task with the nurse? Do you understand what the nurse expects?
  - The right supervision. Is a nurse available to answer questions? Is a nurse available if the person's condition changes or if problems occur?

Your Role in Delegation

- When you agree to perform a task, you are responsible for your own actions. You must complete the task safely. Report to the nurse what you did and the observations you made.
- You should refuse to perform a task when:
  - The task is beyond the legal limits of your role.
  - The task is not in your job description.
  - You were not prepared to perform the task.
  - The task could harm the person.
  - The person's condition has changed.
  - You do not know how to use the supplies or equipment.
  - Directions are not ethical or legal.

413

- Directions are against center policies.
- Directions are unclear or incomplete.
- A nurse is not available for supervision.
- Never ignore an order or request to do something. Tell the nurse about your concerns.

CHAPTER 1 REVIEW QUESTIONS

Circle the BEST answer.

1. Nursing assistants do all the following *except*
   a. Provide quality care
   b. Follow agency policies and procedures
   c. Conduct themselves in an unprofessional manner
   d. Help keep the agency clean and safe

2. Nursing assistants report to
   a. Other nursing assistants
   b. Licensed nurses
   c. The administrator
   d. The medical director

3. All are true about the interdisciplinary health care team *except* that it:
   a. Involves many health care workers
   b. Follows the direction of the physician
   c. Works together to provide coordinated care
   d. Follows the direction of the RN

4. Nursing assistants perform nursing tasks delegated to them by an RN or LPN/LVN.
   a. True
   b. False

5. A resident asks you about his or her medical condition. You
   a. Tell the nurse about the resident's request
   b. Tell the resident what is in his or her medical record
   c. Ignore the question
   d. Tell another nursing assistant about the resident's request

6. You answer the telephone. The doctor starts to give you an order. You
   a. Take the order from the doctor
   b. Politely give your name and title, ask the doctor to wait for the nurse, and promptly find the nurse
   c. Politely ask the doctor to call back later
   d. Ask the doctor if the nurse may call him back

7. You can have your certification revoked for all the following *except*
   a. Substance abuse or dependency
   b. Abandoning a patient or resident
   c. Performing acts beyond the nursing assistant role
   d. Giving safe care

8. When should you refuse a task?
   a. The task is not in your job description
   b. The task is within the legal limits of your role
   c. The directions for the task are clear
   d. A nurse is available for questions and supervision

9. A nurse delegates a task that you did not learn in your training. The task is in your job description. What is your appropriate response to the nurse?
   a. "I cannot do that task."
   b. "I did not learn that task in my training. Can you show me how to do it?"
   c. "I will ask the other nursing assistant to watch me do the task."
   d. "I will ask the other nursing assistant to do the task for me."

10. You are busy with a new resident. It is time for another resident's bath. You may delegate the bath to another nursing assistant.
    a. True
    b. False

Answers to these questions are on p. 479.

CHAPTER 2 RESIDENT RIGHTS, ETHICS, AND LAWS

The Omnibus Budget Reconciliation Act of 1987 (OBRA)
- OBRA is a federal law.
- OBRA requires that nursing centers provide care in a manner and in a setting that maintains or improves each person's quality of life, health, and safety.
- OBRA requires nursing assistant training and competency evaluation.
- Resident rights are a major part of OBRA.

Resident Rights
- Centers must protect and promote resident rights.
- Residents must be free to exercise their rights without interference. If residents are not able to exercise their rights, legal representatives do so for them.

Information
- The right to information includes:
  - Access to medical records, incident reports, contracts, and financial records.
  - Information about his or her health condition.
  - Information about his or her doctor, including name, specialty, and contact information.
- Report any request for information to the nurse.

Refusing Treatment
- The person has the right to refuse treatment.
- A person who does not give consent or refuses treatment cannot be treated against his or her wishes.
- The center must find out what the person is refusing and why.
- Advance directives are part of the right to refuse treatment.
- Report any treatment refusal to the nurse.

Privacy and Confidentiality

- Residents have the right to:
  - Personal privacy. The person's body is not exposed unnecessarily. Only staff directly involved in care and treatments are present. The person must give consent for others to be present. A person has the right to use the bathroom in private. Privacy is maintained for all personal care measures.
  - Visit with others in private—in areas where others cannot see or hear them. This includes phone calls.
  - Send and receive mail without others interfering. No one can open mail the person sends or receives without his or her consent. Mail is given to the person within 24 hours of delivery to the center.
- Information about the person's care, treatment, and condition is kept confidential. So are medical and financial records. Consent is needed to release information to other agencies or persons.

Personal Choice

- Residents have the right to make their own choices. They can:
  - Choose their own doctor.
  - Take part in planning and deciding their care and treatment.
  - Choose activities, schedules, and care based on their preferences.
  - Choose when to get up and go to bed, what to wear, what to eat, and how to spend their time.
  - Choose friends and visitors inside and outside the center.

Grievances

- Residents have the right to voice concerns, ask questions, and complain about treatment or care.
- The center must promptly try to correct the matter.
- No one can punish the person in any way for voicing the grievance.

Work

- The person is not required to work or perform services for the center.
- The person has the right to work or perform services if he or she wants to.
- Residents volunteer or are paid for their services.

Taking Part in Resident and Family Groups

- The resident has the right to:
  - Form and take part in resident and family groups.
  - Take part in social, cultural, religious, and community events. The resident has the right to help in getting to and from events of his or her choice.

Care and Security of Personal Items

- The resident has the right to:
  - Keep and use personal items, such as clothing and some furnishings.
  - Have his or her property treated with care and respect. Items are labeled with the person's name.
- Protect yourself and the center from being accused of stealing a person's property. Do not go through a person's closet, drawers, purse, or other space without the person's knowledge and consent. If you have to inspect closets and drawers, follow center policy for reporting and recording the inspection.

Freedom From Abuse, Mistreatment, and Neglect

- Residents have the right to be free from:
  - Verbal, sexual, physical, or mental abuse.
  - Involuntary seclusion—separating a person from others against his or her will, confining a person to a certain area, keeping the person away from his or her room without consent.
- No one can abuse, neglect, or mistreat a resident. This includes center staff, volunteers, staff from other agencies or groups, other residents, family members, visitors, and legal representatives.

Freedom From Restraint

- Residents have the right not to have body movements restricted by restraints or medications.
- Restraints are used only if required to treat the person's medical symptoms or if necessary to protect the person or others from harm. A doctor's order is needed for restraint use.

Quality of Life

- Residents must be cared for in a manner that promotes dignity and respect for self. Physical, psychological, and mental well-being must be promoted. Review Box 2.2, OBRA-Required Actions That Promote Dignity and Privacy, in your textbook.
- Centers must provide activity programs that promote physical, intellectual, social, spiritual, and emotional well-being. Many centers provide religious services for spiritual health. You assist residents to and from activity programs. You may need to help them with activities.
- Residents have a right to a safe, clean, comfortable, and home-like setting. The center must provide a setting and services that meet the person's needs and preferences. The setting and staff must promote the person's independence, dignity, and well-being.

OMBUDSMAN PROGRAM

- The Older Americans Act requires an ombudsman program in every state.
- Ombudsmen are employed by a state agency. They are not nursing center employees.
- Ombudsmen protect the health, safety, welfare, and rights of residents. They also may investigate and resolve complaints, provide support to resident and family groups, and help the center manage difficult problems.

415

- OBRA requires that the nursing center post the names, addresses, and phone numbers of local and state ombudsmen. This information must be posted where residents can easily see it.

ETHICAL ASPECTS

- Ethics is the knowledge of what is right conduct and wrong conduct. It also deals with choices or judgments about what should or should not be done. An ethical person does not cause a person harm.
- Ethical behavior involves not being prejudiced or biased. To be prejudiced or biased means to make judgments and have views before knowing the facts. You should not judge a person by your values and standards. Also, do not avoid persons whose standards and values differ from your own.
- Ethical problems involve making choices. You must decide what is the right thing to do.

Boundaries

- Professional boundaries separate helpful behaviors from behaviors that are not helpful.
- A boundary crossing is a brief act or behavior outside the helpful zone. The act may be thoughtless or something you did not mean to do.
- A boundary violation is an act or behavior that meets your needs, not the person's. The act or behavior is unethical. Boundary violations include abuse, keeping secrets with a person, or giving a lot of personal information about yourself to another. Review Box 2.3, Code of Conduct for Nursing Assistants, in the textbook.
- Professional sexual misconduct is an act, behavior, or comment that is sexual in nature. It is sexual misconduct even if the person consents or makes the first move.
- To maintain professional boundaries, review Box 2.4, Rules for Maintaining Professional Boundaries. Be alert to boundary signs (acts, behaviors, or thoughts that warn of a boundary crossing or violation).

LEGAL ASPECTS

- Negligence is an unintentional wrong. The negligent person did not act in a reasonable and careful manner. As a result, harm was caused to the person or property of another. The person did not mean to cause harm.
- Malpractice is negligence by a professional person.
- Standards of care are skills, care, and judgments required by a health team member. Standards of care come from laws, including nurse practice acts; center policy and procedure manuals; job descriptions; agency standards; and government agencies, among others.
- You are legally responsible (liable) for your own actions. The nurse is liable as your supervisor.
- Defamation is injuring a person's name and reputation by making false statements to a third person.

Libel is making false statements in print, writing, or through pictures or drawings. Slander is making false statements orally. Never make false statements about a patient, resident, coworker, or any other person.
- False imprisonment is the unlawful restraint or restriction of a person's freedom of movement. It involves threatening to restrain a person, restraining a person, and preventing a person from leaving the center.
- Invasion of privacy is violating a person's right not to have his or her name, photo, or private affairs exposed or made public without giving consent. Review Box 2.6, Protecting the Right to Privacy, in the textbook.
- The Health Insurance Portability and Accountability Act (HIPAA) protects the privacy and security of a person's health information. Protected health information refers to identifying information and information about the person's health care. Direct any questions about the person or the person's care to the nurse.
- Fraud is saying or doing something to trick, fool, or deceive a person. The act is fraud if it does or could cause harm to a person or the person's property.
- Assault is intentionally attempting or threatening to touch a person's body without the person's consent. The person fears bodily harm. Battery is touching a person's body without his or her consent. Protect yourself from being accused of assault and battery. Explain to the person what is to be done and get the person's consent.

Informed Consent

- A person has the right to decide what will be done to his or her body and who can touch his or her body. Consent is informed when the person clearly understands all aspects of treatment.
- Persons who cannot give consent are persons who are under the legal age or are mentally incompetent. Unconscious, sedated, or confused persons also do not give consent. Informed consent is given by a responsible party—wife, husband, daughter, son, legal representative.
- You are never responsible for obtaining written consent.

Reporting Abuse

- Abuse is
  - The willful infliction of injury, unreasonable confinement, intimidation, or punishment that results in physical harm, pain, or mental anguish. To intimidate means to make afraid with threats of force or violence.
  - Depriving the person (or the person's caregiver) of the goods or services needed to attain or maintain well-being.
- Abuse also includes involuntary seclusion.
- Vulnerable adults are persons 18 years old or older who have disabilities or conditions that make them at

risk to be wounded, attacked, or damaged. They have problems caring for or protecting themselves due to:

- A mental, emotional, physical, or developmental disability
- Brain damage
- Changes from aging
- All residents are vulnerable. Older persons and children are at risk for abuse.

- Elder abuse is any knowing, intentional, or negligent act by a person to an older adult. It may include physical abuse, neglect, verbal abuse, involuntary seclusion, financial exploitation, emotional abuse, sexual abuse, or abandonment. Review Box 2.7, Signs of Elder Abuse, in the textbook.
- If you suspect a person is being abused, report your observations to the nurse.

CHAPTER 2 REVIEW QUESTIONS

Circle the BEST answer.

1. Residents have all the following rights *except*
   a. Refusing a treatment
   b. Making a telephone call in private
   c. Choosing activities to attend
   d. Being punished for voicing a grievance

2. OBRA does not require nursing assistant training and competency evaluation.
   a. True
   b. False

3. The person has a right to take part in planning and deciding their care and treatment.
   a. True
   b. False

4. The person is required to work for the center.
   a. True
   b. False

5. A resident offers you a gift certificate for being kind to her. You should
   a. Say "thank you" and accept the gift
   b. Accept the gift and give it to charity
   c. Thank the resident for thinking of you, then explain it is against policy for you to accept the gift
   d. Accept the gift and give it to your daughter

6. To protect a person's privacy, you should do the following *except*
   a. Keep all information about the person confidential
   b. Discuss the person's treatment or diagnosis with the nurse supervising your work
   c. Open the person's mail
   d. Allow the person to visit with others in private

7. What should you do if you suspect an older person is being abused?
   a. Report the situation to the health department.
   b. Notify the nurse and discuss the observations with him or her.
   c. Notify the doctor about the suspected abuse.
   d. Ask the family why they are abusing the person.

8. A resident needs help going to the bathroom. You do not answer her call light promptly. She gets up without help, falls, and breaks a leg. This is an example of
   a. Negligence
   b. Defamation
   c. False imprisonment
   d. Slander

9. Examples of defamation include all the following *except*
   a. Implying or suggesting that a person uses drugs
   b. Saying that a person is insane or mentally ill
   c. Implying that a person steals money from staff
   d. Burning a resident with water that is too hot

10. Which statement about ethics is false?
    a. An ethical person does not judge others by his or her values and standards.
    b. An ethical person avoids persons whose standards and values differ from his or her own.
    c. An ethical person is not prejudiced or biased.
    d. An ethical person does not cause harm to another person.

11. Examples of false imprisonment include all of the following *except*
    a. Threatening to restrain a resident
    b. Restraining a resident without a doctor's order
    c. Treating the resident with respect
    d. Preventing a resident from leaving the agency

12. To protect yourself from being accused of assault and battery, you should explain to the resident what you plan to do before touching him or her and get consent.
    a. True
    b. False

Answers to these questions are on p. 479.

CHAPTER 3 WORK ETHICS

HEALTH, HYGIENE, AND APPEARANCE

- To give safe and effective care, you must be physically and mentally healthy. You need a balanced diet, sleep and rest, good body mechanics, and exercise on a regular basis.
- Personal hygiene needs careful attention. Bathe daily, use deodorant or antiperspirant, and brush your teeth often. Shampoo often. Keep fingernails clean, short, and neatly shaped.
- Review Box 3.1, Practices for a Professional Appearance, in your textbook.
- Always follow the dress code policy at the center where you are employed.

TEAMWORK

- Practice good work ethics—work when scheduled, be cheerful and friendly, perform delegated tasks, be kind to others, and be available to help others.
- Be ready to work when your shift starts. Arrive on your nursing unit a few minutes early. Stay the entire shift. When it is time to leave, report off duty to the nurse.
- A good attitude is needed. Review Box 3.2, Qualities and Traits for Good Work Ethics, in your textbook.
- Gossiping is unprofessional and hurtful. To avoid being a part of gossip:
    - Remove yourself from a group or situation in which gossip is occurring.
    - Do not make or repeat any comment that can hurt another person.
    - Do not make or repeat any comment that you do not know to be true.
    - Do not talk about residents, family members, visitors, coworkers, or the center at home or in social settings.
- Confidentiality means trusting others with personal and private information. The person's information is shared only among health team members involved in his or her care. Agency and coworker information also is confidential.
- Your speech and language must be professional:
    - Do not swear or use foul, vulgar, or abusive language.
    - Do not use slang.
    - Speak softly, gently, and clearly.
    - Do not shout or yell.
    - Do not fight or argue with a resident, family member, visitor, or coworker.
- A courtesy is a polite, considerate, or helpful comment or act.
    - Address others by Miss, Mrs., Ms., Mr., or Doctor. Use a first name only if the person asks you to do so.
    - Say "please" and "thank you." Say "I'm sorry" when you make a mistake or hurt someone.
    - Let residents, families, and visitors enter elevators first.
    - Be thoughtful—compliment others, give praise.
    - Wish the person and family well when they leave the center.
    - Hold doors open for others.
    - Help others willingly when asked.
    - Do not take credit for another person's deeds. Give the person credit for the action.
- Keep personal matters out of the workplace:
    - Make personal phone calls during meals and breaks.
    - Do not let family and friends visit you on the unit.
    - Do not use the agency's computers and other equipment for personal use.
    - Do not take agency supplies for personal use.
    - Do not discuss personal problems at work.
    - Control your emotions.
    - Do not borrow money from or lend money to coworkers.
    - Do not sell things or engage in fundraising at work.
    - Do not have cell phones on while at work.
- Leave for and return from breaks and meals on time. Tell the nurse when you leave and return to the unit.

MANAGING STRESS

- These guidelines can help you reduce or cope with stress:
    - Exercise regularly.
    - Get enough sleep or rest.
    - Eat healthy.
    - Plan personal and quiet time for yourself.
    - Use common sense about what you can do.
    - Do one thing at a time.
    - Do not judge yourself harshly.
    - Give yourself praise.
    - Have a sense of humor.
    - Talk to the nurse if your work or a person is causing too much stress.

HARASSMENT

- Harassment means to trouble, torment, offend, or worry a person by one's behavior or comments. Harassment can be sexual. Or it can involve age, race, ethnic background, religion, or disability.
- You must respect others. Do not offend others by your gestures, remarks, or use of touch. Do not offend others with jokes, photos, or other pictures.

CHAPTER 3 REVIEW QUESTIONS

Circle the BEST answer.

1. You believe you have good work ethics. This means you do the following *except*
   a. Work when scheduled
   b. Act cheerful and friendly
   c. Refuse to help others
   d. Perform tasks assigned by the nurse

2. A nursing assistant is gossiping about a coworker. You should
   a. Stay with the group and listen to what is being said
   b. Repeat the comment to your family
   c. Remove yourself from the group in which gossip is occurring
   d. Repeat the comment to another coworker

3. You want to maintain confidentiality about others. You do the following *except*
   a. Share information about a resident with a nurse who is on another unit
   b. Avoid talking about a resident in the elevator, hallway, or dining area
   c. Avoid talking about coworkers and residents when others are present
   d. Avoid eavesdropping

4. When you are at work, you should do which of the following?
   a. Swear and use foul language
   b. Use slang
   c. Argue with a visitor
   d. Speak clearly and softly

5. To give safe and effective care, you do all of the following *except*
   a. Eat a balanced diet
   b. Get enough sleep and rest
   c. Exercise on a regular basis
   d. Drink too much alcohol

6. While at work, you should do all of the following *except*
   a. Be courteous to others
   b. Make personal phone calls
   c. Admit when you are wrong or make mistakes
   d. Respect others

Answers to these questions are on p. 479.

CHAPTER 4 COMMUNICATING WITH THE HEALTH TEAM

COMMUNICATION

- For good communication:
  - Use words that mean the same thing to you and the receiver of the message.
  - Use familiar words and be brief and concise.
  - Give information in a logical and orderly manner. Give facts and be specific.
  - Speak clearly and look at the other person or people you are communicating with.
  - Ask questions if you do not understand what is said.

THE MEDICAL RECORD

- The medical record is a way for the health team to share information about the person. It is a legal document.
- If you know a person in the agency but you do not give care to that person, you have no right to review the person's chart. To do so is an invasion of privacy.
- Follow your agency's policies about recording in the medical record.

RESIDENT CARE CONFERENCES

- The registered nurse (RN) may conduct a care conference to share information and ideas about the person's care. The RN, nursing assistants, and other health team members take part in the conference.
- The person has the right to take part in care planning conferences. Sometimes the family is involved. The person may refuse actions suggested by the health team.

REPORTING AND RECORDING

- The health team communicates by reporting and recording.

Reporting

- Reporting is the oral account of care and observations.
- Review Box 4.1 Rules for Reporting and Recording in your textbook.

Recording

- Recording, or charting, is the written account of care and observations.
- Review Box 4.1 Rules for Reporting and Recording in your textbook.
- Review the 24-hour clock, Fig. 4.9, in your textbook.

MEDICAL TERMINOLOGY AND ABBREVIATIONS

- Medical terminology and abbreviations are used in health care. Someone may use a word or phrase that you do not understand. If so, ask the nurse to explain its meaning.
- Review Box 4.3, Medical Terminology, in the textbook.
- Use only the abbreviations accepted by the center. If you are not sure that an abbreviation is acceptable, write the term out in full. See the inside of the back cover of the textbook for common abbreviations.

COMPUTERS AND OTHER ELECTRONIC DEVICES

- Computers contain vast amounts of information about a person. Therefore, the right to privacy must be protected. If allowed access, you must follow the agency's policies.
- Review Box 4.5, Using the Center's Computer and Other Electronic Devices, in your textbook.

DEALING WITH CONFLICT

- These guidelines can help you deal with conflict:
  - Ask your supervisor for some time to talk privately about the problem.
  - Approach the person with whom you have the conflict. Ask to talk privately. Be polite and professional.
  - Agree on a time and place to talk.
  - Talk in a private setting. No one should hear you or the other person.
  - Explain the problem and what is bothering you. Give facts and specific behaviors. Focus on the problem. Do not focus on the person.
  - Listen to the person. Do not interrupt.
  - Identify ways to solve the problem. Offer your thoughts. Ask for the coworker's ideas.
  - Set a date and time to review the matter.
  - Thank the person for meeting with you.
  - Carry out the solution.
  - Review the matter as scheduled.

Circle the BEST answer.

1. For good communication, you should do the following *except*
   a. Use words with more than one meaning
   b. Use words familiar to the person or family
   c. Give facts in a brief and concise manner
   d. Give information in a logical and orderly manner

2. When you record in a person's chart, you do the following *except*
   a. Record what you observed and did
   b. Record the person's response to the treatment or procedure
   c. Use abbreviations that are not on the accepted list for the center
   d. Record the time the observation was made or the treatment performed

3. When reporting care and observations to the nurse, you do all of the following *except*
   a. Give the person's name and room and bed numbers
   b. Report only what you observed or did yourself
   c. Report any changes from normal or changes in the person's condition at once
   d. Report any changes from normal or changes in the person's condition at the end of the shift

Answers to these questions are on p. 479.

CHAPTER 5 ASSISTING WITH THE NURSING PROCESS

- The nursing process is the method nurses use to plan and deliver nursing care.
- You play a key role by making observations as you care and talk with the person.
- Observation is using the senses of sight, hearing, touch, and smell to collect information. Box 5.1. in your textbook, Basic Observations, lists the basic observations you need to make and report to the nurse.
- Observations you need to report to the nurse at once are:
  - A change in the person's ability to respond
  - A change in the person's mobility
  - Complaints of sudden, severe pain
  - A sore or reddened area on the person's skin
  - Complaints of a sudden change in vision
  - Complaints of pain or difficulty breathing
  - Abnormal respirations
  - Complaints or signs of difficulty swallowing
  - Vomiting
  - Bleeding
  - Vital signs outside their normal ranges
- Objective data (signs) are seen, heard, felt, or smelled by an observer. For example, you can feel a pulse.

- Subjective data (symptoms) are things a person tells you about that you cannot observe through your senses. For example, you cannot see the person's nausea.
- The nurse delegates tasks to you though assignment sheets. The assignment sheet tells you about each person's care and what tasks are to be done. Talk to the nurse about any unclear assignments.

CHAPTER 5 REVIEW QUESTIONS

Circle the BEST answer.

1. Which statement about observations is *false?*
   a. You make observations as you care and talk with people.
   b. Observation uses the senses of smell, sight, touch, and hearing.
   c. A reddened area on the person's skin is reported to the nurse at once.
   d. You report observations to the doctor.

2. Objective data include all of the following *except*
   a. The person has pain in his abdomen
   b. The person's pulse is 76
   c. The person's urine is dark amber
   d. The person's breath has an odor

Answers to these questions are on p. 479.

CHAPTER 6 UNDERSTANDING THE RESIDENT

CARING FOR THE PERSON

- The whole person needs to be considered when you provide care—physical, social, psychological, and spiritual parts. These parts are woven together and cannot be separated.
- Follow these rules to address persons with dignity and respect:
  - Call persons by their titles—for example, Mrs. Dennison, Mr. Smith, Miss Turner, or Dr. Gonzalez.
  - Do not call persons by their first names unless they ask you to.
  - Do not call persons by any other name unless they ask you to.
  - Do not call persons Grandma, Papa, Sweetheart, Honey, or other name.

BASIC NEEDS

- A need is something necessary or desired for maintaining life and mental well-being.
- According to Maslow, basic needs must be met for a person to survive and function:
  - *Physical needs*—are required for life. They are oxygen, food, water, elimination, rest, and shelter.
  - *Safety and security needs*—relate to feeling safe from harm, danger, and fear.
  - *Love and belonging needs*—relate to love, closeness, affection, and meaningful relationships with others. Family, friends, and the health team can meet love and belonging needs.

- *Self-esteem needs*—relate to thinking well of oneself and to seeing oneself as useful and having value. People often lack self-esteem when ill, injured, older, or disabled.
- *The need for self-actualization*—involves learning, understanding, and creating to the limit of a person's capacity. Rarely, if ever, is this need totally met.

EFFECTS OF ILLNESS AND DISABILITY

- Sickness and injury have physical, psychologic, and social effects.
- Disability is any lost, absent, or impaired physical or mental function.
- Residents are helped to maintain their optimal level of function or the person's highest potential for mental and physical performance.

BEHAVIOR ISSUES

- Many people do not adjust well to illness, injury, and disability. They may have some of the following behaviors:
  - *Anger.* Anger may be communicated verbally and nonverbally. Verbal outbursts, shouting, and rapid speech are common. Some people are silent. Others are uncooperative and may refuse to answer questions. Nonverbal signs include rapid movements, pacing, clenched fists, and a red face. Glaring and getting close to you when speaking are other signs. Violent behaviors can occur.
  - *Demanding behavior.* Nothing seems to please the person. The person is critical of others.
  - *Self-centered behavior.* The person cares only about his or her own needs. The needs of others are ignored. The person becomes impatient if needs are not met.
  - *Aggressive behavior.* The person may swear, bite, hit, pinch, scratch, or kick. Protect the person, others, and yourself from harm.
  - *Withdrawal.* The person has little or no contact with family, friends, and staff. Some people are generally not social and prefer to be alone.
  - *Inappropriate sexual behavior.* Some people make inappropriate sexual remarks or touch others in the wrong way. These behaviors may be on purpose. Or they are caused by disease, confusion, dementia, or medication side effects.
- You cannot avoid persons with unpleasant behaviors or who lose control. Review Box 6.1, Dealing With Behavior Issues, in your textbook.

COMMUNICATING WITH THE PERSON

- For effective communication between you and the person, you must:
  - Understand and respect the patient or resident as a person.

- View the person as a physical, psychological, social, and spiritual human being.
- Appreciate the person's problems and frustrations.
- Respect the person's rights.
- Respect the person's religion and culture.
- Give the person time to understand the information that you give.
- Repeat information as often as needed.
- Ask questions to see if the person understood you.
- Be patient. People with memory problems may ask the same question many times.
- Include the person in conversations when others are present.

Verbal Communication

- When talking with a person, follow these rules:
  - Face the person.
  - Position yourself at the person's eye level.
  - Control the loudness and tone of your voice.
  - Speak clearly, slowly, and distinctly.
  - Do not use slang or vulgar words.
  - Repeat information as needed.
  - Ask one question at a time and wait for an answer.
  - Do not shout, whisper, or mumble.
  - Be kind, courteous, and friendly.
- Use written words if the person cannot speak or hear but can read. Keep written messages brief and concise. Use a black felt pen on white paper and print in large letters.
- Some persons cannot speak or read. Ask questions that have "yes" and "no" answers. A picture board may be helpful.

Nonverbal Communication

- Messages are sent with gestures, facial expressions, posture, body movements, touch, and smell. A person may say one thing but act another way. Watch the person's eyes, hand movements, gestures, posture, and other actions.
- Touch conveys comfort, caring, love, affection, interest, trust, concern, and reassurance. Touch should be gentle. Touch means different things to different people. Some people do not like to be touched.
- People send messages through their body language—facial expressions, gestures, posture, hand and body movements, gait, eye contact, and appearance. Your body language should show interest, enthusiasm, caring, and respect for the person. Often you need to control your body language. Control reactions to odors from body fluids, secretions, or excretions.

Communication Methods

- *Listening* means to focus on verbal and nonverbal communication. You use sight, hearing, touch, and smell.
- *Paraphrasing* is restating the person's message in your own words.

- *Direct questions* focus on certain information. You ask the person something you need to know.
- *Open-ended questions* lead or invite the person to share thoughts, feelings, or ideas. The person chooses what to talk about.
- *Clarifying* lets you make sure that you understand the message. You can ask the person to repeat the message, say you do not understand, or restate the message.
- *Focusing* deals with a certain topic. It is useful when a person wanders in thought.
- *Silence* is a very powerful way to communicate. Silence on your part shows caring and respect for the person's situation and feelings.

Communication Barriers
- *Language.* You and the person must use and understand the same language.
- *Cultural differences.* A person from another country may attach different meanings to verbal and nonverbal communication from what you intended.
- *Changing the subject.* Avoid changing the subject whenever possible.
- *Giving your opinions.* Opinions involve judging values, behavior, or feelings. Let others express feelings and concerns. Do not make judgments or jump to conclusions.
- *Talking a lot when others are silent.* Talking too much is usually because of nervousness and discomfort with silence.
- *Failure to listen.* Do not pretend to listen. It shows lack of caring and interest. You may miss complaints of pain, discomfort, or other symptoms that you must report to the nurse.
- *Pat answers.* "Don't worry." "Everything will be okay." These make the person feel that you do not care about his or her concerns, feelings, and fears.
- *Illness and disability.* Speech, hearing, vision, cognitive function, and body movements may be affected. Verbal and nonverbal communication are affected.
- *Age.* Values and communication styles vary among age-groups.

RESIDENTS WITH DISABILITIES
- Common courtesies and manners apply to any person with a disability. Review Box 6.2, Disability Etiquette, in the textbook.
- The person who is comatose is unconscious and cannot respond to others. Often the person can feel touch and pain. Assume that the person hears and understands you. Use touch and give care gently. Practice these measures:
  - Knock before entering the person's room.
  - Tell the person your name, the time, and the place every time you enter the room.

- Give care on the same schedule every day.
- Explain what you are going to do.
- Tell the person when you are finishing care.
- Use touch to communicate care, concern, and comfort.
- Tell the person what time you will be back to check on him or her.
- Tell the person when you are leaving the room.

FAMILY AND FRIENDS
- If you need to give care when visitors are there, protect the person's right to privacy. Politely ask the visitors to leave the room when you give care. A partner or family member may help you if the patient or resident consents.
- Treat family and visitors with courtesy and respect.
- Do not discuss the person's condition with family and friends. Refer questions to the nurse. A visitor may upset or tire a person. Report your observations to the nurse.

CHAPTER 6 REVIEW QUESTIONS
Circle the BEST answer.
1. While caring for a person, you need to
   a. Consider only the person's physical and social needs
   b. Consider the person's physical, social, psychological, and spiritual needs
   c. Consider only the person's cultural needs
   d. Ignore the person's spiritual needs

2. When referring to residents, you should
   a. Refer to them by their room number
   b. Call them "Honey"
   c. Call them by their first name
   d. Call them by their name and title

3. Based on Maslow's theory of basic needs, which person's needs must be met first?
   a. The person who wants to talk about her granddaughter's wedding
   b. The person who is uncomfortable in the dining room
   c. The person who wants mail opened
   d. The person who asks for more water

4. A person is angry and is shouting at you. You should do the following *except*
   a. Stay calm and professional
   b. Yell so the person will listen to you
   c. Listen to what the person is saying
   d. Report the person's behavior to the nurse

5. A person tries to scratch and kick you. You should
   a. Protect yourself from harm
   b. Argue with the person
   c. Become angry with the person
   d. Refuse to care for the person

6. When speaking with another person, you do all of the following *except*
    a. Position yourself at the person's eye level
    b. Speak slowly, clearly, and distinctly
    c. Shout, mumble, and whisper
    d. Ask one question at a time

7. Which statement about listening is *false?*
    a. You use sight, hearing, touch, and smell when you listen.
    b. You observe nonverbal cues.
    c. You have good eye contact with the person.
    d. You sit back with your arms crossed.

8. Which statement about silence is *false?*
    a. Silence is a powerful way to communicate.
    b. Silence gives people time to think.
    c. You should talk a lot when the other person is silent.
    d. Silence helps when the person is upset and needs to gain control.

9. A person speaks a foreign language. You should do the following *except*
    a. Keep messages short and simple
    b. Use gestures and pictures
    c. Shout or speak loudly
    d. Repeat the message in other words

10. When caring for a person who is comatose, you do the following *except*
    a. Tell the person your name when you enter the room
    b. Explain what you are doing
    c. Use touch to communicate care and comfort
    d. Make jokes about how sick the person is

11. A person is in a wheelchair. You should do all of the following *except*
    a. Lean on a person's wheelchair
    b. Sit or squat to talk to a person in a wheelchair or chair
    c. Think about obstacles before giving directions to a person in a wheelchair
    d. Extend the same courtesies to the person as you would to anyone else

12. A person's daughter is visiting and you need to provide care to the person. You
    a. Expose the person's body in front of the visitor
    b. Politely ask the visitor to leave the room
    c. Decide to not provide the care at all
    d. Discuss the person's condition with the visitor

Answers to these questions are on p. 479.

CULTURE, RELIGION AND SPIRITUALITY

- Culture refers to the characteristics of a group of people. People come from many cultures, races, and nationalities. Family practices, food choices, hygiene habits, clothing styles, and language are part of their culture. The person's culture also influences health beliefs and practices. Review Box 7.1, Guidelines for Relating to Persons from Different Cultures, in your textbook.

- Ethnicity is a classification of people based on national origin and shared culture. Members of these groups often share language, customs, and beliefs.

- Personal space is the distance that people require to comfortably communicate or interact. Persons from some cultures stand very close and may touch each other while communicating. Others may stand farther away. Gestures may have different meanings in different cultures.

- Religion relates to spiritual beliefs, needs, and practices. A person's religion influences health and illness practices. Many may want to pray and observe religious practices. Assist residents to attend religious services as needed. If a person wants to see a spiritual leader or adviser, tell the nurse. Provide privacy during the visit.
    - A person may not follow all the beliefs and practices of his or her culture or religion. Some people do not practice a religion.
    - Respect and accept the person's culture and religion. Learn about practices and beliefs different from your own. Do not judge a person by your standards.

CHAPTER 7 REVIEW QUESTIONS

Circle the BEST answer.

1. Which statement about culture is *false?*
    a. A person's culture influences health beliefs and practices.
    b. You must respect a person's culture.
    c. You should ignore the person's culture while you give his or her care.
    d. You should learn about another person's culture that is different from yours.

2. Which statement about religion and spiritual beliefs is *false?*
    a. A person's religion influences health and illness practices.
    b. You should assist a person to attend services in the nursing center.
    c. Many people find comfort and strength from religion during illness.
    d. A person must follow all beliefs of his or her religion.

Answers to these questions are on p. 479.

GROWTH AND DEVELOPMENT

- Growth refers to the physical changes that are measured and that occur in a steady and orderly manner.
- Development relates to changes in mental, emotional, and social function.
- Growth and development occur in a sequence, order, and pattern. Review Box 9.1, Stages of Growth and Development, in your textbook.

PSYCHOLOGICAL AND SOCIAL CHANGES

- Physical reminders of growing old affect self-esteem and may threaten self-image, feelings of self-worth, and independence.
- People cope with aging in their own way. How they cope depends on their health status, life experiences, finances, education, and social support systems.
- *Retirement.* Many people enjoy retirement. Others are in poor health and have medical bills that can make retirement hard.
- *Reduced income.* Retirement usually means reduced income. The retired person still has expenses. Reduced income may force lifestyle changes. One example is that the person avoids health care or needed medications.
- *Social relationships.* Social relationships change throughout life. Family time helps prevent loneliness, as do hobbies, religious and community events, and new friends.
- *Children as caregivers.* Some older persons feel more secure when their children care for them. Others feel unwanted and useless. Some lose dignity and self-respect. Tensions may occur among the child, parent, and other household members.
- *Death of a partner.* When death occurs, the person loses a lover, friend, companion, and confidant. Grief may be great. The person's life will likely change.

PHYSICAL CHANGES

- Body processes slow down. Energy level and body efficiency decline.
- *The integumentary system.* The skin loses its elasticity, strength, and fatty tissue layer. Wrinkles appear. Dry skin and itching occur. The skin is fragile and easily injured. The person is more sensitive to cold. Nails become thick and tough. Feet may have poor circulation. Fragile skin, poor circulation, and decreased ability to sense heat and cold increase risk of burns. White or gray hair is common and hair thins. Facial hair may occur in women. Hair is drier. The risk of skin cancer increases.
- *The musculoskeletal system.* Muscle and bone strength are lost. Bones become brittle and break easily. Vertebrae shorten. Joints become stiff and painful. Mobility decreases. There is a gradual loss of height. Activity, exercise and diet help prevent bone loss and loss of muscle strength.
- *The nervous system.* Confusion, dizziness, and fatigue may occur. Responses are slower. The risk for falls increases. Forgetfulness increases. Memory is shorter. Events from long ago are remembered better than recent ones. Older persons have a harder time falling asleep. Sleep periods are shorter.
- *The senses.* Hearing and vision losses occur. Taste and smell dull. Touch and sensitivity to pain, pressure, hot, and cold are reduced.
- *The circulatory system.* The heart muscle weakens. Arteries narrow and are less elastic. Poor circulation occurs in many body parts.
- *The respiratory system.* Respiratory muscles weaken. Lung tissue becomes less elastic. Difficult, labored, or painful breathing may occur with activity. The person may lack strength to cough and clear the airway of secretions. Respiratory infections and diseases may develop.
- *The digestive system.* Less saliva is produced. The person may have difficulty swallowing (dysphagia). Indigestion may occur. Loss of teeth and ill-fitting dentures cause chewing problems and digestion problems. Flatulence and constipation can occur. Fewer calories are needed as energy and activity levels decline. More fluids are needed.
- *The urinary system.* Urine is more concentrated. Bladder muscles weaken. Bladder size decreases. Urinary frequency or urgency may occur. Urinary incontinence may occur. The prostate gland enlarges in men. This may cause difficulty urinating or frequent urination. Urinary infections are risks.
- *The reproductive system.* In men, testosterone decreases. An erection takes longer. Orgasm is less forceful. Women experience menopause. Female hormones of estrogen and progesterone decrease. The uterus, vagina, and genitalia shrink (atrophy). Vaginal walls thin. There is vaginal dryness. Arousal takes longer. Orgasm is less intense.

Needing Nursing Center Care

- The person needing nursing center care may suffer some or all of these losses:
  - Loss of identity as a productive member of a family and community
  - Loss of possessions—home, household items, car, and so on
  - Loss of independence
  - Loss of real-world experiences—shopping, traveling, cooking, driving, hobbies
  - Loss of health and mobility
- The person may feel useless, powerless, and hopeless. The health team helps the person cope with loss and improve quality of life.

CHAPTER 9 REVIEW QUESTIONS

Circle the Best answer.

1. Which is a developmental task of late adulthood?
   a. Accepting changes in appearance
   b. Adjusting to decreased strength
   c. Developing a satisfactory sex life
   d. Performing self-care

2. Which statement is *false*?
   a. Physical changes occur with aging.
   b. Energy level and body efficiency decline with age.
   c. Some people age faster than others.
   d. Normal aging means loss of health.

3. As a person ages, the integumentary system changes. Which statement is *false*?
   a. Dry skin and itching occur.
   b. Nails become thick and tough.
   c. Skin disorders decrease with age.
   d. Skin is injured more easily.

4. Which statement is *false* about the musculoskeletal system and aging?
   a. Strength decreases
   b. Vertebrae shorten
   c. Mobility increases
   d. Bone mass decreases

5. Which statement about the nervous system and aging is *false*?
   a. Reflexes slow
   b. Memory may be shorter
   c. Sleep patterns change
   d. Forgetfulness decreases

6. Which statement about the digestive system and aging is *false*?
   a. Appetite decreases
   b. Less saliva is produced
   c. Flatulence and constipation may decrease
   d. Teeth may be lost

7. Which statement about the urinary system and aging is *false*?
   a. Urine becomes more concentrated
   b. Urinary frequency may occur
   c. Urinary urgency may occur
   d. Bladder muscles become stronger

Answers to these questions are on p. 479.

CHAPTER 11 SAFETY

ACCIDENT RISK FACTORS

- *Age.* Older persons are at risk for falls and other injuries.
- *Awareness of surroundings.* People need to know their surroundings to protect themselves from injury.
- *Agitated and aggressive behaviors.* Pain, confusion, fear, and decreased awareness of surroundings can cause these behaviors.

- *Vision loss.* Persons can fall or trip over items. Some have problems reading labels on containers.
- *Hearing loss.* Persons have problems hearing explanations and instructions. They may not hear warning signals or fire alarms. They do not know to move to safety.
- *Impaired smell and touch.* Persons may have trouble detecting smoke or gas odors. Decreased sense of touch may increase risk of burns or other injury.
- *Impaired mobility.* A person may be aware of danger but is unable to move to safety.
- *Medications.* Medications have side effects. Report behavior changes and the person's complaints.

IDENTIFYING THE PERSON

- You must give the right care to the right person. To identify the person:
  - Compare identifying information on the assignment sheet with that on the identification (ID) bracelet.
  - Use two identifiers. Some centers require birth date or another identification number.
  - Some nursing centers have photo ID systems. Use this system safely.
  - Alert and oriented persons may choose not to wear ID bracelets. Follow center policy and the care plan to identify the person.

PREVENTING BURNS

- Smoking, spilled hot liquids, very hot water, and electrical devices are common causes of burns. See Box 11.1 in your textbook for safety measures to prevent burns.

PREVENTING POISONING

- Medications and household products are common poisons. Poisoning in adults may result from carelessness, confusion, or poor vision when reading labels. See Box 11.2 in your textbook for safety measures to prevent poisoning.

PREVENTING SUFFOCATION

- Suffocation is when breathing stops from the lack of oxygen. Death occurs if the person does not start breathing.
- To prevent suffocation, review Box 11.3, Safety Measures to Prevent Suffocation, in your textbook.

PREVENTING EQUIPMENT ACCIDENTS

- All equipment is unsafe if broken, not used correctly, or not working properly. Inspect all equipment before use. Review Box 11.4, Safety Measures to Prevent Equipment Accidents, in the textbook.

WHEELCHAIR AND STRETCHER SAFETY

- Review Box 11.5, Wheelchair and Stretcher Safety, in the textbook.

425

HANDLING HAZARDOUS SUBSTANCES

- A hazardous substance is any chemical in the workplace that can cause harm, such as oxygen, mercury, disinfectants, and cleaning agents.
- Hazardous substance containers must have a warning label. If a label is removed or damaged, do not use the substance. Take the container to the nurse. Do not leave the container unattended.
- Check the Safety Data Sheet (SDS) before using a hazardous substance, cleaning up a leak or spill, or disposing of the substance. Tell the nurse about a leak or spill right away. Do not leave a leak or spill unattended.

FIRE SAFETY

- Faulty electrical equipment and wiring, overloaded electrical circuits, and smoking are major causes of fires.
- Safety measures are needed where oxygen is used and stored:
  - NO SMOKING signs are placed on the door and near the person's bed.
  - The person and visitors are reminded not to smoke in the room.
  - Smoking materials are removed from the room.
  - Electrical items are turned off before being unplugged.
  - Wool blankets and fabrics that cause static electricity are not used.
  - The person wears a cotton gown or pajamas.
  - Electrical items are in good working order.
  - Lit candles and other open flames are not allowed.
  - Materials that ignite easily are removed from the room.
- Review Box 11.7, Fire Prevention Measures, in the textbook.
- Know your center's policies and procedures for fire emergencies. Know where to find fire alarms, fire extinguishers, and emergency exits. Remember the word RACE:
  - R—*rescue*. Rescue persons in immediate danger. Move them to a safe place.
  - A—*alarm*. Sound the nearest fire alarm. Notify the telephone operator.
  - C—*confine*. Close doors and windows. Turn off oxygen or electrical items.
  - E—*extinguish*. Use a fire extinguisher on a small fire.
- Remember the word PASS for using a fire extinguisher:
  - P—*pull* the safety pin.
  - A—*aim* low. Aim at the base of the fire.
  - S—*squeeze* the lever to start the stream.
  - S—*sweep* back and forth (side to side) at the base of the fire.
- Do not use elevators during a fire.

DISASTERS

- A disaster is a sudden catastrophic event. The agency has procedures for disasters that could occur in your area. Follow them to keep patients, residents, visitors, staff, and yourself safe.

WORKPLACE VIOLENCE

- Workplace violence consists of violent acts (including assault or threat of assault) directed toward persons at work or while on duty. Review Box 11.8, Measures to Prevent or Control Workplace Violence, in the textbook.

CHAPTER 11 REVIEW QUESTIONS

Circle the BEST answer.

1. You see a water spill in the hallway. What will you do?
   a. Ask housekeeping to wipe up the spill right away.
   b. Wipe up the spill right away.
   c. Report the spill to the nurse.
   d. Ask the resident to walk around the spill.

2. An electrical outlet in a person's room does not work. What will you do?
   a. Tell the administrator about the problem.
   b. Tell another nursing assistant about the problem.
   c. Try to repair the electrical outlet.
   d. Follow the center's policy for reporting the problem.

3. Accident risk factors include all of the following *except*
   a. Walking without difficulty
   b. Hearing problems
   c. Dulled sense of smell
   d. Poor vision

4. To prevent a person from being burned, you should do the following *except*
   a. Supervise the smoking of persons who are confused
   b. Turn cold water on first; turn hot water off first
   c. Do not let the person sleep with a heating pad
   d. Allow smoking in bed

5. To prevent suffocation, you should do all of the following *except*
   a. Make sure dentures fit properly
   b. Check the care plan for swallowing problems before serving food or liquids
   c. Leave a person alone in a bathtub or shower
   d. Position the person in bed properly

6. Which statement about wheelchair safety is *false?*
   a. Lock the wheels before transferring a resident to or from a wheelchair.
   b. The person's feet should rest on the footplate when you are pushing the wheelchair.
   c. Let the footplates fall back onto a person's legs.
   d. Check for flat or loose tires.

7. Which of the following is *not* a safety measure with oxygen?
   a. NO SMOKING signs are placed on the resident's door and near the bed.
   b. Lit candles and other open flames are permitted in the room.
   c. Electrical items are turned off before being unplugged.
   d. The person wears a cotton gown or pajamas.

8. You have discovered a fire in the nursing center. You should do the following *except*
   a. Rescue persons in immediate danger
   b. Sound the nearest fire alarm
   c. Open doors and windows and keep oxygen on
   d. Use a fire extinguisher on a small fire that has not spread to a larger area

9. When using a fire extinguisher, you do all of the following *except*
   a. Pull the safety pin on the fire extinguisher
   b. Aim at the top of the flames
   c. Squeeze the lever to start the stream
   d. Sweep the stream back and forth

Answers to these questions are on p. 479.

CHAPTER 12 PREVENTING FALLS

- Falls are the most common accidents in nursing centers.
- Most falls occur in resident rooms and bathrooms. Most occur between 1600 (4:00 PM) and 2000 (8:00 PM). Falls are more likely during shift changes.
- Causes for falls are poor lighting, cluttered floors, incorrect bed height, needing to use the bathroom, and out-of-place furniture. So are wet and slippery floors, bathtubs, and showers. Review Box 12.1, Factors Increasing the Risk of Falls, in the textbook.
- Nursing centers have fall prevention programs. Review Box 12.2, Safety Measures to Prevent Falls, in the textbook. The person's care plan also lists measures specific for the person.

BED RAILS

- A bed rail *(side rail)* is a device that serves as a guard or barrier along the side of the bed.
- The nurse and care plan tell you when to raise bed rails. They are needed by persons who are unconscious or sedated with medications. Some confused and disoriented people need them. If a person needs bed rails, keep them up at all times except when giving bedside nursing care.
- Bed rails present hazards. The person can fall when trying to get out of bed. Or the person can get caught, trapped, entangled, or strangled.
- Bed rails are considered restraints if the person cannot get out of bed or lower them without help.

- Bed rails cannot be used unless they are needed to treat a person's medical symptoms. The person or legal representative must give consent for raised bed rails. The need for bed rails is carefully noted in the person's medical record and the care plan. If a person uses bed rails, check the person often. Record when you checked the person and your observations.
- To prevent falls:
  - Never leave the person alone when the bed is raised.
  - Always lower the bed to its lowest position when you are done giving care.
  - If a person does not use bed rails and you need to raise the bed, ask a coworker to stand on the far side of the bed to protect the person from falling.
  - If you raise the bed to give care, always raise the far bed rail if you are working alone.
  - Be sure the person who uses raised bed rails has access to items on the bedside stand and overbed table. The call light, water pitcher and cup, tissues, phone, and TV and light controls should be within the person's reach.

HANDRAILS AND GRAB BARS

- Handrails give support to persons who are weak or unsteady when walking.
- Grab bars provide support for sitting down or getting up from a toilet. They also are used for getting in and out of the shower or tub.

WHEEL LOCKS

- Bed wheels are locked at all times except when moving the bed.
- Wheelchair and stretcher wheels are locked when transferring a person.

TRANSFER/GAIT BELTS

- Use a transfer belt (gait belt) to support a person who is unsteady or disabled. Always follow the manufacturer's instructions. Apply the belt over clothing and under the breasts. The belt buckle is never positioned over the person's spine. Tighten the belt so it is snug. You should be able to slide your open, flat hand under the belt. Tuck the excess strap under the belt. Remove the belt after the procedure.
- Check with the nurse and care plan before using a transfer/gait belt if the person has:
  - A colostomy, ileostomy, gastrostomy, or urostomy
  - A gastric tube
  - Chronic obstructive pulmonary disease
  - An abdominal wound, incision, or drainage tube
  - A chest wound, incision, or drainage tube
  - Monitoring equipment
  - A hernia
  - Other conditions or care equipment involving the chest or abdomen

427

THE FALLING PERSON

- If a person starts to fall, do not try to prevent the fall. You could injure yourself and the person. Ease the person to the floor and protect the person's head. Do not let the person get up before the nurse checks for injuries. An incident report is completed after all falls.

CHAPTER 12 REVIEW QUESTIONS

Circle the BEST answer.

1. Most falls occur in
   a. Resident rooms and bathrooms
   b. Dining rooms
   c. Hallways
   d. Activity rooms

2. Which statement about falls is *false?*
   a. Poor lighting, cluttered floors, and throw rugs may cause falls.
   b. Improper shoes and needing to use the bathroom may cause falls.
   c. Most falls occur between 4:00 PM and 8:00 PM.
   d. Falls are less likely to occur during shift changes.

3. You note the following after a person got dressed. Which is unsafe?
   a. Non skid footwear is worn
   b. Pant cuffs are dragging on the floor
   c. Clothing fits properly
   d. The belt is fastened

4. Which statement about bed rails is *false?*
   a. The nurse and care plan tell you when to raise bed rails.
   b. Bed rails are considered restraints.
   c. You may leave a person alone when the bed is raised and the bed rails are down.
   d. Bed rails can present hazards because people try to climb over them.

5. Which statement about transfer/gait belts is *false?*
   a. To use the belt safely, follow the manufacturer's instructions.
   b. Always apply the belt over clothing.
   c. Tighten the belt so it is very snug and breathing is impaired.
   d. Place the belt buckle off center so it is not over the spine.

6. A person becomes faint in the hallway and begins to fall. You should do the following *except*
   a. Ease the person to the floor
   b. Protect the person's head
   c. Let the person get up before the nurse checks him or her
   d. Help the nurse complete the incident report

Answers to these questions are on p. 479.

CHAPTER 13 RESTRAINT ALTERNATIVES AND SAFE RESTRAINT USE

- The Centers for Medicare and Medicaid Services (CMS) has rules for using restraints. These rules protect the person's rights and safety.
- Restraints may be used only to treat a medical symptom or for the immediate physical safety of the person or others. Restraints may be used only when less restrictive measures fail to protect the person or others. They must be discontinued at the earliest possible time.
- A physical restraint is any manual method or physical or mechanical device, material, or equipment attached to or near the person's body that he or she cannot remove easily and that restricts freedom of movement or normal access to one's body.
- A chemical restraint is a medication that is used for discipline or convenience and not required to treat medical symptoms. The medication or dosage is not a standard treatment for the person's condition.
- Federal, state, and accrediting agencies have guidelines about restraint use. They do not forbid restraint use. They require considering or trying all other appropriate alternatives first.

RESTRAINT ALTERNATIVES

- Knowing and treating the cause of harmful behaviors can prevent restraint use. There are many alternatives to restraints, such as answering the call light promptly. For other alternatives, see Box 13.2, Alternatives to Restraint Use, in the textbook.

SAFE RESTRAINT USE

- Restraints are used only when necessary to treat a person's medical symptoms—physical, emotional, or behavioral problems. Sometimes restraints are needed to protect the person or others.

Physical and Chemical Restraints

- *Physical restraints* are applied to the chest, waist, elbows, wrists, hands, or ankles. They confine the person to a bed or chair or they prevent movement of a body part.
- Some furniture or barriers prevent free movement:
  - Geriatric chairs or chairs with attached trays
  - Any chair placed so close to the wall that the person cannot move
  - Bed rails
  - Sheets tucked in so tightly that they restrict movement
- Medications or medication dosages are *chemical restraints* if they:
  - Control behavior or restrict movement
  - Are not standard treatment for the person's condition

Complications of Restraint Use

- Restraints can cause many complications. Injuries occur as the person tries to get free of the restraint. Injuries also occur from using the wrong restraint, applying it wrong, or keeping it on too long. Cuts, bruises, and fractures are common. The most serious risk is death from strangulation. Review Box 13.1, Risks of Restraint Use, in the textbook.
- Restraints may also affect a person's dignity and self-esteem.

Legal Aspects

- *Restraints must protect the person.* A restraint is used only when it is the best safety measure for the person.
- *A doctor's order is required.* The doctor gives the reason for the restraint, what body part to restrain, what to use, and how long to use it.
- *The least restrictive method is used.* It allows the greatest amount of movement or body access possible.
- *Restraints are used only after other measures fail to protect the person.* Box 13.2 lists alternatives to restraint use.
- *Unnecessary restraint is false imprisonment.* If you apply an unneeded restraint, you could face false imprisonment charges.
- *Consent is required.* The person must understand the reason for the restraint. If the person cannot give consent, his or her legal representative must give consent before a restraint can be used. The doctor or nurse provides the necessary information and obtains the consent.

Safety Guidelines

- Review Box 13.3, Safety Measures for Using Restraints, in the textbook.
- *Observe for increased confusion and agitation.* Restraints can increase confusion and agitation. Restrained persons need repeated explanations and reassurance. Spending time with them has a calming effect.
- *Protect the person's quality of life.* Restraints are used for as short a time as possible. You must meet the person's physical, emotional, and social needs.
- *Follow the manufacturer's instructions.* The restraint must be snug and firm but not tight. You could be negligent if you do not apply or secure a restraint properly.
- *Apply restraints with enough help to protect the person and staff from injury.*
- *Observe the person at least every 15 minutes or more often as noted in the care plan.* Injuries and deaths can result from improper restraint use and poor observation.
- *Remove or release the restraint, reposition the person, and meet basic needs at least every 2 hours or as often as noted in the care plan.* This includes food, fluid, comfort, safety, hygiene, and elimination needs and giving skin care. Perform range of motion exercises or help the person walk.

Reporting and Recording

- Report and record the following:
  - Type of restraint applied
  - Body part or parts restrained
  - Reason for the restraint
  - Safety measures taken
  - Time you applied the restraint
  - Time you removed or released the restraint
  - Care given when restraint was removed
  - Person's vital signs
  - Skin color and condition
  - Condition of the limbs
  - Pulse felt in the restrained part

CHAPTER 13 REVIEW QUESTIONS

Circle the BEST answer.

1. A geriatric chair or a bed rail may be considered a restraint if free movement is restricted.
   a. True
   b. False

2. Which statement about the use of restraints is *false?*
   a. A person may be embarrassed and humiliated when restraints are on.
   b. A person may experience depression and agitation when restraints are on.
   c. Restraints can be used for staff convenience.
   d. Restraints can cause serious injury and death.

3. Restraints can increase a person's confusion and agitation.
   a. True
   b. False

4. The person with a restraint should be observed at least every
   a. 15 minutes
   b. 30 minutes
   c. 1 hour
   d. 2 hours

5. Restraints need to be removed at least every
   a. 1 hour
   b. 2 hours
   c. 3 hours
   d. 4 hours

6. You should record all the following *except*
   a. The type of restraint used
   b. The consent for the restraint
   c. The time you removed the restraint
   d. The care you gave when the restraint was removed

Answers to these questions are on p. 479.

MICROORGANISMS

- A microorganism (microbe) is a small (micro) living plant or animal (organism).
- Some microbes are harmful and can cause infections (pathogens). Others do not usually cause infection (nonpathogens).

Multidrug-Resistant Organisms

- Multidrug-resistant organisms (MDROs) can resist the effects of antibiotics. Such organisms are able to change their structures to survive in the presence of antibiotics. The infections they cause are harder to treat.
- MDROs are caused by doctors prescribing antibiotics when they are not needed (over-prescribing). Not taking antibiotics for the prescribed length of time is also a cause.
- Three common types of MDROs are resistant to many antibiotics:
  - Methicillin-resistant Staphylococcus aureus (MRSA)
  - Vancomycin-resistant Enterococcus (VRE)
  - Clostridium difficile (C. diff or C. difficile)

INFECTION

- An infection is a disease state resulting from the invasion and growth of microbes in the body.
- Review Box 14.1, Signs and Symptoms of Infection, in the textbook.

Infection in Older Persons

- Older persons may not show the normal signs and symptoms of infection. The person may have only a slight fever or no fever at all. Redness and swelling may be very slight. The person may not complain of pain. Confusion and delirium may occur.
- Infections can become life-threatening before the older person has obvious signs and symptoms. Be alert to minor changes in the person's behavior or condition. Review Box 14.1, Signs and Symptoms of Infection, in the textbook. Report any concerns to the nurse at once.

Healthcare-Associated Infection

- A healthcare-associated infection (HAI) is an infection that develops in a person cared for in any setting where health care is given. Hospitals, nursing centers, clinics, and home care settings are examples. HAIs also are called nosocomial infections.
- The health team must prevent the spread of HAIs by:
  - Medical asepsis. This includes hand hygiene.
  - Surgical asepsis.
  - Standard Precautions and Transmission-Based Precautions.
  - The Bloodborne Pathogen Standard.

MEDICAL ASEPSIS

- Asepsis is being free of disease-producing microbes.
- Medical asepsis (clean technique) refers to the practices used to:
  - Remove or destroy pathogens.
  - Prevent pathogens from spreading from one person or place to another person or place.

Common Aseptic Practices

- To prevent the spread of microbes, wash your hands:
  - After urinating or having a bowel movement.
  - After changing tampons or sanitary pads.
  - After contact with your own or another person's blood, body fluids, secretions, or excretions. This includes saliva, vomitus, urine, feces, vaginal discharge, mucus, semen, wound drainage, pus, and respiratory secretions.
  - After coughing, sneezing, or blowing your nose.
  - Before and after handling, preparing, or eating food.
  - After smoking a cigarette, cigar, or pipe.
- Also do the following:
  - Provide all persons with their own linens and personal care items.
  - Cover your nose and mouth when coughing, sneezing, or blowing your nose.
  - Bathe, wash hair, and brush your teeth regularly.
  - Wash fruits and raw vegetables before eating or serving them.
  - Wash cooking and eating utensils with soap and water after use.

Hand Hygiene

- Hand hygiene is the easiest and most important way to prevent the spread of infection. Practice hand hygiene before and after giving care. Review Box 14.2, Rules of Hand Hygiene, in the textbook.

Supplies and Equipment

- Most health care equipment is disposable. Bedpans, urinals, wash basins, water pitchers, and drinking cups are multi-use items. Do not "borrow" them for another person.
- Non disposable items are cleaned and then disinfected. Then they are sterilized.

Other Aseptic Measures

- Review Box 14.3, Aseptic Measures, in the textbook.

ISOLATION PRECAUTIONS

- Isolation precautions prevent the spread of communicable diseases (contagious diseases). They are diseases caused by pathogens that spread easily.
- The CDC's isolation precautions guideline has two tiers of precautions:
  - Standard Precautions
  - Transmission-Based Precautions

Standard Precautions

- Standard Precautions reduce the risk of spreading pathogens and known and unknown infections. Standard Precautions are used for all persons whenever care is given. They prevent the spread of infection from:
  - Blood.
  - All body fluids, secretions, and excretions even if blood is not visible. Sweat is not known to spread infections.
  - Non intact skin (skin with open breaks).
  - Mucous membranes.
- Review Box 14.4, Standard Precautions, in the textbook.

Transmission-Based Precautions

- Some infections require Transmission-Based Precautions. Review Box 14.5, Transmission-Based Precautions, in the textbook.
- Agency policies may differ from those in the book. The rules in Box 14.6 in the textbook, Rules for Isolation Precautions, are a guide for giving safe care.

Protective Measures

- Isolation precautions involve wearing personal protective equipment (PPE)—gloves, a gown, a mask, and goggles or a face shield.
- Removing linens, trash, and equipment from the room may require double-bagging.
- Follow center procedures when collecting specimens and transporting persons.
- Wear gloves whenever contact with blood, body fluids, secretions, excretions, mucous membranes, and non intact skin is likely. Wearing gloves is the most common protective measure used with Standard Precautions and Transmission-Based Precautions. Remember the following when using gloves:
  - The outside of gloves is contaminated.
  - Gloves are easier to put on when your hands are dry.
  - Do not tear gloves when putting them on.
  - You need a new pair for every person.
  - Remove and discard torn, cut, or punctured gloves at once. Practice hand hygiene. Then put on a new pair.
  - Wear gloves once. Discard them after use.
  - Put on clean gloves just before touching mucous membranes or non intact skin.
  - Put on new gloves whenever gloves become contaminated with blood, body fluids, secretions, or excretions. A task may require more than one pair of gloves.
  - Change gloves if interacting with the person involves touching portable computer keyboards or other mobile equipment that is transported from room to room.
  - Put on gloves last when worn with other PPE.
  - Change gloves whenever moving from a contaminated body site to a clean body site.

- Make sure gloves cover your wrists. If you wear a gown, gloves cover the cuffs.
- Remove gloves so the inside part is on the outside. The inside is clean.
- Decontaminate your hands after removing gloves.
- Latex allergies are common and can cause skin rashes. Asthma and shock are more serious problems associated with latex allergies. Report skin rashes and breathing problems at once. If you or a resident has a latex allergy, wear latex-free gloves.
- Gowns must completely cover your neck to your knees. The gown front and sleeves are considered contaminated. A wet gown is contaminated. Gowns are used once. When removing a gown, roll it away from you. Keep it inside out.
- Masks are disposable. A wet or moist mask is contaminated. When removing a mask, touch only the ties or elastic bands. The front of the mask is contaminated.
- The front of goggles or a face shield is contaminated. Use the device's ties, headband, or ear-pieces to remove the device.
- Contaminated items, linens, and trash are bagged to remove them from the person's room. Leak-proof plastic bags are used. They have the *BIOHAZARD* symbol. Double-bagging is not needed unless the outside of the bag is soiled.

Meeting Basic Needs

- Love, belonging, and self-esteem needs are often unmet when Transmission-Based Precautions are used. Visitors and staff often avoid the person. The person may feel lonely, unwanted, and rejected. He or she may feel dirty and undesirable. The person may feel ashamed and guilty for having a contagious disease. You can help the person, family, and staff understand the need for Transmission-Based Precautions and how they affect the person.

BLOODBORNE PATHOGEN STANDARD

- The health team is at risk for exposure to the human immunodeficiency virus (HIV) and the hepatitis B virus (HBV). HIV and HBV are bloodborne pathogens found in the blood.
- The Bloodborne Pathogen Standard is intended to protect you from exposure.
- Staff at risk for exposure to HIV and HBV receive free training.
- *Hepatitis B vaccination.* You can receive the hepatitis B vaccination within 10 working days of being hired. The agency pays for it. If you refuse the vaccination, you must sign a statement. You can have the vaccination at a later date.

Engineering and Work Practice Controls

- *Engineering controls* reduce employee exposure in the workplace. There are special containers for contaminated sharps (needles, broken glass) and specimens. These containers are puncture-resistant, leak-proof, and color-coded in red. They have the *BIOHAZARD* symbol.

- *Work practice controls* reduce exposure risk. All tasks involving blood or other potentially infectious materials (OPIM) are done in ways to limit splatters, splashes, and sprays. Other controls include:
  - Do not eat, drink, smoke, apply cosmetics or lip balm, or handle contact lenses in areas of occupational exposure.
  - Do not store food or drinks where blood or OPIM are kept.
  - Practice hand hygiene after removing gloves.
  - Wash hands as soon as possible after skin contact with blood or OPIM.
  - Never recap, bend, or remove needles by hand.
  - Never shear or break contaminated needles.
  - Discard contaminated needles and sharp instruments (razors) in containers that are closable, puncture-resistant, and leak-proof.

Personal Protective Equipment (PPE)

- This includes gloves, goggles, face shields, masks, laboratory coats, gowns, shoe covers, and surgical caps. For safe handling and use of PPE:
  - Remove PPE before leaving the work area.
  - Remove PPE when a garment becomes contaminated.
  - Place used PPE in marked areas or containers when being stored, washed, decontaminated, or discarded.
  - Wear gloves when you expect contact with blood or OPIM.
  - Wear gloves when handling or touching contaminated items or surfaces.
  - Replace worn, punctured, or contaminated gloves.
  - Never wash or decontaminate disposable gloves for re-use.
  - Discard utility gloves that show signs of cracking, peeling, tearing, or puncturing. Utility gloves are decontaminated for re-use if the process will not ruin them.

Equipment

- Contaminated equipment is cleaned and decontaminated. Decontaminate work surfaces with a proper disinfectant:
  - Upon completing tasks
  - At once when there is obvious contamination
  - After any spill of blood or OPIM
  - At the end of the work shift when surfaces become contaminated

Laundry

- The Occupational and Safety Health Administration (OSHA) requires these measures for contaminated laundry:

- Handle it as little as possible.
- Wear gloves or other needed PPE.
- Bag contaminated laundry where it is used.
- Mark laundry bags or containers with the *BIOHAZARD* symbol for laundry sent off-site.
- Place wet, contaminated laundry in leak-proof containers before transport. The containers are color-coded in red or have the *BIOHAZARD* symbol.

Exposure Incidents

- Report exposure incidents at once. Medical evaluation, follow-up, and required tests are free. Your blood is tested for HIV and HBV. Confidentiality is important.

CHAPTER 14 REVIEW QUESTIONS

Circle the BEST answer.

1. A healthcare-associated infection (nosocomial infection) is
   a. An infection free of disease-producing microbes
   b. An infection that develops in a person cared for in any setting where health care is given
   c. An infection acquired by health care workers
   d. An infection acquired only by older persons

2. Which statement about hand hygiene is *false?*
   a. Hand hygiene is the easiest way to prevent the spread of infection.
   b. Hand hygiene is the most important way to prevent the spread of infection.
   c. Hand hygiene is practiced before and after giving care to a person.
   d. If hands are visibly soiled, hand hygiene can be done with an alcohol-based hand rub.

3. When washing your hands, you should do all of the following *except*
   a. Stand away from the sink so your clothes do not touch the sink
   b. Keep your hands lower than your elbows
   c. Wash your hands for at least 15 seconds
   d. Dry your arms from the forearms to the fingertips

4. Which statement about wearing gloves is *false?*
   a. The insides of gloves are contaminated.
   b. You need a new pair of gloves for each person you care for.
   c. Change gloves when moving from a contaminated body site to a clean body site.
   d. Gloves need to cover your wrists.

5. Which statement is *false?*
   a. Gowns must cover you from your neck to your waist.
   b. A moist mask is contaminated.
   c. The front of goggles is contaminated.
   d. You should wash your hands after removing a gown, mask, or goggles.

6. Which statement about PPE is *false?*
   a. Remove PPE when a garment becomes contaminated.
   b. Wear gloves when handling or touching contaminated items or surfaces.
   c. Wash or decontaminate disposable gloves for re-use.
   d. Remove PPE before leaving the work area.

Answers to these questions are on p. 479.

CHAPTER 15 BODY MECHANICS AND SAFE RESIDENT HANDLING, POSITIONING, AND TRANSFERS

PRINCIPLES OF BODY MECHANICS

- Your strongest and largest muscles are in the shoulders, upper arms, hips, and thighs. Use these muscles to lift and move persons and heavy objects.
- For good body mechanics:
  - Bend your knees and squat to lift a heavy object. Do not bend from your waist.
  - Hold items close to your body and base of support.
- Review Box 15.1, Rules for Body Mechanics, in your textbook.

ERGONOMICS

- Ergonomics is the science of designing a job to fit the worker. The task, work station, equipment, and tools are changed to help reduce stress on the worker's body. The goal is to prevent injury and disorders of the muscles, tendons, ligaments, joints, cartilage, and nervous system.
- Early signs and symptoms of injury include pain, limited joint movement, or soft tissue swelling. Always report a work-related injury as soon as possible. Early attention can help prevent the problem from becoming worse.

POSITIONING THE PERSON

- The person must be properly positioned at all times. Regular position changes and good alignment promote comfort and well-being. Breathing is easier. Circulation is promoted. Pressure injuries and contractures are prevented.
- Whether in bed or in a chair, the person is repositioned at least every 2 hours. To safely position a person:
  - Use good body mechanics.
  - Ask a coworker to help you if needed.
  - Explain the procedure to the person.
  - Be gentle when moving the person.
  - Provide for privacy.
  - Use pillows as directed by the nurse for support and alignment.
  - Provide for comfort after positioning.
  - Place the call light within reach after positioning.

- Complete a safety check before leaving the room.
- **Fowler position** is a semi-sitting position. The head of the bed is raised between 45 and 60 degrees. The knees may be slightly elevated.
- The **supine position (dorsal recumbent position)** is the back-lying position.
- A person in the **prone position** lies on the abdomen with the head turned to one side.
- A person in the **lateral position (side-lying position)** lies on one side or the other.
- For some procedures, the person is placed in a **left side-lying position**.
- Persons who sit in chairs must hold their upper bodies and heads erect. For good alignment:
  - The person's back and buttocks are against the back of the chair.
  - Feet are flat on the floor or wheelchair footplates. Never leave feet unsupported.
  - Backs of the knees and calves are slightly away from the edge of the seat.

PREVENTING WORK-RELATED INJURIES

- Review Box 15.2, Preventing Work-Related Injuries, in your textbook.
- To safely handle, move, and transfer a person, the nurse and health team determine:
  - The person's dependence level (review Box 15.3, Levels of Dependence, in your textbook).
  - The amount of assistance needed.
  - What procedure to use.
  - What equipment is needed.

PROTECTING THE SKIN

- Protect the person's skin from friction and shearing. Both cause infection and pressure injuries To reduce friction and shearing:
  - Roll the person.
  - Use a lift sheet (turning sheet).
  - Use a turning pad, slide board, slide sheet, or large incontinence product.

MOVING PERSONS IN BED

- Determine the person's ability before moving the person. Review Delegations Guidelines: Moving Persons in Bed, in your textbook.
- It is best to have help with older persons and with those who are heavy and hard to move. This protects the person and you from injury.
- You can sometimes move lightweight adults up in bed alone if they can assist and use a trapeze.
- Assist devices are used to reduce shearing and friction. Such assist devices include a drawsheet (lift sheet), flat sheet folded in half, turning pad, slide sheet, and large incontinence product.

TURNING PERSONS

- Turning persons onto their sides helps prevent complications from bedrest. Certain procedures and care measures also require the side-lying position. After the person is turned, position him or her in good alignment. Use pillows as directed to support the person in the side-lying position.
- Logrolling is turning the person as a unit, in alignment, with one motion. The spine is kept straight.

SITTING ON THE SIDE OF THE BED (DANGLING)

- Many older persons become dizzy or faint when getting out of bed too fast. They need to sit on the side of the bed before walking or transferring. Some persons increase activity in stages—bedrest, to sitting on the side of the bed, to sitting in a chair, to walking.
- While dangling, the person coughs and deep breathes. He or she moves the legs back and forth in circles to stimulate circulation.
- Observations to report and record:
  - Pulse and respiratory rates
  - Pale or bluish skin color (cyanosis)
  - Complaints of light headedness, dizziness, or difficulty breathing
  - How well the activity was tolerated
  - The length of time the person dangled
  - The amount of help needed
  - Other observations and complaints

TRANSFERRING PERSONS

- The rules of body mechanics apply during transfers.
- Arrange the room so there is enough space for a safe transfer. Correct placement of the chair, wheelchair, or other device also is needed for a safe transfer.
- Have the person wear non skid footwear for transfers.
- Lock the wheels of the bed, wheelchair, stretcher, or other assist device.
- After the transfer, position the person in good alignment.
- Transfer belts (gait belts) are used to support persons during transfers and reposition persons in chairs and wheelchairs.

Bed to Chair or Wheelchair Transfers

- Safety is important for transfers. In transferring, the strong side moves first. Help the person out of bed on his or her strong side. Help the person from the wheelchair to the bed on his or her strong side.
- The person must not put his or her arms around your neck.
- Chair or wheelchair to bed transfers have the same rules as bed to chair or wheelchair transfers. Transfer the person so that the strong side moves first

Mechanical Lifts

- Persons who cannot help themselves are transferred with mechanical lifts. So are persons who are too heavy for the staff to transfer.
- Before using a mechanical lift, you must be trained in its use. The sling, straps, hooks, and chains must be in good repair. The person's weight must not exceed the lift's capacity. At least two staff members are needed. Always follow the manufacturer's instructions for using the lift.
- Falling from the lift is a common fear. To promote the person's mental comfort, always explain the procedure before you begin. Also show the person how the lift works.

CHAPTER 15 REVIEW QUESTIONS

Circle the BEST answer.

1. To lift and move residents and heavy objects you should
   a. Use the muscles in your lower arms
   b. Use the muscles in your legs
   c. Use the muscles in your shoulders, upper arms, hips, and thighs
   d. Use the muscles in your abdomen

2. For good body mechanics, you should do all of the following *except*
   a. Bend your knees and squat to lift a heavy object
   b. Bend from your waist to lift a heavy object
   c. Hold items close to your body and base of support
   d. Bend your legs; do not bend your back

3. Which statement is *false?*
   a. A person must be properly positioned at all times.
   b. Regular position changes and good alignment promote comfort and well-being.
   c. Regular position changes and good alignment promote pressure injuries and contractures.
   d. When a person is in good alignment, breathing is easier and circulation is promoted.

4. In Fowler position
   a. The head of the bed is flat
   b. The head of the bed is raised to 90 degrees
   c. The head of the bed is raised between 45 and 60 degrees
   d. The head of the bed is raised between 30 and 35 degrees

5. Friction and shearing are reduced by doing all of the following *except*
   a. Rolling the person
   b. Using a lift sheet or turning pad
   c. Using a pillow
   d. Using a slide board or slide sheet

6. After a person is turned, you must position him or her in good alignment.
   a. True
   b. False

7. Many older persons become dizzy or faint when getting out of bed too fast.
   a. True
   b. False

8. You are transferring a person from the bed to a wheelchair. Which statement is *false?*
   a. The person should wear non skid footwear.
   b. The person may put his or her arm around your neck.
   c. You should use a gait/transfer belt.
   d. You should lock the wheelchair wheels.

9. A person has a weak left side and a strong right side. In transferring the person from the bed to the wheelchair, his or her strong (right) side moves first.
   a. True
   b. False

10. Before using a mechanical lift, you do all of the following *except*
    a. Check the sling, straps, and chains to ensure good repair
    b. Check the person's weight to be sure it does not exceed the lift's capacity
    c. Follow the manufacturer's instructions for using the lift
    d. Operate the lift without a coworker

Answers to these questions are on p. 479.

CHAPTER 16 THE RESIDENT'S UNIT

- A resident unit is the personal space, furniture, and equipment provided for the person by the nursing center. Resident units are as personal and home-like as possible.

Comfort

- Age, illness, and activity are factors that affect comfort.
- Temperature, ventilation, noise, odors, and lighting are factors that are controlled to meet the person's needs.

Temperature and Ventilation

- Older persons, and those who are ill, may need higher temperatures for comfort.
- To protect older and ill persons from cool areas and drafts:
  - Make sure they wear the correct clothing.
  - Offer lap robes to cover the legs.
  - Provide enough blankets for warmth and cover them with bath blankets when giving care.
  - Move them from drafty areas.

Odors

- To reduce odors in nursing centers:
  - Empty, clean, and disinfect bedpans, urinals, commodes, and kidney basins promptly.
  - Check to make sure toilets are flushed.
  - Check incontinent people often.
  - Clean persons who are wet or soiled from urine, feces, or wound drainage.
  - Change wet or soiled linens and clothing promptly.
  - Keep laundry containers closed.
  - Follow center policy for wet or soiled linens and clothing.
  - Dispose of incontinence and ostomy products promptly.
  - Remove and seal off trash can liners promptly and transport to soiled utility area.
  - Provide good hygiene to prevent body and breath odors.
  - Use room deodorizers as needed.
- If you smoke, practice hand washing after handling smoking materials and before giving care. Give careful attention to your uniform, hair, and breath because of smoke odors.

Noise

- To decrease noise:
  - Control your voice.
  - Handle equipment carefully and keep equipment in good working order.
  - Answer phones, call lights, and intercoms promptly.

Lighting

- Adjust lighting to meet the person's needs. Glares, shadows, and dull lighting can cause falls, headaches, and eyestrain. A bright room is cheerful. Dim light is better for relaxing and rest. Persons with poor vision need bright light. Always keep light controls within the person's reach.

ROOM FURNITURE AND EQUIPMENT

The Bed

- Beds are raised to give care. They are positioned at the lowest level when not giving care.
- Basic bed positions:
  - *Flat*—the usual sleeping position.
  - *Fowler position*—a semi-sitting position. The head of the bed is raised between 45 and 60 degrees.
  - *High-Fowler position*—a semi-sitting position. The head of the bed is raised between 60 and 90 degrees.
  - *Semi-Fowler position*—the head of the bed is raised 30 degrees. Some centers define semi-Fowler position as when the head of the bed is raised 30 degrees and the knee portion is raised 15 degrees. Know the definition used by your center.
  - *Trendelenburg's position*—the head of the bed is lowered and the foot of the bed is raised. A doctor orders the position.
  - *Reverse Trendelenburg's position*—the head of the bed is raised and the foot of the bed is lowered. A doctor orders the position.

Bed Safety

- *Entrapment* means the person can get caught, trapped, or entangled in spaces created by bed rails, the mattress, the bed frame, or the headboard and footboard. Serious injuries and deaths have occurred from entrapment. If a person is at risk for entrapment, report your concerns to the nurse at once. If a person is caught, trapped, or entangled, try to release the person. Call for the nurse at once.

The Overbed Table and Bedside Stand

- Only clean and sterile items are placed on the over bed table. Never place bedpans, urinals, or soiled linens on the overbed table or on top of the bedside stand.
- Clean the table and bedside stand after using them as a work surface.

Privacy Curtains

- Always pull the curtain completely around the bed before giving care. Privacy curtains do not block sound or conversations.

The Call System

- The call light must always be kept within the person's reach—in the room, bathroom, and shower or tub room. You must:
  - Place the call light on the person's strong side.
  - Remind the person to signal when help is needed.
  - Answer call lights promptly.
  - Answer bathroom and shower or tub room call lights at once.
- Persons with limited hand mobility may need special communication measures.
- Be careful when using the intercom. Remember confidentiality. Persons nearby can hear what you and the person say.

Closet and Drawer Space

- The person must have free access to the closet and its contents. You must have the person's permission to open or search closets or drawers.
- Agency staff can inspect a person's closet or drawers if hoarding is suspected. The person is informed of the inspection and is present when it takes place. Have a coworker present when you inspect a person's closet.

General Rules

- Keep the person's room clean, neat, safe, and comfortable. Follow the rules in Box 16.1, Maintaining the Person's Unit, and Box 16.2, OBRA and CMS Requirements for Resident Rooms.

CHAPTER 16 REVIEW QUESTIONS

Circle the BEST answer.

1. Serious injuries and death have occurred from entrapment.
   a. True
   b. False

2. You should never place bedpans, urinals, or soiled linens on the overbed table.
   a. True
   b. False

3. You should clean the bedside stand if you use it for a work surface.
   a. True
   b. False

4. The following protect a person from drafts *except*
   a. Wearing enough clothing
   b. Lap robes
   c. Using a sheet when giving care
   d. Providing blankets

5. To reduce odors, you do all of the following *except*
   a. Empty bedpans and commodes promptly
   b. Keep laundry containers open
   c. Check to make sure toilets are flushed
   d. Clean persons who are wet or soiled from urine or feces

6. Which statement about the call light is *false?*
   a. The call light must always be within the person's reach.
   b. Place the call light on the person's strong side.
   c. You have to answer the call lights only for residents assigned to you.
   d. Answer call lights promptly.

7. You suspect a person is hoarding food in her closet. Before you inspect the closet, what do you do?
   a. Tell another nursing assistant what you suspect.
   b. Inspect the closet without telling the resident.
   c. Tell the family.
   d. Ask the resident if you can inspect the closet.

Answers to these questions are on p. 479.

CHAPTER 17 BEDMAKING

- Clean, dry, and wrinkle-free linens promote comfort. Skin breakdown and pressure injuries are prevented.
- To keep beds neat and clean:
  - Straighten linens whenever loose or wrinkled and at bedtime.
  - Check for and remove food and crumbs after meals.
  - Check linens for dentures, eyeglasses, hearing aids, sharp objects, and other items.
  - Change linens whenever they become wet, soiled, or damp.
  - Follow Standard Precautions and the Bloodborne Pathogen Standard.

TYPES OF BEDS

- Beds are made in these ways:
  - A closed bed is not used until bedtime. Or the bed is ready for a new resident. Top linens are not folded back.
  - An open bed is in use. Top linens are fan-folded back so the person can get into bed. A closed bed becomes an open bed by fan-folding back the top linens.

- An occupied bed is made with the person in it.
- A surgical bed is made to transfer a person from a stretcher. This bed is also made for persons who arrive by ambulance.

LINENS

- When handling linens and making beds:
  - Practice medical asepsis.
  - Always hold linens away from your body and uniform. Your uniform is considered dirty.
  - Never shake linens.
  - Place clean linens on a clean surface.
  - Never put clean or dirty linens on the floor.
- Collect enough linens. Do not bring unneeded linens into the person's room. Once in the room, extra linens are considered contaminated. They cannot be used for another person.
- Roll each piece of dirty linen away from you. The side that touched the person is inside the roll and away from you.

Making Beds

- When making beds, safety and medical asepsis are important. Use good body mechanics. Follow the rules for safe resident handling, moving, and transfers. Practice hand hygiene before handling clean linens and after handling dirty linens.
- Review Box 17.1, Rules for Bedmaking, in the textbook.

The Occupied Bed

- You make an occupied bed when the person stays in bed. Keep the person in good alignment. Follow restrictions or limits in the person's movement or position. Explain each procedure step to the person before it is done. This is important even if the person cannot respond to you.

CHAPTER 17 REVIEW QUESTIONS

Circle the BEST answer.

1. Once in the person's room, extra linens are considered contaminated. They can be used for another person.
   a. True
   b. False

2. Roll each piece of dirty linen away from you. The side that touched the person is inside the roll.
   a. True
   b. False

3. Wear gloves when removing linens from the person's bed.
   a. True
   b. False

4. To keep beds neat and clean, do the following *except*
   a. Straighten linens whenever loose or wrinkled
   b. Check for and remove food and crumbs after meals
   c. Check linens for dentures, eyeglasses, and hearing aids
   d. Change linens monthly

5. Which statement is *false?*
   a. Practice medical asepsis when handling linens.
   b. Always hold linens away from your body and uniform.
   c. Shake linens to remove crumbs.
   d. Put dirty linens in the dirty laundry bin.

Answers to these questions are on p. 479.

CHAPTER 18 HYGIENE

- Besides cleansing, good hygiene prevents body and breath odors. It is relaxing and increases circulation.
- Culture and personal choice affect hygiene.

DAILY CARE

- Most people have hygiene routines and habits. Hygiene measures are often done before and after meals and at bedtime. You assist with hygiene whenever it is needed. Protect the person's right to privacy and to personal choice.

ORAL HYGIENE

- Oral hygiene keeps the mouth and teeth clean. It prevents mouth odors and infections, increases comfort, and makes food taste better. Mouth care also reduces the risk for cavities and periodontal disease.
- Assist with oral hygiene after sleep, after meals, and at bedtime. Follow the care plan.
- Follow Standard Precautions and the Bloodborne Pathogen Standard.
- Report and record:
  - Dry, cracked, swollen, or blistered lips
  - Mouth or breath odor
  - Redness, swelling, irritation, sores, or white patches in the mouth or on the tongue
  - Bleeding, swelling, or redness of the gums
  - Loose teeth
  - Rough, sharp, or chipped areas on dentures

Brushing and Flossing Teeth

- Flossing removes plaque and tartar from the teeth as well as food from between the teeth. Flossing is usually done after brushing. If done once a day, bedtime is the best time to floss.
- Some persons need help gathering and setting up equipment for oral hygiene. You may have to perform

oral care for persons who are weak, cannot move their arms, or are too confused to brush their teeth.

Mouth Care for the Unconscious Person

- Unconscious persons may breathe with their mouth open, leaving dry mouths and crusting on the tongue and mucous membranes. Oral hygiene keeps the mouth clean and moist. It also helps prevent infection.
- Use sponge swabs to apply the cleaning agent. To prevent cracking of the lips, apply a lubricant to the lips. Check the care plan.
- To prevent aspiration by the unconscious person:
  - Position the person on one side with the head turned well to the side.
  - Use only a small amount of fluid to clean the mouth.
  - Do not insert dentures. Dentures are not worn when the person is unconscious.
- When giving oral hygiene, keep the person's mouth open with a padded tongue blade.
- Mouth care is given at least every 2 hours. Follow the nurse's direction and the care plan.

Denture Care

- Mouth care is given and dentures are cleaned as often as natural teeth. Dentures are usually removed at bedtime and stored in a container with cool water or denture solution.
- Dentures are slippery when wet. Hold them firmly. During cleaning, hold them over a basin of water lined with a towel. Use a cleaning agent and follow the manufacturer's instructions.
- Hot water causes dentures to lose their shape. If dentures are not worn after cleaning, store them in a container with cool water or a denture soaking solution.
- Label the denture cup with the person's name, room number, and bed number. Report lost or damaged dentures to the nurse at once. Losing or damaging dentures is negligent conduct.
- Many people do not like being seen without their dentures. Privacy is important. If you clean dentures, return them to the person as quickly as possible.
- Persons with partial dentures have some natural teeth. They need to brush and floss the natural teeth.

BATHING

- Bathing cleans the skin. The mucous membranes of the genital and anal areas are cleaned as well. A bath is refreshing and relaxing. Circulation is stimulated and body parts are exercised. You have time to talk to the person. You also can make observations.
- Review Box 18.1, Rules for Bathing, in the textbook.
- Soap dries the skin. Therefore, older persons usually need a complete bath or shower twice a week. Partial baths are taken on the other days. Some bathe daily but not with soap. Thorough rinsing is needed when using soap. Lotions and oils keep the skin soft.

- Water temperature for complete bed baths and partial bed baths is between 110 °F and 115 °F. Older persons have fragile skin and need lower water temperatures. Measure water temperature according to center policy.
- Report and record:
  - The color of the skin, lips, nail beds, and sclera
  - The location and description of rashes
  - Dry skin
  - Bruises or open areas
  - Pale or reddened areas, especially over bony parts
  - Drainage or bleeding from wounds or body openings
  - Swelling of the feet and legs
  - Corns or calluses on the feet
  - Skin temperature
  - Complaints of pain or discomfort
- Use caution when applying powders. Do not use powders near persons with respiratory disorders. Do not sprinkle or shake powder onto the person. To safely apply powder:
  - Turn away from the person.
  - Sprinkle a small amount onto your hands or a cloth.
  - Apply the powder in a thin layer.
  - Make sure powder does not get on the floor. Powder is slippery and can cause falls.

The Complete Bed Bath

- The complete bed bath involves washing the person's entire body in bed. Complete bed baths are given to persons who cannot bathe themselves. Bed baths are usually needed by persons who are unconscious, paralyzed, in casts or traction, or weak from illness or injury.
- Water temperature should be between 110° F and 115° F.
- A towel bath uses an oversized towel that is soaked in water and cleaning, skin-softening, and drying agents. A bag bath is a commercially prepared product that contains pre moistened washcloths. Each washcloth is used for a different body part.

The Partial Bath

- The partial bath involves bathing the face, hands, axillae (underarms), back, buttocks, and perineal area. You assist the person as needed. Most need help washing the back.

Tub Baths and Showers

- Falls, burns, and chilling from water are risks. Review Box 18.2, Safety Measures for Tub Baths and Showers, in the textbook.
- A tub bath can cause a person to feel faint, weak, or tired. The person may need a transfer bench, a tub with a side entry door, a wheelchair or stretcher lift, or a mechanical lift to get in and out of the tub.
- Some people can use a regular shower. Have the person use the grab bars for support during the shower. Use a bath mat if the shower does not have non skid

surfaces. Never let weak or unsteady persons stand in the shower. They may need to use shower chairs, shower stalls or cabinets, or shower trolleys. Some shower rooms have two or more stations. Protect the person's privacy. Properly screen and cover the person.

- Water temperature for tub baths and showers is usually 105°F. Report and record dizziness and light headedness.

THE BACK MASSAGE

- The back massage relaxes muscles and stimulates circulation.
- Massages are given after the bath and with evening care. You also can give back massages at other times, such as after repositioning a person.
- Observe the skin for breaks, bruises, reddened areas, and other signs of skin breakdown.
- Lotion reduces friction during the massage. It is warmed before applying.
- Use firm strokes. Keep your hands in contact with the person's skin.
- After the massage, apply some lotion to the elbows, knees, and heels.
- Back massages are dangerous for persons with certain heart diseases, back injuries, back surgeries, skin diseases, and some lung disorders. Check with the nurse and the care plan before giving back massages to persons with these conditions.
- Do not massage reddened bony areas. Reddened areas signal skin breakdown and pressure injuries. Massage can lead to more tissue damage.
- Wear gloves if the person's skin is not intact. Always follow Standard Precautions and the Bloodborne Pathogen Standard.
- Report and record skin breakdown, redness, and bruising.

PERINEAL CARE

- Perineal care involves cleaning the genital and anal areas. It is done daily during the bath and whenever the area is soiled with urine or feces. The person does perineal care if able.
- Perineal and perineum are not common terms. Most people understand privates, private parts, crotch, genitals, or the area between the legs. Use terms the person understands.
- Standard Precautions, medical asepsis, and the Bloodborne Pathogen Standard are followed.
- Work from the cleanest area to the dirtiest—commonly called cleaning from "front to back." On a woman, clean from the urethra (cleanest) to the anal (dirtiest) area. On a male, start at the meatus of the urethra and work outward.

- Use warm water. Use washcloths, towelettes, cotton balls, or swabs according to center policy. Rinse thoroughly. Pat dry. Water temperature is usually 105°F–109°F.
- Report and record:
  - Bleeding, redness, swelling, discharge, irritation
  - Complaints of pain or burning
  - Signs of urinary or fecal incontinence
  - Signs of skin breakdown
  - Odors

CHAPTER 18 REVIEW QUESTIONS

Circle the BEST answer.

1. Oral hygiene does all of the following *except*
   a. Keeps the mouth and teeth clean
   b. Prevents mouth odors and infections
   c. Decreases comfort
   d. Makes food taste better

2. When giving oral hygiene, you should report and record all of the following *except*
   a. Dry, cracked, swollen, or blistered lips
   b. Redness, sores, or white patches in the mouth
   c. Bleeding, swelling, or redness of the gums
   d. The number of fillings a person has

3. A person is unconscious. When you do mouth care, you do all of the following *except*
   a. Use only a small amount of fluid to clean the mouth
   b. Use your fingers to keep the mouth open
   c. Explain what you are doing
   d. Give mouth care at least every 2 hours

4. To prevent damage to dentures during cleaning, hold dentures over a basin of water lined with a towel.
   a. True
   b. False

5. Bathing does all of the following *except*
   a. Cleanses the skin
   b. Stimulates circulation
   c. Makes a person tense
   d. Permits you to observe the person's skin

6. The water temperature for a complete bed bath is
   a. 102°F–108°F
   b. 110°F–115°F
   c. 115°F–120°F
   d. 120°F–125°F

7. Which statement is *false?*
   a. Use powder near persons with respiratory disorders.
   b. Before applying powder, check with the nurse and the care plan.
   c. Before applying powder, sprinkle a small amount of powder onto your hands.
   d. Apply powder in a thin layer.

8. Which statement is *false?*
   a. A back massage relaxes and stimulates circulation.
   b. Massages are given after the bath and with evening care.
   c. You can observe the person's skin before beginning the massage.
   d. You should use cold lotion for the massage.

9. When giving female perineal care, you should work from the urethra to the anal area.
   a. True
   b. False

10. When giving male perineal care, start at the meatus and work outward.
    a. True
    b. False

Answers to these questions are on p. 479.

CHAPTER 19 GROOMING

- Hair care, shaving, and nail and foot care prevent infection and promote comfort. They also affect love, belonging, and self-esteem needs.

HAIR CARE

- The nursing process reflects the person's culture, personal choice, skin and scalp condition, health history, and self-care ability. You assist with hair care as needed.

Brushing and Combing Hair

- Brushing and combing prevent tangled, matted hair.
- When brushing and combing hair, start at the scalp and brush or comb to the hair ends.
- Never cut hair for any reason. Tell the nurse if you think the person's hair needs to be cut.
- Special measures are needed for curly, coarse, and dry hair. Check the care plan.
- When giving hair care, place a towel across the person's back and shoulders to protect garments from falling hair. If the person is in bed, give hair care before changing the linens and pillowcase.

Shampooing

- Shampooing frequency depends on the person's needs and preferences. Usually, shampooing is done weekly on the person's bath or shower day.
- Hair is dried and styled as quickly as possible after the shampoo.
- During shampooing, report and record:
  - Scalp sores
  - Flaking
  - Itching
  - Presence of nits or lice
  - Patches of hair loss or hair falling out in patches
  - Very dry or very oily hair

- Matted or tangled hair
- How the person tolerated the procedure
- Keep shampoo away from and out of eyes. Have the person hold a washcloth over the eyes.
- Wear gloves if the person has scalp sores.
- Follow Standard Precautions and the Bloodborne Pathogen Standard.

SHAVING

- Review Box 19.1, Rules for Shaving, in your textbook.

Caring for Mustaches and Beards

- Wash and comb mustaches and beards daily and as needed. Ask the person how to groom his mustache or beard.
- Never trim a mustache or beard without the person's consent.

Shaving Legs and Underarms

- Many women shave their legs and underarms. This practice varies among cultures. Legs and underarms are shaved after bathing when the skin is soft.

NAIL AND FOOT CARE

- Nail and foot care prevent infection, injury, and odors.
- Nails are easier to trim and clean right after soaking or bathing.
- Use nail clippers to cut fingernails. Never use scissors. Use extreme caution to prevent damage to nearby tissues.
- Follow center policy for cutting or trimming fingernails or toenails.
- Report and record:
  - Reddened, irritated, or calloused areas
  - Breaks in the skin
  - Corns on top of and between the toes
  - Very thick nails
  - Loose nails
- Always follow center policy for nail care. You do not cut or trim toenails if a person has diabetes or poor circulation to the legs and feet or takes medications that affect blood clotting. Also, do not cut or trim toenails if the person has very thick nails or ingrown toenails. The nurse or podiatrist cuts toenails and provides foot care for these persons.
- When doing foot care, check between the toes for cracks and sores. If left untreated, a serious infection could occur.
- The feet of persons with decreased sensation or circulatory problems may easily burn because they do not feel hot temperatures.
- After soaking, apply lotion to the feet. Because the lotion can cause slippery feet, help the person put on non skid footwear before you transfer the person or let the person walk.

CHANGING CLOTHING AND HOSPITAL GOWNS

- Garments are changed after the bath and whenever wet or soiled.
- When changing clothing:
  - Provide for privacy.
  - Encourage the person to do as much as possible.
  - Let the person choose what to wear. Make sure the right undergarments are chosen.
  - Remove clothing from the strong or "good" (unaffected) side first.
  - Put clothing on the weak (affected) side first.
  - Support the arm or leg when removing or putting on a garment.

CHAPTER 19 REVIEW QUESTIONS

Circle the BEST answer.

1. Hair care, shaving, and nail and foot care prevent infection and promote comfort.
   a. True
   b. False

2. If a person's hair is matted, you may cut the hair.
   a. True
   b. False

3. When giving hair care, place a towel across the person's back and shoulders to protect garments from falling hair.
   a. True
   b. False

4. You should wear gloves when shampooing a person who has scalp sores.
   a. True
   b. False

5. A person takes an anticoagulant. Therefore, he shaves with a blade razor.
   a. True
   b. False

6. Never trim a mustache or beard without the person's consent.
   a. True
   b. False

7. Mustaches and beards need daily care.
   a. True
   b. False

8. A person has diabetes. You can cut his or her toenails.
   a. True
   b. False

9. Fingernails are cut with
   a. Scissors
   b. Nail clippers
   c. An emery board
   d. A nail file

10. Which statement is *false?*
    a. Provide privacy when a person is changing clothes.
    b. Most residents wear street clothes during the day.
    c. Let the person choose what to wear.
    d. You may tear a person's clothing.

Answers to these questions are on p. 479.

CHAPTER 20 NUTRITION AND FLUIDS

- Food and water are necessary for life. A poor diet and poor eating habits:
  - Increase the risk for infection and acute and chronic diseases
  - Cause healing problems
  - Affect physical and mental function, increasing the risk for accidents and injuries

BASIC NUTRITION

- Nutrition is the process involved in the ingestion, digestion, absorption, and use of foods and fluids by the body. Good nutrition is needed for growth, healing, and body functions.
- Food and fluid contain nutrients. A *nutrient* is a substance that is ingested, digested, absorbed, and used by the body.

Nutrients

- A well-balanced diet ensures an adequate intake of essential nutrients.
- *Protein*—is needed for tissue growth and repair. Sources include meat, fish, poultry, eggs, milk and milk products, cereals, beans, peas, and nuts.
- *Carbohydrates*—provide energy and fiber for bowel elimination. They are found in fruits, vegetables, breads, cereals, and sugar.
- *Fats*—provide energy, add flavor to food, and help the body use certain vitamins. Sources include meats, lard, butter, shortening, oils, milk, cheese, egg yolks, and nuts.
- *Vitamins*—are needed for certain body functions. The body stores vitamins A, D, E, and K. Vitamin C and the B complex vitamins must be ingested daily.
- *Minerals*—are needed for bone and tooth formation, nerve and muscle function, fluid balance, and other body processes.
- *Water*—is needed for all body processes.

FACTORS AFFECTING EATING AND NUTRITION

- *Culture and religion.* Culture influences dietary practices, food choices, and food preparation. Selecting, preparing, and eating food often involve religious practices. A person may follow all, some, or none of the dietary practices of his or her faith.

441

- *Finances.* People with limited incomes may buy cheaper food. Diets may lack protein and certain vitamins and minerals.
- *Appetite.* Illness, medications, anxiety, pain, and depression can cause loss of appetite. Unpleasant sights, thoughts, and smells are other causes.
- *Personal choice.* Food likes and dislikes are influenced by foods served in the home. Usually, food likes expand with age and social experiences.
- *Body reactions, allergies and illness.* People usually avoid foods that cause allergic reactions. They also avoid foods that cause nausea, vomiting, diarrhea, indigestion, gas, or headaches. Appetite usually decreases during illness and recovery from injuries. However, nutritional needs are increased.
- *Chewing and swallowing problems.* Mouth, teeth, and gum problems can affect chewing. Foods with soft bulk may be ordered for those with chewing problems. Many health problems can affect swallowing and a dysphagia diet may be required.
- *Disability.* Disease or injury can affect the hands, wrists, and arms. Assist devices let the person eat independently.
- *Age.* Taste and smell dull, appetite decreases, and secretion of digestive juices decreases. Avoid foods that are hard to digest.

OBRA DIETARY REQUIREMENTS

- OBRA has requirements for food served in nursing centers:
  - Each person's nutritional and dietary needs are met.
  - The person's diet is well-balanced. It is nourishing and tastes good. Food is well-seasoned.
  - Food is appetizing. It has an appealing aroma and is attractive.
  - Hot food is served hot. Cold food is served cold.
  - Food is served promptly.
  - Food is prepared to meet each person's needs. Some people need food cut, ground, or chopped. Others have special diets ordered by the doctor.
  - Other foods are offered if the person refused the food served. Substituted food must have a similar nutritional value to the first foods served.
  - Each person receives at least three meals a day. A bedtime snack is offered.
  - The center provides needed adaptive equipment and utensils.

SPECIAL DIETS

The Sodium-Controlled Diet

- A sodium-controlled diet decreases the amount of sodium in the body. The diet involves:
  - Omitting high-sodium foods. Review Box 20.4, High-Sodium Foods, in the textbook.
  - Not adding salt when eating.
  - Limiting the amount of salt used in cooking.

Diabetes Meal Planning

- Diabetes meal planning is for people with diabetes. It involves the person's food preferences and calories needed. It also involves eating meals and snacks at regular times.
- Serve the person's meals and snacks on time to maintain a certain blood sugar level.
- Always check what was eaten. Tell the nurse what the person did and did not eat. If not all the food was eaten, between-meal nourishment is needed. The nurse tells you what to give. Tell the nurse about changes in the person's eating habits.

The Dysphagia Diet

- Dysphagia means difficulty swallowing. Food thickness is changed to meet the person's needs. Review Box 20.5, Dysphagia Diet, in the textbook.
- You may need to feed a person with dysphagia. To promote the person's comfort:
  - Know the signs and symptoms of dysphagia. Review Box 20.6 in the textbook.
  - Feed the person according to the care plan.
  - Follow aspiration precautions. Review Box 20.7 in the textbook.
  - Report changes in how the person eats.
  - Report choking, coughing, or difficulty breathing during or after meals. Also report abnormal breathing or respiratory sounds. Report these observations at once.

FLUID BALANCE

- Fluid balance is needed for health. The amount of fluid taken in (input) and the amount of fluid lost (output) must be equal. If fluid intake exceeds fluid output, body tissues swell with water (edema).
- Dehydration is a decrease in the amount of water in body tissues. Fluid output exceeds intake. Common causes are poor fluid intake, vomiting, diarrhea, bleeding, excess sweating, and increased urine production.

Normal Fluid Requirements

- An adult needs 1500 mL of water daily to survive. About 2000–2500 mL of fluid per day is needed for normal fluid balance. Water requirements increase with hot weather, exercise, fever, illness, and excess fluid loss.
- Older persons may have a decreased sense of thirst. Their bodies need water, but they may not feel thirsty. Offer fluids according to the care plan.

Special Fluid Orders

- The doctor may order the amount of fluid a person can have in 24 hours. Intake and output (I&O) records are kept.
- *Encourage fluids.* The person drinks an increased amount of fluid.

- *Restrict fluids.* Fluids are limited to a certain amount.
- *Nothing by mouth (NPO).* The person cannot eat or drink.
- *Thickened liquids.* All liquids are thickened, including water.

INTAKE AND OUTPUT

- All fluids taken by mouth are measured and recorded—water, milk, and so forth. So are foods that melt at room temperature—ice cream, sherbet, pudding, gelatin, and Popsicles.
- Output includes urine, vomitus, diarrhea, and wound drainage.

Measuring Intake and Output

- To measure intake and output, you need to know:
  - 1 ounce (oz) equals 30 mL
  - A pint is about 500 mL
  - A quart is about 1000 mL
  - The serving sizes of bowls, dishes, cups, pitchers, glasses, and other containers
- An I&O record is kept at the bedside. Record I&O measurements in the correct column. Amounts are totaled at the end of the shift. The totals are recorded in the person's chart.
- The urinal, commode, bedpan, or specimen pan is used for voiding. Remind the person not to void in the toilet. Also remind the person not to put toilet tissue into the receptacle.

MEETING FOOD AND FLUID NEEDS

Preparing for Meals

- Preparing residents for meals promotes their comfort:
  - Assist with elimination needs.
  - Provide oral hygiene. Make sure dentures are in place.
  - Make sure eyeglasses and hearing aids are in place.
  - Make sure incontinent persons are clean and dry.
  - Position the person in a comfortable position.
  - Assist with hand washing.

Serving Meals

- Food is served in containers that keep foods at the correct temperature. Hot food is kept hot. Cold food is kept cold.
- Prompt serving keeps food at the correct temperature.

Feeding the Person

- Serve food and fluid in the order the person prefers. Offer fluids during the meal.
- Use teaspoons to feed the person.
- Persons who need to be fed are often angry, humiliated, and embarrassed. Some are depressed or refuse to eat. Let them do as much as possible. If strong

enough, let them hold milk or juice glasses. Never let them hold hot drinks.
- Tell the visually impaired person what is on the tray. Describe what you are offering. For persons who feed themselves, use the numbers on the clock for the location of foods.
- Many people pray before eating. Allow time and privacy for prayer.
- Meals provide social contact with others. Engage the person in pleasant conversations. Also, sit facing the person.
- Report and record:
  - The amount and kind of food eaten
  - Complaints of nausea or dysphagia
  - Signs and symptoms of dysphagia
  - Signs and symptoms of aspiration
- The person will eat better if not rushed.
- Wipe the person's hands, face, and mouth as needed during the meal.

Between-Meal Snacks

- Many special diets involve between-meal snacks. These snacks are served upon arrival on the nursing unit. Follow the same considerations and procedures for serving meal trays and feeding persons.

Calorie Counts

- Calorie records are kept for some people. On a flow sheet, note what the person ate and how much. A nurse or dietitian converts these portions into calories.

Providing Drinking Water

- Patients and residents need fresh drinking water. Follow the agency's procedure for providing fresh water.
- Water glasses and pitchers can spread microbes. To prevent the spread of microbes:
  - Label the water pitcher with the person's name and room and bed numbers.
  - Do not touch the rim or inside of the water glass, cup, or pitcher.
  - Do not let the ice scoop touch the rim or inside of the water glass, cup, or pitcher.
  - Place the ice scoop in the holder or on a towel, not in the ice container or dispenser.
  - Make sure the person's water pitcher and cup are clean and free of cracks and chips.

CHAPTER 20 REVIEW QUESTIONS

Circle the BEST answer.

1. A person is on a sodium-controlled diet. Which statement is *true?*
   - a. High-sodium foods are allowed.
   - b. Salt is added at the table.
   - c. Pretzels and potato chips are a good snack.
   - d. The amount of salt used in cooking is limited.

2. A person is a diabetic. You should do all of the following *except*
   a. Serve his meals and snacks late
   b. Always check his tray to see what he ate
   c. Tell the nurse what he ate and did not eat
   d. Provide a between-meal snack as the nurse directs

3. A person has dysphagia. You should do all of the following *except*
   a. Report choking and coughing during a meal at once
   b. Report difficulty in breathing during a meal at the end of the shift
   c. Report changes in how the person eats
   d. Follow aspiration precautions

4. Older persons have a decreased sense of thirst.
   a. True
   b. False

5. When feeding a person, you do all of the following *except*
   a. Use a teaspoon to feed the person
   b. Offer fluids during the meal
   c. Let the person do as much as possible
   d. Stand so you can feed two people at once

6. A person is visually impaired. You do all of the following *except*
   a. Tell the person what is on the tray
   b. Use the numbers on a clock to tell the person the location of food
   c. If feeding the person, describe what you are offering
   d. Let the person guess what is served

7. A person is on intake and output. He just ate ice cream. This is recorded as intake.
   a. True
   b. False

8. A person drank a pint of milk at lunch. You know he drank
   a. 250 mL of milk
   b. 350 mL of milk
   c. 500 mL of milk
   d. 750 mL of milk

9. The soup bowl holds 6 ounces. A person ate all of the soup. You record his intake as
   a. 50 mL
   b. 120 mL
   c. 180 mL
   d. 200 mL

Answers to these questions are on p. 479.

NORMAL URINATION

- Healthy adults produce about 1500 mL of urine a day.
- The frequency of urination is affected by amount of fluid intake, habits, availability of toilet facilities, activity, work, and illness. People usually void at bedtime, after sleep, and before meals. Some people void every 2–3 hours. The need to void at night disturbs sleep. Review Box 22.1, Rules for Normal Urination, in the textbook.
- Observe urine for color, clarity, odor, amount, and particles. Normal urine is pale yellow, straw-colored, or amber. It is clear with no particles. A faint odor is normal.
- Some foods and medications affect urine color. Ask the nurse to observe urine that looks or smells abnormal.
- Report the following urinary problems:
  - Dysuria—painful or difficult urination
  - Hematuria—blood in the urine
  - Nocturia—frequent urination at night
  - Oliguria—scant amount of urine; less than 500 mL in 24 hours
  - Polyuria—abnormally large amounts of urine
  - Urinary frequency—voiding at frequent intervals
  - Urinary incontinence—the involuntary loss or leakage of urine
  - Urinary urgency—the need to void at once

Bedpans

- Follow Standard Precautions and the Bloodborne Pathogen Standard when handling bedpans, urinals, commodes, and their contents.
- Thoroughly clean and disinfect bedpans, urinals, and commodes after use.

Urinals

- Some men need support when standing to use the urinal.
- You may have to place and hold the urinal for some men.
- Remind men to hang urinals on bed rails and to signal after using them.

URINARY INCONTINENCE

- Urinary incontinence is the involuntary loss or leakage of urine.
- If urinary incontinence is a new problem, tell the nurse at once.
- Incontinence is embarrassing. Garments are wet, and odors develop. Skin irritation, infection, and pressure injuries are risks. The person's pride, dignity, and self-esteem are affected. Social isolation, loss of independence, and depression are common.

- Good skin care and dry garments and linens are essential. Promoting normal urinary elimination prevents incontinence in some people. Other people may need bladder training.
- Review Box 22.2, Nursing Measures for Person with Urinary Incontinence, in the textbook.
- Caring for persons with incontinence is stressful. Remember, the person does not choose to be incontinent. If you find yourself short-tempered and impatient, talk to the nurse at once. Kindness, empathy, understanding, and patience are needed.

CATHETERS

- A straight catheter drains the bladder and then is removed.
- An indwelling catheter (retention or Foley catheter) is left in the bladder and drains urine constantly into a drainage bag.
- The catheter must not pull at the insertion site. Hold the catheter securely during catheter care. Then properly secure the catheter. Also make sure the tubing is not under the person. Besides obstructing urine flow, lying on the tubing is uncomfortable. It can also cause skin breakdown.
- Follow Standard Precautions and the Bloodborne Pathogen Standard. Review Box 22.3, Caring for Persons With Indwelling Catheters, in the textbook.
- Report and record:
  - Complaints of pain, burning, irritation, or the need to void
  - The color, clarity, odor of urine, or particles in the urine
  - Urine leaking at the insertion site

Drainage Systems

- A closed drainage system is used for indwelling catheters. The drainage bag hangs from the bed frame, chair, or wheelchair. It must not touch the floor. The bag is always kept lower than the person's bladder. Do not hang the drainage bag on a bed rail.
- If the drainage system is disconnected accidentally, tell the nurse at once. Do not touch the ends of the catheter or tubing. Do the following:
  - Practice hand hygiene. Put on gloves.
  - Wipe the end of the tube with an antiseptic wipe.
  - Wipe the end of the catheter with another antiseptic wipe.
  - Do not put the ends down. Do not touch the ends after you clean them.
  - Connect the tubing to the catheter.
  - Discard the wipes into a biohazard bag.
  - Remove the gloves. Practice hand hygiene.
- Check with the nurse and care plan about when to empty and measure the urine in the drainage bag. Follow Standard Precautions and the Bloodborne Pathogen Standard.

- A leg bag is a drainage system that attaches to the thigh or calf. Empty and measure a leg bag when it is half full.
- Report and record:
  - The amount of urine measured
  - The color, clarity, and odor of urine
  - Particles or blood in the urine or cloudy urine
  - Complaints of pain, burning, irritation, or the need to urinate
  - Drainage system leaks

Condom Catheters

- Condom catheters are often used for incontinent men. They are also called external catheters, Texas catheters, and urinary sheaths.
- These catheters are changed daily after perineal care.
- To apply a condom catheter, follow the manufacturer's instructions. Thoroughly wash and dry the penis before applying the catheter.
- Some condom catheters are self-adhering. Other catheters are secured in place with elastic tape in a spiral manner. Never use adhesive tape to secure catheters. It does not expand. Blood flow to the penis is cut off, injuring the penis.
- When removing or applying a condom catheter, report and record the following observations to the nurse at once.
  - Reddened or open areas on the penis
  - Swelling of the penis
  - Color, clarity, and odor of urine
  - Particles in the urine
  - Blood in the urine
  - Cloudy urine

BLADDER TRAINING

- Bladder training helps some persons with urinary incontinence. Control of urination is the goal. Bladder control promotes comfort and quality of life. It also increases self-esteem. You assist with bladder training as directed by the nurse and the care plan.

CHAPTER 22 REVIEW QUESTIONS

Circle the BEST answer.
1. Which statement is false?
   a. Normal urine is yellow, straw-colored, or amber.
   b. Urine with a strong odor is normal.
   c. A person normally voids 1500 mL a day.
   d. Observe urine for color, clarity, odor, amount, and particles.

2. Which observation does not need to be reported to the nurse promptly?
   a. Complaints of urgency
   b. Burning on urination
   c. Painful or difficult urination
   d. Clear amber urine

445

3. Which statement is false?
   a. Incontinence is embarrassing.
   b. Caring for persons with incontinence may be stressful.
   c. Incontinence is a personal choice.
   d. Be kind and patient to persons who are incontinent.

4. A person with a catheter complains of pain. You should notify the nurse at once.
   a. True
   b. False

5. Which statement is false?
   a. The urinary drainage system should hang from the bed frame or chair.
   b. The urinary drainage system should hang on a bed rail.
   c. The urinary drainage system must be off the floor.
   d. The urine drainage system must be kept lower than the person's bladder.

6. Which statement is false?
   a. Condom catheters are changed daily.
   b. Follow the manufacturer's instructions when applying a condom catheter.
   c. Use adhesive tape to secure a condom catheter in place.
   d. Report and record open or reddened areas on the penis at once.

7. The goal of bladder training is to
   a. Allow the person to use the toilet
   b. Keep the catheter
   c. Gain control of urination
   d. Decrease self-esteem

Answers to these questions are on p. 479.

CHAPTER 23 BOWEL ELIMINATION

NORMAL BOWEL ELIMINATION

Observations

- Stools are normally brown, soft, formed, moist, and shaped like the rectum. They have a normal odor caused by bacterial action in the intestines. Certain food and medications cause odors.
- Carefully observe stools before disposing of them. Observe and report the color, amount, consistency, odor, and shape of stools. Also, observe and report the presence of blood or mucus, frequency of defecation, and any complaints of pain or discomfort.

FACTORS AFFECTING BOWEL ELIMINATION

- *Privacy.* Bowel elimination is a private act.
- *Habits.* Many people have a bowel movement after breakfast. Defecation is easier when a person is relaxed.
- *Diet—high-fiber foods.* Fiber helps prevent constipation.

- *Diet—other foods.* Some foods cause constipation. Other foods cause frequent stools or diarrhea.
- *Fluids.* Drinking 6–8 glasses of water daily promotes normal bowel elimination. Warm fluids—coffee, tea, hot cider, warm water—increase peristalsis.
- *Activity.* Exercise and activity maintain muscle tone and stimulate peristalsis.
- *Medications.* Medications can prevent constipation or control diarrhea. Some have diarrhea or constipation as side effects.
- *Disability.* Some people cannot control bowel movements. A bowel training program is needed.
- *Aging.* Older persons are at risk for constipation. Some older persons lose bowel control and have fecal incontinence.
- To provide comfort and safety during bowel elimination, review Box 23.1, Safety and Comfort During Bowel Elimination, in the textbook. Follow Standard Precautions and the Bloodborne Pathogen Standard.

COMMON PROBLEMS

- Common problems include constipation, fecal impaction, diarrhea, fecal incontinence, and flatulence.

Constipation

- Constipation is the passage of a hard, dry stool.
- Common causes of constipation are a low fiber diet and ignoring the urge to defecate. Other causes include decreased fluid intake, inactivity, medications, aging, and certain diseases.
- Dietary changes, fluids, and activity prevent or relieve constipation. Medications and enemas also help relieve constipation.

Fecal Impaction

- A fecal impaction is the prolonged retention and buildup of feces in the rectum.
- Fecal impaction results if constipation is not relieved. The person cannot defecate. Liquid feces pass around the hardened fecal mass in the rectum. The liquid feces seep from the anus.
- Abdominal discomfort, abdominal distention, nausea, cramping, and rectal pain are common. Older persons have poor appetite or confusion. Some persons have a fever. Report these signs and symptoms to the nurse.

Diarrhea

- Diarrhea is the frequent passage of liquid stools.
- The need to have a bowel movement is urgent. Some people cannot get to a bathroom in time. Abdominal cramping, nausea, and vomiting may occur.
- Assist with elimination needs promptly, dispose of stools promptly, and give good skin care. Liquid stools irritate the skin as does frequent wiping with toilet paper. Skin breakdown and pressure injuries are risks.

- Follow Standard Precautions and the Bloodborne Pathogen Standard when in contact with stools.
- Report signs of diarrhea at once. Ask the nurse to observe the stool.

Fecal Incontinence

- Fecal incontinence is the inability to control the passage of feces and gas through the anus.
- Fecal incontinence affects the person emotionally. Frustration, embarrassment, anger, and humiliation are common. The person may need:
  - Bowel training
  - Help with elimination after meals and every 2–3 hours
  - Incontinence products to keep garments and linens clean
  - Good skin care

Flatulence

- Flatulence is the excessive formation of gas or air in the stomach and intestines.
- Causes include swallowing air while eating and drinking and bacterial action in the intestines. Other causes may be gas-forming foods, constipation, bowel and abdominal surgeries, and medications that decrease peristalsis.
- If flatus is not expelled, the intestines distend (swell or enlarge from the pressure of gases). Abdominal cramping or pain, shortness of breath, and a swollen abdomen occur. "Bloating" is a common complaint. Exercise, walking, moving in bed, and the left side-lying position often produce flatus. Enemas and medications may be ordered.

BOWEL TRAINING

- Bowel training has two goals:
  - To gain control of bowel movements.
  - To develop a regular pattern of elimination. Fecal impactions, constipation, and fecal incontinence are prevented.
  - Factors that promote elimination are part of the care plan and bowel training program.

ENEMAS

- An enema is the introduction of fluid into the rectum and lower colon.
- Doctors order enemas:
  - To remove feces
  - To relieve constipation, fecal impaction, or flatulence
  - To clean the bowel of feces before certain surgeries and diagnostic procedures
- Review Box 23.2, Safety and Comfort Measures for Giving Enemas, in the textbook.

The Person with an Ostomy

- Sometimes part of the intestines is removed surgically. An ostomy is sometimes necessary. An ostomy is a surgically-created opening. The opening is called a stoma. The person wears a pouch over the stoma to collect stools and flatus.
- Stools irritate the skin. Skin care prevents skin breakdown around the stoma. It prevents stools from having contact with the skin. The skin barrier is part of the pouch or a separate device.
- The pouch has an adhesive backing that is applied to the skin. Some pouches are secured to ostomy belts.
- The pouch is changed every 3–7 days and when it leaks. Frequent pouch changes can damage the skin.
- Many pouches have a drain at the bottom that closes with a clip, clamp, or wire closure. The drain is opened to empty the pouch. The drain is wiped with toilet tissue before it is closed.

CHAPTER 23 REVIEW QUESTIONS

Circle the BEST answer.
1. Which statement is *false*?
   a. Lack of privacy can prevent defecation.
   b. Low-fiber foods promote defecation.
   c. Drinking 6–8 glasses of water daily promotes normal bowel elimination.
   d. Exercise stimulates peristalsis.

2. Which of the following does *not* prevent constipation?
   a. A high-fiber diet
   b. Increased fluid intake
   c. Exercise
   d. Ignoring the urge to defecate

3. A person has fecal incontinence. You should do all of the following *except*
   a. Be patient
   b. Help with elimination after meals
   c. Provide good skin care
   d. Scold the person for being incontinent

4. The preferred position for an enema is the
   a. Left side-lying position
   b. Prone position
   c. Supine position
   d. Trendelenburg's position

Answers to these questions are on p. 479.

CHAPTER 24 EXERCISE AND ACTIVITY

BEDREST

- The doctor may order bedrest to treat a health problem.

Complications of Bedrest

- Pressure injuries, constipation, and fecal impactions can result. Urinary tract infections and renal calculi (kidney stones) can occur. So can blood clots and pneumonia.

447

- The musculoskeletal system is affected by lack of exercise and activity. These complications must be prevented to maintain normal movement:
  - A contracture is the lack of joint mobility caused by abnormal shortening of a muscle. Common sites are the fingers, wrists, elbows, toes, ankles, knees, and hips. The person is permanently deformed and disabled.
  - Atrophy is the decrease in size or the wasting away of tissue. Tissues shrink in size.
- Orthostatic hypotension (postural hypotension) is abnormally low blood pressure when the person suddenly stands up. The person is dizzy and weak and has spots before the eyes. Fainting can occur. To prevent orthostatic hypotension, have the person change slowly from a lying or sitting position to a standing position.

Positioning
- Supportive devices are often used to support and maintain the person in a certain position:
  - *Bedboards*—are placed under the mattress to prevent the mattress from sagging.
  - *Footboards*—are placed at the foot of mattresses to prevent plantar flexion that can lead to footdrop.
  - *Trochanter rolls*—prevent the hips and legs from turning outward (external rotation).
  - *Hip abduction wedges*—keep the hips abducted.
  - *Hand rolls or hand grips*—prevent contractures of the thumb, fingers, and wrist.
  - *Splints*—keep the elbows, wrists, thumbs, fingers, ankles, and knees in normal position.
  - *Bed cradles*—keep the weight of top linens off the feet and toes.

RANGE OF MOTION EXERCISES
- Range of motion (ROM) exercises involve moving the joints through their complete range of motion. They are usually done at least two times a day.
- *Active ROM*—exercises are done by the person.
- *Passive ROM*—someone moves the joints through their range of motion.
- *Active-assistive ROM*—the person does the exercises with some help.
- Review Box 24.2, Joint Movements, in the textbook.
- Range of motion exercises can cause injury if not done properly. Practice these rules:
  - Exercise only the joints the nurse tells you to exercise.
  - Expose only the body part being exercised.
  - Use good body mechanics.
  - Support the part being exercised.
  - Move the joint slowly, smoothly, and gently.
  - Do not force a joint beyond its present range of motion.
  - Do not force a joint to the point of pain.

- Ask the person if he or she has pain or discomfort.
- Perform ROM exercises to the neck only if allowed by center policy.

AMBULATION
- Ambulation is the act of walking.
- Follow the care plan when helping a person walk. Use a gait (transfer) belt if the person is weak or unsteady. The person uses handrails along the wall. Always check the person for orthostatic hypotension.
- When you help the person walk, walk to the side and slightly behind the person on the person's weak side. Encourage the person to use the handrail on his or her strong side.

Walking Aids
- A cane is held on the strong side of the body. The cane tip is about 6–10 inches to the side of the foot. It is about 6–10 inches in front of the foot on the strong side. The grip is level with the hip. To walk:
  - Step A: The cane is moved forward 6–10 inches.
  - Step B: The weak leg (opposite the cane) is moved forward even with the cane.
  - Step C: The strong leg is moved forward and ahead of the cane and the weak leg.
- A walker gives more support than a cane. Wheeled walkers are common. They have wheels on the front legs and rubber tips on the back legs. The person pushes a wheeled walker about 6–8 inches in front of his or her feet.
- Braces support weak body parts, prevent or correct deformities, or prevent joint movement. A brace is applied over the ankle, knee, or back. Skin and bony points under braces are kept clean and dry. Report redness or signs of skin breakdown at once. Also report complaints of pain or discomfort.

CHAPTER 24 REVIEW QUESTIONS

Circle the BEST answer.

1. To prevent orthostatic hypotension, you should
   a. Move a person from the lying position to the sitting position quickly
   b. Move a person from the sitting position to the standing position quickly
   c. Move a person from the lying or sitting position to a standing position slowly
   d. Keep the person in bed

2. Exercise helps prevent contractures and muscle atrophy.
   a. True
   b. False

3. When performing ROM exercises, you should force a joint to the point of pain.
   a. True
   b. False

4. A person's left leg is weaker than his right. The person holds the cane on his right side.
    a. True
    b. False

Answers to these questions are on p. 479.

CHAPTER 25 COMFORT, REST, AND SLEEP

- Comfort is a state of well-being. Many factors affect comfort.

PAIN

- Pain or discomfort means to ache, hurt, or be sore. Pain, comfort, or discomfort is subjective. You cannot see, hear, touch, or smell pain or discomfort. You must rely on what the person says.
- Report the person's complaints of pain and your observations to the nurse.
- Review Box 25.3, Nursing Measures to Promote Comfort and Relieve Pain, in the textbook.

Factors Affecting Pain

- *Past experience.* The severity of pain, its cause, how long it lasted, and if relief occurred all affect the person's current response to pain.
- *Anxiety.* Pain and anxiety are related. Pain can cause anxiety. Anxiety increases how much pain the person feels. Reducing anxiety helps lessen pain.
- *Rest and sleep.* Pain seems worse when a person is tired or restless.
- *Attention.* The more a person thinks about pain, the worse it seems.
- *Personal and family duties.* Often pain is ignored when there are children to care for. Some deny pain if a serious illness is feared.
- *The value or meaning of pain.* To some people, pain is a weakness. For some persons, pain means avoiding daily routines and people.
- *Support from others.* Dealing with pain is often easier when family and friends offer comfort and support. Just being nearby helps. Facing pain alone is hard for persons.
- *Culture.* Culture affects pain responses. Non–English-speaking persons may have problems describing pain.
- *Illness.* Some diseases cause decreased pain sensations.
- *Age.* Older persons may have decreased pain sensations. They may not feel pain, or it may not feel severe. The person is at risk for undetected disease or injury. Chronic pain may mask new pain.
- *Persons with dementia.* Persons with dementia may not be able to complain of pain. Changes in usual behavior may signal pain. Loss of appetite also signals pain. Report any changes in a person's usual behavior to the nurse.

Signs and Symptoms

- You cannot see, hear, touch, or smell the person's pain. Rely on what the person tells you. Promptly report any information you collect about pain. Use the person's exact words when reporting and recording pain. The nurse needs the following information:
  - *Location.* Where is the pain?
  - *Onset and duration.* When did the pain start? How long has it lasted?
  - *Intensity.* Ask the person to rate the pain. Use a pain scale.
  - *Description.* Ask the person to describe the pain.
  - *Factors causing pain.* Ask when the pain started and what the person was doing.
  - *Factors affecting pain.* Ask what makes the pain better and what makes it worse.
  - *Vital signs.* Increases often occur with acute pain. They may be normal with chronic pain.
  - *Other signs and symptoms.* Dizziness, nausea, vomiting, weakness, numbness, and tingling.
- Review Box 25.2, Signs and Symptoms of Pain, in the textbook.

PROMOTING SLEEP

- Sleep is a basic need. Tissue healing and repair occur during sleep. Sleep lowers stress, tension, and anxiety. It refreshes and renews the person. The person regains energy and mental alertness. The person thinks and functions better after sleep.

Factors Affecting Sleep

- *Illness.* Illness increases the need for sleep.
- *Nutrition.* Sleep needs increase with weight gain. Foods with caffeine prevent sleep.
- *Exercise.* People tire after exercise. Being tired helps people sleep well. Exercise before bedtime interferes with sleep. Exercise is avoided 2 hours before bedtime.
- *Environment.* People adjust to their usual sleep settings.
- *Medications and other substances.* Sleeping pills promote sleep. Medications for anxiety, depression, and pain may cause the person to sleep.
- *Emotional problems.* Fear, worry, depression, and anxiety affect sleep.

Sleep Disorders

- Insomnia is a chronic condition in which the person cannot sleep or stay asleep all night.
- Sleep deprivation means that the amount and quality of sleep are decreased. Sleep is interrupted.
- Sleepwalking is when the person leaves the bed and walks about. If a person is sleepwalking, protect the person from injury. Guide sleepwalkers back to bed. They startle easily. Awaken them gently.
- Sleep apnea is when a person temporarily stops breathing for short periods during the night. Sleep apnea has

449

different causes. A doctor may order a continuous positive airway pressure (CPAP) mask for the person with sleep apnea.

Promoting Sleep

- The person chooses the measures that help promote sleep. Review Box 25.6, Nursing Measures to Promote Sleep, in the textbook for other measures.

CHAPTER 25 REVIEW QUESTIONS

Circle the BEST answer.

1. A person complains of pain. You will do all of the following *except*
   a. Ask where the pain is
   b. Ask when the pain started
   c. Ask what the intensity of the pain is on a scale of 1–10
   d. Ask what he or she is complaining about

2. Persons with dementia may not complain of pain. Which of the following might be a signal of pain for a person with dementia?
   a. Illness
   b. Mental alertness
   c. Loss of appetite
   d. Forgetfulness

3. You can promote rest for a person by doing all of the following *except*
   a. Ask the person if he or she would like coffee or tea
   b. Place the call light within reach
   c. Provide a quiet setting
   d. Follow the person's routines and rituals before rest

4. To promote sleep for a person, you should do all of the following *except*
   a. Follow the person's wishes
   b. Follow the care plan
   c. Follow the person's rituals and routines before bedtime
   d. Tell the person when to go to bed

Answers to these questions are on p. 479.

CHAPTER 26 OXYGEN NEEDS AND RESPIRATORY THERAPIES

ALTERED RESPIRATORY FUNCTION

- Hypoxia means that cells do not have enough oxygen.
- Restlessness, dizziness, and disorientation are signs of hypoxia.
- Review Box 26.1, Signs and Symptoms of Hypoxia, in the textbook. Report signs and symptoms of hypoxia to the nurse at once. Hypoxia is life-threatening.

Abnormal Respirations

- Adults normally have 12–20 respirations per minute. They are quiet, effortless, and regular. Both sides of the chest rise and fall equally. Report these observations at once:
  - *Tachypnea*—rapid breathing. Respirations are 20 or more per minute.
  - *Bradypnea*—slow breathing. Respirations are fewer than 12 per minute.
  - *Apnea*—lack or absence of breathing.
  - *Hypoventilation*—respirations are slow, shallow, and sometimes irregular.
  - *Hyperventilation*—respirations are rapid and deeper than normal.
  - *Dyspnea*—difficult, labored, or painful breathing.
  - *Cheyne-Stokes respirations*—respirations gradually increase in rate and depth. Then they become shallow and slow. Breathing may stop for 10–20 seconds.
  - *Orthopnea*—breathing deeply and comfortably only when sitting.
  - *Biot respirations*—rapid and deep respirations followed by 10–30 seconds of apnea.
  - *Kussmaul respirations*—very deep and rapid respirations.

PROMOTING OXYGENATION

Positioning

- Breathing is usually easier in semi-Fowler and Fowler positions. Persons with difficulty breathing often prefer the orthopneic position (sitting up and leaning over a table to breathe).
- Positioning changes are needed every 2 hours to keep secretions from pooling.

Deep Breathing and Coughing

- Deep breathing moves air into most parts of the lungs. Coughing removes mucus. Deep breathing and coughing are usually done every 2 hours while the person is awake.

Incentive Spirometry

- With incentive spirometry, the person is encouraged to inhale until reaching a preset volume of air and holding the air for 3 seconds. Improved lung function is the goal.

ASSISTING WITH OXYGEN THERAPY

Oxygen Devices

- A nasal cannula allows eating and drinking. Tight prongs can irritate the nose. Pressure on the ears and cheekbones is possible.
- A simple face mask covers the nose and mouth. Talking and eating are hard to do with a mask. Listen carefully. Moisture can build up under the mask. Keep the face clean and dry. Masks are removed for eating. Usually oxygen is given by cannula during meals.

Oxygen Flow Rates

- When giving care and checking the person, always check the flow rate. Tell the nurse at once if it is too high or too low. A nurse or respiratory therapist will adjust the flow rate.

Oxygen Safety

- You do not give oxygen. You assist the nurse in providing safe care.
- Review Box 26.3, Safety Rules for Oxygen Therapy, in your textbook.

CHAPTER 26 REVIEW QUESTIONS

Circle the BEST answer.

1. Which statement is *false?*
   a. Restlessness, dizziness, and disorientation are signs of hypoxia.
   b. Hypoxia is life threatening.
   c. Report signs and symptoms of hypoxia at the end of the shift.
   d. Anything that affects respiratory function can cause hypoxia.

2. Adults normally have
   a. 8–10 respirations per minute
   b. 12–20 respirations per minute
   c. 10–12 respirations per minute
   d. 20–24 respirations per minute

3. Dyspnea is
   a. Difficult, labored, or painful breathing
   b. Slow breathing with fewer than 12 respirations per minute
   c. Rapid breathing with 24 or more respirations per minute
   d. Lack or absence of breathing

4. Which statement about positioning is *false?*
   a. Breathing is usually easier in semi-Fowler or Fowler position.
   b. Persons with difficulty breathing often prefer the orthopneic position.
   c. Position changes are needed at least every 4 hours.
   d. Follow the person's care plan for positioning preferences.

5. A person has a nasal cannula. Which statement is *false?*
   a. You will leave the nasal cannula on while the person is eating.
   b. You will watch the nose area for irritation.
   c. You will watch the ears and cheekbones for skin breakdown.
   d. You will take the nasal cannula off while the person is eating.

Answers to these questions are on p. 479.

VITAL SIGNS

- Accuracy is essential when you measure, record, and report vital signs. If unsure of your measurements, promptly ask the nurse to take them again.
- Report the following at once:
  - Any vital sign that is changed from a prior measurement
  - Vital signs above or below the normal range

BODY TEMPERATURE

- Thermometers are used to measure temperature. It is measured using the Fahrenheit (F) and centigrade or Celsius (C) scales.
- Temperature sites are the mouth, rectum, axilla (underarm), tympanic membrane (ear), and temporal artery (forehead).
- Review Box 27.1, Temperature Sites, in the textbook.
- Normal ranges for body temperatures vary by site:
  - Oral: 97.6 °F–99.6 °F
  - Rectal: 98.6 °F–100.6 °F
  - Axillary: 96.6 °F–98.6 °F
  - Tympanic membrane: 97.6 °F–99.6 °F
  - Temporal artery: 97.6 °F–99.6 °F
- Older persons have lower body temperatures than younger persons.

Electronic Thermometers

- Most electronic thermometers are designed to measure temperatures at the oral or axillary site.
- A separate thermometer or probe is used for rectal temperatures and the thermometer or probe is always color-coded red.
- Tympanic membrane thermometers are gently inserted into the ear. The temperature is measured in 1–3 seconds. These thermometers are not used if there is ear drainage.
- Temporal artery thermometers measure body temperature at the temporal artery in the forehead. These thermometers measure body temperature in 3–4 seconds. Follow the manufacturer's instructions for using, cleaning, and storing the device.
- Infrared thermometers are helpful because they use a noncontact method of measuring body temperature.

PULSE

Pulse Rate

- The pulse rate for adults (12 years and older) is between 60 and 100 beats per minute. Report these abnormal rates to the nurse at once:
  - *Tachycardia*—the heart rate is more than 100 beats per minute.

- *Bradycardia*—the heart rate is less than 60 beats per minute.

Rhythm and Force of the Pulse

- The rhythm of the pulse should be regular. Report and record an irregular pulse rhythm.
- Report and record if the pulse force is strong, full, bounding, weak, thready, or feeble.

Taking Pulses

- The radial pulse is used for routine vital signs. Do not use your thumb to take a pulse. Count the pulse for 30 seconds and multiply by 2 if center policy permits. If the pulse is irregular, count it for 1 minute. Report and record if the pulse is regular or irregular.
- The apical pulse is on the left side of the chest slightly below the nipple. Count the apical pulse for 1 minute.

RESPIRATIONS

- The healthy adult has 12–20 respirations per minute. Respirations are normally quiet, effortless, and regular. Both sides of the chest rise and fall equally.
- Count respirations when the person is at rest. Count respirations right after taking a pulse.
- Count respirations for 30 seconds and multiply the number by 2 if center policy permits. If an abnormal pattern is noted, count the respirations for 1 minute.
- Report and record:
  - The respiratory rate
  - Equality and depth of respirations
  - If the respirations were regular or irregular
  - If the person has pain or difficulty breathing
  - Any respiratory noises
  - An abnormal respiratory pattern

BLOOD PRESSURE

Normal and Abnormal Blood Pressures

- Blood pressure has normal ranges:
  - *Systolic pressure* (upper number)—less than 120 mm Hg
  - *Diastolic pressure* (lower number)—less than 80 mm Hg
- Hypertension—can be classified as elevated, stage 1, stage 2, or hypertensive crisis. Report any elevated blood pressure measurements to the nurse.
- Hypotension—when the systolic blood pressure is below 90 mm Hg and the diastolic pressure is below 60 mm Hg. Report a systolic pressure below 90 mm Hg. Also report a diastolic pressure below 60 mm Hg.
- Review Box 27.3, Guidelines for Measuring Blood Pressure, in your textbook.

CHAPTER 27 REVIEW QUESTIONS

Circle the BEST answer.

1. Which statement about taking a rectal temperature is *false?*
   a. The bulb end of the thermometer needs to be lubricated.
   b. The person is placed in the left side-lying position.
   c. Privacy is important.
   d. The normal range is 97.6 °F–99.6 °F.

2. Which pulse rate should you report at once?
   a. A pulse rate of 52 beats per minute
   b. A pulse rate of 60 beats per minute
   c. A pulse rate of 76 beats per minute
   d. A pulse rate of 100 beats per minute

3. Which statement is *false?*
   a. An irregular pulse is counted for 1 minute.
   b. You may use your thumb to take a radial pulse rate.
   c. The radial pulse is usually used to count a pulse rate.
   d. Tachycardia is a fast pulse rate.

4. Which blood pressure should you report?
   a. 119/70 mm Hg
   b. 88/62 mm Hg
   c. 110/70 mm Hg
   d. 92/68 mm Hg

Answers to these questions are on p. 479.

CHAPTER 31 WOUND CARE

- A wound is a break in the skin or mucous membrane.
- The wound is a portal of entry for microbes. Infection is a major threat. Wound care involves preventing infection and further injury to the wound and nearby tissues.

SKIN TEARS

- A skin tear is a break or rip in the outer layers of the skin.
- Skin tears are caused by friction, shearing, pulling, or pressure on the skin. Falls or bumping a hand, arm, or leg on any hard surface can cause a skin tear. Beds, bed rails, chairs, wheelchair footplates, and tables are dangers. So is holding the person's arm or leg too tight, removing tape or adhesives, pulling buttons or zippers across the skin, or jewelry hitting the skin.
- Skin tears are painful. They are portals of entry for microbes. Wound complications can develop. Tell the nurse at once if you cause or find a skin tear.
- Review Box 31.2, Measures to Prevent Skin Tears, in the textbook.

VASCULAR ULCERS

- *Vascular ulcers* are open sores on the lower legs or feet. They are caused by decreased blood flow through the arteries or veins.
- Review Box 31.3, Measures to Prevent Vascular Ulcers, in the textbook.
- *Venous ulcers (stasis ulcers)* are open sores on the lower legs or feet. They are caused by poor blood flow through the veins. The lower legs and inner aspect of the ankles are common sites for venous ulcers.
- *Arterial ulcers* are open wounds on the lower legs or feet caused by poor arterial blood flow. They are found between the toes, on top of the toes, and on the outer side of the ankle.
- A *diabetic foot ulcer* is an open wound on the foot caused by complications from diabetes. When nerves are affected, the person can lose sensation in a foot or leg. The person may not feel pain, heat, or cold. Therefore, the person may not feel a cut, blister, burn, or other trauma to the foot. Infection and a large sore can develop. When blood flow to the foot decreases, tissues and cells do not get needed oxygen and nutrients. A sore does not heal properly. Tissue death (gangrene) can occur.

Prevention and Treatment

- Check the person's feet and legs every day. Report any sign of a problem to the nurse at once. Follow the care plan to prevent and treat circulatory ulcers.

Compression Stockings

- Compression stockings also are called elastic, anti-embolism or anti-embolic (AE) stockings. They also are called TED hose.
- The person usually has two pairs of stockings. One pair is washed; the other pair is worn.
- Stockings should not have twists, creases, or wrinkles after you apply them.
- Stockings are applied before the person gets out of bed.

WARM AND COLD APPLICATIONS

Warm Applications

- Heat relieves pain, relaxes muscles, promotes healing, reduces tissue swelling, and decreases joint stiffness.

Complications

- High temperatures can cause burns. Report pain, excessive redness, and blisters at once. Also observe for pale skin.
- Metal implants pose risks. Pacemakers and joint replacements are made of metal. Do not apply heat to an implant area.

Cold Applications

- Cold applications reduce pain, prevent swelling, and decrease circulation and bleeding.

Complications

- Complications include pain, burns, blisters, and poor circulation. Burns and blisters occur from intense cold. They also occur when dry cold is in direct contact with the skin.

Applying Warm and Cold

- Protect the person from injury during warm and cold applications. Review Box 31.8, Rules for Applying Warm and Cold, in the textbook.

CHAPTER 31 REVIEW QUESTIONS

Circle the BEST answer.

1. All of the following can cause a skin tear *except*
   a. Friction and shearing
   b. Holding a person's arm or leg too tight
   c. Rings, watches, and bracelets
   d. Trimmed, short nails

2. A person is diabetic. Which statement is *false?*
   a. The person may not feel pain in her feet.
   b. The person may not feel heat or cold in her feet.
   c. You need to check her feet weekly for foot problems.
   d. The person is at risk for diabetic foot ulcers.

3. Which statement about elastic stockings is *false?*
   a. Compression stockings are also called anti-embolic stockings.
   b. Compression stockings should be wrinkle-free after being applied.
   c. A person usually has two pairs of compression stockings.
   d. Compression stockings are applied after a person gets out of bed.

4. Complications from a warm application include all of the following *except*
   a. Excessive redness
   b. Blisters
   c. Pale skin
   d. Cyanotic (bluish) nail beds

5. When applying warm or cold, you should do all of the following *except*
   a. Ask the nurse what the temperature of the application should be
   b. Cover dry warm or cold applications before applying them
   c. Observe the skin every 2 hours
   d. Know how long to leave the application in place

Answers to these questions are on p. 479.

453

CHAPTER 32 PRESSURE INJURIES

- A pressure injury is localized damage to the skin and/or underlying tissue. Pressure injuries usually occur over a bony prominence—the back of the head, shoulder blades, elbows, hips, spine, sacrum, knees, ankles, heels, and toes.
- *Decubitus ulcer, bed sore, pressure sore*, and *pressure ulcer* are other terms for pressure injury.
- A pressure injury is any lesion caused by unrelieved pressure. Shearing and friction are contributing factors to skin breakdown leading to pressure injuries. Risk factors include immobility, breaks in the skin, poor circulation to an area, moisture, dry skin, and irritation by urine and feces.

Persons at Risk

- Persons at risk for pressure injuries are those who:
  - Are confined to a bed or chair
  - Need some or total help in moving
  - Are agitated or have involuntary muscle movements
  - Have loss of bowel or bladder control
  - Are exposed to moisture
  - Have poor nutrition
  - Have poor fluid balance
  - Have lowered mental awareness
  - Have problems sensing pain or pressure
  - Have circulatory problems
  - Are older
  - Are obese or very thin
  - Refuse care

Pressure Injury Stages

- In persons with light skin, a reddened bony area is the first sign of a pressure injury. In persons with dark skin, a bony area may appear different from the surrounding area. The area may feel warm or cool. The person may complain of pain, burning, tingling, or itching in the area.
- Figure 31.4 in the textbook shows the stages of pressure injuries.
- Box 32.2 in the textbook describes pressure injuries.

Prevention and Treatment

- Preventing pressure injuries is much easier than trying to heal them. Review Box 32.3, Measures to Prevent Pressure Injuries, in the textbook.
- The person at risk for pressure injuries may be placed on a foam, air, alternating air, gel, or water mattress.
- Protective devices are often used to prevent and treat pressure injuries and skin breakdown. Protective devices include:
  - Bed cradle
  - Heel and elbow protectors
  - Heel and foot elevators
  - Gel or fluid-filled pads and cushions
  - Alternating air mattress overlays
  - Special beds
  - Other equipment—pillows, trochanter rolls, and footboards

CHAPTER 32 REVIEW QUESTIONS

Circle the BEST answer.

1. You may expect to find a pressure injury at all of the following sites *except*
   a. Back of the head
   b. Elbow
   c. Top of the thigh
   d. Toes

2. Which of the following is not a protective device used to prevent and treat pressure injuries?
   a. Heel elevator
   b. Bed cradle
   c. Drawsheet
   d. Elbow protector

3. Pressure injuries can occur on the ears.
   a. True
   b. False

4. Pressure injuries never occur over a bony prominence.
   a. True
   b. False

Answers to these questions are on p. 480.

CHAPTER 33 HEARING, SPEECH, AND VISION PROBLEMS

HEARING LOSS

- Hearing loss is not being able to hear the range of sounds associated with normal hearing. Deafness is the most severe form of hearing loss.
- Obvious signs and symptoms of hearing loss include:
  - Speaking too loudly
  - Leaning forward to hear
  - Turning and cupping the better ear toward the speaker
  - Answering questions or responding inappropriately
  - Asking for words to be repeated
  - Asking others to speak louder or to speak more slowly and clearly
  - Having trouble hearing over the phone
  - Finding it hard to follow conversations when two or more people are talking
  - Turning up the TV, radio, or music volume so loud that others complain
  - Thinking that others are mumbling or slurring words
  - Having trouble understanding women and children
- Persons with hearing loss may wear hearing aids or lip-read (speech-read). They watch facial expressions, gestures, and body language. Some people learn American Sign Language (ASL). Others may have hearing assistance dogs.

- Review Box 33.1, Measures to Promote Hearing, in the textbook.
- Hearing aids are battery-operated. If they do not seem to work properly:
  - Check if the hearing aid is on. It has an on and off switch.
  - Check the battery position.
  - Insert a new battery if needed.
  - Clean the hearing aid. Follow the nurse's direction and the manufacturer's instructions.
- Hearing aids are turned off when not in use. The battery is removed.
- Handle and care for hearing aids properly. If lost or damaged, report it to the nurse at once.

SPEECH DISORDERS

- *Aphasia.* Aphasia is the total or partial loss of the ability to use or understand language. It results from damage to parts of the brain responsible for language. Stroke, head injury, brain infarctions and cancer are common causes. *Expressive aphasia* relates to difficulty expressing or sending out thoughts. Thinking is clear, but the person has difficulty or cannot speak the words.
- *Apraxia.* The person with apraxia of speech cannot use the speech muscles to produce understandable speech. The person understands speech and knows what to say. However, the brain cannot coordinate the speech muscles to form words. Apraxia is caused by damage to the motor speech area of the brain.
- *Dysarthria.* Difficult or poor speech caused by damage to the nervous system. Mouth and face muscles are affected. Slurred speech, hoarseness, or drooling are problems that can occur.

EYE DISORDERS

- *Glaucoma.* Glaucoma results when fluid builds up in the eye and causes pressure on the optic nerve. The optic nerve is damaged. Vision loss with eventual blindness occurs. Medications and surgery can control glaucoma and prevent further damage to the optic nerve. Prior damage cannot be reversed.
- *Cataract.* Cataract is a clouding of the lens in the eye. Signs and symptoms include cloudy, blurry, or dimmed vision. Persons may also be sensitive to light and glares or see halos around lights. Poor vision at night and double vision in one eye are other symptoms. Surgery is the only treatment. Review the list of post operative care measures on p. 480 in the textbook.
- *Age-related macular degeneration (AMD).* AMD is blurring of central vision. Onset is gradual and painless. AMD is the leading cause of blindness in persons 60 years and older. Risk factors include cardiovascular disease, smoking, and obesity. Treatment, such as laser surgery, may slow or stop the progression of the disease.

Impaired Vision and Blindness

- Birth defects, accidents, and eye diseases are among the many causes of impaired vision and blindness. Impaired vision and blindness are also complications of some diseases.
- Review Box 33.4, Caring for Blind and Visually Impaired Persons, in the textbook.

Corrective Lenses

- Clean eyeglasses daily and as needed.
- Protect eyeglasses from loss or damage. When not worn, put them in their case.
- Contact lenses are cleaned, removed, and stored according to the manufacturer's instructions.

CHAPTER 33 REVIEW QUESTIONS

Circle the BEST answer.
1. A person is hard-of-hearing. You do all of the following *except*
   a. Face the person when speaking
   b. Speak clearly, distinctly, and slowly
   c. Use facial expressions and gestures to give clues
   d. Use long sentences

2. A person has taken his hearing aid out for the evening. You do all of the following *except*
   a. Make sure the hearing aid is turned off
   b. Keep the battery in the hearing aid
   c. Place the hearing aid in a safe place
   d. Handle the hearing aid carefully

3. A person is blind. You do all of the following *except*
   a. Identify yourself when you enter her room
   b. Describe people, places, and things thoroughly
   c. Rearrange her furniture without telling her
   d. Encourage her to do as much for herself as possible

4. Fluid buildup in the eye that causes pressure on the optic nerve is
   a. Cataract
   b. Cerumen
   c. Glaucoma
   d. Tinnitus

Answers to these questions are on p. 480.

CHAPTER 34 CANCER, IMMUNE SYSTEM, AND SKIN DISORDERS

CANCER

- Cancer is the second leading cause of death in the United States.
- Review Box 34.1, Some Signs and Symptoms of Cancer, in the textbook.
- Surgery, radiation therapy, and chemotherapy are the most common treatments.

- Persons with cancer have many needs. They include:
  - Pain relief or control
  - Rest and exercise
  - Fluids and nutrition
  - Preventing skin breakdown
  - Preventing bowel problems (constipation, diarrhea)
  - Dealing with treatment side effects
  - Psychological and social needs
  - Spiritual needs
  - Sexual needs
- Anger, fear, and depression are common. Some surgeries are disfiguring. The person may feel unwhole, unattractive, or unclean. The person and family need support.
- Talk to the person. Do not avoid the person because you are uncomfortable. Use touch and listening to show that you care.
- Spiritual needs are important. A spiritual leader may provide comfort.

IMMUNE SYSTEM DISORDERS

- The immune system protects the body from microbes, cancer cells, and other harmful substances. It defends against threats inside and outside the body.

Acquired Immunodeficiency Syndrome

- Acquired immunodeficiency syndrome (AIDS) is caused by a virus. The virus is spread through body fluids—blood, semen, vaginal secretions, and breast milk. The human immunodeficiency virus (HIV) is not spread by saliva, tears, sweat, sneezing, coughing, insects, or casual contact.
- Persons with AIDS are at risk for pneumonia, tuberculosis, Kaposi's sarcoma (a cancer), and nervous system damage.
- To protect yourself and others from the virus, follow Standard Precautions and the Bloodborne Pathogen Standard.
- Review Box 34.3, Caring for the Person With AIDS, in the textbook.
- Older persons also get AIDS. They may get and spread HIV through sexual contact and intravenous (IV) drug use. Aging and some diseases can mask the signs and symptoms of AIDS. Older persons are less likely to be tested for HIV/AIDS.

CHAPTER 34 REVIEW QUESTIONS

Circle the BEST answer.
1. A person with cancer may need all the following *except*
   a. Pain relief or control
   b. Avoidance from you
   c. Fluids and nutrition
   d. Psychological support

2. Which statement about HIV is *false?*
   a. HIV is spread through body fluids.
   b. Standard Precautions and the Bloodborne Pathogen Standard are followed.
   c. Older persons cannot get and spread HIV.
   d. Older persons are less likely to be tested for HIV/AIDS.

3. The immune system defends against threats inside and outside the body.
   a. True
   b. False

Answers to these questions are on p. 480.

CHAPTER 35 NERVOUS SYSTEM AND MUSCULOSKELETAL DISORDERS

NERVOUS SYSTEM DISORDERS

Stroke

- Stroke is also called a brain attack or cerebrovascular accident (CVA). It is the third leading cause of death in the United States. Review Box 35.1, Warning Signs of Stroke, in the textbook.
- The effects of stroke include:
  - Loss of face, hand, arm, leg, or body control
  - *Hemiplegia*—paralysis on one side of the body
  - Changing emotions (crying easily or mood swings, sometimes for no reason)
  - Difficulty swallowing (dysphagia)
  - Aphasia or slowed or slurred speech
  - Changes in sight, touch, movement, and thought
  - Impaired memory
  - Urinary frequency, urgency, or incontinence
  - Loss of bowel control or constipation
  - Depression and frustration
- The health team helps the person regain the highest possible level of function. Review Box 35.2, Care of the Person With a Stroke, in the textbook.

Parkinson's Disease

- Parkinson's disease is a slow, progressive disorder with no cure. Persons over the age of 50 are at risk. Signs and symptoms become worse over time. They include:
  - *Tremors*—often start in one finger and spread to the whole arm. Pill-rolling movements—rubbing the thumb and index finger—may occur. The person may have trembling in the hands, arms, legs, jaw, and face.
  - *Rigid, stiff muscles*—in the arms, legs, neck, and trunk.
  - *Slow movements*—the person has a slow, shuffling gait.
  - *Stooped posture and impaired balance*—it is hard to walk. Falls are a risk.
  - *Mask-like expression*—the person cannot blink and smile. A fixed stare is common.
- Other signs and symptoms that develop over time include swallowing and chewing problems,

constipation, and bladder problems. Sleep problems, depression, and emotional changes (fear, insecurity) can occur. So can memory loss and slow thinking. The person may have slurred, monotone, and soft speech. Some people talk too fast or repeat what they say.

- Medications are ordered to treat and control the disease. Exercise and physical therapy improve strength, posture, balance, and mobility. Therapy is needed for speech and swallowing problems. The person may need help with eating and self-care. Safety measures are needed to prevent falls and injury.

Multiple Sclerosis

- Multiple sclerosis (MS) is a chronic disease. The myelin (which covers nerve fibers) in the brain and spinal cord is destroyed. Nerve impulses are not sent to and from the brain in a normal manner. Functions are impaired or lost. There is no cure.
- Symptoms usually start between the ages of 20 and 40. Signs and symptoms depend on the damaged area. They may include vision problems, muscle weakness in the arms and legs, and balance problems that affect standing and walking. Tingling, prickling, or numb sensations may occur. Also, partial or complete paralysis and pain may occur.
- Persons with MS are kept active as long as possible and as independent as possible. Skin care, hygiene, and range of motion (ROM) exercises are important. So are turning, positioning, and deep breathing and coughing. Bowel and bladder elimination is promoted. Injuries and complications from bedrest are prevented.

Spinal Cord Injury

- Spinal cord injuries can permanently damage the nervous system. Common causes are stab or gunshot wounds, motor vehicle crashes, falls, and sports injuries.
- The higher the level of injury, the more functions are lost:
  - Lumbar injuries—sensory and muscle function in the legs is lost. The person has paraplegia—paralysis in legs and lower trunk.
  - Thoracic injuries—sensory and muscle function below the chest is lost. The person has paraplegia.
  - Cervical injuries—sensory and muscle function of the arms, legs, and trunk is lost. Paralysis in the arms, legs, and trunk is called quadriplegia or tetraplegia.
- Review Box 35.3, Care of Persons With Paralysis, in the textbook.

MUSCULOSKELETAL DISORDERS

Arthritis

- Arthritis means joint inflammation.
- *Osteoarthritis (degenerative joint disease).* The fingers, spine (neck and lower back), and

weight-bearing joints (hips, knees, and feet) are often affected. Treatment involves pain relief, heat applications, exercise, rest and joint care, weight control, and a healthy lifestyle. Falls are prevented. Help is given with activities of daily living (ADL) as needed. Toilet seat risers are helpful when hips and knees are affected. So are chairs with higher seats and armrests. Some people need joint replacement surgery.

- *Rheumatoid arthritis.* Rheumatoid arthritis (RA) causes joint pain, swelling, stiffness, and loss of function. Joints are tender, warm, and swollen. Fatigue and fever are common. The person does not feel well. The person's care plan may include rest balanced with exercise, proper positioning, joint care, weight control, measures to reduce stress, and measures to prevent falls. Medications are ordered for pain relief and to reduce inflammation. Heat and cold applications may be ordered. Some persons need joint replacement surgery. Emotional support is needed. Persons with RA need to stay as active as possible. Give encouragement and praise. Listen when the person needs to talk.

CHAPTER 35 REVIEW QUESTIONS

Circle the BEST answer.

1. The person had a stroke. Care includes all of the following *except*
   a. Place the call light on the person's strong side
   b. Reposition the person every 2 hours
   c. Perform ROM exercises as ordered
   d. Place objects on the affected side

2. The person with hemiplegia
   a. Is paralyzed on one side of the body
   b. Has both arms paralyzed
   c. Has both legs paralyzed
   a. Has all extremities paralyzed

3. The person with multiple sclerosis should be kept active as long as possible.
   a. True
   b. False

4. The person has paralysis in the legs and lower trunk. This is called
   a. Quadriplegia
   b. Paraplegia
   c. Hemiplegia
   d. Tetraplegia

5. Fever is a common symptom of osteoarthritis.
   a. True
   b. False

Answers to these questions are on p. 480.

CARDIOVASCULAR DISORDERS

Hypertension

- In hypertension, the resting blood pressure is too high. Normal blood pressure for an adult is less than 120 mm Hg systolic and less than 80 mm Hg diastolic. Hypertension is caused by a narrowing of the blood vessels and may first be detected with blood pressure measurements.
- Lifestyle changes can often lower blood pressure. A diet low in salt and fat, a healthy weight, and regular exercise are needed.

Angina

- Angina is chest pain. It is from reduced blood flow to part of the heart muscle. Chest pain is described as tightness, pressure, squeezing, or burning in the chest. Pain can occur in the shoulders, arms, neck, jaw, or back. The person may be pale, feel faint, and perspire. Dyspnea is common. Nausea, fatigue, and weakness may occur. Some persons complain of "gas" or indigestion.
- Rest often relieves symptoms in 3–15 minutes. Chest pain lasting longer than a few minutes and not relieved by rest and nitroglycerin may signal heart attack. The person needs emergency care.

Myocardial Infarction

- Myocardial infarction (MI) also is called heart attack, acute myocardial infarction (AMI), and acute coronary syndrome (ACS).
- Blood flow to the heart muscle is suddenly blocked. Part of the heart muscle dies. MI is an emergency. Sudden cardiac death (sudden cardiac arrest) can occur.
- Review Box 36.2, Signs and Symptoms of Myocardial Infarction, in the textbook.

Heart Failure

- Heart failure or congestive heart failure (CHF) occurs when the heart is weakened and cannot pump normally. Blood backs up. Tissue congestion occurs.
- Medications are given to strengthen the heart. They also reduce the amount of fluid in the body. A sodium-controlled diet is ordered. Oxygen is given. Semi-Fowler position is preferred for breathing. Intake and output (I&O), daily weight, compression stockings, and range of motion exercises are part of the care plan.

RESPIRATORY DISORDERS

Chronic Obstructive Pulmonary Disease

- Two disorders are grouped under chronic obstructive pulmonary disease (COPD). They are chronic bronchitis and emphysema. These disorders obstruct airflow. Lung function is gradually lost.

- *Chronic bronchitis.* Bronchitis means inflammation of the bronchi. Chronic bronchitis occurs after repeated episodes of bronchitis. Smoking is the major cause. Smoker's cough in the morning is often the first symptom of chronic bronchitis. Over time, the cough becomes more frequent. The person has difficulty breathing and tires easily. The person must stop smoking. Oxygen therapy and breathing exercises are often ordered. If a respiratory tract infection occurs, the person needs prompt treatment.
- *Emphysema.* In emphysema, the alveoli enlarge and become less elastic. They do not expand and shrink normally when breathing in and out. Air becomes trapped when exhaling. Smoking is the most common cause. The person has shortness of breath and a cough. Sputum may contain pus. Fatigue is common. The person works hard to breathe in and out. Breathing is easier when the person sits upright and slightly forward. The person must stop smoking. Respiratory therapy, breathing exercises, oxygen, and medication therapy are ordered.

Asthma

- In asthma, the airway becomes inflamed and narrow. Extra mucus is produced. Dyspnea results. Wheezing and coughing are common. So are pain and tightening in the chest. Asthma usually is triggered by allergies. Other triggers include air pollutants and irritants, smoking and second-hand smoke, respiratory tract infections, exertion, and cold air. Asthma is treated with medications. Severe attacks may require emergency care.

Influenza

- Influenza is a respiratory infection. The following may signal flu in older persons: changes in mental status; worsening of other health problems; a body temperature below the normal range; fatigue; decreased appetite and fluid intake. Treatment includes increased fluids and rest. Thorough and frequent hand hygiene is stressed. The CDC recommends the flu vaccine for all persons over the age of six months, but especially those who are 50 years of age and older; have chronic diseases; reside in nursing centers or other long-term care centers; or have contact with persons at high risk for flu complications.

Pneumonia

- Pneumonia is an inflammation and infection of lung tissue. Bacteria, viruses, and other microbes are causes.
- High fever, chills, painful cough, chest pain on breathing, and rapid pulse occur. Shortness of breath and rapid breathing also occur. Cyanosis may be present. Sputum is thick and white, green, yellow, or rust-colored. Other signs and symptoms are nausea, vomiting, headache, tiredness, and muscle aches.
- Medications are ordered for infection and pain. Fluid intake is increased. Intravenous therapy and oxygen

may be needed. Semi-Fowler position eases breathing. Rest is important. Standard Precautions are followed. Isolation precautions are used depending on the cause.

COVID-19

- COVID-19 is caused by a virus called SARS-Co-V-2. It is part of the coronavirus family.
- It spreads quickly through droplets that project through the mouth or nose when you breathe, cough, or speak.
- Signs and symptoms can include fever, cough, sore throat, nasal congestion, diarrhea, and fatigue.
- Special precautions are taken with PPE and isolation to prevent the spread of infection. The CDC recommends people ages six months and older getting the COVID-19 vaccine and boosters.

Tuberculosis

- Tuberculosis (TB) is a bacterial infection in the lungs. TB is spread by airborne droplets with coughing, sneezing, speaking, singing, or laughing. Those who have close, frequent contact with an infected person are at risk. TB is more likely to occur in close, crowded areas. Age, poor nutrition, and human immunodeficiency virus (HIV) infection are other risk factors.
- Signs and symptoms are tiredness, loss of appetite, weight loss, fever, and night sweats. Cough and sputum production increase over time. Sputum may contain blood. Chest pain occurs.
- Medications for TB are given. Standard Precautions and isolation precautions are needed. The person must cover the mouth and nose with tissues when sneezing, coughing, or producing sputum. Tissues are flushed down the toilet, placed in a BIOHAZARD bag, or placed in a paper bag and burned. Hand washing after contact with sputum is essential.

CHAPTER 36 REVIEW QUESTIONS

Circle the BEST answer.

1. Which statement about angina is *false?*
   a. Angina is chest pain.
   b. The person may be pale and perspire.
   c. Rest often relieves the symptoms.
   d. You do not report angina to the nurse.

2. A person has heart failure. You do all of the following *except*
   a. Measure intake and output
   b. Measure weight daily
   c. Promote a diet that is high in salt
   d. Restrict fluids as ordered

3. Which position is usually best for the person with pneumonia?
   a. Semi-Fowler
   b. Prone
   c. Supine
   d. Trendelenburg's

4. A bacterial infection in the lungs is
   a. Asthma
   b. Bronchitis
   c. Tuberculosis
   d. Emphysema

Answers to these questions are on p. 480.

CHAPTER 37 DIGESTIVE AND ENDOCRINE DISORDERS

DIGESTIVE DISORDERS

Gastroesophageal Reflux Disease (GERD)

- In gastroesophageal reflux disease (GERD), stomach contents flow back from the stomach into the esophagus. The acid in the stomach contents can irritate and inflame the esophagus lining. Heartburn is the most common symptom of GERD. Heartburn is a burning sensation in the chest and sometimes the throat. Heartburn that occurs more than twice a week is a signal that the person may have GERD.
- Large meals and lying down after eating can cause gastric reflux. Certain foods such as citrus fruits, chocolate, caffeine drinks, fried, fatty, or spicy foods, garlic, onions, and tomato-based foods can also cause gastric reflux. Medications and lifestyle changes can help alleviate symptoms.

Vomiting

- These measures are needed:
  - Follow Standard Precautions and the Bloodborne Pathogen Standard.
  - Turn the person's head well to one side. This prevents aspiration.
  - Place a kidney basin under the person's chin.
  - Move vomitus away from the person.
  - Provide oral hygiene.
  - Observe vomitus for color, odor, and undigested food. If it looks like coffee grounds, it contains undigested blood. This signals bleeding. Report your observations.
  - Measure, report, and record the amount of vomitus. Also record the amount on the intake and output (I&O) record.
  - Save a specimen for laboratory study.
  - Dispose of vomitus after the nurse observes it.
  - Eliminate odors.
  - Provide for comfort.

Diverticular Disease

- Small pouches, called diverticulum, can develop in the colon. This condition is called diverticulosis. About half of persons over the age of 60 have this condition. Diverticulitis occurs when feces enters the pouches and they can become infected or inflamed. The person has abdominal pain and tenderness in the lower left abdomen. Fever, nausea, vomiting, chills, cramping, and constipation are common

- Treatment includes low-residue, low-fiber diet and antibiotics. Surgery is needed for severe disease, obstruction, or ruptured pouches.

Hepatitis

- Hepatitis is an inflammation of the liver. It can be mild or cause death. Signs and symptoms are listed in Box 37.2 in the textbook. Some people do not have symptoms.
- Protect yourself and others. Follow Standard Precautions and the Bloodborne Pathogen Standard. Isolation precautions are ordered as necessary. Assist the person with hygiene and hand washing as needed.

THE ENDOCRINE SYSTEM

Diabetes

- In this disorder the body cannot produce or use insulin properly. Insulin is needed for glucose to move from the blood into the cells. Sugar builds up in the blood. Cells do not have enough sugar for energy and cannot function.
- Diabetes must be controlled to prevent complications. Complications include blindness, renal failure, nerve damage, and damage to the gums and teeth. Heart and blood vessel diseases are other problems. They can lead to stroke, heart attack, and slow healing. Foot and leg wounds and ulcers are very serious.
- Good foot care is needed. Corns, blisters, calluses, and other foot problems can lead to an infection and amputation.
- Blood glucose is monitored for:
  - *Hypoglycemia*—low sugar in the blood.
  - *Hyperglycemia*—high sugar in the blood.
- Review Table 37.1 in the textbook for the causes, signs, and symptoms of hypoglycemia and hyperglycemia. Both can lead to death if not corrected. You must call for the nurse at once if the person has hypoglycemia or hyperglycemia.

CHAPTER 37 REVIEW QUESTIONS

Circle the BEST answer.
1. A person is vomiting. You should do all of the following *except*
   a. Follow Standard Precautions and the Bloodborne Pathogen Standard
   b. Keep the person supine
   c. Provide oral hygiene
   d. Observe vomitus for color, odor, and undigested food

2. A person with diabetes is trembling, sweating, and feels faint. You
   a. Tell the nurse immediately
   b. Tell the nurse at the end of the shift
   c. Tell another nursing assistant
   d. Ignore the symptoms

3. All of the following are signs and symptoms of hepatitis except
   a. Itching
   b. Diarrhea
   c. Skin rash
   d. Increased appetite

Answers to these questions are on p. 480.

CHAPER 38 URINARY AND REPRODUCTIVE DISORDERS

URINARY SYSTEM DISORDERS

Urinary Tract Infections (UTIs)

- UTIs are common. Catheters, poor perineal hygiene, immobility, and poor fluid intake are common causes.

Prostate Enlargement

- The prostate grows larger as a man grows older. This is called benign prostatic hyperplasia (BPH). The enlarged prostate presses against the urethra. This obstructs urine flow through the urethra. Bladder function is gradually lost. Most men in their 60s and older have some symptoms of BPH.

REPRODUCTIVE DISORDERS

Sexually Transmitted Infections

- A sexually transmitted infection (STI) is spread by oral, vaginal, or anal sex. Some people do not have signs and symptoms or are not aware of an infection. Others know but do not seek treatment because of embarrassment or other reasons. Standard Precautions and the Bloodborne Pathogen Standard are followed.

CHAPTER 38 REVIEW QUESTIONS

Circle the BEST answer.
1. Which statement is *false?*
   a. Older persons are at high risk for urinary tract infections.
   b. Skin irritation and infection can occur if urine leaks onto the skin.
   c. Benign prostatic hypertrophy may cause urinary problems in women.
   d. Some people may not be aware of having a sexually transmitted infection.

2. An STI is spread by oral, vaginal, or anal sex.
   a. True
   b. False

3. A person with an STI always has signs and symptoms.
   a. True
   b. False

Answers to these questions are on p. 480.

CHAPTER 39 MENTAL HEALTH DISORDERS

- The whole person has physical, social, psychological, and spiritual parts. Each part affects the other.
- Mental health means the person copes with and adjusts to everyday stresses in ways accepted by society.
- Mental disorder is a disturbance in the ability to cope with or adjust to stress. Behavior and function are impaired. Mental disorder, emotional illness, and psychiatric disorder also mean mental illness.

ANXIETY DISORDERS

- Anxiety is a vague, uneasy feeling in response to stress. The person may not know why he or she feels anxious or the cause of the anxiety. The person senses danger or harm—real or imagined. Some anxiety is normal. Review Box 39.1, Signs and Symptoms of Anxiety, in the textbook.
- Coping and defense mechanisms are used to relieve anxiety. Review Box 39.2, Defense Mechanisms, in the textbook.
- Some common anxiety disorders include panic disorder, phobias, obsessive-compulsive disorder, and post-traumatic stress disorder.
- *Panic disorder*. Panic is an intense and sudden feeling of fear, anxiety, terror, or dread. Onset of panic in panic disorder is sudden with no obvious reason. The person cannot function. Signs and symptoms of anxiety are severe.
- *Phobias*. Phobia means an intense fear. The person has an intense fear of an object, situation, or activity that may have little or no actual danger. The person avoids what is feared. When faced with the fear, the person has high anxiety and cannot function.
- *Obsessive-compulsive disorder (OCD)*. An obsession is a recurrent, unwanted thought, idea, or image. Compulsion is repeating an act over and over again. The act may not make sense, but the person has much anxiety if the act is not done. Some persons with OCD also have depression, eating disorders, substance abuse, and other anxiety disorders.
- *Posttraumatic stress disorder (PTSD)*. PTSD occurs after a terrifying ordeal. The ordeal involved physical harm or the threat of physical harm. Review Box 39.3, Signs and Symptoms of Posttraumatic Stress Disorder, in the textbook. Flashbacks are common. A flashback is reliving the trauma in thoughts during the day and in nightmares during sleep. During a flashback, the person may lose touch with reality. He or she may believe that the trauma is happening all over again. Signs and symptoms usually develop about 3 months after the harmful event. Or they may emerge years later. PTSD can develop at any age.

SCHIZOPHRENIA

- *Schizophrenia* means split mind. It is a severe, chronic, disabling brain disorder that involves:
- *Psychosis*—a state of severe mental impairment. The person does not view the real or unreal correctly.
- *Delusion*—a false belief.
- *Hallucination*—seeing, hearing, smelling, or feeling something that is not real.
- *Paranoia*—a disorder of the mind. The person has false beliefs (delusions). He or she is suspicious about a person or situation.
- *Delusion of grandeur*—an exaggerated belief about one's importance, wealth, power, or talents.
- *Delusion of persecution*—the false belief that one is being mistreated, abused, or harassed.
- The person with schizophrenia has problems relating to others. He or she may be paranoid. The person may have difficulty organizing thoughts. Responses are inappropriate. Communication is disturbed. The person may withdraw. Some people regress to an earlier time or condition. Some persons with schizophrenia attempt suicide.

MOOD DISORDERS

- Mood disorders involve feelings, emotions, and moods.

Bipolar Disorder

- The person with bipolar disorder has severe extremes in mood, energy, and ability to function. There are emotional lows (depression) and emotional highs (mania). This disorder is also called manic-depressive illness. This disorder must be managed throughout life. Review Box 39.4, Signs and Symptoms of Bipolar Disorder, in the textbook. Bipolar disorder can damage relationships and affect school or work performance. Some people are suicidal.

Major Depression

- Depression involves the body, mood, and thoughts. Symptoms affect work, study, sleep, eating, and other activities. The person is very sad.
- Depression is common in older persons. They have many losses—death of family and friends, loss of health, loss of body functions, loss of independence. Loneliness and the side effects of some medications also are causes. Review Box 39.5, Signs and Symptoms of Depression in Older Persons, in the textbook. Depression in older persons is often overlooked or a wrong diagnosis is made.

SUBSTANCE ABUSE AND ADDICTION

Alcoholism

- Alcohol affects alertness, judgment, coordination, and reaction time. Over time, heavy drinking damages the brain, central nervous system, liver, heart, kidneys, and stomach. It causes changes in the heart and blood vessels. It also can cause forgetfulness and confusion. Alcoholism is a chronic disease. There is no cure. However, alcoholism can be treated. Counseling and medications are used to help the person stop drinking. The person must avoid all alcohol to avoid a relapse.

461

- Alcohol effects vary with age. Even small amounts can make older persons feel "high." Older persons are at risk for falls, vehicle crashes, and other injuries from drinking. Mixing alcohol with some medications can be harmful or fatal. Alcohol also makes some health problems worse.

SUICIDE

- Suicide means to kill oneself.
- People think about suicide when they feel hopeless or when they cannot see solutions to their problems. Suicide is most often linked to depression, alcohol or substance abuse, or stressful events. Review Box 39.6, Risk Factors for Suicide, in the textbook.
- Older persons are at higher risk for suicide than younger persons. White males age 75 and older have the highest risk.
- If a person mentions or talks about suicide, take the person seriously. Call for the nurse at once. Do not leave the person alone.

CARE AND TREATMENT

- Treatment of mental health disorders involves having the person explore his or her thoughts and feelings. This is done through psychotherapy and behavior, group, occupational, art, and family therapies. Often medications are ordered.
- The care plan reflects the person's needs. The physical, safety and security, and emotional needs of the person must be met.
- Communication is important. Be alert to nonverbal communication.

CHAPTER 39 REVIEW QUESTIONS

Circle the BEST answer.

1. A person may not know why anxiety occurs.
   a. True
   b. False

2. Panic is an intense and sudden feeling of fear, anxiety, terror, or dread.
   a. True
   b. False

3. A person with an obsessive-compulsive disorder has a ritual that is repeated over and over again.
   a. True
   b. False

4. A person talks about suicide. You must do all of the following *except*
   a. Call the nurse at once
   b. Stay with the person
   c. Leave the person alone
   d. Take the person seriously

5. Which statement about depression in older persons is *false?*
   a. Depression is often overlooked in older persons.
   b. Depression rarely occurs in older persons.
   c. Loneliness may be a cause of depression in older persons.
   d. Side effects of some medications may cause depression in older persons.

6. Which statement is *false?*
   a. Communication is important when caring for a person with a mental health disorder.
   b. You should be alert to nonverbal communication when caring for a person with a mental health disorder.
   c. The care plan reflects the needs of the person.
   d. The focus is only on the person's emotional needs.

Answers to these questions are on p. 480.

CHAPTER 40 CONFUSION AND DEMENTIA

- Changes in the brain and nervous system occur with aging. Review Box 40.1, Changes in the Nervous System from Aging, in the textbook.
- Changes in the brain can affect cognitive function—memory, thinking, reasoning, ability to understand, judgment, and behavior.

CONFUSION

- Confusion has many causes. Diseases, infections, hearing and vision loss, brain injury, and medication side effects are some causes.
- When caring for the confused person:
  - Follow the person's care plan.
  - Provide for safety.
  - Face the person and speak clearly.
  - Call the person by name every time you are in contact with him or her.
  - State your name. Show your name tag.
  - Give the date and time each morning. Repeat as needed during the day and evening.
  - Explain what you are going to do and why.
  - Give clear, simple directions and answers to questions.
  - Ask clear, simple questions. Give the person time to respond.
  - Keep calendars and clocks with large numbers in the person's room.
  - Have the person wear eyeglasses and hearing aids as needed.
  - Use touch to communicate.
  - Place familiar objects and pictures within the person's view.
  - Provide newspapers, magazines, TV, and radio. Read to the person if appropriate.
  - Discuss current events with the person.
  - Maintain the day-night cycle.

- Provide a calm, relaxed, and peaceful setting.
- Follow the person's routine.
- Break tasks into small steps when helping the person.
- Do not rearrange furniture or the person's belongings.
- Encourage the person to take part in self-care.
- Be consistent.

DEMENTIA

- Dementia is the loss of cognitive function that interferes with routine personal, social, and occupational activities.
- Dementia is not a normal part of aging. Most older people do not have dementia.
- Some early warning signs include problems with dressing, cooking, and driving, as well as getting lost in familiar places and misplacing items.
- Alzheimer disease is the most common type of permanent dementia.

ALZHEIMER DISEASE

- Alzheimer disease (AD) is a brain disease. Memory, thinking, reasoning, judgment, language, behavior, mood, and personality are affected.

Signs of AD

- The classic sign of AD is gradual loss of short-term memory. Warning signs include:
  - Asking the same questions over and over again.
  - Repeating the same story—word for word, again and again.
  - Forgetting activities that were once done regularly with ease.
  - Losing the ability to pay bills or balance a checkbook.
  - Getting lost in familiar places. Or misplacing household objects.
  - Neglecting to bathe or wearing the same clothes over and over again. Meanwhile, the person insists that a bath was taken or that clothes were changed.
  - Relying on someone else to make decisions or answer questions that he or she would have handled.
- Review Box 40.5, Signs of Alzheimer Disease, in the textbook for other signs of AD.

Behaviors

- The following behaviors are common with AD:
  - *Wandering*. Persons with AD are not oriented to person, place, and time. They may wander away from home and not find their way back. The person cannot tell what is safe or dangerous.
  - *Sundowning*. With sundowning, signs, symptoms, and behaviors of AD increase during hours of darkness

- *Hallucinations*. The person with AD may see, hear, or feel things that are not real.
- *Delusions*. People with AD may think they are some other person. A person may believe that the caregiver is someone else.
- *Catastrophic reactions*. The person reacts as if there is a disaster or tragedy.
- *Agitation and restlessness*. The person may pace, hit, or yell.
- *Aggression and combativeness*. These behaviors include hitting, pinching, grabbing, biting, or swearing.
- *Repetitive behaviors*. Persons with AD repeat the same motions over and over again.
- *Communication problems*. Persons with AD have trouble remembering things. They may have trouble remembering what they wanted to say or they may have trouble with attention or difficulty understanding the meaning of some words.
- *Screaming*. Persons with AD may scream to communicate.
- *Rummaging and hiding things*. The person may hide items, lose them, or throw them away. Or the person may be searching for an item but cannot tell you why. Keep harmful products out of reach. Make sure eyeglasses, hearing aids, and dentures are safe.

CARE OF PERSONS WITH AD AND OTHER DEMENTIAS

- People with AD do not choose to be forgetful, incontinent, agitated, or rude. Nor do they choose to have other behaviors, signs, and symptoms of the disease. The disease causes the behaviors.
- Safety, hygiene, nutrition and fluids, elimination, and activity needs must be met. So must comfort and sleep needs. Review Box 40.9, Care of Persons With AD and Other Dementias, in the textbook.
- The person can have other health problems and injuries. However, the person may not recognize pain, fever, constipation, incontinence, or other signs and symptoms. Carefully observe the person. Report any change in the person's usual behavior to the nurse.
- Infection is a risk. Provide good skin care, oral hygiene, and perineal care after bowel and bladder elimination.
- Supervised activities meet the person's needs and cognitive abilities.
- Impaired communication is a common problem. Avoid giving orders, wanting the truth, and correcting the person's errors.
- Always look for dangers in the person's room and in the hallways, lounges, dining areas, and other areas on the nursing unit. Remove the danger if you can.
- Every staff member must be alert to persons who wander. Such persons are allowed to wander in safe areas.

The Family

- The family may have physical, emotional, social, and financial stresses. The family often feels hopeless. No matter what is done, the person only gets worse. Anger and resentment may result. Guilt feelings are common.
- The family is an important part of the health team. They may help plan the person's care. For many persons, family members provide comfort. The family also needs support and understanding from the health team.

CHAPTER 40 REVIEW QUESTIONS

Circle the BEST answer.

1. Cognitive function involves all of the following *except*
   a. Memory and thinking
   b. Reasoning and understanding
   c. Personality and mood
   d. Judgment and behavior

2. When caring for a confused person, you do all of the following *except*
   a. Provide for safety
   b. Maintain the day-night schedule
   c. Keep calendars and clocks in the person's room
   d. Ask difficult-to-understand questions and give complex directions

3. Which statement about dementia is *false?*
   a. Dementia is a normal part of aging.
   b. The person may have changes in personality.
   c. Alzheimer disease is the most common type of permanent dementia.
   d. The person may have changes in behavior.

4. When caring for persons with AD, you do all of the following *except*
   a. Provide good skin care
   b. Talk to them in a calm voice
   c. Observe them closely for unusual behavior
   d. Allow personal choice in wandering

Answers to these questions are on p. 480.

CHAPTER 42 REHABILITATION AND RESTORATIVE NURSING CARE

- A disability is any lost, absent, or impaired physical or mental function.
- Rehabilitation is the process of restoring the person to his or her highest possible level of physical, psychological, social, and economic function. The focus is on improving abilities. This promotes function at the highest level of independence.

REHABILITATION AND THE WHOLE PERSON

- Rehabilitation takes longer in older persons. Changes from aging affect healing, mobility, vision, hearing, and other functions. Chronic health problems can slow recovery.

Physical Aspects

- Rehabilitation starts when the person first seeks health care Complications, such as contractures and pressure injuries , are prevented.
- *Elimination.* Bowel or bladder training may be needed. Fecal impaction, constipation, and fecal incontinence are prevented.
- *Self-care.* Self-care for activities of daily living (ADL) is a major goal. Self-help devices are often needed.
- *Mobility.* The person may need crutches, a walker, a cane, a brace, or a wheelchair.
- *Nutrition.* The person may need a dysphagia diet or enteral nutrition, or other nutritional adjustments.
- *Communication.* Speech therapy and communication devices may be helpful.
- *Mechanical ventilation.* Some persons need mechanical ventilation. Some may need to learn to breathe without the machine or they may need to learn to live with lifelong mechanical ventilation.

Psychological and Social Aspects

- A disability can affect function and appearance. Self-esteem and relationships may suffer. The person may feel unwhole, useless, unattractive, unclean, or undesirable. The person may deny the disability. The person may expect therapy to correct the problem. He or she may be depressed, angry, and hostile.
- Successful rehabilitation depends largely on the person's attitude. The person must accept his or her limits and be motivated. The focus is on abilities and strengths. Despair and frustration are common. Progress may be slow. Old fears and emotions may recur.
- Remind persons of their progress. They need help accepting disabilities and limits. Give support, reassurance, and encouragement. Spiritual support helps some people. Psychological and social needs are part of the care plan.

THE REHABILITATION TEAM

- Rehabilitation is a team effort. The person is the key member. The health team and family help the person set goals and plan care. All help the person regain function and independence.

Your Role

- Every part of your job focuses on promoting the person's independence. Preventing decline in function also is a goal. Review Box 42.2, Assisting with Rehabilitation and Restorative Care, in the textbook.

Quality of Life

- To promote quality of life:
  - *Protect the right to privacy.* The person relearns old skills or practices new skills in private. Others do not need to see mistakes, falls, spills, clumsiness, anger, or tears.

- *Encourage personal choice.* This gives the person control.
- *Protect the right to be free from abuse and mistreatment.* Sometimes improvement is not seen for weeks. Repeated explanations and demonstrations may have little or no results. You and other staff and family may become upset and short-tempered. However, no one can shout, scream, or yell at the person. Nor can they call the person names or hit or strike the person. Unkind remarks are not allowed. Report signs of abuse or mistreatment.
- *Learn to deal with your anger and frustration.* The person does not choose loss of function. If the process upsets you, discuss your feelings with the nurse.
- *Encourage activities.* Provide support and reassurance to the person with the disability. Remind the person that others with disabilities can give support and understanding.
- *Provide a safe setting.* The setting must meet the person's needs. The overbed table, bedside stand, and call light are moved to the person's strong side.
- *Show patience, understanding, and sensitivity.* The person may be upset and discouraged. Give support, encouragement, and praise when needed. Stress the person's abilities and strengths. Do not give pity or sympathy.

CHAPTER 42 REVIEW QUESTIONS

Circle the BEST answer.
1. Successful rehabilitation depends largely on the person's attitude.
   a. True
   b. False

2. A person with a disability may be depressed, angry, and hostile.
   a. True
   b. False

3. A person needs rehabilitation. You should do all of the following *except*
   a. Let the person relearn old skills in private
   b. Let the person practice new skills in private
   c. Encourage the person to make choices
   d. Shout at the person

4. You saw a family member hit and scream at a person. You need to report your observations to the nurse.
   a. True
   b. False

5. A person has a weak left arm. You will
   a. Place the call light on his left side
   b. Place the call light on his right side
   c. Give him sympathy
   d. Give him pity

Answers to these questions are on p. 480.

CHAPTER 44 BASIC EMERGENCY CARE
First Aid
- First aid is the care given to an ill or injured person before medical help arrives.
- The goals of first aid are to prevent death and to prevent injuries from becoming worse.
- In nursing centers, a nurse decides when to activate the Emergency Medical Services (EMS) system.
- Be familiar with how this is done in your facility.
- Know where first aid equipment is stored (emergency cart, automated external defibrillator (AED), first aid kit, etc.)

SUDDEN CARDIAC ARREST
- Sudden cardiac arrest (SCA) is when the heart stops suddenly and without warning.
- There are three major signs of SCA:
  No response
  No breathing
  No pulse
- In some centers, nursing assistants are trained in CPR and expected to start performing CPR in case of sudden cardiac arrest. In other centers, this is performed only by the nurses. Know the policy at your center.
- Know how to quickly determine if the resident has a DNR (Do Not Resuscitate) status or should have CPR performed.
- Follow the directions of the nurse.

Choking
- Choking or foreign-body airway obstruction (FBAO) occurs when a foreign body obstructs the airway. Air cannot pass through the air passages to the lungs. The body does not get enough oxygen. This can lead to cardiac arrest.
- Choking often occurs during eating. A large, poorly chewed piece of meat is the most common cause. Other common causes include laughing and talking while eating.
- With *mild airway obstruction*, some air moves in and out of the lungs. The person is conscious. Usually, the person can speak. Often forceful coughing can remove the object.
- With *severe airway obstruction*, the conscious person clutches at the throat—the "universal sign of choking." The person has difficulty breathing. Some persons cannot breathe, speak, or cough. The person appears pale and cyanotic. Air does not move in and out of the lungs. If the obstruction is not removed, the person will die. Severe airway obstruction is an emergency.
- Use abdominal thrusts to relieve severe airway obstruction. Chest thrusts are used for very obese persons and pregnant women.
- Call for help when a person has an obstructed airway. Report and record what happened, what you did, and the person's response.

Hemorrhage

- **Hemorrhage** is the excessive loss of blood in a short amount of time. It can be internal or external bleeding.
    - *For internal bleeding:*
        Activate the EMS system.
        Keep the person warm, flat and quiet until help arrives.
        Do not give fluids.
    - *For external bleeding:*
        Apply a sterile or clean dressing over the wound and apply direct pressure with your fingers or hand.
        If the bleeding does not stop, pack the wound with clean material.
        If bleeding continues, correctly apply a tourniquet, if available.

Fainting

- **Fainting** is the sudden loss of consciousness from an inadequate blood supply to the brain. Dizziness, perspiration, and blackness before the eyes are warning signs. The person looks pale. The pulse is weak. Respirations are shallow if consciousness is lost.
- Emergency care for fainting includes the following:
    - Have the person sit or lie down before fainting occurs.
    - If sitting, the person bends forward and places the head in between the knees.
    - If the person is lying down, raise the legs.
    - Loosen tight clothing (belts, ties, scarves, collars and so on).
    - Keep the person lying down if fainting has occurred. Raise the legs.
    - Do not let the person get up until symptoms have subsided for about 5 minutes.
    - Help the person to a sitting position after recovery from fainting.

Shock

- **Shock** results when organs and tissues do not get enough blood. Blood loss, heart attack (myocardial infarction), burns and severe infection are common causes. Signs and symptoms include the following:
    - Low or falling blood pressure
    - Rapid and weak pulse
    - Rapid respirations
    - Cold, moist, and pale skin
    - Thirst
    - Restlessness
    - Confusion and loss of consciousness as shock worsens
- Shock is possible in any person who is acutely ill or severely injured. Follow the rules in Box 44.1. Keep the person lying down, maintain and open airway, and control bleeding. Begin CPR if cardiac arrest occurs.

Stroke

- **Stroke** (cerebrovascular accident) occurs when the brain is suddenly deprived of its blood supply. Usually, only part of the brain is affected. A stroke may be caused by a thrombus, an embolus, or hemorrhage if a blood vessel in the brain ruptures.
- Signs of a stroke vary. They depend on the size and location of brain injury. Loss of consciousness or semiconsciousness, rapid pulse, labored respirations, high blood pressure, facial drooping, and hemiplegia (paralysis on one side of the body) are signs of a stroke. The person may have slurred speech or aphasia (the inability to have normal speech). Remember the acronym **FAST**. (**F**—facial drooping, **A**—arm drifting downward, **S**—speech slurred, **T**—time to call 9-1-1). Loss of vision in one eye, unsteadiness, and falling are also signs. Seizures may occur.
- Emergency care includes the following:
    - Follow the rules in Box 44.1. This includes activating the EMS system.
    - Position the person in the recovery position on the affected side (see Fig. 44.17). The affected side is limp, and the cheek appears puffy.
    - Raise the head without flexing the neck.
    - Loosen tight clothing (belts, ties, scarves, collars and so on).
    - Keep the person quiet and warm.
    - Reassure the person.

Seizures

Seizures (convulsions) are violent and sudden contractions or tremors of muscle groups. Movements are uncontrolled. The person may lose consciousness. Seizures are caused by an abnormality in the brain. Causes include head injury during birth or from trauma, high fever, brain tumors, poisoning, and nervous system disorders or infections. Lack of blood flow to the brain, seizure disorders, and epilepsy are other causes.

- **Emergency Care for Seizures**
- You cannot stop a seizure. However, you can protect the person from injury.
    - Follow the rules in Box 44.1. This includes activating the EMS system.
    - Do not leave the person alone.
    - Lower the person to the floor. This protects the person from falling.
    - Turn the person gently onto one side. This will help the person breathe.
    - Clear the area around the person of anything hard or sharp.
    - Note the time the seizure started.
    - Place something soft and flat under the person's head (Fig. 44.24). It prevents the person's head from striking the floor. You can use a pillow, a cushion, or a folded blanket, towel, or jacket.
    - Remove eyeglasses.

- Loosen tight jewelry and clothing around the person's neck (ties, scarves, collars and necklaces are examples).
- Time the seizure. Call 9-1-1 if the seizure lasts longer than 5 minutes (Box 44.2).
- Do not put any objects or your fingers between the person's teeth. The person can bite down on your fingers during the seizure.
- Do not try to stop the seizure or control the person's movements.
- Make sure the mouth is clear of food, fluids, and saliva after the seizure.
- Stay with the person until the seizure ends and the person is fully awake. Help the person sit in a safe place. Comfort the person and speak calmly.

CHAPTER 44 REVIEW QUESTIONS

Circle the BEST answer.

1. Which of the following is *not* a major sign of sudden cardiac arrest (SCA)?
   a. No response
   b. High blood pressure
   c. No breathing
   d. No pulse

2. Which statement about mild airway obstruction is *false?*
   a. Some air moves in and out of the lungs.
   b. The person is conscious.
   c. Usually the person cannot speak.
   d. Forceful coughing will often remove the object.

3. The "universal sign of choking" is
   a. Clutching at the chest
   b. Clutching at the throat
   c. Not being able to talk
   d. Not being able to breathe

4. Which of the following is *not* a sign or symptom of shock?
   a. Rapid, weak pulse
   b. Low blood pressure
   c. Warm, dry, reddened skin
   d. Rapid respirations

5. Which is correct care for a person having a seizure?
   a. Leave them alone to provide privacy.
   b. Place a tongue blade in their mouth.
   c. Try to hold their limbs down.
   d. Turn the person gently onto one side and place something soft under the head.

Answers to these questions are on p. 480

CHAPTER 45 END-OF-LIFE CARE

End-of life care describes the support and care given during the time surrounding death. Sometimes death is sudden. Often it is expected. Some people gradually fail. End-of-life care may involve days, weeks, or months.

You will help meet the dying person's physical, psychological, social and spiritual needs. Therefore, you must understand the dying process. Then you can approach the dying person with care, kindness and respect.

Terminal Illness
Many illnesses and diseases have no cure. Some injuries are so serious that the body cannot function. Recovery is not expected. The disease or injury ends in death.

Palliative Care
Palliative care involves relieving or reducing the intensity of uncomfortable symptoms without producing a cure. The person receives care to relieve symptoms and their illness is also treated. The intent is to improve the person's quality of life and provide support for the family. This type of care is for anyone with a long-term illness that will cause death. Settings include hospitals, nursing centers, and the person's home.

Hospice Care
Hospice care focuses on the physical, emotional, social, and spiritual needs of dying persons and their families. Often the person has less than 6 months to live. No attempts are made to cure the person. It is not concerned with cure or life-saving measures. Pain relief and comfort are stressed. The goal is to improve the dying person's quality of life. Hospitals, nursing centers, and home care agencies offer hospice care.

The Stages of Dying
Dr. Elisabeth Kübler-Ross described five stages of dying. They also are known as the "stages of grief". *Grief* is the person's response to loss.
- Stage 1: Denial
- Stage 2: Anger
- Stage 3: Bargaining
- Stage 4: Depression
- Stage 5: Acceptance

Dying persons do not always pass through all five stages. A person may never get beyond a certain stage. Some move back and forth between stages.

Physical Needs
- Dying may take a few minutes, hours, days or weeks. Body processes slow. The person is weak. Changes occur in levels of consciousness. To the extent possible, independence is allowed. As the person weakens, basic needs are met. The person may depend on others for basic needs and activities of daily living. Every effort is made to promote physical and psychologic comfort. The person is allowed to die in peace and with dignity.

Advance Directives
- An **advance direct**ive is a document stating a person's wishes about health care when that person cannot make his or her own decisions. It lets others know the

type of care he or she wants if seriously ill or dying. Advance directives usually forbid certain care if there is no hope of recovery. Living wills and durable power of attorney for health care are common advance directives. For terminally ill person, doctors often write Do Not Resuscitate (DNR) or No Code orders. The person will not be resuscitated. The person is allowed to die with peace and dignity. The orders are written after consulting with the person and family.

Signs of Death

In the weeks before death, the following may occur:

- Restlessness and agitation
- Shortness of breath (dyspnea)
- Depression
- Anxiety
- Drowsiness
- Confusion
- Constipation or incontinence
- Nausea
- Loss of appetite
- Healing problems
- Swelling in the hands, feet, or other body areas
- Pauses in breathing

  As death nears, these signs may occur fast or slowly:

- Movement, muscle tone and sensation are lost. This usually starts in the feet and legs. When mouth muscles relax, the jaw drops. The mouth may stay open. The facial expression is often peaceful.
- Peristalsis and other gastrointestinal functions slow down. Abdominal distention, fecal incontinence, nausea, and vomiting are common.
- Body temperature rises. The person feels cool or cold, looks pale, and perspires heavily.
- Circulation fails. The pulse is fast or slow, weak, and irregular. Blood pressure starts to fall.

- The respiratory system fails. Slow or rapid shallow respirations are observed. Mucus collects in the airway. Breathing sounds are noisy and gurgling—commonly called the *death rattle*.
- Pain decreases as the person loses consciousness. However, some people are conscious until the moment of death.
- Hearing is one of the last functions lost. Many people hear until the moment of death. Even unconscious persons may hear.

The signs of death include no pulse, no respirations, and no blood pressure. The pupils are fixed and dilated.

CHAPTER 45 REVIEW QUESTIONS

1. Hospice care is concerned with cure and life-saving measures.
   a. True
   b. False

2. The dying person tells you "I just want to live long enough to see my great-grandchild born." What stage of dying is this?
   a. Denial
   b. Anger
   c. Bargaining
   d. Acceptance

3. Which is *not* an example of an advance directive?
   a. Doctor's order for an antibiotic
   b. Living will
   c. Durable power of attorney for health care
   d. Do Not Resuscitate (DNR) order

4. Hearing is one of the last functions lost during the dying process.
   a. True
   b. False

Answers to these questions are on p. 480

Practice Examination 1

Answers to this exam are available on Evolve Student Resources.

This test contains 75 questions. For each question, circle the BEST answer.

1. A nurse asks you to give a person his medication when he is done in the bathroom. Your response to the nurse is
   A. "I will give the medication for you."
   B. "I will ask the other nursing assistant to give the medication."
   C. "I am sorry but I cannot give that medication. I will let you know when he is out of the bathroom."
   D. "I refuse to give that medication."

2. An ethical person
   A. Does not judge others
   B. Avoids persons whose standards and values are different from his or hers
   C. Is prejudiced and biased
   D. Causes harm to another person

3. You smell alcohol on the breath of a coworker. You
   A. Ignore the situation
   B. Tell the coworker to get counseling
   C. Take a break and drink some alcohol, too
   D. Tell the nurse at once

4. A person's call light goes unanswered. He gets out of bed and falls. His leg is broken. This is
   A. Neglect
   B. Emotional abuse
   C. Physical abuse
   D. Malpractice

5. Your mom asks you about a person on your unit. How should you respond?
   A. "She is walking better now that she is receiving physical therapy."
   B. "I'm sorry but I cannot talk about her. It is unprofessional and violates her privacy and confidentiality."
   C. "Don't tell anyone I told you but she is getting worse."
   D. "She has been very sad recently and needs visitors."

6. You are going off duty. The nursing assistant coming on duty is on the unit with you. A person puts her call light on. Your response is
   A. "I'm ready to go. I will let you answer that light."
   B. "I've been here all day so I am not answering that light."
   C. "No one helped me answer lights when I came on duty."
   D. "I will answer that light so you can get organized for the shift."

7. When recording in the medical record, you
   A. Write in pencil
   B. Spell words incorrectly
   C. Use only center-approved abbreviations
   D. Record what your coworker did

8. You are answering the phone in the nurses' station. You
   A. Answer in a rushed manner
   B. Give a courteous greeting
   C. End the conversation and hang up without saying good-bye
   D. Give confidential information about a resident to the caller

9. A person who was admitted to the nursing center yesterday does not feel safe. You
   A. Are rude as you care for the person
   B. Ignore the person's requests for information
   C. Show the person around the nursing center
   D. Act rushed as you care for the person

10. A person is angry and is shouting at you. You should
    A. Yell back at the person
    B. Stay calm and professional
    C. Put the person in a room away from others
    D. Call the family

11. When speaking with another person, you
    A. Use medical terms that may not be familiar to the person
    B. Mumble your words as you talk
    C. Ask several questions at a time
    D. Speak clearly and distinctly

12. To use a transfer or gait belt safely, you should
    A. Ignore the manufacturer's instructions
    B. Leave the excess strap dangling
    C. Apply the belt over bare skin
    D. Apply the belt under the breasts

13. When you are listening to a person, you
    A. Look around the room
    B. Sit with your arms crossed
    C. Act rushed and not interested in what the person is saying
    D. Have good eye contact with the person

14. When caring for a person who is comatose, you
    A. Make jokes about how sick the person is
    B. Care for the person without talking to him or her
    C. Explain what you are doing to him or her
    D. Discuss your problems with the other nursing assistant in the room with you

469

15. You need to give care to a person when a visitor is present. You
    A. Politely ask the visitor to leave the room
    B. Do the care in the presence of the visitor
    C. Expose the person's body in front of the visitor
    D. Rudely tell the visitor where to wait while you care for the person
16. A person tells you he wants to talk with a minister. You
    A. Ignore the request
    B. Tell the nurse
    C. Ask what the person wants to discuss with the minister
    D. Tell the person there is no need to talk with a minister
17. When you care for a person who has a restraint, you
    A. Observe the person every 15 minutes
    B. Remove the restraint and reposition the person every 4 hours
    C. Apply the restraint tightly
    D. Apply the restraint incorrectly
18. As a person ages
    A. The skin becomes less dry
    B. Muscle strength increases
    C. Reflexes are faster
    D. Bladder muscles weaken
19. A person you are caring for touches your buttocks several times. You
    A. Tell the person you like being touched
    B. Ask the person not to touch you again
    C. Tell the person's daughter
    D. Tell the person's girlfriend
20. You are transporting a person in a wheelchair. You
    A. Pull the chair backward
    B. Let the person's feet touch the floor
    C. Push the chair forward
    D. Rest the footplates on the person's leg
21. You cannot read the person's name on the identification (ID) bracelet. You
    A. Tell the nurse so a new bracelet can be made
    B. Ignore the fact that you cannot read the name
    C. Ask another nursing assistant to identify the person
    D. Tell the family the person needs a new ID bracelet
22. The universal sign of choking is
    A. Holding your breath
    B. Clutching at the throat
    C. Having difficulty breathing
    D. Coughing
23. A person is on a diabetic diet. You
    A. Serve the person's meals late
    B. Let the person eat whenever he or she is hungry
    C. Sometimes check the tray to see what was eaten
    D. Tell the nurse about changes in the person's eating habits

24. With mild airway obstruction
    A. The person is usually unconscious
    B. The person cannot speak
    C. Forceful coughing often does not remove the object
    D. Forceful coughing often can remove the object
25. To relieve severe airway obstruction in a conscious adult, you do
    A. Abdominal thrusts
    B. Back thrusts
    C. Chest compressions
    D. A finger sweep
26. Faulty electrical equipment
    A. Can be used in a nursing center
    B. Should be given to the nurse
    C. Should be taken home by you for repair
    D. Should be used only with alert persons
27. A warning label has been removed from a hazardous substance container. You
    A. May use the substance if you know what is in the container
    B. Leave the container where it is
    C. Take the container to the nurse and explain the problem
    D. Tell another nursing assistant about the missing label
28. A person's beliefs and values are different from your views. What should you do?
    A. Refuse to care for the person
    B. Delegate care to another nursing assistant
    C. Tell the nurse about your concerns
    D. Tell the person how you feel
29. You find a person smoking in the nursing center. You should
    A. Ignore the situation
    B. Tell the person to leave
    C. Tell another nursing assistant
    D. Ask the person to put the cigarette out and show him or her where smoking is permitted
30. During a fire, the first thing you do is
    A. Rescue persons in immediate danger
    B. Sound the nearest fire alarm
    C. Close doors and windows to confine the fire
    D. Extinguish the fire
31. A person with Alzheimer disease has increased restlessness and confusion as daylight ends. You
    A. Try to reason with the person
    B. Ask the person to tell you what is bothering him or her
    C. Provide a calm, quiet setting late in the day
    D. Complete his or her treatments and activities late in the day
32. To prevent suffocation, you should
    A. Make sure dentures fit loosely
    B. Cut food into large pieces
    C. Make sure the person can chew and swallow the food served
    D. Ignore loose teeth or dentures

470

33. When using a wheelchair, you should
    A. Lock both wheels before you transfer a person to and from the wheelchair
    B. Lock only one wheel before you transfer a person to and from the wheelchair
    C. Let the person's feet touch the floor when the chair is moving
    D. Let the person stand on the footplates
34. A person begins to fall while you are walking him or her. You should
    A. Try to prevent the fall
    B. Ease the person to the floor
    C. Yell at the person for falling
    D. Tell the nurse at the end of the shift
35. A person has a restraint on. You know that
    A. Restraints are used for staff convenience
    B. Death from strangulation is a risk factor when using a restraint
    C. Restraints may be used to punish a person
    D. A written nurse's order is required for a restraint
36. Before feeding a person, you
    A. Tell the other nursing assistant
    B. Go to the restroom
    C. Wash your hands
    D. Tell the nurse
37. When wearing gloves, you remember to
    A. Wear them several times before discarding them
    B. Wear the same ones from room to room
    C. Wear gloves with a tear or puncture
    D. Change gloves when they become contaminated with urine
38. When washing your hands, you
    A. Use hot water
    B. Let your uniform touch the sink
    C. Keep your watch at your wrist
    D. Keep your hands and forearms lower than your elbows
39. You need to move a box from the floor to the counter in the utility room. You
    A. Bend from your waist to pick up the box
    B. Hold the box away from your body as you pick it up
    C. Bend your knees and squat to lift the box
    D. Stand with your feet close together as you pick up the box
40. The nurse asks you to place a person in Fowler position. You
    A. Put the bed flat
    B. Raise the head of the bed between 45 and 60 degrees
    C. Raise the head of the bed between 80 and 90 degrees
    D. Raise the head of the bed 15 degrees
41. You accidentally scratch a person. This is
    A. Neglect
    B. Negligence
    C. Malpractice
    D. Physical abuse
42. You positioned a person in a chair. For good body alignment, you
    A. Have the person's back and buttocks against the back of the chair
    B. Leave the person's feet unsupported
    C. Have the backs of the person's knees touch the edge of the chair
    D. Have the person sit on the edge of the chair
43. You need to transfer a person with a weak left leg from the bed to the wheelchair. You
    A. Get the person out of bed on the left side
    B. Get the person out of bed on the right side
    C. Keep the person in bed
    D. Ask the person which side moves first
44. A person tries to scratch and kick you. You should
    A. Protect yourself from harm
    B. Argue with the person
    C. Become angry with the person
    D. Ignore the person
45. When moving a person up in bed
    A. Window coverings may be left open so people can look in
    B. Body parts may be exposed
    C. Ask the person to help
    D. Ask the person to lie still
46. For comfort, most older persons prefer
    A. Rooms that are cold
    B. Restrooms that smell of urine
    C. Loud talking and laughter in the nurses' station
    D. Lighting that meets their needs
47. Call lights are
    A. Placed on the person's strong side
    B. Answered when time permits
    C. Kept on the bedside table
    D. Kept on the person's weak side
48. A nurse asks you to inspect a person's closet. You
    A. Tell the nurse you cannot do this
    B. Inspect the closet when the person is in the dining room
    C. Ask the person if you can inspect his or her closet
    D. Tell the nurse to inspect the closet
49. When changing bed linens, you
    A. Hold the linens close to your uniform
    B. Shake the sheet when putting it on the bed
    C. Take only needed linens into the person's room
    D. Put dirty linens on the floor
50. To use a fire extinguisher, you
    A. Keep the safety pin in the extinguisher
    B. Direct the hose or nozzle at the top of the fire
    C. Squeeze the lever to start the stream
    D. Sweep the stream at the top of the fire
51. When doing mouth care for an unconscious person, you
    A. Do not need to wear gloves
    B. Give mouth care at least every 2 hours
    C. Place the person in a supine position
    D. Keep the mouth open with your fingers

52. A person is angry because he did not get to the activity room on time because a coworker did not come to work. How should you respond to him?
    A. "It's not my fault. A coworker called off today and we are short-staffed."
    B. "I'm sorry you were late for activities. I will try to plan better."
    C. "I am doing the best I can."
    D. "I'm just too busy."
53. You are asked to clean a person's dentures. You
    A. Use hot water
    B. Hold the dentures firmly and line the basin with a towel
    C. Wrap the dentures in tissues after cleaning
    D. Store the dentures in a denture cup with the person's room number on it
54. When bathing a person, you notice a rash that was not there before. You
    A. Do nothing
    B. Tell the person
    C. Tell the nurse and record it in the medical record
    D. Tell the person's daughter
55. When washing a person's eyes, you
    A. Use soap
    B. Clean the eye near you first
    C. Wipe from the inner aspect to the outer aspect of the eye
    D. Wipe from the outer aspect to the inner aspect of the eye
56. When giving a back massage, you
    A. Use cold lotion
    B. Use light strokes
    C. Massage reddened bony areas
    D. Look for bruises and breaks in the skin
57. You need to give perineal care to a female. You
    A. Separate the labia and clean downward from front to back
    B. Separate the labia and clean upward from back to front
    C. Wear gloves only if there is drainage
    D. Only use water
58. When giving a person a tub bath or shower, you
    A. Do not give the person a call light
    B. Turn the hot water on first, then the cold water
    C. Stay within hearing distance if the person can be left alone
    D. Direct water toward the person while adjusting the water temperature
59. A person is on an anticoagulant. You
    A. Use a safety razor
    B. Use an electric razor
    C. Let him grow a beard
    D. Let him choose which type of razor to use

60. A person with a weak left arm wants to remove his or her sweater. You
    A. Let the person do it without any assistance
    B. Help the person remove the sweater from his or her right arm first
    C. Help the person remove the sweater from his or her left arm first
    D. Tell the person to keep the sweater on
61. When talking with a person, you should call the person
    A. "Honey"
    B. By his or her first name
    C. By his or her title—for example, Mr., Mrs., Dr., Miss, etc.
    D. "Grandpa" or "Grandma"
62. A person has an indwelling catheter. You
    A. Let the person lie on the tubing
    B. Disconnect the catheter from the drainage tubing every 8 hours
    C. Secure the catheter to the lower leg
    D. Measure and record the amount of urine in the drainage bag
63. A person needs to eat a diet that contains carbohydrates. Carbohydrates
    A. Are needed for tissue repair and growth
    B. Provide energy and fiber for bowel elimination
    C. Add flavor to food and help the body use certain vitamins
    D. Are needed for nerve and muscle function
64. You are taking a rectal temperature with a thermometer. You
    A. Insert the thermometer before lubricating it
    B. Leave the privacy curtain open
    C. Leave the thermometer in place for 10 minutes
    D. Hold the thermometer in place
65. A person has a blood pressure (BP) of 86/58 mm Hg. You
    A. Report the BP to the nurse at once
    B. Record the BP but do not tell the nurse
    C. Ask the unit secretary to tell the nurse
    D. Retake the BP in 30 minutes before telling the nurse
66. On which person would you take an oral temperature?
    A. An unconscious person
    B. A person receiving oxygen
    C. A person who breathes through his or her mouth
    D. A conscious person
67. When caring for a person who is blind or visually impaired, you
    A. Offer the person your arm and have the person walk a half step behind you
    B. Do as much for the person as possible
    C. Shout at the person when talking with him or her
    D. Touch the person before indicating your presence
68. You are caring for a person with dementia. You
    A. Misplace the person's clothes
    B. Choose the activities the person attends
    C. Send personal items home
    D. Let the family make choices if the person cannot

69. When caring for a person with a disability, you
    A. Can shout or scream at the person
    B. Can hit or strike the person
    C. Can call the person names
    D. Discuss your anger with the nurse
70. While bathing a person, you
    A. Keep doors and windows open
    B. Wash from the dirtiest areas to the cleanest areas
    C. Encourage the person to help as much as possible
    D. Rub the skin dry
71. When a person is dying
    A. Assume that the person can hear you
    B. Oral care is done every 5 hours
    C. Skin care is done weekly
    D. Reposition the person every 3 hours
72. A person is on intake and output. You
    A. Measure only liquids such as water and juice
    B. Measure ice cream and gelatin as part of intake
    C. Measure intravenous (IV) fluids
    D. Measure tube feedings
73. A person has been on bedrest. You need to have the person walk. What will you do first?
    A. Help the person move quickly.
    B. Have the person dangle before getting out of bed.
    C. Have the person sit in a chair.
    D. Walk with the person as soon as he or she gets out of bed.
74. Your ring accidentally causes a skin tear on an elderly person. You
    A. Tell yourself to be more careful the next time
    B. Tell the nurse at once
    C. Do nothing
    D. Hope no one finds out
75. To protect a person's privacy, you should
    A. Keep all information about the person confidential
    B. Discuss the person's treatment with another nursing assistant in the lunchroom
    C. Open the person's mail
    D. Keep the privacy curtain open when providing care to the person

Practice Examination 2

Answers to this exam are available on Evolve Student Resources.

This test contains 75 questions. For each question, circle the BEST answer.

1. You can refuse to do a delegated task when
   A. You are too busy
   B. You do not like the task
   C. The task is not in your job description
   D. It is the end of the shift

2. Mr. Smith does not want lifesaving measures. You
   A. Explain to Mr. Smith why he should have lifesaving measures
   B. Respect his decision
   C. Explain to Mr. Smith's family why lifesaving measures are needed
   D. Tell your friend about Mr. Smith's decision

3. You are walking by a resident's room. You hear a nurse shouting at a person. This is
   A. Battery
   B. Malpractice
   C. Verbal abuse
   D. Neglect

4. When communicating with a foreign-speaking person, you
   A. Speak loudly or shout
   B. Use medical terms the person may not understand
   C. Use words the person seems to understand
   D. Speak quickly and mumble

5. To protect a person from getting burned, you
   A. Allow smoking in bed
   B. Turn hot water on first, then cold water
   C. Assist the person with drinking or eating hot food
   D. Let the person sleep with a heating pad

6. To prevent equipment accidents, you should
   A. Use two-pronged plugs on all electrical devices
   B. Follow the manufacturer's instructions
   C. Wipe up spills when you have time
   D. Use unfamiliar equipment without training

7. To prevent a person from falling, you should
   A. Ignore call lights
   B. Use throw rugs on the floor
   C. Keep the bed in a high position
   D. Use grab bars in showers

8. You need to wash your hands
   A. Before you document a procedure
   B. After you remove gloves
   C. After you talk with a person
   D. After you talk with a coworker

9. You need to turn a heavy person in bed. You
   A. Do the procedure alone
   B. Keep the privacy curtain open
   C. Ask the person to lie still
   D. Use good body mechanics

10. When transferring a person from a bed to a wheelchair, you never
    A. Ask a coworker to help you
    B. Use a transfer or gait belt
    C. Have the person put his or her arms around your neck
    D. Lock the wheels on the wheelchair

11. When making a bed, you
    A. Keep the bed in the low position
    B. Wear gloves when removing linens
    C. Raise the head of the bed
    D. Raise the foot of the bed

12. To give perineal care to a male, you
    A. Use a circular motion and work toward the meatus
    B. Use a circular motion and start at the meatus and work outward
    C. Wear gloves only if there is drainage
    D. Use only water

13. A person with a weak left arm wants to put his or her sweater on. You
    A. Let the person do it without any assistance
    B. Help the person put the sweater on his or her right arm first
    C. Help the person put the sweater on his or her left arm first
    D. Tell the person to keep the sweater off

14. A person has an indwelling catheter. You
    A. Let the drainage bag touch the floor
    B. Keep the drainage bag higher than the bladder
    C. Hang the drainage bag on a bed rail
    D. Have the drainage bag hang from the bed frame or chair

15. A person needs to eat a diet that contains protein. Protein
    A. Is needed for tissue repair and growth
    B. Provides energy and fiber for bowel elimination
    C. Adds flavor to food and helps the body use certain vitamins
    D. Is needed for nerve and muscle function

16. Older persons
    A. Have an increased sense of thirst
    B. Need less water than younger persons
    C. May not feel thirsty
    D. Seldom need to have water offered to them

17. A person is NPO. You
    A. Post a sign in the bathroom
    B. Keep the water pitcher filled at the bedside
    C. Remove the water pitcher and glass from the room
    D. Provide oral hygiene every day
18. A person drank 3 oz of milk at lunch. He or she drank
    A. 30 mL
    B. 60 mL
    C. 90 mL
    D. 120 mL
19. When feeding a person, you
    A. Offer fluids at the end of the meal
    B. Use forks
    C. Do not talk to the person
    D. Allow time for chewing and swallowing
20. You need to do range of motion (ROM) exercises to a person's right shoulder. You
    A. Force the joint beyond its present ROM
    B. Move the joint quickly
    C. Force the joint to the point of pain
    D. Support the part being exercised
21. A person has a weak left leg. The person should
    A. Hold the cane in his or her left hand
    B. Hold the cane in his or her right hand
    C. Hold the cane in either hand
    D. Use a walker
22. To promote comfort and relieve pain, you
    A. Keep wrinkles in the bed linens
    B. Position the person in good alignment
    C. Talk loudly to the person
    D. Make sudden and jarring movements of the bed or chair
23. A person is receiving oxygen through a nasal cannula. You
    A. Turn the oxygen higher when he or she is short of breath
    B. Fill the humidifier when it is not bubbling
    C. Check behind the ears and under the nose for signs of irritation
    D. Remove the cannula when the person goes to the dining room
24. When taking an apical pulse, count the pulse for
    A. 1 minute
    B. 30 seconds
    C. 2 minutes
    D. 1 minute 30 seconds
25. When taking a person's pulse, you
    A. Use the brachial pulse
    B. Take the pulse for 30 seconds if it is irregular
    C. Tell the nurse if the pulse is less than 60
    D. Use your thumb to take a pulse
26. You are counting respirations on a person. You
    A. Tell the person you are counting his or her respirations
    B. Count for 1 minute if an abnormal breathing pattern is noted
    C. Report a rate of 16 to the nurse at once
    D. Count for 30 seconds if an abnormal breathing pattern is noted

27. You are taking blood pressures on people assigned to you. An older person has a blood pressure (BP) of 188/96 mm Hg. You
    A. Report the BP to the nurse at once
    B. Finish taking all the blood pressures before telling the nurse
    C. Retake the BP in 30 minutes before telling the nurse
    D. Ask the unit secretary to tell the nurse about the BP
28. When assisting a person with their meal, you should do all of the following *except*
    A. Check the ID bracelet with the dietary card
    B. Drape a clothes protector across the person's chest
    C. Stand next to the person
    D. Practice hand hygiene
29. A person has been admitted to the nursing center recently. You
    A. Look through his or her belongings
    B. Ignore his or her questions
    C. Speak in a gentle, calm voice
    D. Enter the person's room without knocking
30. When taking a person's height and weight, you
    A. Let the person wear shoes
    B. Have the person void before being weighed
    C. Weigh the person at different times of the day
    D. Balance the scale every 6 months
31. A person is bedfast. To prevent pressure injuries, you
    A. Reposition the person at least every 3 hours
    B. Massage reddened areas
    C. Let heels and ankles touch the bed
    D. Keep the skin free of moisture from urine, stools, or perspiration
32. A person has a hearing problem. When talking with the person, you
    A. Keep the TV or radio on
    B. Shout
    C. Face the person
    D. Speak quickly
33. When caring for a person who is blind or visually impaired, you
    A. Place furniture and equipment where the person walks
    B. Keep the lights off
    C. Explain the location of food and beverages
    D. Rearrange furniture and equipment
34. You are caring for a person with dementia. You
    A. Share information about the person's care
    B. Share information about the person's condition
    C. Protect confidential information
    D. Expose the person's body when you provide care
35. When caring for a confused person, you
    A. Call the person "Honey"
    B. Do not need to explain what you are doing
    C. Ask clear, simple questions
    D. Remove the calendar from the person's room

475

36. A person with Alzheimer disease likes to wander. You
    A. Keep the person in his or her room
    B. Restrain the person
    C. Argue with the person who wants to leave
    D. Exercise the person as ordered
37. Restorative nursing programs
    A. Help maintain the lowest level of function
    B. Promote self-care measures
    C. Focus on the disability, not the person
    D. Help the person lose strength and independence
38. When caring for a person with a disability, you
    A. Focus on his or her limitations
    B. Expect progress in a rehabilitation program to be fast
    C. Remind the person of his or her progress in the rehabilitation program
    D. Deny the disability
39. After a person dies, you
    A. Can expose his or her body unnecessarily
    B. Can discuss the person's diagnosis with your family
    C. Can talk about the family's reactions to your friends
    D. Respect the person's right to privacy
40. You enter a person's room and find a fire in the wastebasket. Your first action is to
    A. Remove the person from the room
    B. Close the door
    C. Call for help
    D. Activate the fire alarm
41. You leave a person lying in urine and he or she develops a bedsore. This is
    A. Fraud
    B. Neglect
    C. Assault
    D. Battery
42. A nurse asks you to place a medication and a sterile dressing on a small foot wound. You
    A. Agree to do the task
    B. Ask another nursing assistant to do the task
    C. Politely tell the nurse you cannot do that task
    D. Report the nurse to the director of nursing
43. You observe that a person's urine is foul-smelling and dark amber. Your first action is to
    A. Tell the other nursing assistant
    B. Tell the person
    C. Tell the nurse
    D. Record the observation
44. A daughter asks you for water for her mom. Your response is
    A. "I am not caring for your mom. I will get her nursing assistant for you."
    B. "I do not have time to do that."
    C. "That's not my job."
    D. "I will be happy to do that."

45. A person has a restraint on. You
    A. Observe the person for breathing and circulation complications every 30 minutes
    B. Know that unnecessary restraint is false imprisonment
    C. Use the most restrictive type of restraint
    D. Know that restraints decrease confusion and agitation
46. The nurse asks you to place a person in the supine position. You
    A. Elevate the head of the bed 45 degrees
    B. Elevate the foot of the bed 15 degrees
    C. Place the person on his or her back with the bed flat
    D. Place the person on his or her abdomen
47. The most important way to prevent or avoid spreading infection is to
    A. Wash your hands
    B. Cover your nose when coughing
    C. Use disposable gloves
    D. Wear a mask
48. You are eating lunch and a nursing assistant begins to gossip about another person. You
    A. Join the conversation and talk about the person
    B. Remove yourself from the group
    C. Tell your roommate about the gossip you heard at lunch
    D. Tell another nursing assistant about the gossip you heard
49. When moving a person up in bed, you should
    A. Raise the head of the bed
    B. Ask the person to keep his or her legs straight
    C. Cause friction and shearing
    D. Ask a coworker to help you
50. A person is on a sodium-controlled diet. This means
    A. Canned vegetables are omitted from his or her diet
    B. Salt may be added to food at the table
    C. Large amounts of salt are used in cooking
    D. Ham is eaten regularly
51. Compression stockings
    A. Are applied after a person gets out of bed
    B. Should not have wrinkles or creases after being applied
    C. Come in one size only
    D. Are forced on the person
52. While walking, the person begins to fall. You
    A. Call for help
    B. Reach for a chair
    C. Ease the person to the floor
    D. Ask a visitor to help
53. Before bathing a person, you should
    A. Offer the bedpan or urinal
    B. Partially undress the person
    C. Raise the head of the bed
    D. Open the privacy curtain

54. When taking a rectal temperature, you insert the thermometer
    A. ½ inch
    B. 1.5 inches
    C. 2 inches
    D. 2.5 inches
55. Touch
    A. Is a form of nonverbal communication
    B. Is a form of verbal communication
    C. Means the same thing to everyone
    D. Should be used for all persons
56. You may share information about a person's care and condition to
    A. The staff caring for the person
    B. The person's daughter
    C. Your family members
    D. The volunteer in the gift shop
57. A person tells you he or she has pain upon urination. You
    A. Tell the nurse
    B. Let the nurse document this information
    C. Ask the person to tell you if it happens again
    D. Tell the person's son
58. A person's culture and religion are different from yours. You
    A. Laugh about the person's customs
    B. Tell your family about the person's customs
    C. Ask the person to explain his or her beliefs and practices to you
    D. Tell the person his or her beliefs and customs are silly
59. You need to wear gloves when you
    A. Do range of motion exercises
    B. Feed a person
    C. Give perineal care
    D. Walk a person
60. An older person is normally alert. Today he or she is confused. What should you do?
    A. Ask the person why he or she is confused
    B. Ignore the confusion
    C. Check to see if the person is confused later in the day
    D. Tell the nurse
61. While walking with a person, he tells you he feels faint. What do you do first?
    A. Have the person sit down
    B. Call for the nurse
    C. Open the window
    D. Ask the person to take a deep breath
62. You are asked to encourage fluids for a person. You
    A. Increase the person's fluid intake
    B. Decrease the person's fluid intake
    C. Limit fluids to meal times
    D. Keep fluids where the person cannot reach them
63. Communication fails when you
    A. Use words the other person understands
    B. Talk too much
    C. Let others express their feelings and concerns
    D. Talk about a topic that is uncomfortable

64. During bathing, a person may
    A. Decide what products to use
    B. Be exposed in the shower room
    C. Have visitors present without his or her permission
    D. Have no personal choices
65. People in late adulthood need to
    A. Adjust to increased income
    B. Adjust to their health being better
    C. Develop new friends and relationships
    D. Adjust to increased strength
66. When measuring blood pressure, you should do the following except
    A. Apply the cuff to a bare upper arm
    B. Turn off the TV
    C. Locate the brachial artery
    D. Use the arm with an intravenous (IV) infusion
67. You find clean linens on the floor in a person's room. You
    A. Use the linens to make the bed
    B. Return the linens to the linen cart
    C. Put the linens in the laundry
    D. Tell the nurse
68. When doing mouth care on an unconscious person, you
    A. Use a large amount of fluid
    B. Position the person on his or her side
    C. Do the task without telling the person what you are doing
    D. Insert his or her dentures when done
69. When brushing or combing a person's hair, you
    A. Cut matted or tangled hair
    B. Encourage the person to do as much as possible
    C. Style the hair as you want
    D. Perform the task weekly
70. When providing nail and foot care, you
    A. Cut fingernails with scissors
    B. Trim toenails for a diabetic person
    C. Trim toenails for a person with poor circulation
    D. Check between the toes for cracks and sores
71. An indwelling catheter becomes disconnected from the drainage system. You
    A. Reconnect the tubing to the catheter quickly without gloves
    B. Tell the nurse at once
    C. Get a new drainage system
    D. Touch the ends of the catheter
72. Urinary drainage bags are
    A. Hung on the bed rail
    B. Emptied and measured at the end of each shift
    C. Kept on the floor
    D. Kept higher than the person's bladder
73. A person needs a condom catheter applied. You remember to
    A. Apply it to a penis that is red and irritated
    B. Use adhesive tape to secure the catheter
    C. Use elastic tape to secure the catheter
    D. Act in an unprofessional manner

74. For comfort during bowel elimination
   A. Have the person use the bedpan rather than the bathroom or commode if possible
   B. Permit visitors to stay
   C. Keep the door and privacy curtain open
   D. Leave the person alone if possible

75. You are transferring a person with a weak right side from the wheelchair to the bed. You
   A. Place the wheelchair on the left side of the bed
   B. Place the wheelchair on the right side of the bed
   C. Keep the person in the wheelchair
   D. Ask the person which side moves first

Answers to Review Questions in Textbook Chapters Review

Note: Review questions included for selected chapters only based on competency evaluation requirements.

CHAPTER 1
1. c
2. b
3. b
4. a
5. a
6. b
7. d
8. a
9. b
10. b

CHAPTER 2
1. d
2. b
3. a
4. b
5. c
6. c
7. b
8. a
9. d
10. b
11. c
12. a

CHAPTER 3
1. c
2. c
3. a
4. d
5. d
6. b

CHAPTER 4
1. a
2. c
3. d

CHAPTER 5
1. d
2. a

CHAPTER 6
1. b
2. d
3. d
4. b
5. a
6. c
7. d
8. c
9. c
10. d
11. a
12. b

CHAPTER 7
1. c
2. d

CHAPTER 9
1. b
2. d
3. c
4. c
5. d
6. c
7. d

CHAPTER 11
1. b
2. d
3. a
4. d
5. c
6. c
7. b
8. c
9. b

CHAPTER 12
1. a
2. d
3. b
4. c
5. c
6. c

CHAPTER 13
1. a
2. c
3. a
4. a
5. b
6. b

CHAPTER 14
1. b
2. d
3. d
4. a
5. a
6. c

CHAPTER 15
1. c
2. b
3. c
4. c
5. c
6. a
7. a
8. b
9. a
10. d

CHAPTER 16
1. a
2. a
3. a
4. c
5. b
6. c
7. d

CHAPTER 17
1. b
2. a
3. a
4. d
5. c

CHAPTER 18
1. c
2. d
3. b
4. a
5. c
6. b
7. a
8. d
9. a
10. a

CHAPTER 19
1. a
2. b
3. a
4. a
5. b
6. a
7. a
8. b
9. b
10. d

CHAPTER 20
1. d
2. a
3. b
4. a
5. d
6. d
7. a
8. c
9. c

CHAPTER 22
1. b
2. d
3. c
4. a
5. b
6. c
7. c

CHAPTER 23
1. b
2. d
3. d
4. a

CHAPTER 24
1. c
2. a
3. b
4. a

CHAPTER 25
1. d
2. c
3. a
4. d

CHAPTER 26
1. c
2. b
3. a
4. c
5. d

CHAPTER 27
1. d
2. a
3. b
4. b

CHAPTER 31
1. d
2. c
3. d
4. d
5. c

CHAPTER 32
1. c
2. c
3. a
4. b

CHAPTER 33

1. d
2. b
3. c
4. c

CHAPTER 34

1. b
2. c
3. a

CHAPTER 35

1. d
2. a
3. a
4. b
5. b

CHAPTER 36

1. d
2. c
3. a
4. c

CHAPTER 37

1. b
2. a
3. d

CHAPTER 38

1. c
2. a
3. b

CHAPTER 39

1. a
2. a
3. a
4. c
5. b
6. d

CHAPTER 40

1. c
2. d
3. a
4. d

CHAPTER 42

1. a
2. a
3. d
4. a
5. b

CHAPTER 44

1. b
2. c
3. b
4. c
5. d

CHAPTER 45

1. b
2. c
3. a
4. a

NOTES